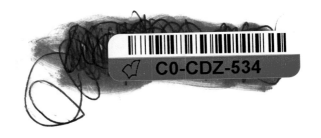

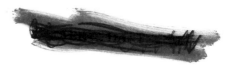

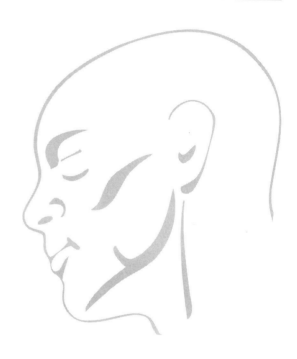

Atlas of
Craniofacial Trauma

ROBERT H. MATHOG, M.D.
Professor and Chairman
Department of Otolaryngology
Wayne State University
Chief of Otolaryngology
Harper Hospital and
Detroit Receiving Hospital
Detroit, Michigan

Illustrations by
William Loechel

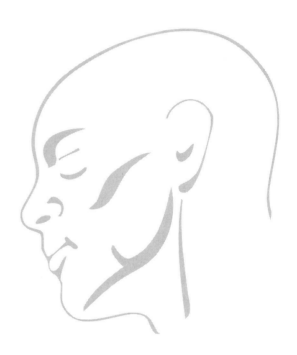

Atlas of Craniofacial Trauma

W.B. SAUNDERS COMPANY
Harcourt Brace Jovanovich, Inc.
Philadelphia London Toronto Montreal Sydney Tokyo

W. B. SAUNDERS COMPANY
Harcourt Brace Jovanovich, Inc.

The Curtis Center
Independence Square West
Philadelphia, PA 19106

Library of Congress Cataloging-in-Publication Data

Mathog, Robert H.

    Atlas of craniofacial trauma / Robert H. Mathog. p. cm.

    ISBN 0–7216–3204–1

    1. Face—Fractures—Atlases.   2. Skull—Fractures—Atlases.

I. Title.

[DNLM: 1. Maxillofacial injuries—atlases.   2. Skull injuries—
    atlases.   WU 17 M432a]

RD523.M3725   1992

617.1′56—dc20

DNLM/DLC   91-14268

Editor: Jennifer Mitchell
Designer: Ellen Bodner-Zanolle
Production Manager: Kenneth Neimeister
Manuscript Editor: Jeanne M. Carper
Illustration Coordinator: Cecilia Roberts
Indexer: Kathy Garcia

Atlas of Craniofacial Trauma   ISBN 0–7216–3204–1

Last digit is the print number: 9   8   7   6   5   4   3   2   1

To my family, my wife, Deena, and our children, Tiby, Heather, Lauren, and Jason, who patiently provided me with emotional support and time to complete this atlas.

Consultants

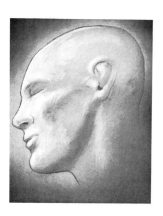

RICHARD ARDEN, M.D.
Assistant Professor, Department of Otolaryngology, Wayne State University, Detroit, Michigan

RAMON BERGUER, M.D., Ph.D.
Professor, Department of Surgery, Wayne State University; Chief, Division of Vascular Surgery, Wayne State University and Harper-Grace Hospitals; Director, Acute Stroke Unit, Harper-Grace Hospitals, Detroit, Michigan

BRIAN W. BLAKELY, M.D.
Department of Otolaryngology, Wayne State University, Detroit, Michigan

FRANCIS G. LeVEQUE, D.D.S.
Clinical Assistant Professor, Department of Otolaryngology, Wayne State University; Clinical Assistant Professor, Department of Oral Medicine, University of Detroit Dental School; Chief of Dentistry, Harper-Grace Hospitals, Detroit, Michigan

ROBERT BRUCE MacINTOSH, D.D.S.
Clinical Professor, Department of Oral and Maxillofacial Surgery, University of Detroit, School of Dentistry, Detroit, Michigan

MARK T. MARUNICK, D.D.S.
Assistant Professor, Department of Otolaryngology; Head, Maxillofacial Prosthodontia, Harper-Grace Hospitals, Detroit, Michigan

L. MURRAY THOMAS, M.D.
Professor, Department of Neurosurgery, Wayne State University; Former Chairman, Department of Neurosurgery, Wayne State University, Detroit, Michigan

Preface

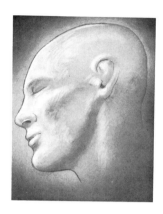

There is much interest in craniofacial trauma. Many people drive or ride in automobiles and play sports, and these activities often lead to accidents and injury to the head and neck region. New textbooks and articles have been published carefully documenting the exciting advances in diagnostic and treatment modalities. Cost-effective treatment methods and ways to prevent these injuries are foci of research activity.

At present, there are many methods to analyze and treat patients with head and neck injuries. Imaging studies such as computed tomographic (CT) and magnetic resonance scans clearly define skeletal and soft tissue abnormalities. Electrodiagnostic techniques help determine temporary or permanent neurologic deficits. The surgeon has many new approaches and methods available to reinforce or repair damaged tissues. Nonreactive alloplastic implants, free vascularized grafts, and tissue expanders are all recent additions to the surgical armamentarium. Wire fixation is no longer the only method of stabilization, and there are a number of reliable fixation plates of different size and composition.

This atlas is an attempt to provide a series of selected time-proven methods that, in the hands of the author, have been successful in the treatment of craniofacial injury. Each section reviews the pathophysiology of the injury and indications for surgery. The usual format is to illustrate a "typical" injury and then describe what is considered to be an appropriate technique. Modifications, options, and alternatives are provided to give some breadth to the management protocol. Methods to make the procedures easier and ways to prevent and treat complications are also included. The atlas is not intended to be comprehensive, but it does highlight common injuries and one or several chosen methods that will work for that specific situation.

One of the guidelines of this atlas is to provide simple, expedient methodology. With the advent of new techniques, it is tempting to try new approaches and apply new procedures, but these should only be used if they will truly help the patient. A technique should not cause additional morbidity. There is no excuse for a prolonged operative time, unless the surgeon can be assured that the result that can be achieved, in terms of form and function, is an improvement over that which can be achieved by a simpler approach. Over-operation must be avoided.

It should also be noted that this atlas uses consultants to discuss several associated injuries. Although there are many practitioners who can cross specialties, for the most part, the specialists provide an advantage in the management of complex multisystem injuries that often affect the head and neck region. Dentists, orthodontists, oral surgeons, and prosthodontists add invaluable expertise with regard to dental health, tooth stabilization, and occlusal status. For patients with cranial injury, the neuro-surgeon plays an important part of the treatment program. Ophthalmologic consultation is essential when there is eye involvement. Laryngologists and otologists are important for evaluation and treatment of laryngeal and temporal bone trauma. The vascular surgeon is also invaluable when the injury involves one of the great vessels of the neck. Craniofacial trauma demands a multidisciplinary approach, and for this reason, we have used consultants liberally to describe their role in the treatment of the patient.

This atlas is written to provide management protocols for the head and neck trauma patient. The methods should help in the training of students, residents, and fellows, and hopefully, the alternative and modified techniques will be of interest to the active practitioner. A base of information is thereby established, setting up future challenges for improvements in patient care.

Acknowledgments

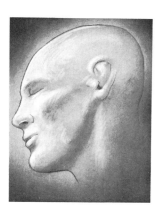

This atlas of craniofacial trauma could not have been written and illustrated if it were not for the kind support and assistance of many individuals. I am indebted to them.

My associate, William Loechel, was a continual inspiration. Mr. Loechel spent at least 1½ years drawing figures to accompany the text. He is commended on his attention to anatomic detail. On several occasions he discarded illustrations "that just might not be right." Many times he would pick up a more difficult method of illustration so as "not to bore the reader." His determination to achieve perfection and take no shortcuts must be acknowledged.

The consultants are well-known and respected practitioners, leaders, and investigators in their specialties. I trust them and use them in my practice. I am honored to have worked with them, and I deeply respect their time and effort.

For my secretary, Sandra White, there is a special appreciation. I am grateful to her for her many hours of dedication in the development of this manuscript.

Contents

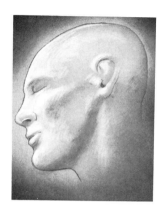

part
one

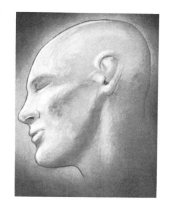

Emergency
Measures

section I

Airway

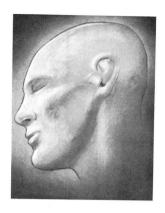

chapter 1

Control of the Airway by Reduction of Facial Fractures or Pharyngeal Intubation

A patent airway with adequate respiration is critical for life processes. Once it is established, attention can be devoted to the cardiovascular, gastrointestinal, neurologic, and other important systems.

In the patient with craniofacial injury, the available options include clearing of secretions, oro- or nasopharyngeal intubation, tracheostomy, or cricothyrotomy. Determining which method is best applied requires an understanding of the respiratory difficulty, site and severity of the injury, level of consciousness, cervical spine stability, and the immediate and long-term objectives. The methods of establishing an airway are highly specialized, and because of the urgency of the situation, they must be performed expediently.

All patients must be treated as if they have a cervical spine injury, and until they are cleared by physical and radiographic examination, the neck must be stabilized. For the obtunded patient in whom blood and secretions are collecting in the pharyngeal portion of the airway, the pharynx can be cleared with a Yankauer suction tube. If the patient still shows evidence of obstruction at a high level within the airway, a naso- and/or oropharyngeal intubation can be performed. Sometimes reduction of retrodisplaced facial fractures is indicated. If these methods do not secure the airway and assist with respiration, then oro- or nasotracheal intubation, cricothyrotomy, and/or tracheostomy must be considered (see Chapters 2, 3, and 4).

PROCEDURE

A–C The head and neck of the patient should be stabilized by an assistant, but if no one is available, sandbags can be strategically placed to restrict movement. The pharynx is inspected with a headlight and tongue blade and cleared of secretions with a Yankauer suction tube. If the patient is obtunded and still having respiratory difficulty, the mandible and/or maxilla should be reduced with digital manipulation. The body or parasymphysis of the mandible should be grasped and lifted forward. Alternatively, the lower jaw can be thrust upward with pressure exerted from behind the angles. The maxilla, if retrodisplaced, should be reduced by placing an index finger behind the palate and pulling anteriorly. Im-

3

pacted fractures may require special hooks or disimpaction forceps (see Chapter 32).

D,E The patient is then immediately reevaluated. If the airway still is not adequate, pharyngeal intubation should be considered. For the nasal route, the nose is sprayed with ¼% oxymetazoline hydrochloride (Neo-Synephrine); a nasopharyngeal tube is then coated with an antibiotic ointment, and the tube is inserted through the nares into the nasopharynx. For oral intubation, a plastic airway, generally used for anesthesia, can be inserted through the mouth and behind the base of the tongue.

Success is ensured by improvements in the clinical and laboratory evaluations of respiration. Failure to observe normal chest movement and airflow, corroborated by abnormal blood gases, should prompt consideration of other procedures (see Chapters 2 through 4). Also, the oro- or nasopharyngeal airways should be considered temporary, and if the patient is unable to be extubated in a short period of time, alternative methods must be implemented.

PITFALLS

1. Problems with the upper airway should be approached systematically. One should first appreciate that there may be an injury to the cervical spine and that all maneuvers should be carried out with stabilization of the neck. Initially secretions should be cleared and the facial fractures reduced. Only after these measures have failed is it necessary to insert the naso- or oropharyngeal airway.

2. Remember that the pharyngeal airway is a temporary device. Nasopharyngeal tubes or oropharyngeal airways are often extruded and are easily blocked with blood and pharyngeal secretions. Long-term usage should be avoided.

3. Usually the patient can be temporarily ventilated with positive pressure while the surgeon checks for spinal injuries. Any patient who does not resume unassisted respiration should be considered a candidate for oro- or nasotracheal intubation, cricothyrotomy, or tracheostomy.

COMPLICATIONS

1. The main complication of oro- or nasopharyngeal intubation is failure to achieve adequate respiration. This will become evident if there is still labored and noisy breathing, retraction of the chest, poor aeration of the lungs on auscultation and less than optimal blood gas levels. In such situations, the surgeon can try to replace the tube and again clear secretions, but if this fails, alternative methods of airway control should be considered.

2. Aspiration is a common problem in the obtunded patient with a naso- or oropharyngeal airway. This complication can be prevented by keeping the airway clean or, alternatively, converting to cuffed endotracheal intubation. If aspiration has already occurred, tracheobronchial cleansing and administration of antibiotics are important methods of treatment.

3. Occasionally the cervical spine has been destabilized by the injury, and if the neck is flexed or turned too abruptly, there can be damage to the spinal cord. The surgeon should always be aware of this possibility and keep the patient's neck in a neutral position. If the patient is to be intubated, an assistant should stabilize the neck during the maneuver. Cervical spine radiographs should be obtained as soon as possible to help in the evaluation.

4. Insertion of the oro- or nasopharyngeal airway can cause bleeding. Often this bleeding stops in a few minutes, but if it continues, the surgeon should consider placing packing around the nasal tube and/or cauterizing the bleeding sites. If pharyngeal bleeding persists, tracheostomy and direct control of bleeding with cauterization and/or packing are procedures of choice.

CONTROL OF THE AIRWAY

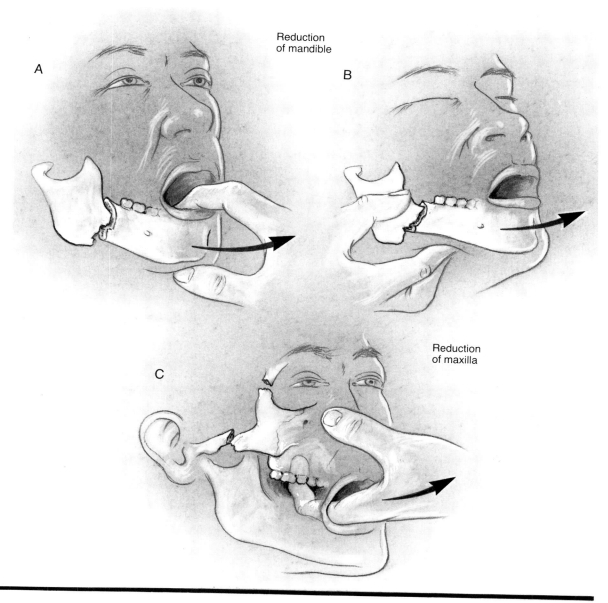

Reduction
of mandible

A

B

Reduction
of maxilla

C

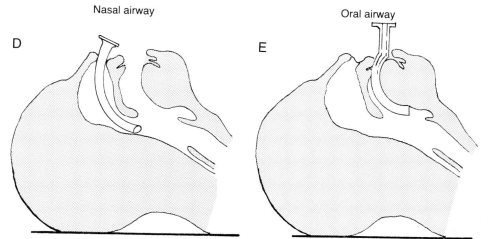

Nasal airway

D

Oral airway

E

chapter 2

Establishing an Airway With Nasotracheal or Orotracheal Intubation
Alternative Techniques Using "Blind" and Nasopharyngoscopic Methods

INDICATIONS

Tracheal intubation is an excellent emergency technique with which to establish a controlled airway. It is easily performed and is an efficient method of ventilation. It also provides an opportunity to stabilize the patient and examine the sites and degree of injury.

The main indications for tracheal intubation are breathing difficulty even after oro- and/or nasopharyngeal intubation or a known functional obstruction involving the pharynx and/or larynx. Intubation should also be considered in patients with obvious closed head injury (or other associated injuries) necessitating assisted ventilation. Caution must be exercised when there is a suspected cervical spine injury.

Nasotracheal intubation is more difficult to perform than orotracheal intubation but is better tolerated by the patient and provides for a longer period of airway control. Evaluation of occlusion is also possible. Furthermore, after orotracheal intubation, the patient tends to struggle and may bite the tube. However, both oro- and nasotracheal intubation techniques are excellent methods in stabilizing the patient for a tracheostomy.

PROCEDURE

The positioning of the patient is very important for the tracheal intubation procedure. Unless there is evidence to the contrary, the possibility of cervical spine instability should be assumed and precautions taken to stabilize the head and neck. In most patients, the neck should be slightly flexed and the head slightly extended. A stethoscope should be attached to the patient's chest to listen for adequacy of breath sounds.

A–D For the orotracheal intubation, the mouth and pharynx should be sprayed with a topical anesthetic and the pharynx suctioned and cleared of blood and secretions. The individual who is performing the procedure should be standing at the patient's head. A straight-blade laryngoscope is then introduced into the right side of the oral cavity, and the tongue is pushed to the left. The blade is inserted further, and when the epiglottis is visualized, the blade is pushed under it into the vestibule of the larynx and into the trachea. If a curved blade is used, the end of the scope will project into the vallecula. Elevation of the epiglottis with the blade will demonstrate the vocal cords, and the tube can be introduced into the trachea. A No. 7 or 8 orotracheal cuffed tube (with or without a stylet) can be inserted. The tube is hooked up to a ventilator bag, and breath sounds are checked. The cuff is then injected with air to an optimal pressure, and the tube is secured to the face with adhesive solutions and plastic tape. Alternatively, a gauze strap can be tied around the tube and then around the head.

E For the nasal intubation, the nose should be sprayed with a vasoconstrictive agent. If the patient is alert, the nose and pharynx should also be prepared with a topical anesthetic. A No. 7 or 8 nasotracheal tube is then passed through the nose and into the pharynx. The mouth is opened, and after suctioning the pharynx, the laryngoscope is introduced into the airway. Using a special forceps (Magill), the tube is grasped and placed into the glottic chink. As in oral intubation, the adequacy of the airway should be checked, the cuff inflated, and the tube secured with tape to the face.

Postoperatively, cuff pressures must be checked and occasionally relieved to avoid necrosis at the site of contact of the cuff with the wall of the trachea. Secretions should be removed as necessary and the

INTUBATION TECHNIQUES

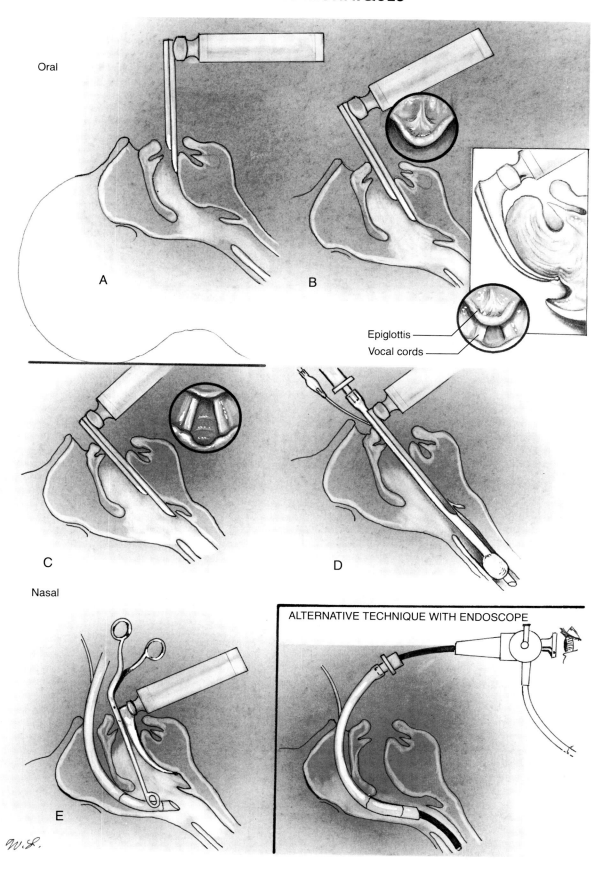

Oral

A

B

Epiglottis

Vocal cords

C

D

Nasal

E

ALTERNATIVE TECHNIQUE WITH ENDOSCOPE

W.S.

oral cavity kept clean with mouthwashes and suctioning. Prophylactic antibiotics are recommended. Tension on the tube by respirator tubing should be minimized. The tube should not be retained for more than 5 to 10 days, as longer periods of intubation can produce inflammation and cicatrization of the trachea. For prolonged intubation, a tracheostomy should be considered (see Chapter 4).

PITFALLS

1. If the patient's cervical spine status is not known, the head should be slightly extended and the neck slightly flexed. Abrupt and excessive movements of the neck should be avoided. With these precautions, the risk of damage is minimal.

2. If possible, avoid tracheal intubation in patients with laryngeal injury. Placement of the tube can cause additional damage to the soft tissues and can confound the diagnosis and treatment of the condition. If time permits, the patient should undergo a routine tracheostomy.

3. Do not use the upper dentition as a fulcrum for the laryngoscope. Undue pressure can cause tooth fractures, and portions of the tooth can potentially enter the airway. Placing a moist 4 × 4 gauze pad on the upper alveolus can help prevent this complication.

4. Be prepared for regurgitation of stomach contents during the intubation and for the possibility of aspiration. If time permits, the stomach should be preliminarily emptied with a nasogastric tube. If any material is aspirated into the lungs, the upper respiratory tract should be suctioned and irrigated with normal saline solution.

5. Long-term tracheal intubation should be avoided, as it is associated with potential subglottic stenosis and granuloma formation of the vocal cords. If the patient requires intubation for more than 5 to 10 days, a tracheostomy should be considered.

6. Postintubation care is extremely important. The patient should be watched carefully for displacement of the tube and accumulation of secretions. Suctioning must be performed using aseptic techniques. Cuff pressure must be maintained below levels that would cause necrosis of the adjacent tracheal wall. Ideally the cuff should be deflated for a few minutes every 1 to 2 hours.

7. If the patient receives assisted ventilation, the ventilation tubes must not put undue tension on the intubation tubes. Such pressures can lead to necrosis of the nasal ala and/or septum and cause damage along other portions of the respiratory tract.

COMPLICATIONS

1. Spinal cord injury is possible, especially if the vertebrae are unstable and displaced during the intubation. To avoid this problem, it is advisable to evaluate the neck with radiographs and physical examination. If satisfactory radiographs cannot be obtained, the neck should be stabilized by an assistant while the intubation is being performed. Maintaining a neutral position will often prevent additional injury. Blind or flexible laryngoscopic intubation should be considered (see later).

2. Tooth fractures can occur by the scope striking the tooth and/or alveolus. To avoid this complication, the laryngoscope should be introduced into the mouth and pressure exerted by lifting the laryngoscope up against the tongue and mandible. Fulcrum-like effects should be avoided. If a tooth should become fractured, the fragments should be collected and the fracture treated as described in Chapter 22.

3. Occasionally the laryngoscope and/or intubation tube injure the arytenoid and displace it from its joint. Following such an occurrence, the arytenoid will appear rotated, the patient's voice will be changed, and there can be a risk of aspiration. Early recognition of the complication provides an opportunity to replace the arytenoid to its normal position; later repairs are generally unsuccessful.

4. Crusting, displacement, or kinking of the tube can cause further problems with obstruction. Thus the patient should receive humidified oxygen, and aseptic suctioning should be performed to collect accumulated secretions. The patient must be watched closely for displacement and kinking of the tube.

5. Subglottic stenosis, although uncommon, is most often observed following long-term intubation. It is believed to develop secondarily to pressure necrosis caused by twisting and tension on the tube and by excessive cuff or tube tip pressures. Such a situation often develops in patients who are obtunded or who do not, or cannot, respond to pain; infection and reintubation are also contributory factors. Many of these conditions can be minimized or avoided. Cuff pressures and tube position should be checked repeatedly, and the patient should be maintained on antibiotics. The tube should be replaced by a tracheostomy after 5 to 10 days.

6. Vocal cord granulomas can also develop as a result of intubation. Although it is suggested that repeated motion and trauma by the tube on the vocal cords is significant, the factors that cause this problem are generally unknown. Granulomas are best treated with excision using laser or microsurgical techniques. Voice rest should be implemented. Repeated trauma should be avoided.

7. Sinusitis involving the maxilla and/or other

paranasal sinuses is common following nasal intubation. The complication is difficult to avoid, but if it should occur, secretions should be cultured and appropriate antibiotics started. Usually the sinuses clear when the intubation tube is removed. If the tube needs to be in place for long periods of time, it may be more prudent to perform a tracheostomy.

ALTERNATIVE TECHNIQUES USING "BLIND" AND NASOPHARYNGOSCOPIC METHODS

If there is a possibility that neck extension may cause damage to the cervical spine or it is difficult to open the patient's mouth, then "blind" intubation should be considered. The technique is often difficult to perform, and if it causes additional trauma, the patient may have increased respiratory problems.

For the "blind" intubation, the patient is placed in the same position used for the direct technique. The nares and pharynx are prepared with topical anesthesia. The tube is then inserted through the nose into the pharynx. When the breath sounds are the loudest and/or condensation is observed on the tube with breathing, the tube is advanced. The patient will usually cough as the tube strikes and passes the vocal cords. Ventilation is checked by movement of air and by breath sounds that are evident on auscultation.

The nasopharyngoscope can also be used for this type of intubation. The end of the fiberoptic laryngoscope is first placed through the endotracheal tube, and both are inserted through one side of the nose. The fiberoptic scope should be advanced to identify the laryngeal structures. When the glottis is visualized, the scope should be inserted into the upper trachea. The endotracheal tube is then passed over the scope into the trachea, and the scope removed. Postoperative management is the same as for patients intubated with other techniques.

chapter 3

Treatment of Respiratory Difficulty With Cricothyrotomy

INDICATIONS

Cricothyrotomy is indicated for life-threatening situations in which the equipment or expertise to perform intubation is not available or the laryngopharynx is so distorted that intubation would be difficult, if not impossible, to perform. The procedure should be considered when there is insufficient time for tracheostomy. However, cricothyrotomy has limitations, and because it can cause progressive damage to the cricoid and subglottic area, it should be converted as soon as possible to tracheostomy.

PROCEDURE

A–E The cricothyrotomy is truly an emergency procedure. The position of the cricoid cartilage and cricothyroid membrane should be determined by palpation, and the larynx should be stabilized between the thumb and index finger. If time permits, the cricothyroid membrane can be marked and the area infiltrated with 2% lidocaine. A horizontal incision (about 2 to 3 cm) is then made with a No. 15 knife blade, cutting through the skin, subcutaneous tissues, the cricothyroid membrane and respiratory mucosa. Once into the airway, the opening can be enlarged with a small Kelly clamp. A No. 4 tracheostomy tube can then be inserted and tied to the neck with sutures and/or straps.

Postoperatively the cricothyrotomy wound should be cleaned with 3% hydrogen peroxide. The airway should be kept free of secretions, and prophylactic antibiotics (i.e., penicillin or erythromycin) should be administered. Ideally the patient is soon stabilized, and in 24 to 48 hours a tracheostomy should be performed. The cricothyrotomy tube can then be removed.

PITFALLS

1. Because cricothyrotomy is associated with a high degree of laryngeal and subglottic injury, it should only be performed when other methods are not applicable (see Chapters 1, 2, and 4). To avoid complications, the cricothyrotomy should be converted to a tracheostomy within 24 to 48 hours after the initial procedure.

2. Cricothyrotomy requires accurate placement of the knife, and thus obliteration of the anatomic landmarks with overinjection of a local anesthetic should be avoided. If there is some concern about the position of the cricothyroid membrane, a 16- or 18-gauge needle can be inserted. Once air is aspirated, an incision can be made around the needle and the opening enlarged into the airway.

3. The cricothyroid membrane is small, and a tube should not be forced into it, as this will injure the cricoid cartilage. Usually a No. 4 (rarely, a No. 6) tracheostomy tube fits and will maintain the airway until a more permanent method can be applied.

COMPLICATIONS

1. Cricoid injury and subglottic stenosis are common complications following cricothyrotomy. The damage can be minimized by accurate placement of the incision, a small indwelling tube, and a limited time of intubation. Because the procedure is usually performed in life-threatening situations, the surgeon should wait until the patient has been stabilized and then convert the cricothyrotomy to a tracheostomy. The sooner the tracheostomy is performed, the less chance there is of subglottic damage. Conversion of the airway ideally should take place within 24 to 48 hours of the initial procedure.

2. Cricothyrotomy places the patient at risk for the same problems that can occur with any type of intubation. The airway must be maintained with suction, and infection should be kept to a minimum with local wound care and prophylactic antibiotics. Bleeding is rare and usually can be stopped with cauterization and/or judicious use of packing.

CRICOTHYROTOMY

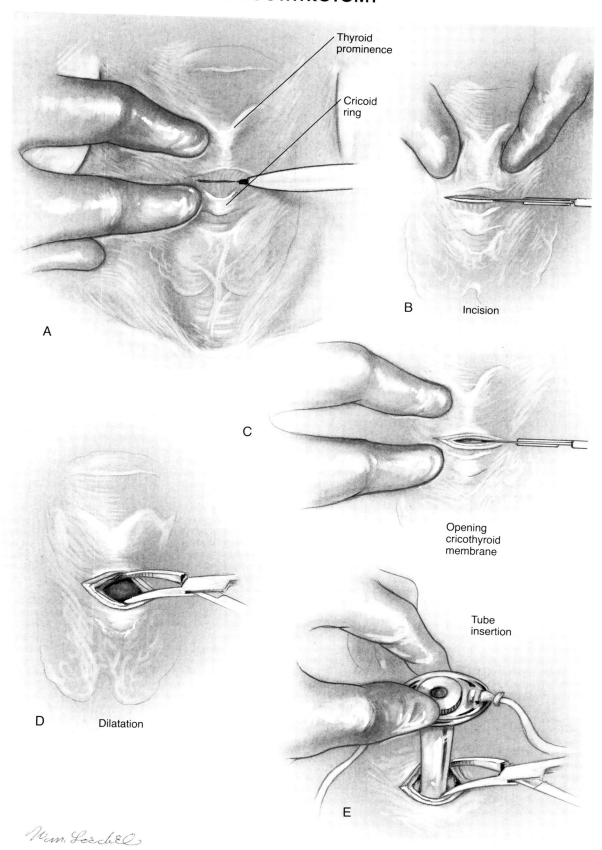

Thyroid prominence

Cricoid ring

A

B   Incision

C   Opening cricothyroid membrane

D   Dilatation

Tube insertion

E

chapter 4

Tracheostomy
Alternative Technique in Children

INDICATIONS

Tracheostomy should be considered in any patient who has sustained craniofacial injury and is not exchanging a sufficient amount of air. However, if the condition of the patient is critical and speed is important, then an emergency cricothyrotomy (see Chapter 3) is performed.

In most patients, the possibility of cervical spine injury should be assumed and the stability of the neck maintained while establishing an airway. First there should be an attempt to clear secretions and blood from the pharynx and manually reduce the facial fractures that may be obstructing the airway. In the obtunded patient, an oral or nasal airway should be inserted. If these measures fail to improve breathing, then oral intubation must be considered. Nasotracheal intubation may be indicated when the patient's mouth cannot be adequately opened or in preparation for a procedure that requires occlusal evaluation and adjustments.

Tracheostomy is indicated when intubation is required for more than 5 days or when complex facial fractures require multiple procedures and repeated intubations. The procedure is helpful to relate occlusal surfaces to each other and should be considered when there is a subsequent risk of aspiration. Tracheostomy is a reasonable treatment option when packing of the nose is combined with intermaxillary fixation. The procedure is elective, and for emergency situations in which time is critical, cricothyrotomy or intubation should be used.

PROCEDURE

Ideally tracheostomy should be performed in the operating room. An initial tracheal intubation is preferred, with the patient either sedated or controlled with a general anesthetic. If the patient is alert and oriented but the situation is such that intubation of the airway may pose a risk, the tracheostomy should be performed under local anesthesia.

A–C The patient should be positioned so that there is a "safe" slight extension of the neck and prominence of the laryngeal cartilages. Useful landmarks are the thyroid lamina projections, the cricoid ring, and the suprasternal notch. Usually an incision is designed horizontally in a crease halfway between the cricoid and suprasternal notch. The width of the incision is determined by the degree of anticipated difficulty. Usually a 3- to 4-cm incision is sufficient, but a larger 4- to 6-cm incision should be used in patients with short, thick necks and in situations in which speed is important. The area of incision should be infiltrated with 1% or 2% lidocaine; the anesthesiologist should approve the use of 1:100,000 epinephrine, which can be helpful for the control of bleeding.

D,E The incision is carried through the subcutaneous tissues. The anterior jugular veins are ligated with 3–0 silk sutures. The investing layer of fascia is cleaned to expose the fine fibrous septum between the strap muscles (sternohyoid and sternothyroid). This septum is incised, and the strap muscles are displaced laterally with Army-Navy retractors. The lower portion of the thyroid gland should be exposed and, beneath it, the pretracheal fat and fascia. The inferior thyroid veins are divided and ligated with fine silk sutures.

F Using a clamp or peanut dissector, the soft tissues overlying the trachea are teased apart. The thyroid isthmus is elevated superiorly with blunt dissection. The surgeon should then be able to visualize the upper tracheal rings and at least palpate the cricoid arch. A cricoid hook is subsequently inserted between the first and second or the second and third rings to stabilize the airway. An incision through the trachea, preferably between the second and third tracheal rings, is made with a small curved knife blade.

G,H The opening is enlarged by resection of a ring. Usually the lower ring is grasped with an Allis clamp, and the anterior portion of the ring is excised with

TRACHEOSTOMY

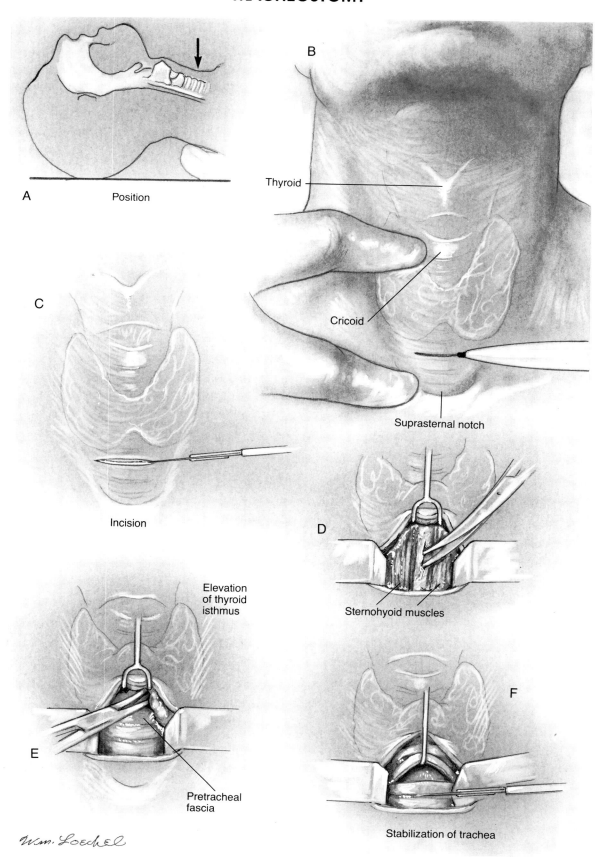

A   Position

B

Thyroid

Cricoid

Suprasternal notch

C

Incision

D

Sternohyoid muscles

Elevation
of thyroid
isthmus

E

Pretracheal
fascia

F

Stabilization of trachea

Wm. Loechel

heavy scissors. The endotracheal tube is advanced to the upper part of the tracheal incision. A tracheostomy tube is then inserted by rotating the tube 90° to the midline and rotating it back into the trachea. There is also the option of widening the airway with a Trousseau dilator before inserting the tube.

Once assured that the tube is in the airway by suctioning secretions and observing for exchange of air, the surgeon should secure the tube to the neck with umbilical tape. Additional fixation is obtained by attaching the tube directly to the skin with 2–0 silk sutures. The neck should then be gently flexed and the tapes tied with a square knot. A gauze dressing is placed under the flanges of the tube.

Tracheostomy care requires close observation and periodic suctioning for secretions that accumulate within the airway. A postoperative chest radiograph should be performed to ensure that the lungs are well aerated and that there are no intrathoracic complications such as pneumothorax or atelectasis. The cuff of the tracheostomy tube should be inflated according to the directions that accompany the tube. Cuff deflation with suctioning should be performed every hour. The tube should be changed between 4 and 7 days after the tracheostomy and then every other week as needed. The tracheostomy wound should be kept clean with frequent dressing changes.

Decannulation can be carried out when the tracheostomy tube has fulfilled its purpose and the patient is able to breath without assisted respiration. The patient should also be free of aspiration and able to cough out tracheal secretions. There should be no evidence of upper airway obstruction.

The procedure for decannulation should be initiated by changing the cuffed tube to a noncuffed tube and then by changing the noncuffed tube to a tube of smaller size. When a No. 4 or 6 tube size is reached, the tube can then be plugged with a finger and the patient checked for airflow through the nasal or oral airway. If satisfactory airflow is observed, the tube can be plugged for 24 hours and removed thereafter. The wound is then covered with a petrolatum gauze dressing and allowed to close by secondary intention.

PITFALLS

1. Recognition of landmarks and anatomic layers is an important part of the surgery. The incision should be long enough to provide adequate exposure. Bright lighting should be available from a source located on the forehead or nasoglabella region.

2. The procedure is best performed with patient cooperation and a local anesthetic block, but if the patient cannot lie still, a general anesthetic is preferred. An agitated, struggling patient makes the procedure extremely difficult and dangerous.

3. Check for pulsations in the suprasternal notch. An abnormally high innominate artery can be injured at the time of dissection, or it can later bleed from pressure necrosis exerted by the bend, cuff, or tip of the tracheostomy tube. Excessive extension of the neck should be avoided, as this can elevate the innominate artery from the chest into the lower portion of the neck.

4. Use vasoconstrictive agents whenever possible to reduce bleeding. Small vessels should be treated with cauterization and/or ligation.

5. Cutting through the thyroid can often cause a bloody field and postoperative bleeding. Thus elevation of the thyroid isthmus by blunt dissection is preferred over division and ligation of the gland.

6. The trachea should be stabilized while incising the tracheal wall. The trachea can be isolated and held in position with a vein retractor pulling upward beneath the thyroid isthmus or with a tracheal hook secured between the first and second rings. The hook can be used to keep the trachea from moving; it also improves exposure by elevating the trachea toward the surface of the wound.

7. Although there is much controversy as to the best tracheal opening, we prefer, in adult patients, to remove an anterior portion of the third ring. If more exposure is needed, a Trousseau dilator is inserted, and the walls of the trachea are displaced laterally. Extension of the horizontal incisions may also be helpful. In children, a vertical cut through the second, third, and fourth rings provides an adequate opening (see later).

8. If there is concern that the tracheostomy tube may become dislodged, silk sutures can be applied through the lateral portion of the tracheal rings. These sutures are then tied in loops and secured with tape to the skin of the neck. If the tube should become dislodged, pulling up on the sutures will elevate and secure the trachea for reinsertion of the tube.

9. In attaching the tracheostomy tape, make sure that the head is flexed. If tape is placed around the neck when the neck is extended, the tape will loosen when the head returns to the flexed position. The tracheostomy tube can then slip out of the trachea. The tracheostomy tube can also be secured to the skin of the neck with 2–0 black silk sutures.

10. Avoid a tight closure of the tracheostomy incision. On coughing, air can enter into the tissues and cause a subcutaneous and mediastinal dissection.

11. A chest radiograph should be performed postoperatively to check the position of the tube and

TRACHEOSTOMY *(Continued)*

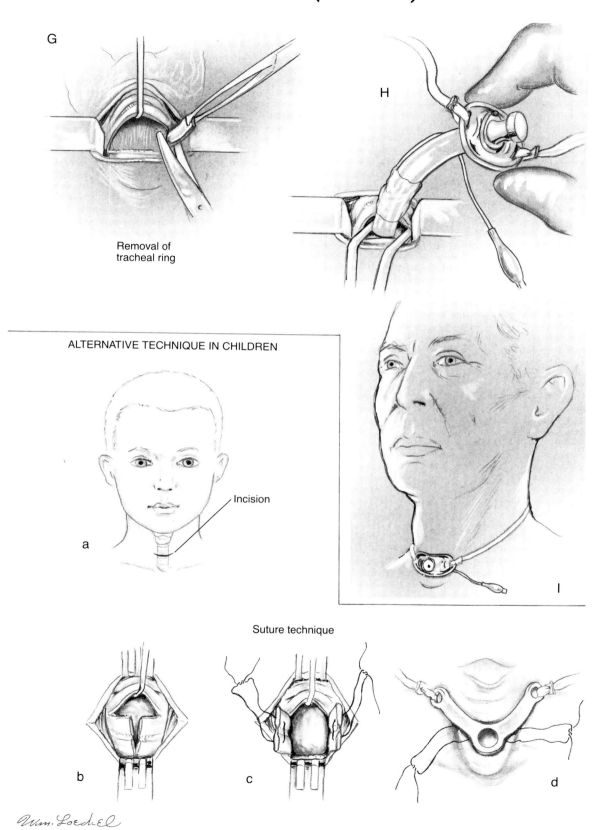

G

Removal of
tracheal ring

H

ALTERNATIVE TECHNIQUE IN CHILDREN

Incision

a

I

Suture technique

b

c

d

Wm. Loechel

aeration of the lungs. A tracheostomy can cause pneumothorax and/or atelectasis, and an early diagnosis is helpful in the treatment of these complications.

12. Check the tracheostomy tube for pulsations and/or obstruction of the mainstem bronchi. A tube that is too short may enter into the pretracheal tissues and be partially obstructed. A tube that is too long will project from the soft tissues of the neck. Pulsations may indicate that the tube is resting near the innominate artery. Should any of these conditions develop, the tube should be changed to one of appropriate size and position.

COMPLICATIONS

1. Postoperative obstructive phenomena should alert the surgeon to the possibility that the tube and/or cuff are not properly positioned. If obstruction is associated with inflation of the cuff, the cuff may be covering the end of the tube, and the tube and cuff should be replaced. Occasionally the tube is too short and is partially inserted into the mediastinal space anterior to the trachea. In such a situation, the tube size and contour should be corrected. Finally, the airway should be checked for obstructive crusts and secretions. This problem can be prevented by cleaning the inner cannula and maintaining high humidity in the airway. Suctioning is also important to prevent secretions from collecting and drying out. Airway patency can be checked by observing the exchange of air or by examining the airway with a fiberoptic endoscope.

2. Early bleeding following tracheostomy usually indicates failure of cauterization and/or ligation to control bleeding from a vessel of the neck or thyroid gland. Oozing of blood around the tube can often be controlled by placing ½- to 1-inch gauze packing into the wound. If this does not stop the bleeding, the patient should be returned to the operating room to have the wound explored and bleeding controlled.

3. Postoperative pneumothorax can occur from overzealous retraction and direct injury to the pleura. If this complication develops, immediate insertion of a chest tube must be considered.

4. Atelectasis can also be a problem in the postoperative period. This can usually can be treated by suctioning, irrigation, and positive pressure respiration. Occasionally there is obstruction from a tube that is too long and enters one of the mainstem bronchi. If such a situation develops, the tube should be changed and the position of the tube monitored by chest radiograph.

5. Subcutaneous emphysema can occur, especially if the patient is coughing and soft tissue closure around the tube is too tight. Although air can be diverted into the pleura and mediastinum, rarely is there any compression of the airway or spread of infection. Once the air is observed in the tissues, precipitating forces should be corrected.

6. Infection of the wound site, bronchitis, and pneumonia are all possibilities following the tracheostomy. To avoid these sequelae, the tube should be kept clean with proper tracheobronchial care. Cultures should be obtained and appropriate antibiotic treatment instituted.

7. Injury to the esophagus, carotid artery, and innominate artery at the time of surgery can be prevented by accurate, relatively atraumatic techniques. If any of these anatomic structures are damaged, appropriate consultation and therapy should be immediately instituted.

8. One of the most feared delayed complications is erosion of the innominate artery. This problem can be avoided by keeping the dissection superior to the innominate vessels and by avoiding cuff pressures and/or suctioning that will destroy the anterior tracheal wall adjacent to the vessel. Many times the patient will have a sudden, small amount of bleeding. This "sentinel" bleed should alert the surgeon to the possibility of tracheal erosion, and emergency measures should be instituted. The trachea should be examined with fiberoptic endoscopy, and if it is apparent that bleeding is coming from the region of the innominate artery, the region of bleeding should be tamponed with finger or cuff pressure. Ultimately, ligation of the innominate artery or bypass surgery must be considered.

9. Tracheal stenosis can develop as a result of tracheal wall injury occurring directly from the tracheostomy tube, cuff, and/or tip pressure (see Chapters 101 through 105). Infection also plays a major contributory role. In the case of early stenosis, removal of granulation tissues and dilatation with a bronchoscope or an indwelling T tube can be considered. If the stenosis becomes mature and does not respond to dilatation, then tracheal resection should be considered.

ALTERNATIVE TECHNIQUE IN CHILDREN

a Modifications in the tracheostomy technique are required in children. Generally children's tissues are very pliable, and coughing can raise the pleura into the neck region. For these reasons, the surgeon must be careful with the retractors; the tracheostomy also should be kept as high as possible, away from the thorax. However, a tracheostomy that is too high should be avoided, as postoperative subglottic narrowing and stenosis can result.

b–d The tracheal rings in children are soft, and the tracheostomy tube can usually be inserted through a vertical incision of two or three rings of the trachea (second, third, and fourth rings). The opening is secured with 3–0 black silk sutures, which are placed through rings lateral to the tracheal incision, tied in loops, and subsequently secured with adhesive solutions and tape to the neck. These sutures are also helpful in stabilizing and exposing the trachea and are immediately available should the tube become dislodged.

Postoperative care and decannulation are performed in a fashion similar to that used in adults. Pediatric tracheostomy tubes are usually pliable and do not require cuffs. Nevertheless, many of the complications that occur following adult tracheostomy can also occur in children.

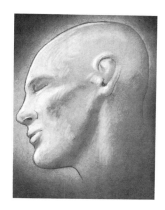

chapter 5

Control of Bleeding
Alternative Technique of Posterior Packs

INDICATIONS

Management priorities in the critically injured patient are to establish an airway and control bleeding. The preferred order of emergency care is to ensure ventilation and soon after to stop the bleeding and restore blood volume. The patient should be evaluated for other associated injuries and disorders that can contribute to the bleeding. If the patient is in stable condition, the surgeon can diagnose and plan the treatment of the facial damage.

In a patient in whom there is evidence of blood loss (i.e., hypotension, oliguria, tachycardia, and gross bleeding), an intravenous large-bore (No. 16 or larger) catheter should be inserted into one of the antecubital veins and blood drawn for type and crossmatch. A balanced salt solution is administered; this should be helpful in expanding the blood volume. However, blood is preferred, and the appropriate matched type should be administered as soon as possible.

Most bleeding sites in the head and neck region can be controlled with digital pressure, clamping of vessels, and/or packing. Nosebleeds are common with naso-orbital, maxillary, and nasal fractures, and if bleeding does not stop, the nose should be packed with ½-inch antibiotic-soaked gauze. Bleeding from the ear, which often accompanies temporal bone injuries, can be treated with cotton or gauze packs. Bleeding from the pharynx requires simultaneous control of respiration, and once this is achieved, the pharynx can be tamponed with vaginal packing. Damage to the larger vessels (i.e., carotid artery and jugular vein) can be initially controlled with digital pressure, but definitive treatment can be difficult, and it is important to consult immediately with a vascular surgeon (see Chapter 106).

PROCEDURE

Packing of the nose is best performed when bleeding has diminished and the structures of the nose can be visualized. This also provides an opportunity to examine the damage to the lateral walls and septum.

A The nose should first be sprayed with ¼% oxymetazoline hydrochloride (Neo-Synephrine). Eight small cotton pledgets, soaked in 8 mL of 4% cocaine solution containing five drops of 1:10,000 epinephrine, are strategically placed throughout the nasal cavity. For optimal effects, pledgets should be positioned in the nasal vault, behind the middle turbinate, on the floor, and along the septum. The pledgets should be retained for at least 5 minutes.

B Bacitracin gauze, which can be used for packing, is prepared from ½-inch gauge moistened with bacitracin ointment. After the pledgets are removed from the nose, the packing is inserted in layers with a bayonet or Hartmann forceps. The first loop is placed directly on the floor; additional loops are layered horizontally against one another, and blood is suctioned as necessary to observe the orientation of the loops. Once the vault is packed, the loops can be directly inserted into the vestibule of the nose.

Ideally both sides of the nose should be packed, or the septum will be pushed to one side, and compression will be released. Adhesive tape can be applied across the nose to hold the dressings in place. The patient should be placed on antibiotics (i.e., penicillin or erythromycin). The airway should be evaluated for obstruction, and if necessary, oxygen should be administered or an alternative airway considered. Packing should be removed at 3 to 5 days, and at that time, the nose should be sprayed with ¼% oxymetazoline hydrochloride. Saline douches should be used to provide a physiologic wash and to prevent crusts from forming.

PITFALLS

1. If the nasal bones are fractured, it may be more prudent to reduce the nasal fracture before packing the nares (see Chapter 46). Such action may avoid subsequent surgery to the nose and still control bleeding.

2. Beware of making the initial loops of packing too long or too loose. Loops of packing can fall into the pharynx; when this occurs, the patient will start gagging. If such a situation develops, the surgeon can cut off the excess loops in the pharynx and/or remove the gauze and repack the nose.

3. Avoid overpacking the nose, which can cause displacement of nasal or facial fractures. If this should occur, the bones should be reduced digitally into an anatomic position and the excess packing removed.

4. If bleeding is not controlled by anteriorly placed nasal packs, then the surgeon should consider either adding more packing or administering posterior packs (see later). Maxillary ligation is difficult to perform in acutely traumatized patients and should be avoided.

5. Most patients with nasal packing can usually breathe quite well through the oral cavity. However, if the oropharynx is compromised, there may be an obstruction, and an airway may need to be established. In these cases, oral intubation or tracheostomy should be performed.

6. In most cases, epistaxis can be controlled with light packs. As an alternative, prefabricated tampons coated with bacitracin ointment can be used.

COMPLICATIONS

1. Usually persistent bleeding is the result of inadequate packing. This can be corrected by repacking and/or additional packing. Only rarely is arterial ligation necessary. If bleeding continues, it is possible that the patient has a blood dyscrasia that should be evaluated and treated as soon as possible.

2. Excessive bleeding can lead to hypotension and inadequate perfusion of vital organs. Thus bleeding must be brought under immediate control, intravenous lines established, and preparations made for blood replacement. Electrocardiograms and catheterization for monitoring central venous pressure and urinary output are important adjunctive procedures. Ventilation should be evaluated, and because ventilatory insufficiency can compound the problems created by blood loss, respiration should be normalized as soon as possible.

3. Packing of the nose can cause displacement of facial fractures and confound the definitive treatment. To avoid this, nasomaxillary fractures should be reduced and manipulated into anatomic position (see Chapters 1 and 42). If there is too much packing, several loops of packing should be removed and the fragments of bone once again reset into proper alignment.

4. Overpacking of the nose can infrequently cause necrosis, loss of tissue, and scar formation. These complications can be avoided by packing just enough to control bleeding and by removing the packs in 3 to 5 days. Prophylactic antibiotics are helpful in reducing the degree of damage.

ALTERNATIVE TECHNIQUE OF POSTERIOR PACKS

Posterior packs are indicated in those patients who have bleeding from the posterior nares or nasopharynx and/or who do not have control of bleeding with the anterior pack method described previously. The posterior pack technique requires patient cooperation; sedation or general anesthesia may be necessary.

a—c The nose should be prepared with ¼% oxy-

CONTROL OF BLEEDING

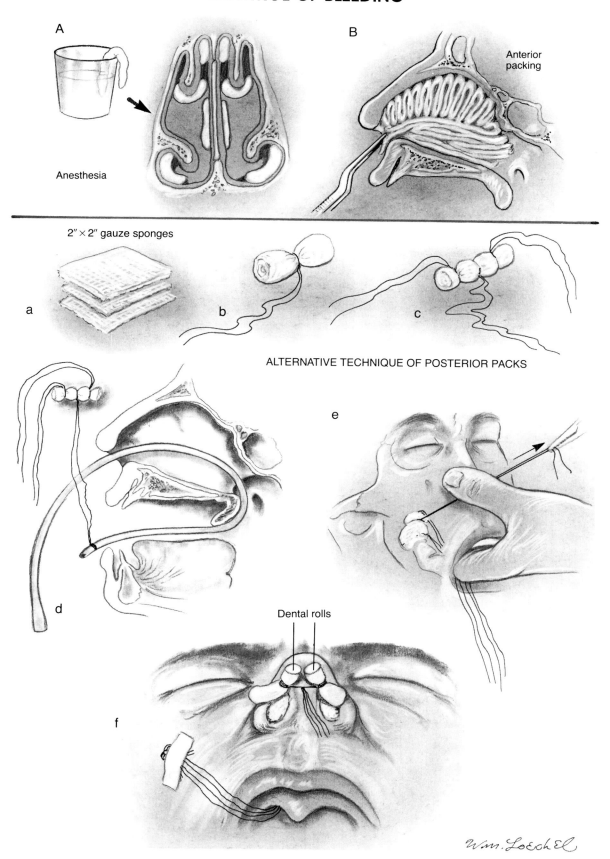

A

Anesthesia

B

Anterior packing

2″ × 2″ gauze sponges

a

b

c

ALTERNATIVE TECHNIQUE OF POSTERIOR PACKS

d

e

Dental rolls

f

Wm. Loechel

metazoline hydrochloride and 4% cocaine containing epinephrine, as with the anterior packs. Two or three 2-in. × 2-in. gauze sponges are rolled into a tampon. An assistant then holds the sponges as the physician ties a length of 2–0 silk around the center of the roll. The ends of the silk should be left long. The ends of the tampon are then tied with additional lengths of 2–0 silk. These strands are placed 5 mm from the edge, and the knots are positioned so that the strands are in a direction opposite to that of the central silks. The tampon is coated with bacitracin. A second tampon is similarly prepared.

d–f Two 8-gauge French catheters are then passed through the nose (one on the right, the other on the left) and into the pharynx. With use of a headlight and tongue blade, the catheters are pulled out through the mouth and secured to the center strings. The catheters are pulled and the tampons guided into the posterior nares with the surgeon's finger. The tampons will fold as they become lodged in the posterior nares. The central silk strands are pulled tightly along the floor of the nose; the ends of the other strands are left dangling from the side of the mouth, to be later secured to the cheeks with tape. The nose is subsequently packed anteriorly with gauze, and the silk strands are tied over the gauze or a small dental roll that is placed over the gauze packing.

Postoperatively the patient should be treated with antibiotics. The columella and ala of the nose should be inspected for pressure necrosis, and if this occurs, the tightness of the silk strands should be adjusted. Because the packing can affect the airway by pressing down on the soft palate, the patient should be evaluated for signs of respiratory difficulty. Evaluation of blood gases will help in assessing adequate oxygenation and CO_2 exchange.

part
two

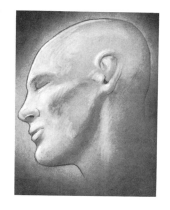

Mandibular
Fractures

section I

Classification and Pathophysiology of Mandibular Fractures

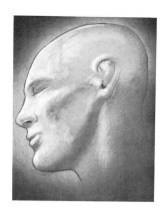

chapter 6

General Considerations

Patients with mandibular fractures can present with a myriad of signs and symptoms related to the type of fracture, pull of muscles of mastication, and the preexisting dentition. Swelling, tenderness, and ecchymoses are often accompanied intraorally by fractured teeth, lacerations, and exposure of bone fragments. Speech and swallowing are impaired, and saliva collects in dependent areas. In severe cases, the tongue is displaced posteriorly and can be associated with respiratory obstruction. The patient complains of pain, and with displacement of the fracture, there is an inability to occlude and approximate the upper jaw to the lower one. Premature contact of the molars often causes an open bite deformity. Unilateral injuries may cause deviation of the jaw and a crossbite appearance. To recognize these conditions, the surgeon must have a complete understanding of the types of fracture and of those pathophysiologic processes that produce each clinical picture. This information is also essential in designing the best treatment program.

CLASSIFICATION

A Fractures of the mandible are classified according to both anatomic location and the specific characteristics of the fracture. Most adult fractures are classified according to the area of involvement (i.e., coronoid, ramus, angle, body, and parasymphysis). The most common areas of injury are the condyle, angle, body, and parasymphysis; rarely is the coronoid process involved. The alveolar ridge fracture is a subtype that can occur in one or several regions. Mandibular fractures may be isolated or multiple and unilateral or bilateral.

B Other descriptions of mandibular fractures consider the extent of injury. In the *simple* fracture, the mucosa and skin are intact. When the fracture is *compound* (or *open*), there is an exposure of bone, either into the oral cavity or extraorally, by way of a laceration or avulsion. The *greenstick* fracture, which often occurs in children, is an incomplete fracture in

MANDIBULAR FRACTURES

A

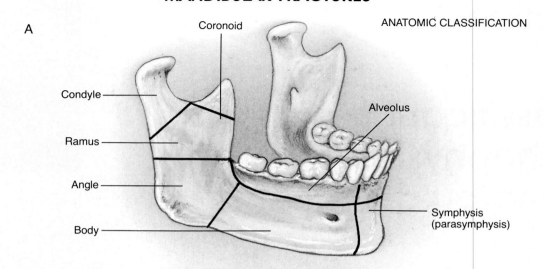

Coronoid

Condyle

Ramus

Angle

Body

Alveolus

Symphysis
(parasymphysis)

B   CLASSIFICATION BY TYPE OF FRACTURE

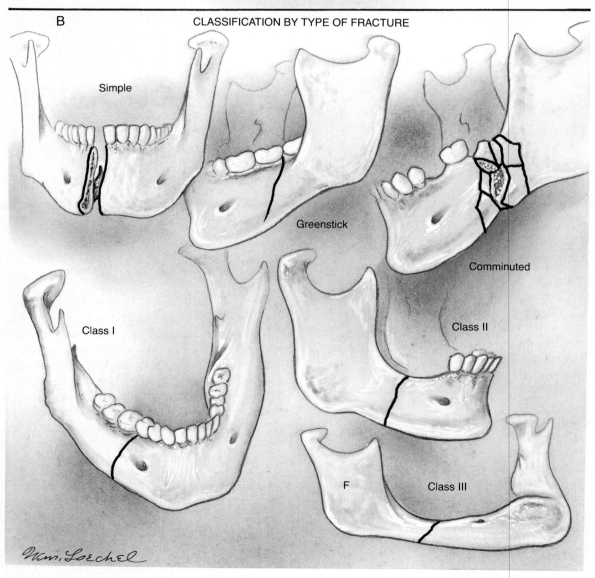

Simple

Greenstick

Comminuted

Class I

Class II

F   Class III

26

which only one cortical surface is involved. The *comminuted* type is characterized by several small fragments of bone. The fractures can also be *complex,* in which the fracture is in continuity with fractures of other areas of the mandible, or *complicated,* in which the fracture involves both the mandible and maxilla.

The presence or absence of teeth can also provide an important classification. A class I fracture has teeth on both sides of the fracture line (dentulous), a class II fracture has teeth on one side (partially edentulous), and a class III fracture (endentulous) has no teeth adjacent to the sides of the fracture. Often class III fracture patients are completely edentulous.

STABILITY CONCEPTS

The various directions and planes of fracture, coupled with the forces exerted by the muscles of mastication, affect displacement and either assist or interfere with the stability of fixation. Other factors that can affect stability are the presence of contralateral or ipsilateral fractures, comminution, and the presence or absence of teeth. In general, fractures that are deemed unstable (or unfavorable) are best treated with open methods of reduction and fixation, whereas those that are stable (or favorable) are usually managed with conservative techniques.

C *Fracture lines* can be extremely important, especially if they allow the muscle groups to pull the fragments from each other. The body and the anterior portion of the angle are depressed by the digastric, geniohyoid, genioglossus, and mylohyoid muscles. The ascending ramus and the upper portion of the angle are elevated by the temporalis and masseter muscles and, to some extent, by the medial and lateral pterygoid muscles.

D An angle fracture that is directed from the posterior part of the angle anteriorly to the third molar is usually displaced and relatively unstable. A vertically directed angle fracture that traverses from the posterior portion of the body superiorly to the third molar tends to be held in a normal position. In the horizontal plane, the pterygoid muscles are unopposed, and if a fracture extends from the lateral part of the angle anteriorly to the inner cortex, the posterior segment will be unstable and displaced inward. Fractures from the lateral portion of the angle directed posteriorly to the inner cortex will be pulled together.

E At the parasymphysis, a relatively vertical line of fracture predisposes to instability. The digastric and mylohyoid muscles tend to pull the hemimandible downward, causing one half of the jaw to be distracted from the other. Obliquity of the fracture may or may not lead to instability; this will depend on the direction of the fracture and on whether the mylohyoid muscle brings the fragments together or apart.

F At the condyle, the line of fracture also determines the degree of instability. Because the lateral pterygoid muscle inserts high into the neck of the condyle and into the capsule of the temporomandibular joint, high fractures are associated with minimal displacement. On the other hand, fractures in the subcondylar area are often associated with medial dislocation of the head and neck of the condyle.

G *Multiplicity of fractures* is also a factor in determining stability and treatment options. Parasymphyseal fractures commonly occur with angle or condylar fractures of the opposite side. Angle fractures are often seen with opposite condyle, parasymphysis, or body fractures. These multiple fractures can also be associated with a depression and rotation of the intervening segment. If the fractures happen to be ipsilateral, as in a parasymphyseal and subcondylar fracture, then the mylohyoid and pterygoid muscles tend to rotate and pull the fragments medially. The same effect can be seen in ipsilateral, parasymphyseal, and angle fractures. For these reasons, multiple fractures commonly lead to unfavorable forces at the fracture site.

Comminuted fractures of the angle also tend to cause instability. Several fractures in the area of the angle will tend to prevent "locking" of the fragments. Internal and/or external fixation thus becomes important in developing a solid union.

H *Loss of teeth* also creates additional stability problems. Second or third molar contacts on the posterior segment prevent upward rotation of the posterior fragment. When these teeth are missing (on either the upper or lower jaw) there is no "stop," and the posterior fragment tends to be more mobile. Occasionally a molar is involved with the fracture, and when the tooth is loose and carious or devitalized from injury to the pulp and/or root, the surgeon must extract the tooth and then select an appropriate method to treat the destabilized segment.

Completely edentulous patients present even more of a problem. For this condition, there is no dentition with which to guide the "fit" of the upper and lower jaws. Also, the option of using the upper dentition to stabilize the lower (through intermaxillary fixation) is not available, and other methods of fixation must be used.

STABILITY CONCEPTS

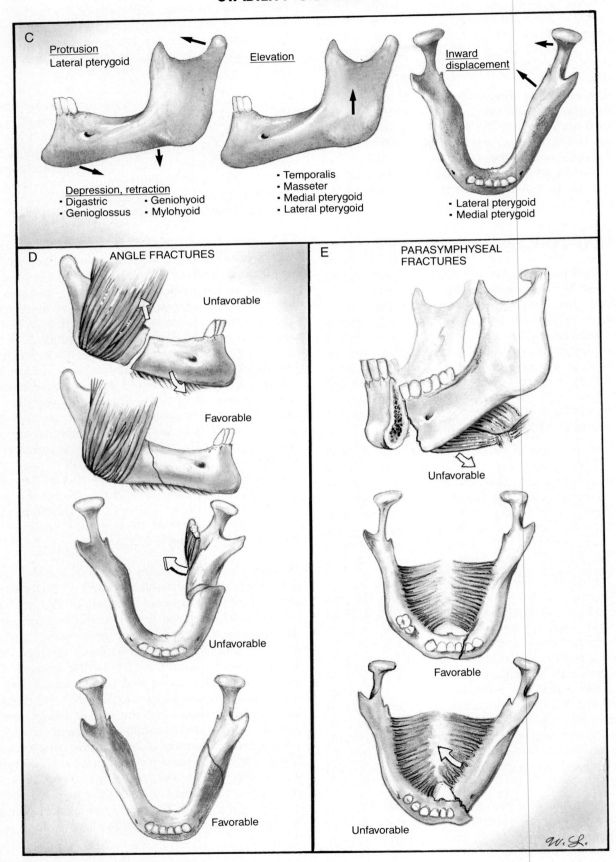

C

Protrusion
Lateral pterygoid

Elevation

Inward displacement

Depression, retraction
- Digastric   - Geniohyoid
- Genioglossus   - Mylohyoid

- Temporalis
- Masseter
- Medial pterygoid
- Lateral pterygoid

- Lateral pterygoid
- Medial pterygoid

D   ANGLE FRACTURES

Unfavorable

Favorable

Unfavorable

Favorable

E   PARASYMPHYSEAL FRACTURES

Unfavorable

Favorable

Unfavorable

STABILITY CONCEPTS *(Continued)*

F

CONDYLAR FRACTURES

Unfavorable

Favorable

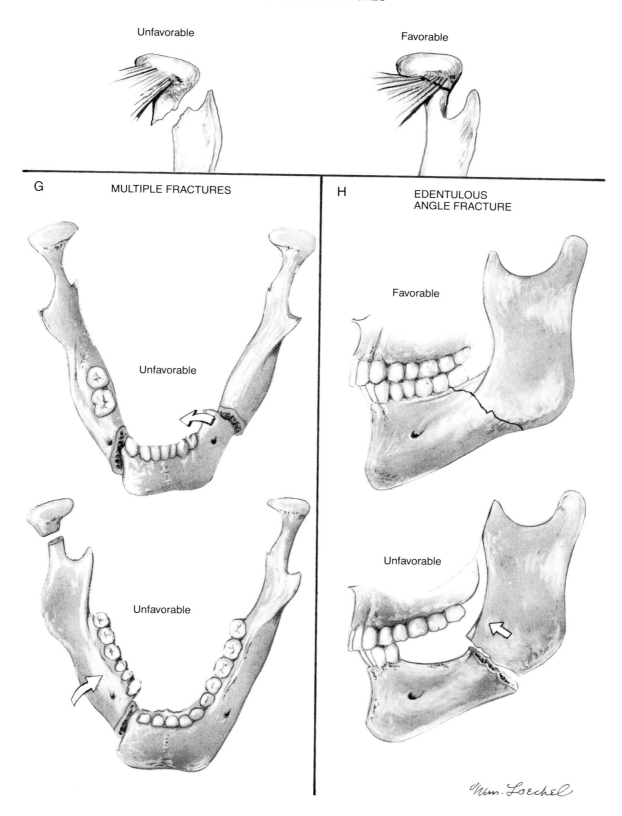

G   MULTIPLE FRACTURES

Unfavorable

Unfavorable

H   EDENTULOUS
ANGLE FRACTURE

Favorable

Unfavorable

Wm. Loechel

PEDIATRIC CONSIDERATIONS

Fractures of the mandible are treated more conservatively in children than in adults because of the growth characteristics of the jaw and the risk of injury to developing teeth. Healing of bones is very efficient in children, and even if the fragments are not lined up perfectly, there can be rapid healing across the gaps, with new bone formation and a remodeling that restores normal anatomic configuration.

I In children, the surgeon must also be aware of the growth of the mandible. Essentially, the ramus and body are remodeled by resorption and deposition processes, whereas the rest of the jaw elongates in response to growth at the condylar region. Injury to the growth area (center) can occur with condylar trauma, and to avoid further damage, open reduction and fixation of the condyle should be avoided. If there is damage, the jaw will have limited growth, especially in the condyle-ramus region. This can cause a dysfunction, and later the jaw, on opening, will deviate to the side of the injury.

The temporomandibular joint can also be indirectly affected. In such patients, there can be a fibrous fixation of the joint and secondary growth deficits. The complication can develop rapidly in children, and early mobilization of the jaw should be attempted to prevent this from occurring. The mandible should be held in intermaxillary fixation for no more than 2 weeks, and if it is necessary to add additional fixation, it should be performed at intermittent periods. Occasionally patients can be treated in a "halfway" manner with loose rubber bands, allowing them a limited use of the joint.

J,K Knowledge of the anatomy and position of teeth is also important. If holes are drilled in the lower portion of the mandible for screws or plates, there can be injury to the primordium of the teeth. For these reasons, the objective in children is to align the fragments in the best manner possible without injury to the growth potential of teeth.

Specific methods that should be applied in children include the following:

1. Avoid open techniques (i.e., interosseous wiring and plating).
2. Consider the use of lingual splints.
3. Intermaxillary fixation can be maintained, but the surgeon must be certain to place the ligatures around sound teeth. Strategically placed Ivy loops are excellent alternatives to the arch bar technique.
4. Avoid prolonged fixation, especially if there is a suspicion of injury to the condyle or temporomandibular joint.

PEDIATRIC MANDIBLES

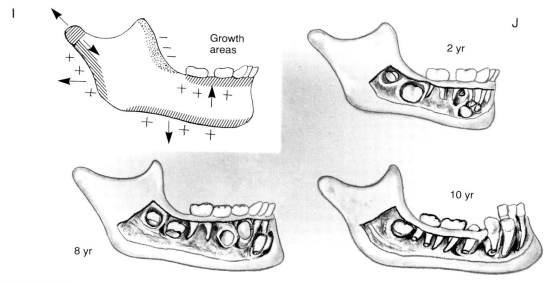

I

Growth areas

J

2 yr

8 yr

10 yr

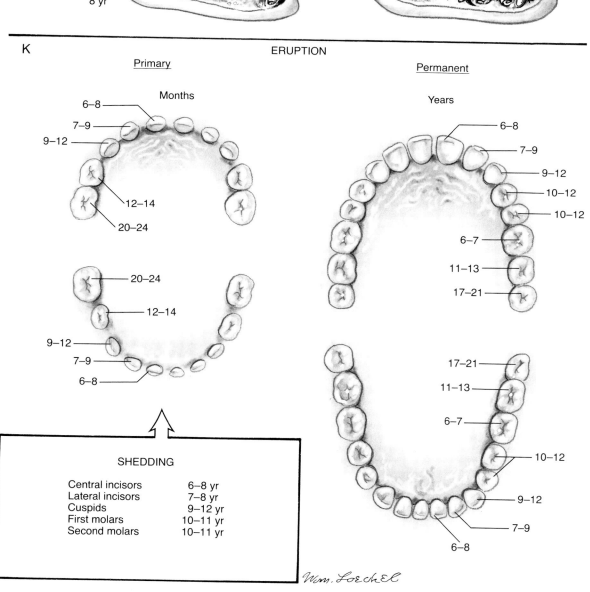

K

ERUPTION

Primary

Months

6–8
7–9
9–12
12–14
20–24

20–24
12–14
9–12
7–9
6–8

Permanent

Years

6–8
7–9
9–12
10–12
10–12
6–7
11–13
17–21

17–21
11–13
6–7
10–12
9–12
7–9
6–8

SHEDDING

Central incisors	6–8 yr
Lateral incisors	7–8 yr
Cuspids	9–12 yr
First molars	10–11 yr
Second molars	10–11 yr

Wm. Loechel

31

section II

Condylar Fractures

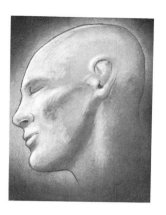

chapter 7

Closed Reduction for
Simple Dislocation of the Condyle
Alternative Technique of Condyloplasty
for Recurrent Dislocation

INDICATIONS

Acute dislocation of the condylar head from the temporomandibular joint without fracture is not common but can develop from any sudden, forceful opening of the jaw. During the dislocation, the condyle usually rotates forward, breaking the adjacent ligaments. The head of the condyle, under the pull of the pterygoid muscles, then leaves the glenoid fossa, crosses the articular eminence, and becomes locked in front of it. The dislocation is often bilateral. It is associated with pain and difficulty in management of the saliva, speech, and swallowing. The condition can become chronic and recurrent if not treated appropriately.

PROCEDURE

A–C Reduction of the condylar head can be achieved with manual pressure exerted at the angle of the jaw. The muscles of the patient should be relaxed, and pain should be controlled by intramuscular administration of 50 to 75 mg of meperidine 30 minutes prior to the reduction. To achieve the correct force for reduction, the surgeon should stand behind the seated patient. The surgeon's thumbs should then be placed at the junction of the body of the ramus just lateral to the molar dentition. The jaw is pushed down while rotating the chin upward. Constant pressure will eventually break the "spasms," but this process may take 5 to 10 minutes. Alternatively, reduction can be performed from the front, but the surgeon will have to use more thumb and hand pressure. During the postreduction period, excursion of the jaw should be limited. The patient should be placed on a liquid diet and told to avoid any chewing of foods for at least 10 days. Pain can be controlled with analgesics.

PITFALLS

1. Be sure that the condylar dislocation is not part of a fracture of the condyle and/or glenoid fossa. Such injuries can be associated with damage to the auditory system and intracranial complications. These problems should be recognized and treated accordingly.

2. A search for factors leading to occlusal disharmony is often beneficial. Some patients have a myofascial pain syndrome or may be taking drugs, such as phenothiazides, that induce extrapyramidal effects and spasms of the muscles of mastication. Such a condition should be referred to the neurologist for appropriate control.

3. Proper sedation will expedite the reduction process. Meperidine has both pain control and sedative effects. The addition of diazepam can promote relaxation of the spastic musculature.

4. Reduction of the dislocation in a noncompliant, noncooperative patient is difficult, and in such situations, general anesthesia is preferred.

COMPLICATIONS

1. Recurrence of the dislocation is easy to diagnose because of the characteristic history. Intermaxillary fixation will limit movement of the condyle and encourage fibrosis of the capsule, but results are quite variable. Frequently something more definitive must be done. Shortening of the capsule with a "pants-over-vest" technique is helpful (see later). Enlargement of the articular eminence with an allo-graft or autogenous bone graft may control anterior excursion of the condyle. In the noncompliant patient, removal of the lateral third of the articular eminence may be the more prudent course.

2. Injury to the meniscus can occur as a result of temporomandibular joint dislocation and/or fracture involving the condylar head. Several types of injury can be defined: inflammation, complete or partial severing of the meniscus from its attachments, or tearing of the meniscus itself. Inflammation alone is diagnosed when the pain responds to analgesics and jaw motion improves within 10 days. The more severe injuries associated with tearing will have persistence of trismus, deviation of the jaw on opening of the mouth, and limitation of excursion of the head of the condyle. The inflammatory condition is treated with a soft diet and analgesics. More serious injury to the joint is treated with intraoral splints and jaw exercises. If conservative approaches are unsuccessful, the surgeon must consider surgical reattachment (or reconstruction) of the soft tissues, meniscectomy, or prosthetic substitution. For indications and details of these procedures, the reader is referred to Chapter 29 and appropriate oral surgery texts.

ALTERNATIVE TECHNIQUE OF CONDYLOPLASTY FOR RECURRENT DISLOCATION

Chronic dislocation may be treated simply by strengthening the loosened capsule over the condylar head and neck. This method is conservative, and therefore, if it is not successful, the surgeon can proceed to a more aggressive approach. Exposure is similar to that obtained in Chapter 10. The capsule is identified and tightened by simply plicating the lower portion of the capsule over the upper portion and securing the plication with two 3–0 nonabsorbable mattress sutures. Excursion of the mandible is limited for 2 weeks, and the patient is subsequently treated with active opening and closing exercises.

TREATMENT OF CONDYLAR DISLOCATION

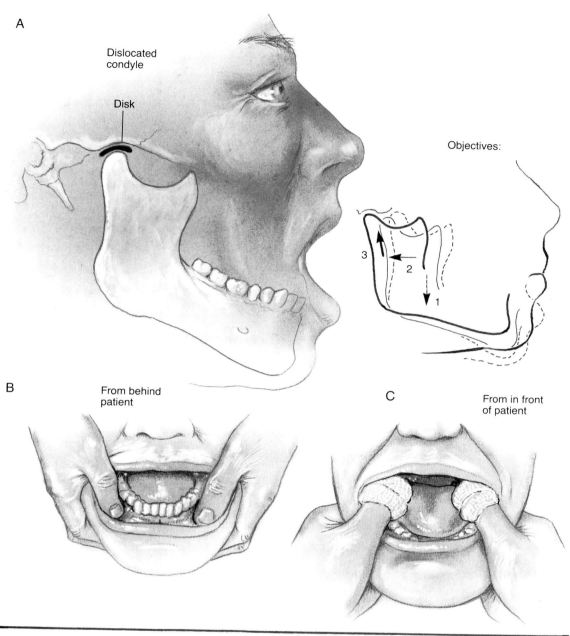

A

Dislocated condyle

Disk

Objectives:

3   2   1

B   From behind patient

C   From in front of patient

ALTERNATIVE TECHNIQUE OF CONDYLOPLASTY

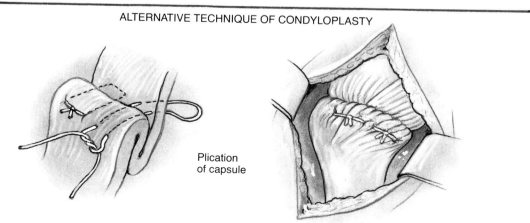

Plication of capsule

Closed Reduction and Immobilization of Condylar Fractures With Intermaxillary Fixation

Alternative Techniques of Ivy Loops and Molar Wafers

In Consultation With Mark T. Marunick, DDS

INDICATIONS

Most condylar fractures can be treated with closed methods of intermaxillary fixation. Contact of the teeth in the molar region drives the mandible downward; this, together with the anterior medial pull of the pterygoid muscles, tends to reduce the fracture. There can also be a remodeling of the condylar neck that reestablishes normal anatomic relationships. In adults with an intact dentition, intermaxillary fixation is carried out with arch bars or Ivy loops; in the edentulous patient, these arch bars can be secured to dentures, which, in turn, are secured to the upper and lower jaws and to each other by intermaxillary fixation. In children, fixation need only be temporary and is often achievable with strategic placement of Ivy loops.

TECHNIQUE

Intermaxillary fixation with arch bars can be carried out using general or local/topical anesthesia. Good lighting is important. An assistant is necessary to help in retraction of the lips and cheeks and to aid in the suctioning of blood and saliva from the field.

A,B For usual fixation, a pliable Erich arch bar is satisfactory. These bars are designed with small hooks that should be directed toward the gums on each dental arch. The bar can be cut to the correct size by placing the bar on half of the arch and counting the number of hooks. The bar is then cut at twice the number of hooks to cover the entire arch. The posterior portion of the bar should be bent inward to avoid unnecessary injury to the mucosa.

C,D The arch bar can be applied first to either the upper or lower jaw. Regardless of which jaw is selected, the bar should initially be affixed to the first premolar tooth. For this technique, a six-inch length of 25- or 26-gauge stainless steel wire is passed above the bar and between the teeth in the interdental space to the lingual surface. The wire is then fed back between the teeth so that it exits below the bar on the buccal surface. The wire is then twisted down across the bar and tooth in a clockwise diagonal fashion and is secured as high as possible on the crown by pushing the wire with a Freer elevator toward the gum line. The curvature on the crown will keep the wire from being displaced toward the occlusal surface of the tooth. All wires should be pulled while twisting in the same direction (i.e., clockwise). The wires should be temporarily left long and secured with a clamp to help in the retraction of the lip.

E After the bar is attached to the premolar of one side, it is then affixed to the first premolar on the opposite side. It is important that the bar be held firmly against the dental arch so that when the second wire is placed, there is no space between the arch bar and the teeth. Subsequently the bar is secured to the other molars and to the canine teeth.

F Because the canine tooth is cone-shaped, special techniques must be applied. As described by Dingman and Natvig (1964), the wire should be passed above the arch bar toward the lingual surface and returned around the tooth (still above the arch bar) to the buccal or lateral surface. One end of the wire is then looped around the arch bar, and the ends are twisted horizontally around the tooth. These techniques can also be used when there is an isolated molar next to an edentulous area or when the sur-

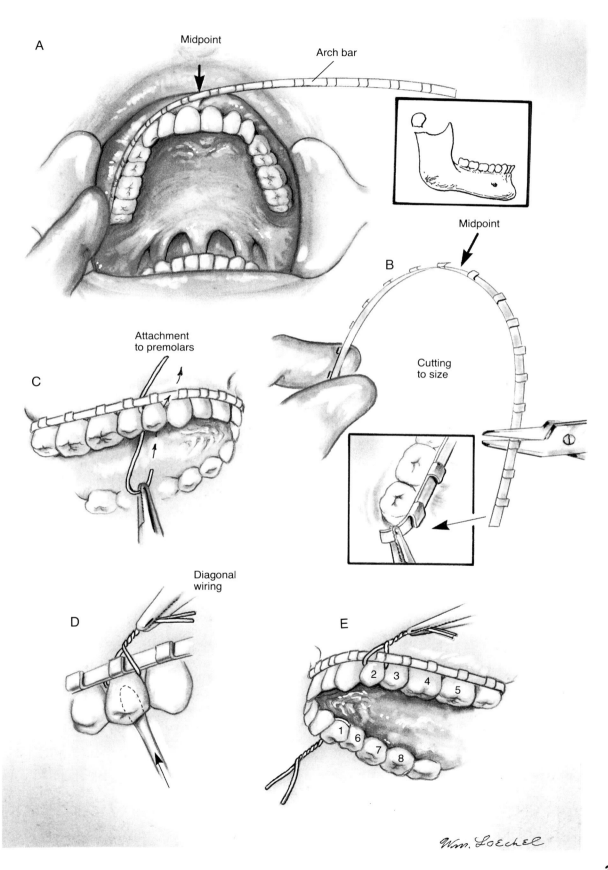

A

Midpoint

Arch bar

Midpoint

B

Cutting to size

Attachment to premolars

C

Diagonal wiring

D

E

Wm. Loechel

geon is forced to use the incisors for additional fixation.

G,H During the process of applying the wires, there is a tendency for the wire to stretch. This can cause some loosening, and to avoid this problem, the surgeon should twist the wires tightly once more later in the procedure. Alternatively, the wire can be prestretched prior to use. The twisted ends of the wire are cut at 1.0 to 1.5 cm, and with the same clockwise rotation, the wire is turned with a hemostat into a sharp curve directed toward the gingival mucous membrane. The other (upper or lower) arch bar is applied in a similar fashion.

I Arch bars can be secured to each other with elastic bands or wires. Elastic bands can be made easily by cutting a No. 14 elastic catheter into thin sections. The elastic bands have the advantage of providing for dynamic reduction and are easily adjusted by incorporating more or fewer loops on the bars. Wires will occasionally need to be tightened or removed and replaced in new positions. There is more difficulty in removing the wire if the patient vomits in the postoperative period.

J,K As the rubber bands or wires are applied, occlusion should be checked in the molar region. Wear facets should be in contact with one another, and centric occlusion should be established. Excessive traction should be avoided on the incisors, as such forces can cause a partial or complete extraction of the teeth.

Postoperative radiographs are useful in evaluating the reduction and fixation. Hygiene of the teeth and gingiva is maintained with a water irrigation device or gentle brushing. When the arch bars are to be removed (2 to 6 weeks later), the bands are first taken off, and the patient is asked to bite on a tongue blade. If there is discomfort at this time or during the next week, or if jaw movement does not return to normal, then the patient must be reevaluated for malunion, delayed union, or nonunion.

PITFALLS

1. Avoid injury to the interdental papillae. Try to pass wires between the teeth, rather than through the gingiva. This will keep the teeth healthier during the period of fixation and avoid permanent injury to the periodontia.

2. Check the arch bar for slippage postoperatively. On occasion, the wires will loosen; when this occurs, they should be tightened with additional turns. If they are not tightened, the arch bar can become dislodged from the dentition.

3. Avoid wire ligatures around the incisors, as

they can pull the incisors from their sockets. However, if there are many missing teeth and the incisors can help with the fixation, they should be used. In such a case, the vertical traction should be kept to a minimum.

4. If a segment of jaw is edentulous, it is possible to bridge this gap with a strong arch bar and a more secure ligature to the remaining teeth. Often this can be accomplished with a heavier Jelenko bar and a Dingman wire ligature applied to the premolar or molar teeth.

5. The surgeon must be sure that the condylar fracture is not associated with another fracture. If this should occur, one or both fractures will usually require open stabilization.

6. Be careful when applying arch bars in children with deciduous teeth, as the bar can prematurely extract the tooth. The teeth should thus be carefully studied for maturity (Chapter 6). Alternatively, Ivy loops can be secured to selected groups to maintain adequate intermaxillary fixation (see later).

7. Arch bar fixation for condylar fractures should be limited to just enough time for healing to take place. If the time of fixation is prolonged, ankylosis can result. In children, intermaxillary fixation should be removed in 2 weeks, and in adults, within 4 weeks. When intermaxillary fixation is used for other types of mandibular (e.g., condyle, body) and maxillary fractures, the arch bars should be retained for 4 to 6 weeks in children and 6 to 8 weeks in adults.

8. If wires are used to attach the bars to each other, the surgeon has to be prepared for possible postoperative vomiting and the need for an emergency cutting of the wires. In anticipation of such an event, wire cutters should be available at the bedside.

COMPLICATIONS

1. Injury to the condyle is often associated with tearing of the ligamentous capsule and/or displacement or tearing of the meniscus of the temporomandibular joint. Often, appropriate fixation and reduction will provide for satisfactory healing. If this does not occur, the surgeon must reevaluate the injury and treat the condition. Management includes nighttime head bandages, soft diet, and analgesics; in other patients, it may be necessary to consider interocclusal splints and even reconstruction of the joint space.

2. Displacement of the condyle can result in bony auditory canal wall fractures and/or penetration of the middle fossa. An accurate diagnosis is essential if appropriate treatment for these complicating injuries is to be provided (see Chapter 6).

3. Failure of the condyle to heal will lead to a

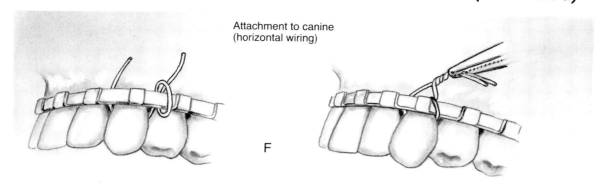

Attachment to canine
(horizontal wiring)

F

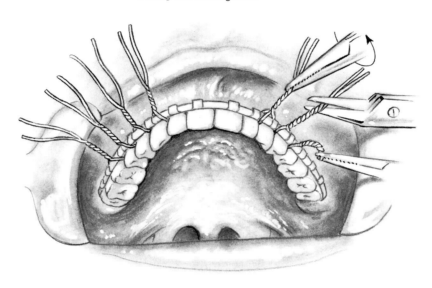

Cutting and twisting ends

G

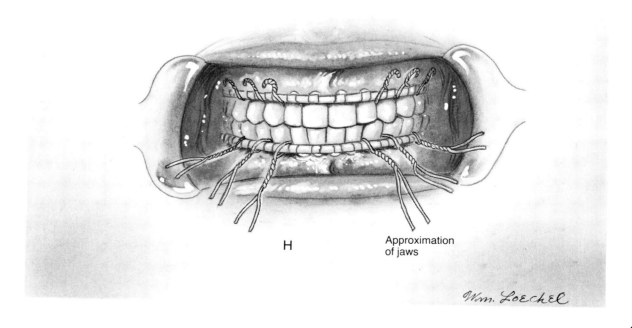

H

Approximation
of jaws

Wm. Loechel

I

Elastic band traction in occlusion

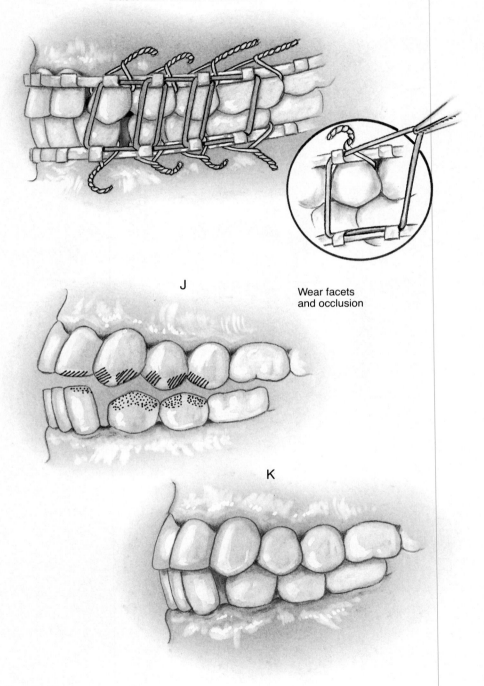

J

Wear facets
and occlusion

K

Wm. Loechel

nonunion or pseudarthrosis. If the fracture is high, the pseudarthrosis will have negligible effects. It may cause short periods of pain and, on opening, a deviation of the jaw to the affected side. However, if nonunion complicates mastication and causes excessive pain, exploration of the condyle and condylectomy or reconstruction of the joint must be considered (see Chapter 29).

4. Ankylosis of the condyle is a serious complication and may lead to failure of growth of the mandible in children and/or major dysfunction of the jaw. In the adult, mastication is usually impaired, and as a result of inability to open the mouth, problems with oral intake resulting in inadequate nutrition may develop.

Ankylosis can be treated with several techniques. Early, the surgeon should attempt jaw prying by sequential placement of increasing numbers of tongue blades between the dental arches. If this is unsatisfactory, then surgical intervention is necessary. If the joint has been irreversibly damaged, it is possible to restore it with a new joint surface made of metal or plastic. If the entire joint has been destroyed, condylectomy or a planned pseudarthrosis may be advisable. In some patients, condylectomy and reconstruction with rib graft or a prosthesis is desirable (see Chapter 29).

ALTERNATIVE TECHNIQUE OF IVY LOOPS

The Ivy loop is an important alternative method for closed reduction and fixation. Although it is not as strong as the arch bar, it is useful in selectively bringing occlusal pairs of teeth together. It is used in children who have a mixed dentition, in partially edentulous patients who will have additional forms of fixation, and in individuals who need temporary occlusion while other methods (i.e., biphase or plates) are being applied.

a,b The Ivy loop is constructed of a 25- or 26-gauge stainless steel wire. The wire is cut to approximately 16 cm. It is then wound around the tip of a small clamp, and a small loop is formed with two to three twists of the end of the wire. The ends are inserted between two suitable teeth. Each wire is wrapped around the neck of the adjoining tooth, and the wire is brought out to the labial/buccal surface.

c—e A mesial wire is then inserted through the loop, and both wires are twisted around the more distal tooth. A Freer elevator should be used to push the wire closer to the neck of the tooth while addi-

tional twists are applied to the wire. A final tightening occurs when the loop is grasped with a needle holder, pulled laterally, and twisted one to two turns around the external wire.

f Additional Ivy loops are placed on opposing pairs of occluding teeth. The jaws can be held in fixation by applying fine wire ligatures (No. 28) through the eyelets (loops).

The loops must be checked often for displacement of the wires, and if this occurs, appropriate adjustments should be made. The dentition must be kept clean with a soft toothbrush or water irrigation device.

ALTERNATIVE TECHNIQUE OF MOLAR WAFERS

If the condyle does not become reduced with time, adjunctive reduction techniques can be considered. Radiographs should be obtained 2 weeks following reduction and fixation. If the condyle is still displaced, an interocclusal acrylic wafer can be made and placed between the molars to provide additional downward traction on the mandible.

a,b The wafer can be fabricated in two ways. The best (and preferred) method is to make stone dental casts (see Chapter 9) and fabricate the wafer on these casts. The wafer is built up approximately 2 to 5 mm to provide more downward stress on the posterior fragments. To achieve these relationships, the casts should be mounted on an articulator and the articulator adjusted to increase the vertical distance between the teeth. The casts are then coated with petrolatum.

c—e The acrylic, in a viscous state, is adapted to the lower cast, and the articulation is closed to the predetermined vertical opening. After polymerization, trimming, and adjustment, the splint is placed into the mouth and held by intermaxillary fixation.

If the surgeon is seeking a reduction only, a splint can be designed so that an incline is exerted on the posterior dentition. However, this splint should be used for only 7 to 10 days.

f A rapid, but less exact, method is to make a splint directly on the teeth. This can be accomplished by applying petrolatum to the posterior maxillary and mandibular molars, having the patient bite down on the viscous material, removing the material, and allowing it to harden. Excess acrylic can be trimmed from the splint. The splint should be secured tightly with intermaxillary fixation.

ALTERNATIVE TECHNIQUE OF IVY LOOPS

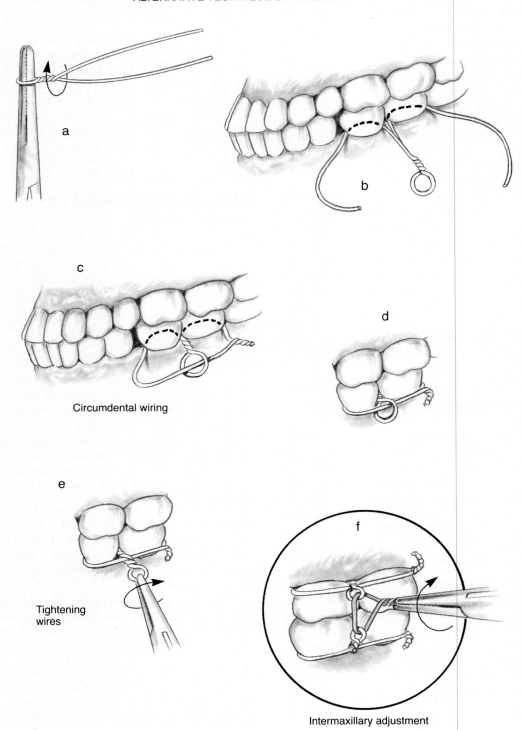

a

b

c

Circumdental wiring

d

e

Tightening wires

f

Intermaxillary adjustment

INTERMAXILLARY FIXATION FOR CONDYLAR FRACTURE *(Continued)*

ALTERNATIVE TECHNIQUE OF INTEROCCLUSAL WAFER

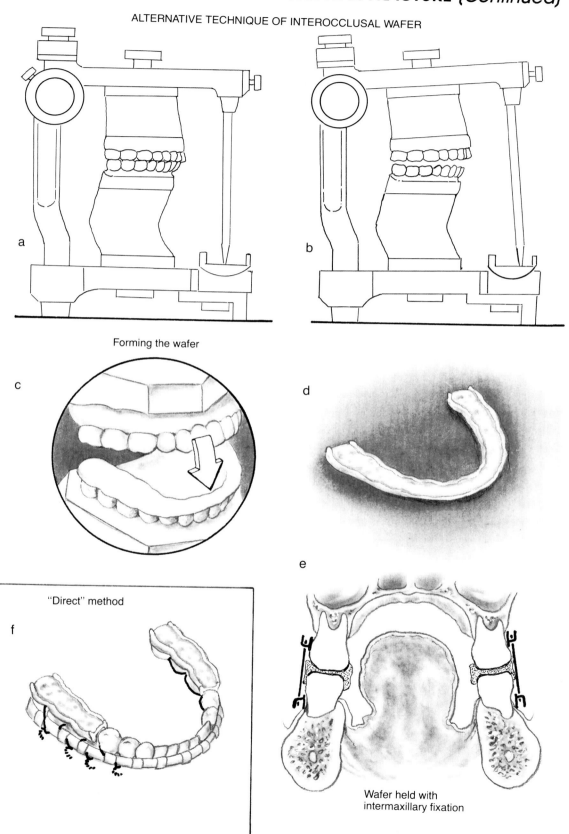

a

b

Forming the wafer

c

d

e

"Direct" method

f

Wafer held with
intermaxillary fixation

Closed Reduction of Condylar Fractures in the Edentulous Patient With Circummandibular and Circumzygomatic Splint Fixation

In Consultation With Mark T. Marunick, DDS

INDICATIONS

Simple isolated condylar fractures can often be treated with intermaxillary fixation or Ivy loops. However, if the patient is edentulous, it becomes necessary to use other fixation methods. Most commonly, the dentures are secured to the mandible and the zygoma by circumosseous wiring and then to each other with intermaxillary wires. For patients who do not have dentures, there is the option of making splints (Gunning type), which are also secured to the upper and lower jaws. The period of fixation is variable, depending on the age of the individual. In children, fixation is employed for a 2-week period; in adults, it is used for a 2- to 4-week period. Consultation and collaboration with a maxillofacial prosthodontist to fabricate and apply these devices are highly recommended.

PROCEDURES

Preparation of the Splint

The splint is made from either an autopolymerizing or a thermoplastic acrylic resin. Most dental laboratories will make the splint, provided they are given satisfactory casts, appropriate instructions, and authorization. The principal aspects of the technique are discussed in the text that follows.

To make the impressions, stock plastic dental or metal edentulous impression trays are used. In selecting trays, the lower tray is identified by its U shape, which provides space for the tongue. The upper tray is ovoid or square to cover the region of the hard palate. The selected trays should fit the alveolus comfortably.

A–D The impression is made using type I, normal-set, alginate material mixed to the manufacturer's specifications. Equal parts by volume of water and powder are mixed in a flexible bowl until the mixture is uniform and smooth. The material is then placed into the upper tray with a spatula to the height of the flanges of the tray. Prior to mixing the alginate, the oral cavity is rinsed with water and dried with 2 in. × 2 in. cotton gauze pads that are placed in the buccal and lingual sulci. The lips are lubricated with petrolatum. The gauze pads are removed, and the loaded tray is centered over the edentulous ridge and carefully seated. Digital pressure is maintained until the mixture "sets" (approximately 3 minutes). The tray is then removed and the impression inspected. If the impression is acceptable, it is washed, wrapped in a moist paper towel, and placed into a plastic bag. The lower impression is made and handled in a similar fashion. When making the impressions, care must be taken to minimize extrusion of impression material from the posterior part of the tray. This can elicit a gag reflex and pose a risk of aspiration.

E–G The material chosen for the cast (made from the impression) can be plaster, stone, or combinations of the two. Ideally the stone (or plaster) should be mixed with the correct water-to-stone ratio and spatulated under vaccuum before pouring with the aid of a vibrator. If these instruments are not available, the stone and water can be hand-mixed in a flexible bowl with a spatula. To minimize voids, the mixed stone should be carefully placed in the impression in small increments on a vibrator, or alternatively, the handle of the tray can be tapped on the top of the table. When the stone has set, the impres-

SPLINT FABRICATION

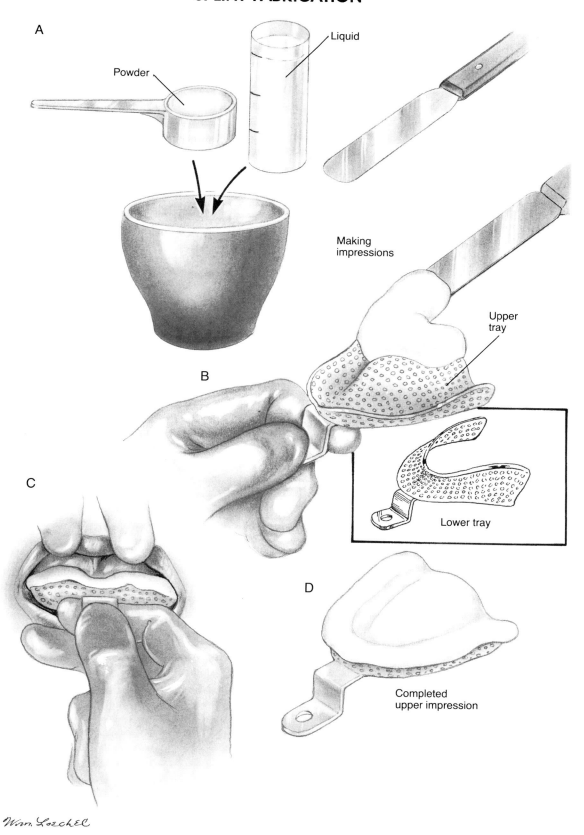

A

Powder

Liquid

Making
impressions

Upper
tray

B

C

Lower tray

D

Completed
upper impression

Wm. Loechel

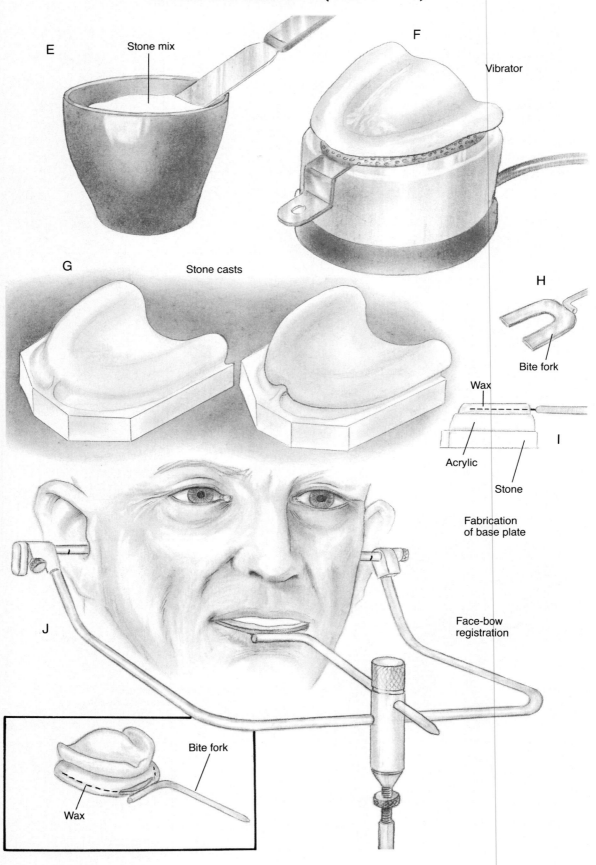

E   Stone mix

F   Vibrator

G   Stone casts

H   Bite fork

Wax

Acrylic

Stone

I

Fabrication
of base plate

Face-bow
registration

J

Bite fork

Wax

SPLINT FABRICATION (Continued)

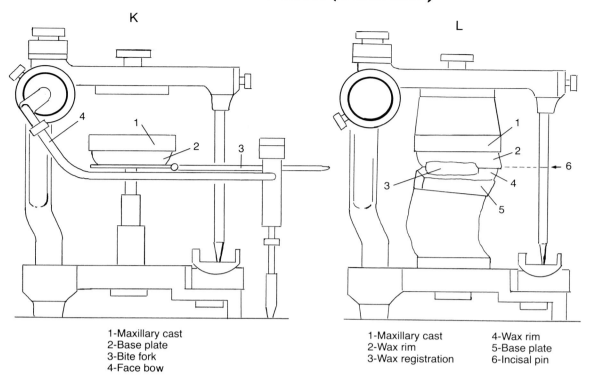

K

1-Maxillary cast
2-Base plate
3-Bite fork
4-Face bow

L

1-Maxillary cast
2-Wax rim
3-Wax registration
4-Wax rim
5-Base plate
6-Incisal pin

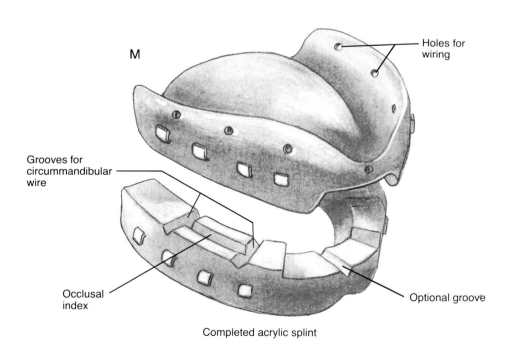

M

Holes for wiring

Grooves for circummandibular wire

Occlusal index

Optional groove

Completed acrylic splint

sion is separated from the cast, and the cast is trimmed appropriately.

H–J The next step is to coat the cast with petrolatum and to fabricate autopolymerizing acrylic resin baseplates. The stone cast must be carefully evaluated to limit the extension of the baseplates where tissues were displaced by the impression. Wax rims are placed on the baseplates, and these same baseplates are used for face-bow registration. The face-bow is then transferred to the articulator. An appropriate clinically determined occlusal vertical dimension and centric position are recorded and used to relate the casts.

K–M With the cast and baseplate on the articulator, the baseplates can be waxed to the appropriate design. To expedite intermaxillary fixation, arch bars are imbedded into the labial aspect of the wax rims. Lateral stability is provided by grooves placed on the top of the lower wax rim; extensions are then waxed on the upper rim so that when it is occluded with the lower, the extensions engage the grooves, relate the two splints to one another, and prevent lateral displacement. Separate grooves are also placed on the lower rim to aid in circummandibular wiring of the lower splint. The anterior portions of the wax rims are cut away, providing access for the intake of food and liquids. The separate upper and lower splints are processed in acrylic resin, finished, and polished. Holes are placed in the flanges of the upper splint, several on each side, for circumzygomatic wiring. The splints should be checked and adjusted in the mouth prior to surgical placement.

Denture Preparation

A–F For those patients with adequate dentures, the preparation process is quite easy. If damaged, the dentures should be repaired with an autopolymerizing acrylic resin. A channel can be cut in the labial aspect of the base of the denture just above the teeth in the upper denture and below the teeth in the lower denture. The channel should be large enough to accommodate a segment of arch bar, which is properly positioned and secured with autopolymerizing acrylic resin. Access to the loops must be maintained. If the flange is too thin, shallow recesses can be cut and stainless steel wire loops secured with autopolymerizing acrylic resin. Grooves or holes are placed on the occlusal surfaces of the lower denture to facilitate circummandibular wiring. Anterior teeth should be removed for intake of food and liquids. Holes are drilled, several on each side of the flanges of the upper denture, to allow circumzygomatic wiring. With such modifications to

the dentures, most patients will require new dentures after healing.

If the teeth are not made out of porcelain, a more expedient option is available. After the denture is repaired, an arch bar can be directly applied to the denture with loops of 26-gauge wire. Usually two sets of holes placed in the molar regions are sufficient to hold the wires, which are secured diagonally to the arch bar. In making the holes, the surgeon must be certain that the holes are not placed near the gingiva of the alveolus. A wire through this area can cause damage to the mucosa, and such wires should not be in contact with the jaw.

Application of Splint or Denture

A–D The methods for applying the splints and dentures are similar. For attachment to the mandible, a small incision through the skin is made beneath the jaw, and a passing awl or large needle is passed to the gingivolingual sulcus. A 24- or 25-gauge stainless steel wire is attached to the end of the awl. The instrument is then pulled down along the inside of the mandible, rotated around the mandible, and pushed out through the gingivobuccal sulcus. The wire is removed from the awl, pulled back and forth to seat on the mandible, and subsequently secured through the preformed hole or groove in the splint. The procedure is performed in an identical fashion on the opposite side of the jaw. One or two wires per side can be applied. The wires are then twisted, cut to size, and bent onto the external surface of the prosthesis.

E For the upper denture or upper part of the splint, a passing awl is placed through a small stab incision made above the zygomatic arch and passed on the medial surface of the zygoma to the upper gingivobuccal sulcus near the area of the first molar. A 25- or 26-gauge wire is attached to the awl, and the awl is pulled to the level of the arch. At the superior border of the arch, the awl is rotated downward, lateral to the arch, carrying the wire into the oral/buccal cavity. Clamps are then placed on the wire, and with a sawing motion, the wire is seated as far anteriorly as possible on the zygoma.

F The ends of the circumzygomatic wire are held with a clamp and twisted on each other to form a loop within the oral/buccal cavity. A second loop of 28-gauge wire is attached to the molar flanges, and the 25-gauge circumzygomatic wire is affixed through this loop.

G Often circumzygomatic wires are sufficient to secure the prosthesis, but if the prosthesis or denture is loose, it is necessary to place additional drop wires

DENTURE PREPARATION

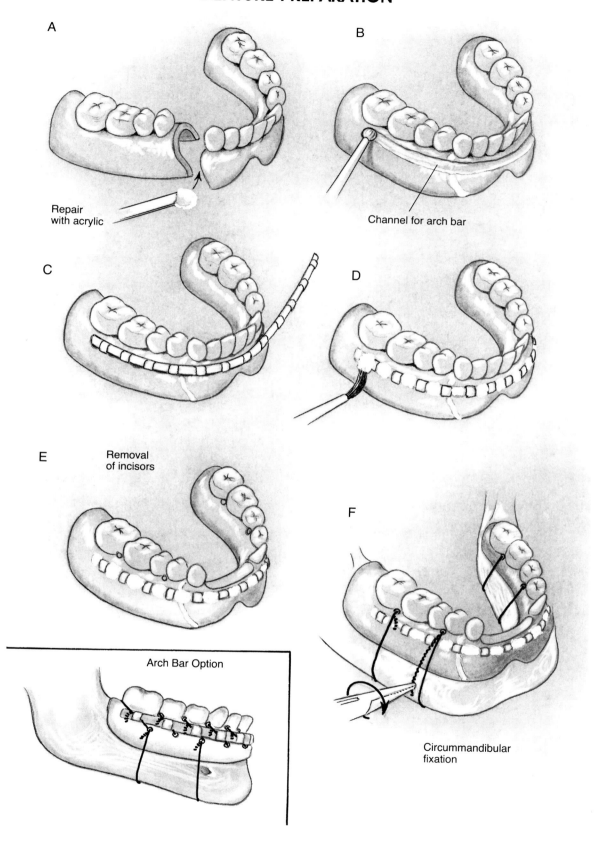

A

Repair with acrylic

B

Channel for arch bar

C

D

E Removal of incisors

F

Arch Bar Option

Circummandibular fixation

in the region of the anterior nasal spine. For this procedure, a small incision is made in the gingivolabial sulcus through the frenulum, and the periosteum is elevated off the anterior nasal spine. A small hole is then made through the spine, and a 26-gauge wire is dropped through this hole and passed through holes in the anterior flange of the denture or splint. The splint is thus secured at three points to provide maximum fixation.

H For fixation between splints or dentures, elastic bands can be applied to the arch bars (see Chapter 8). Occasionally Gunning splints are made as one unit composed of both upper and lower segments, but this limits options in adjustment and should be avoided.

Postoperative Care

Splints and dentures are kept as clean as possible by daily use of a soft toothbrush and/or a water irrigation device. Additional oral hygiene is effected by chlorhexidine oral rinses. Patients are maintained for 5 to 7 days on penicillin (or erythromycin). Patients should be seen weekly to check occlusal relationships, fixation, and reduction. The period of fixation will depend on the age of the patient. Radiographic evaluation should be performed after reduction and prior to the removal of the prosthesis.

PITFALLS

1. The denture or splint can efface the surface of the mandible. This complication often results when there is a laceration or avulsion of the alveolar ridge. Occasionally the prosthesis does not fit properly and may cause an erosion. If this occurs, the prosthesis should be relined with tissue conditioner liner material.

2. For the prosthesis to fit firmly, the circummandibular and circumzygomatic wires must be placed appropriately. The circumzygomatic wires should be dropped as perpendicular as possible; for this to occur, they must be placed anteriorly on the zygomatic arch. The hook or hole for attachment to the upper prosthesis must also be sufficiently posterior to obtain the proper direction of pull of the wire. The anterior nasal spine is useful for providing anterior fixation, but if the anterior nasal spine is small, wires can be dropped from the piriform aperture. For the lower jaw attachment, circummandibular wires can be applied.

3. Check the prosthesis weekly to see if there is any pain or increased mobility of the prosthesis or denture. If increased mobility is noted, the wires should be tightened. Radiographs may be helpful in evaluating for bone healing.

4. The denture is often ruined during the procedure. Moreover, oral relationships will have changed, and for these reasons, patients may have to have a new set of dentures.

COMPLICATIONS

1. Erosion of mucosa with exposure of the mandible and resulting osteomyelitis is one of the most feared complications. If the patient complains of atypical pain, swelling, or redness around the jaw area, the prosthesis must be removed and the area inspected. This complication is prevented by a good fit of the prosthesis and a padding of gutta-percha or tissue conditioner material.

2. Because fixation of a splint or denture is not as tight as that using direct osseous methods, there is a possibility of developing a nonunion or malunion. If this occurs in the subcondylar area, a pseudarthrosis may cause minimal functional sequelae. Failure to heal in other parts of the jaw must be dealt with accordingly.

3. Nonunion (pseudarthrosis), ankylosis, and temporomandibular joint dysfunctions are potential complications. These conditions are addressed in Chapters 25 through 29.

APPLICATION OF SPLINTS

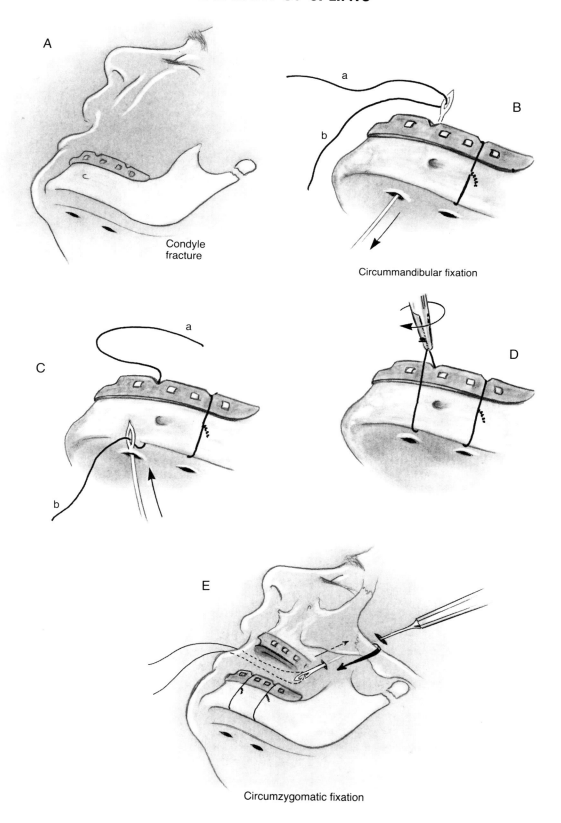

A

Condyle fracture

B

Circummandibular fixation

a

b

C

a

b

D

E

Circumzygomatic fixation

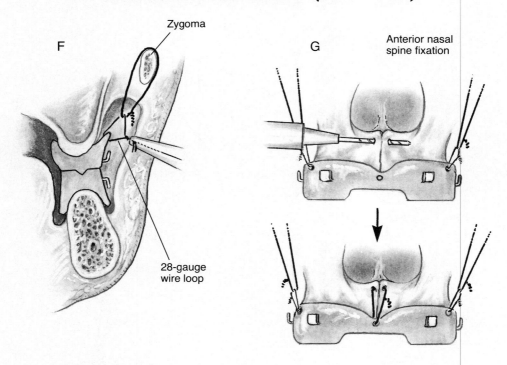

F

Zygoma

28-gauge
wire loop

G

Anterior nasal
spine fixation

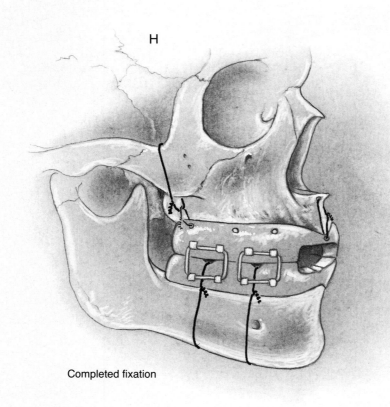

H

Completed fixation

Wm. Loechel

chapter 10

Open Reduction of Condylar Fractures With External Pin Fixation
Alternative Technique Using Interosseous Wires

INDICATIONS

Open reduction may be indicated in patients with severely injured and displaced condylar fractures and in patients with a combination of maxillary and condylar fractures. The technique should be considered when the condyle is subluxated almost completely in a medial direction at right angles to the neck or when it is displaced in the opposite direction, projecting laterally from the zygoma. Exploration should be performed when there are foreign bodies, such as bullets or glass fragments, in or near the joint space. Open reduction should be considered when closed methods are unsuccessful in reduction of the fracture. This can occur especially in edentulous patients with bilateral condylar fractures or in patients with multiple ipsilateral fractures. Of the many methods that are available, external pin fixation has the advantage of direct approximation of fragments with limited trauma to bone and soft tissue. It also provides for a relatively rigid fixation with mobility of the joint during the healing process.

TECHNIQUE

In preparation for open reduction of the condyle and external pin fixation, the upper and lower jaws should be placed into optimal occlusal relationships. Downward digital pressure on the permanent molar region will help in the reduction process. In the dentulous patient, short-term or routine intermaxillary fixation should be obtained with arch bars or Ivy loops (see Chapter 8). In the edentulous patient, the relationships should be evaluated and the jaws manipulated into the best reduced position. The surgeon should also outline with a marking solution the angle of the jaw, the zygomatic arch, and the expected position of the facial nerve as it exits the stylomastoid foramen.

A The incision is made in a preauricular crease line from the lobule to the zygoma. If additional exposure is needed, the incision can be extended several centimeters upward and curved into the temporal hairline. Just anterior to the incision, the superficial temporal artery and vein will be evident, and to prevent troublesome bleeding, the vessels should be identified and ligated.

B The dissection should be performed in such a way as to avoid risk of injury to the main trunk and divisions of the facial nerve. The parotid gland should be separated from the tragus, carefully avoiding extension of the incision inferiorly beyond the "tragal pointer." The dissection should be continued upward to the periosteum of the zygomatic process of the temporal bone and extended no farther forward than a line drawn approximately one half the distance from the tragus to the outer canthus of the eye. The periosteum of the zygoma can then be followed inferiorly, just anterior to the tympanic plate, to expose the capsule of the temporomandibular joint. The elevation of tissues should be extended to the neck of the condyle to expose the fracture site. Staying lateral to the condyle should avoid damage to the middle meningeal, deep auricular, and anterior tympanic arteries, which are on the deep aspect of the bone.

C–E If the fracture is not already reduced, the condyle should be grasped with a Kocher clamp and held securely in the proper position. A small incision should then be made through the skin just lateral to the area selected for fixation. A threaded Kirschner (Steinmann) pin, $5/64$ inch in diameter, is placed through the incision and drilled into the neck of the condyle with a K-wire minidriver. In most patients, a second pin can be applied through a separate incision. Biphase pins are subsequently applied in a standard fashion to the other fragments of the jaw. All pins are secured with an acrylic bar (see Chapter 14).

OPEN REDUCTION OF CONDYLAR FRACTURE

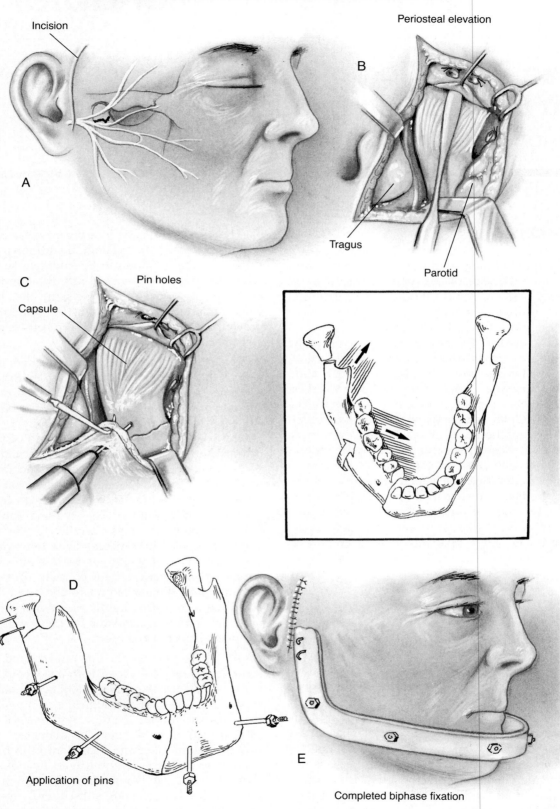

Incision

Periosteal elevation

B

A

Tragus

Parotid

C

Pin holes

Capsule

D

Application of pins

E

Completed biphase fixation

Wm. Loechel

PITFALLS

1. The open technique should be avoided in patients with fractures confined to the intracapsular head of the condyle. This type of injury is made worse by opening the capsule and growth centers within the area can be adversely affected.

2. To avoid injury to the facial nerve, the surgeon must understand the location of the nerve and its branches. The nerve exits the stylomastoid foramen, which will be several centimeters deep to the tragal pointer. The branch going to the forehead travels across the zygomatic arch between the lateral canthus of the eye and midportion of the arch. Thus by keeping the dissection posterior to the middle portion of the arch and above the tragal pointer, the nerve can be protected.

3. A dissection deep to the condylar neck can injure branches of the maxillary artery, and fairly brisk bleeding may occur. This problem can be avoided by elevating only those tissues that are lateral to the condyle. If the surgeon must work on the deep aspect of the condyle, the dissection should be performed subperiosteally.

4. At least two pins inserted into the condyle are necessary for stabilization. If only one pin is used, the fragment will tend to rotate. The pin will also become loose and be separated from the fragment.

5. Kirschner pins, being relatively sharp, can catch on objects and cause damage to the patient. Thus these pins should be bent over or covered with pieces of cork or vacuum container tube tops.

6. Avoid undue pressure on the pins. Patients should be reminded not to sleep on the pin side and to avoid any physical contact sports.

COMPLICATIONS

1. Nonunion is possible, especially if the pins are displaced from their original position. If this is suspected either clinically or radiographically in the postoperative period, the surgeon can reoperate and reinsert the pins; removal of the pins and acceptance of the nonunion or pseudarthrosis can also be considered.

2. Infection of the fracture site is a possibility, but the fracture usually heals with conservative measures (i.e., antibiotics, drainage, and continued immobilization).

3. Salivary fistula has been described following removal of the pins. The abnormal salivary flow will usually stop in time without any specific treatment.

4. Scars from the biphase fixation may require revision. These can be prevented by placing the incisions in crease lines.

5. Facial nerve injury is an uncommon sequela. If damage is suspected as a result of blunt injury (e.g., pressure from a retractor), then watchful waiting is encouraged. However, if disruption of the nerve is suspected and confirmed by neurodiagnostic testing, the nerve must be explored and repair accomplished (see Chapter 107).

ALTERNATIVE TECHNIQUE USING INTEROSSEOUS WIRES

a–c An alternative technique for open reduction and fixation of condylar fractures is interosseous wire stabilization. The exposure is the same as that obtained with the pin method. The dissection should again be kept lateral to the condylar neck and head region. Small drill holes, using a 0.035-inch wire with a K-wire minidriver, are made at the proximal and distal ends of the condylar and ramus fragments. The deeper tissues are protected with a malleable retractor. A 28-gauge stainless steel wire is placed through the hole in the condyle. The deeper part of the wire is picked up with a small clamp and pulled out laterally. A 30-gauge wire loop is then inserted through the hole in the ramus to pick up the end of the 28-gauge wire and bring the wire through the hole. The wire is then twisted in a clockwise fashion to secure the fragments, cut, and twisted down on the surface of the condyle. The technique is useful in keeping the fragments close together, but it will not provide a fixation as secure as that provided by the pin method described previously.

ALTERNATIVE TECHNIQUE USING INTEROSSEOUS WIRES

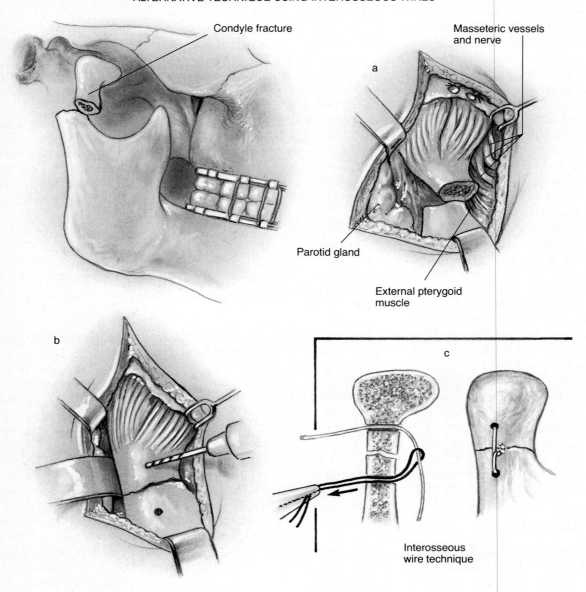

Condyle fracture

a

Masseteric vessels
and nerve

Parotid gland

External pterygoid
muscle

b

c

Interosseous
wire technique

section III

Coronoid Fractures

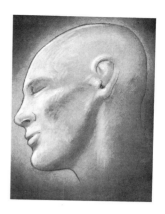

chapter 11

Closed and Open Treatment of Coronoid Fractures
Alternative Technique of Coronoidectomy

INDICATIONS

Coronoid fractures are extremely rare. They often produce minimal symptomatology and can be easily missed on radiographic evaluation. Usually there are transient pain and swelling, but if the coronoid is displaced and comes in contact with the zygoma, limitation of jaw movement can result. Most coronoid fractures can be managed with close observation. Fractures characterized by displacement and/or continuation of pain should be treated with intermaxillary fixation.

TECHNIQUE

Either Erich arch bars or Ivy loops can be used for the fixation. The procedure can be performed using general anesthesia and nasotracheal intubation or local anesthesia with sedation. The methods for applying the arch bars or Ivy loops are described in Chapter 8.

A The jaws can be held together with either elastic bands or loops of 28-gauge stainless steel wire. A postoperative radiograph should be obtained at 10 days, and fixation should be maintained for 6 weeks. Examinations should be carried out weekly for displacement of bars and/or breaks in the fixation devices. Dental hygiene is maintained with gentle brushing and/or with a water irrigation device.

B Intermaxillary fixation is removed at 6 weeks. The patient is then tested, and if there are no problems, the fixation can be removed. Active exercise with application of tongue blades between the incisors will help expand the interincisor distances.

PITFALLS

1. Following fixation, the position of the coronoid should be improved. If radiographs do not confirm reduction of the fracture, it may be necessary to perform an open reduction. Removal of the coronoid

(see later) may be warranted and is more easily performed than a direct wiring procedure.

2. Following removal of intermaxillary fixation, there will be some limitation of jaw movement. Active exercises are encouraged. The tongue blade technique, in which the jaws are pried open with an increasing number of tongue blades between the incisors, is helpful.

3. Coronoid fractures are rare, but when they do occur, they are often associated with zygomatic and maxillary fractures. This relationship can predispose to a malposition of the fragments and ankylosis. To prevent this from occurring, all facial fractures must be recognized and treated appropriately.

4. The edentulous patient with a coronoid fracture usually can be treated with a soft diet and analgesics. However, if a closed reduction becomes necessary, then application of dentures, splints, and intermaxillary fixation must be considered. These techniques are described in Chapter 9. Postoperative care is similar to that used in the treatment of other types of mandibular fractures.

COMPLICATIONS

1. Malunion with fixation to the zygoma is a debilitating complication. If this develops early, it is possible that the jaw can be opened with tongue blades interposed between the incisors and 40 mg/mL of triamcinolone injected into the coronoid/ramus area. If this technique is not successful, a coronoidectomy should be performed.

2. Malunion of the coronoid can also cause problems with denture placement. Projections of the coronoid should be shaved transorally and the denture refitted for proper occlusion.

ALTERNATIVE TECHNIQUE OF CORONOIDECTOMY

a,b A transoral open approach to the coronoid process is a direct, simple method to treat malunion of the coronoid process or a marked displacement of the coronoid fracture. Usually the procedure is performed using general anesthesia. To control bleeding, the coronoid/ascending ramus area should be infiltrated with 1% or 2% lidocaine containing 1:100,000 epinephrine. Exposure is obtained by placing an interocclusal bite block on the opposite side. The coronoid can usually be palpated with the mouth open, and an incision is then made over the prominence of this process and the adjoining ramus. A Joseph elevator is used to elevate the periosteum and the attachment of the temporalis muscle. The coronoid is then removed piecemeal with bone-cutting rongeurs. The bite block is removed, and jaw mobility is tested. The incision is subsequently closed with several 2–0 chromic sutures.

Postoperatively the patient is treated with a 3- to 5-day course of penicillin (or erythromycin). For the first day, the patient is given liquids; then the diet is advanced as tolerated. The patient should be evaluated for contracture in the area of surgery, and if this occurs, intralesional steroids should be injected and jaw-opening exercises instituted.

TREATMENT OF CORONOID FRACTURES

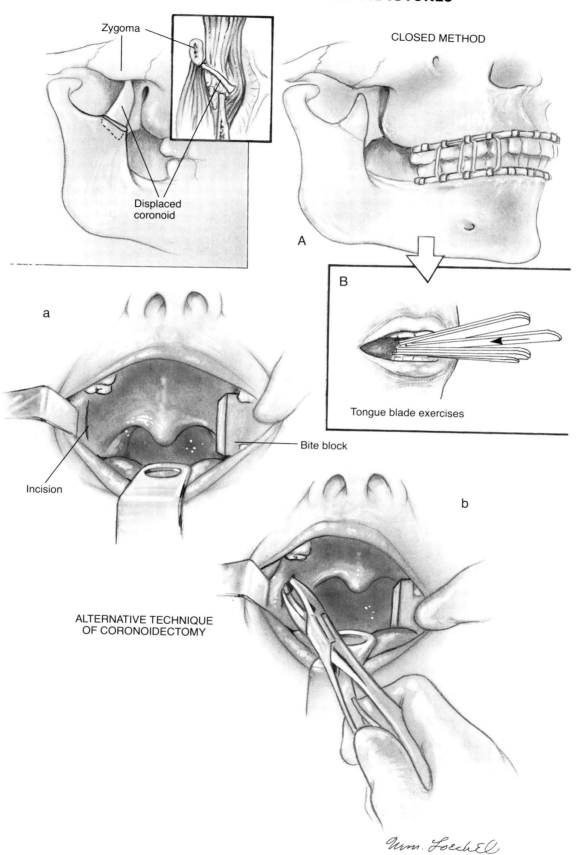

Zygoma

Displaced coronoid

CLOSED METHOD

A

B

Tongue blade exercises

a

Incision

Bite block

b

ALTERNATIVE TECHNIQUE
OF CORONOIDECTOMY

Wm. Loechel

section IV

Ascending Ramus

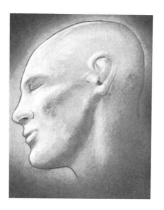

chapter 12

Closed and Open Treatment of Ascending Ramus Fractures

INDICATIONS

Fractures isolated to the ramus of the mandible are uncommon. The ramus is protected by the zygoma and by a "sling" of the pterygoid and masseter muscles. Moreover, displacement of the fracture fragments is usually minimal, and the majority of the fractures can be managed by closed techniques. An open method is necessary only if there are multiple fragments or marked displacement of the fragments.

TECHNIQUE

The ramus fracture is traditionally treated by intermaxillary fixation with Erich arch bars or Ivy loops. The technique is identical to that described for the condylar fracture (see Chapter 8).

A If the ramus must be opened for fixation, the same exposure applicable to the angle fracture should be used (see Chapters 13 and 14). The technique is modified by elevating the periosteum of the mandible

to a higher level. The fracture can then be easily stabilized by a single plate (compression or noncompression) across the fracture line. Wiring techniques are difficult, because exposure adequate to pull the wire from the medial aspect laterally would require a distraction of the fragments.

B For intermaxillary fixation, the jaws are held together with elastic bands or loops of 28-gauge wire. Antibiotics are administered for 5 days. Fixation is checked radiographically, and dental health is maintained by appropriate prophylaxis. Intermaxillary fixation can be removed at 6 weeks.

PITFALLS

1. Intermaxillary fixation often reduces the ramus fracture and provides sufficient fixation for satisfactory healing. If there is displacement of the fragments on a postoperative radiograph, then an open method must be considered.

2. Comminuted ramus fractures in dentulous patients are ideally treated with intermaxillary fixation. However, if the patient is edentulous, other methods must be considered. Marked comminution can be managed by an open technique and application of titanium mesh (see Chapter 27) or, alternatively, by application of the biphase apparatus (see Chapter 14). For the latter technique, screws or pins should be placed on stable proximal and distal segments and the external fixation device used to cradle and hold the fragments in appropriate position.

TREATMENT OF RAMUS FRACTURE

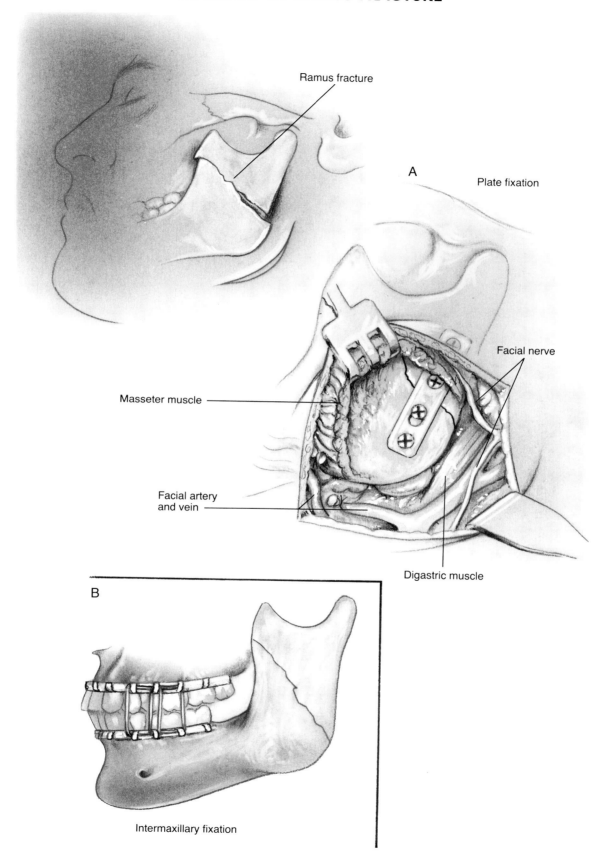

Ramus fracture

A

Plate fixation

Facial nerve

Masseter muscle

Facial artery
and vein

Digastric muscle

B

Intermaxillary fixation

section V

Mandibular Angle Fractures

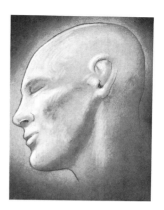

chapter 13

Open Reduction of Angle Fractures With the Luhr Self-Tapping Plate System
Alternative Techniques Using Interosseous Wiring and Intermaxillary Fixation, Eccentric Dynamic Compression Plates, and Lag Screws

INDICATIONS

The plating technique has become one of the more popular methods for open reduction and fixation of angle fractures. It is particularly useful for edentulous patients with unfavorable lines of fracture and/or multiple fractures. The method is also applicable when there is limited comminution of fragments such that the small pieces of bone can be wedged between solid pieces of ramus and body. A major advantage of the technique is that it provides for early oral intake (especially helpful in elderly and/or debilitated patients), and for early mobilization of the condyle, to avoid ankylosis.

TECHNIQUE

A Ideally, dental occlusion and normal jaw relationships should be obtained through temporary arch bar or Ivy loop fixation. A 5-cm curvilinear incision in a crease line is marked at two to three finger breadths below the angle of the mandible. The line is injected with 1% lidocaine containing 1:100,000 epinephrine. The surgeon should wait 10 minutes for maximal vasoconstriction.

B The dissection is carried through the subcutaneous tissues and platysma to the superficial fascia. Just anterior to the sternocleidomastoid muscle, the surgeon should identify the cervical branch of the facial nerve. More superiorly, the marginal mandibular branch of the facial nerve can be noted and preserved. A helpful technique is to identify a branch of the anterior or posterior facial vein system. Because the marginal branch lies superficial to these structures, elevation of the vein during the superior dissection should theoretically protect the structure.

C, D The fascia overlying the submandibular gland is incised inferior to the marginal mandibular nerve, and the dissection is continued beneath the fascia toward the lower margin of the angle of the mandible. The periosteum is stripped on the inferior and outer surfaces of the mandible to demonstrate the fracture line. The masseter muscle is elevated with the periosteum, helping to relieve some of the forces displacing the posterior fragment. The fracture is reduced with small Lane or Dingman bone clamps.

E A Vitallium Luhr compression plate with at least four holes is then fitted so that two holes are placed to each side of the fracture. The plate should be oriented perpendicular to the fracture at least 5 to 7 mm above the inferior border of the mandible and held into position either manually or with a special plate holder. Depending on the line of the fracture, curved or straight plates can be used. It is important that the plate have the same contour as the surface of the mandible; this can be achieved with bending clamps.

The compression plate is secured by drilling a hole at the outer edge of the eccentric compression hole with a 2.1-mm-diameter drill bit. The hole should encompass both cortices. Protection of soft tissues is achieved with an inferiorly placed malleable retractor.

F The depth of the drill hole is measured with a special device, and a 2.7-mm Vitallium screw of appropriate length, held with a screw holder, is then inserted with a Phillips wrench. The screw is tightened just enough to hold the plate in approximate position.

G Attention is then turned to the opposite fragment, and the procedure is repeated, with application of the screw to the outside of the other inner eccentric compression hole. Both screws are tightened completely so that compression is obtained on the fragments. Application of two additional screws, placed through the holes at the outer portion of the plate, stabilizes the system (fixation screws). If one of the screw holes should be stripped during the procedure, the screw can be replaced with a larger diameter screw.

H The periosteum is approximated over the fracture site with several 3–0 chromic sutures. The platysma

is closed with an absorbable suture and the skin with a nonabsorbable suture. If the wound is not dry, drains should be placed and utilized for 24 to 48 hours. The patient is placed on prophylactic antibiotics (i.e., penicillin or erythromycin) for 5 to 7 days and encouraged to use a soft diet. Postreduction radiographs are obtained, with weekly follow-up maintained for 6 to 8 weeks.

PITFALLS

1. Severe comminution can prevent secure placement of screws. In such cases a longer plate should be used with a longer incision. If the patient has teeth and the bone comminution is extensive, the surgeon should consider the possibility of intermaxillary fixation. In the edentulous individual, an internal splint or external pin fixation may be desirable. The mandibular reconstruction plate may also be used (see Chapter 14).

2. Infection can have a serious detrimental effect on healing. Open reduction and fixation with plating techniques should be delayed until infection is brought under control.

3. Over- or undercompression can cause displacement of the fragments from each other. If this occurs, the plate should be reapplied in a new position. If the condition cannot be corrected, the physician must consider an eccentric dynamic compression plate or relocation of the plate with a simple tension band at the alveolar margin (see later discussion and Chapter 15).

4. An oblique fracture can cause the compression screw to push away the deeper segment. In such a situation, the physician should change the position of the plate or consider the lag screw technique described later.

COMPLICATIONS

1. The compression plate technique is "unforgiving." If the mandible is placed in an inaccurate position, malunion will result.

2. Screws can penetrate the inferior alveolar nerve and cause pain and hypoesthesia. If such a situation develops, the screws and plate must be removed.

3. Some plates are associated with increased sensitivity, especially when exposed to cold temperatures. When the bone is sufficiently healed, the plates should be removed.

4. As with all fractures, infections can occur. Adequate drainage, antibiotics, and removal of devitalized teeth should encourage healing. If the infection does not respond to these maneuvers, debridement,

COMPRESSION PLATING OF ANGLE FRACTURE

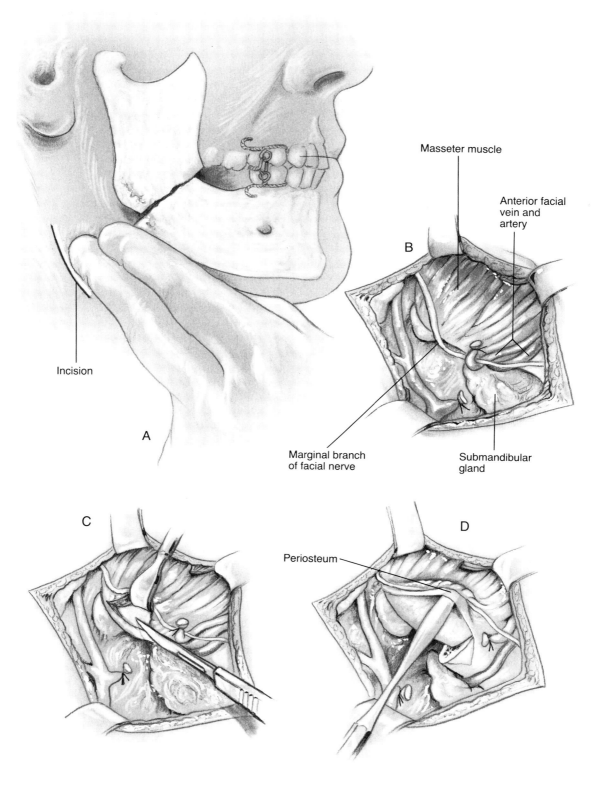

Incision

A

Masseter muscle

Anterior facial vein and artery

B

Marginal branch of facial nerve

Submandibular gland

C

D

Periosteum

Elevation of masseter muscle

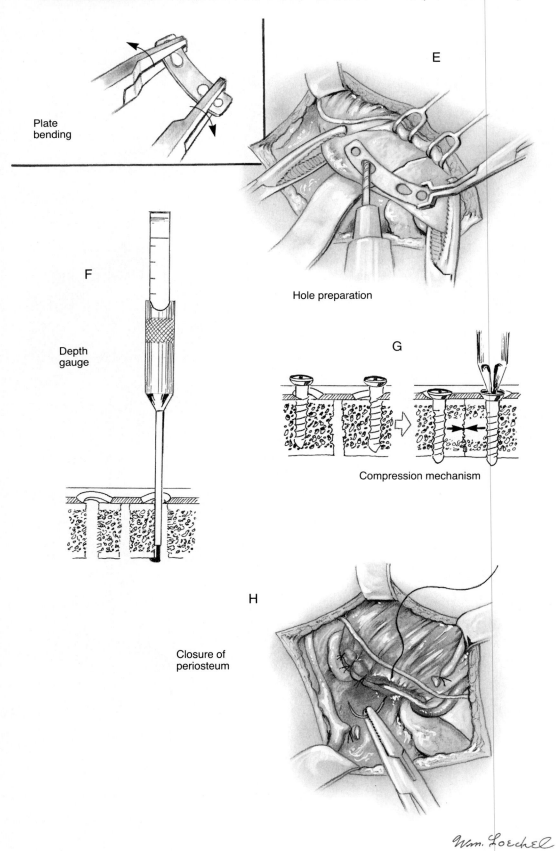

Plate
bending

E

Hole preparation

F

Depth
gauge

G

Compression mechanism

H

Closure of
periosteum

Wm. Loechel

removal of the plate, and external fixation must be considered.

ALTERNATIVE TECHNIQUE USING INTEROSSEOUS WIRING

a Interosseous wires (No. 26) can be applied after intermaxillary fixation. The technique is described in the repair of fractures of the body of the mandible (see Chapter 16). For the angle fracture, it is important to place the wires so that they are perpendicular to the line of fracture. If there should be an oblique component, the wire should be passed perpendicularly through both cortices. A figure-of-eight design is occasionally helpful, but usually more stability can be obtained with two sets of horizontally placed wires.

ALTERNATIVE TECHNIQUE USING ECCENTRIC DYNAMIC COMPRESSION PLATES

b The Arbeitsgemeinschaft fur Osteosynthesefragen (AO) eccentric dynamic compression plate is described in Chapter 15. For the angle fracture, the two inside screws are applied first, followed by the two outside screws. An alternative method is to use a tension plate near the alveolar border in combination with a simple four-hole compression plate.

ALTERNATIVE TECHNIQUE USING LAG SCREWS

c The lag screw technique can be useful for the oblique horizontally directed fractures. First the outer segment of bone is drilled with a 2.7-mm drill. The hole should be accurate, and to avoid wobbling, a drill guide should be used. The drill bit will jerk as it penetrates the inner cortex; at this point drilling should be stopped. Subsequently a 2-mm drill bit is applied, again with a guide, and a hole is made through the inner cortex. The deep hole is then tapped. A gauge is used to measure the depth, and a screw slightly larger than 2 mm is applied. Tightening the screw forces the outer fragment against the head; the deep fragment is then brought up into contact with the outer fragment.

TREATMENT OF ANGLE FRACTURES

ALTERNATIVE TECHNIQUE OF INTEROSSEOUS WIRING

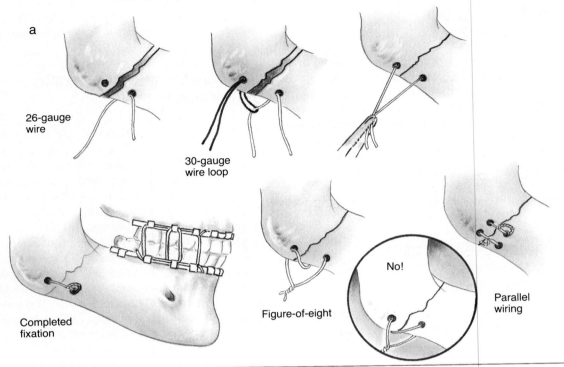

a

26-gauge wire

30-gauge wire loop

Completed fixation

Figure-of-eight

No!

Parallel wiring

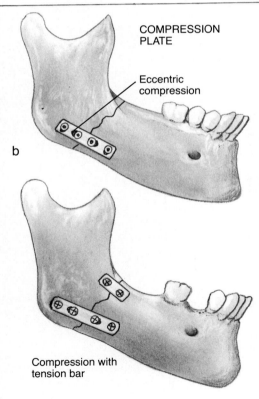

b

COMPRESSION PLATE

Eccentric compression

Compression with tension bar

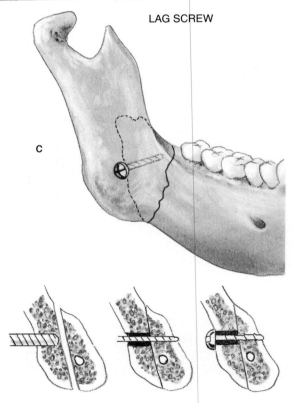

c

LAG SCREW

chapter 14

Open Reduction of Angle Fractures With External Biphase Pin Fixation
Alternative Techniques Using Biphase Compression, Titanium Mesh, and Reconstruction Plates

INDICATIONS

The biphase technique is particularly useful for comminuted or multiple fractures of the angle of the mandible in the edentulous patient. Usually very small pieces of bone can be stabilized between more solid segments of the mandible. Larger pieces of bone can be pinned and maintained in relatively stable position. The technique is also useful in patients who have infected fracture sites in which foreign body implants are to be avoided and splinting is necessary for healing to take place. Other important advantages are that the pin fixation apparatus can be rapidly applied, the patient's mouth can be opened in the early postoperative period, and oral intake can be instituted at an early time. For these reasons, the technique should be a primary consideration in debilitated and/or elderly patients.

TECHNIQUE

A–C The approach is similar to that described in Chapter 13. If there are opposing pairs of teeth, they should be put into occlusion with an appropriate method of intermaxillary fixation. Parts of the body and ascending ramus should be exposed. The attached periosteum should be left undisturbed, and all of the fragments of the intervening comminuted angle should be manipulated into normal anatomic position. Pin holes are subsequently mapped out along the body, angle, and ramus of the mandible so that at least two pin holes are placed in solid bone proximal and distal to the line of the fracture.

D A small stab incision is made in a crease line over the planned placement of each pin. Using a headlight and a medium, narrow-bladed Cottle speculum for visualization, the deeper tissues are spread with a hemostat in the direction of the facial nerve. On exposure of the cortex of the mandible, the periosteum is elevated with a Joseph elevator, and using a minidriver with a drill bit for a ⁵⁄₆₄-inch screw, a hole is made through both cortices. Irrigation with normal saline avoids excessive heating of the bone.

While maintaining visualization of the hole, a special ⁵⁄₆₄-inch pin/screw with a hexagonal head and machine screw end is applied to the hole. Different lengths are available. The screw will encounter some resistance at the outer cortical bone, some loosening in the cancellous bone, and then resistance again as it becomes secure in the inner cortex.

The same procedure is carried out for placement of each pin. In most cases, bleeding from the cortex will stop after a few minutes. The pins should always be oriented perpendicular to the cortex of the mandible and at least 2 to 3 cm apart to obtain maximal stability.

E The pins are secured to each other with metal bars and universal joints. As the fragments are realigned, the bars are adjusted and stabilized in a desired position.

F The acrylic bar that will replace the metal bar is fabricated with autopolymerizing denture acrylic (5 to 10 minutes setting time) or with the slower-setting cranioplasty material (10 to 20 minutes). The acrylic is made by mixing appropriate amounts of powder and liquid. It is then poured into a form bar treated with petrolatum to prevent sticking and allowed to "cure." Usually a small piece of acrylic held in the hand and rolled into a ball will, at some point in time, begin to harden. This is a cue for removal of the bar and application to the pins. The acrylic is best removed from the tray by lifting the band beneath the acrylic or cutting it free with a large (No. 12) knife blade. In this semisoft condition, the acrylic is positioned over the outer machine threads of the

BIPHASE PIN FIXATION OF ANGLE FRACTURE

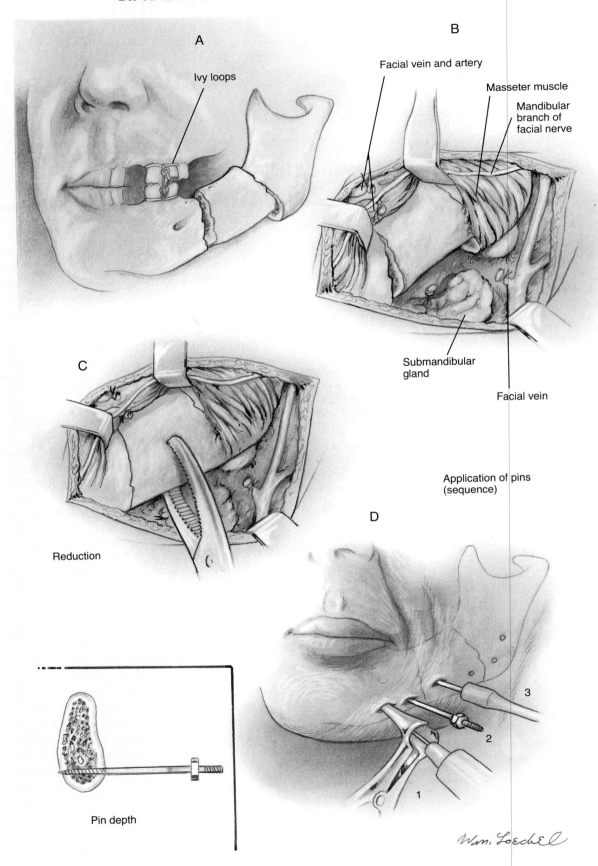

A

Ivy loops

B

Facial vein and artery

Masseter muscle

Mandibular branch of facial nerve

Submandibular gland

Facial vein

C

Reduction

Application of pins (sequence)

D

1

2

3

Pin depth

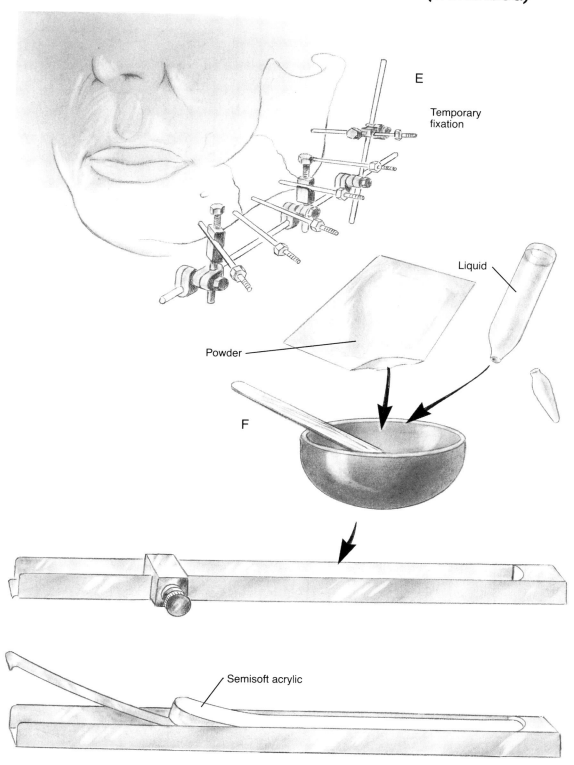

E

Temporary fixation

Liquid

Powder

F

Semisoft acrylic

pins. Washer nuts are then secured to the end of the screws and twisted down so that they are flush with the surface of the acrylic. The acrylic gets hot during the self-curing process, and to avoid injury to the bone and/or soft tissues, the pins should be covered with several turns of petrolatum gauze. When the acrylic is completely hardened, the metal bars can be removed.

The wound is closed in layers as described in Chapter 13. Patients are treated prophylactically with antibiotics, and the acrylic bar is maintained until healing is complete (usually in 6 to 8 weeks). The area around the pin is kept clean with 3% hydrogen peroxide and daily application of antibiotic ointment. At 6 to 8 weeks, radiographs are obtained, and if there is evidence of union, the bar can be removed. Segments of the bar are cut with a Gigli saw, and each segment is rotated counterclockwise (with the screw) for removal from the bone. Bacitracin ointment is applied to the wound.

G A more rapid, optional method for reconstruction uses a polyvinyl tube. For this procedure, a No. 8 endotracheal tube is cut to size and placed over the end of the pins. Using a No. 15 knife blade, holes are then made where the pins come in contact with the tube and also directly on the opposite side of the tube. The tube is then placed over the screws so that the first hole goes over the pin and the second penetrates the free machine end of the pin. The acrylic is pushed through the tube with a large-bore syringe. Usually the acrylic flows through some of the small holes and through the other end, but the dripping can be controlled with a piece of gauze and finger pressure. When the acrylic stops flowing, the surgeon can attend to other portions of the procedure.

PITFALLS

1. A sufficient number of pins (at least two) must be placed to stabilize the fragments. If there are multiple fragments or fractures are found in the opposite body or angle, the surgeon may have to use two bars or an endotracheal tube technique that provides for a lengthened bar.

2. Beware of pins that are too long and penetrate too far beyond the inner cortex. Such pins can enter the mucosa of the mouth and cause contamination of the fracture.

3. The atrophic edentulous mandible can be a problem, and this technique should be avoided in such patients. The bone may be so thin that the pins cannot obtain a sufficient hold for stability. It is also difficult to obtain perpendicular placement of the pin, and multiple attempts may injure the bone.

Unsatisfactory placement of pins or instability predisposes to nonunion or malunion.

4. The biphase technique will leave scars and should be avoided if optimal cosmetic results are desired.

5. If the fracture is characterized by comminution, the solid pieces of body and ramus should be fixed with the biphase technique and the smaller angle fragments molded into an optimal position. A titanium mesh tray or reconstruction plate can also provide stability; these should be considered as alternative techniques (see later).

COMPLICATIONS

1. Biphase pins will cause scars; these may require secondary scar revision.

2. Facial nerve injury, although rare, can occur. Remember to spread tissues in the direction of the nerve to protect them from drill trauma.

3. Salivary fistulas have been reported but will usually subside with time.

4. If pins are not applied accurately, the fragments may rotate, predisposing to nonunion or malunion. Once this condition is recognized, the pins should be reset so that fragments are in an optimal position.

ALTERNATIVE TECHNIQUE USING BIPHASE COMPRESSION

a If the angle is severely comminuted, it can be opened to expose the body and ramus and intervening small fragments. The fragments are subsequently molded into position, and biphase pins are placed in the ascending ramus and body. Using external rods for stabilization, the small fragments can be wedged (compressed) into the defect. After the acrylic bar has been constructed, the periosteum is brought over the fragments and the wound closed in layers.

ALTERNATIVE TECHNIQUE USING MESH FIXATION

b In cases where comminution is extensive and the fragments are very small, the body, ramus, and intervening fragments can also be fixed with titanium mesh. This procedure, as applied to the nonunion, is described in detail in Chapter 27. The jaw should be ideally stabilized with arch bars or Ivy loop intermaxillary fixation. The mesh should be cut to size, and with the aid of special cutting and bending instruments, it should be molded to the contour of the jaw. The mesh is held into position with multiple self-tapping small titanium screws.

BIPHASE PIN FIXATION OF ANGLE FRACTURE *(Continued)*

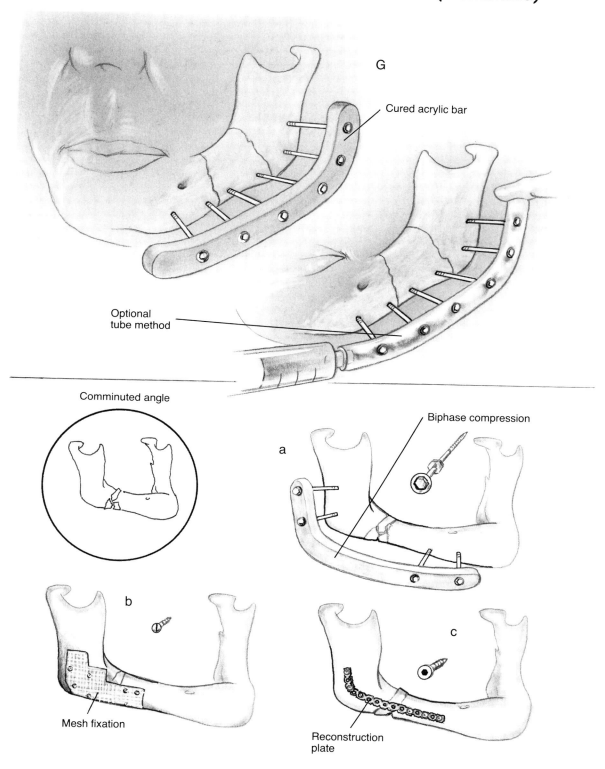

G

Cured acrylic bar

Optional
tube method

Comminuted angle

Biphase compression

a

b

Mesh fixation

c

Reconstruction
plate

ALTERNATIVE TECHNIQUES

ALTERNATIVE TECHNIQUE USING A RECONSTRUCTION PLATE

C Another way to treat the comminuted angle fracture is with a reconstruction plate. This technique has the advantage of directly screwing the larger fragments into position. The plates should be applied so that there are at least three to four screws in the body and an additional three to four screws in the ramus. The bend of the plate must conform to the anatomy of the mandible; this can be achieved with special bending bars or pliers. Large pieces of comminuted bone can be secured directly by the plate, whereas smaller pieces can be molded onto the internal surface of the plate and held in position by a tight approximation of periosteum and adjoining soft tissues. The periosteum is brought over the plate and the wound closed in layers.

chapter 15

Open Intraoral Approach for Angle Fractures Using Interosseous Wiring and Intermaxillary Fixation
Alternative Techniques Using Compression and Noncompression Plate Fixation

INDICATIONS

The intraoral approach may occasionally be indicated when it is important to avoid external scars and potential injury to the marginal mandibular nerve. The technique is also useful when the surgeon must remove a molar tooth from the fracture site and, in doing so, essentially perform the elevation of the periosteum required for the exposure of the fracture. On the other hand, the method requires special instrumentation. It provides limited exposure and, in general, does not provide a fixation as secure as that achieved with the lateral external approach.

TECHNIQUE

A Arch bars should be applied and the fractures manually reduced to achieve normal occlusal relationships. The fracture can be exposed while the jaws are in intermaxillary fixation, but better exposure can be obtained by taking the patient out of intermaxillary fixation and applying a medium-sized bite block to the opposite side.

The alveolus is infiltrated with 1% lidocaine containing 1:100,000 epinephrine. An incision is then carried out along the oblique ridge of the mandible and extended into the buccal sulcus near the second molar. The periosteum is elevated off both sides of the mandible to expose the fracture.

B A stab incision is made externally, just posterior to the area of the fracture. The tissues are spread bluntly in the direct of the facial nerve with a small clamp. A special drill guide is inserted, and a hole is created through both cortices just posterior to the fracture line. Alternatively, the drill hole can be made with a dental offset drill.

C—E Working intraorally, a 25-gauge stainless steel wire is placed through the hole, and using the awl technique described in Chapter 9, the wire is advanced around the inferior edge of the mandible and back to the alveolar surface. The wire, ligated in this fashion, will bring the fragments together. If the surgeon chooses, it is possible to drill two holes at the same level, 1.5 cm from the fracture site, and insert a mattress wire through each of the fragments. The wires should be twisted to bring the fragments into close approximation.

Following fixation of the fragments, the arch bars are tightened and the periosteum is closed with 3–0 chromic sutures. The patient is treated for 5 days with penicillin (or erythromycin), and a radiograph is obtained to verify reduction. Dental hygiene can be maintained with frequent brushings or applications of a water irrigation device. The patient is evaluated weekly, and in 6 weeks, if there is clinical stability, the arch bars can be removed.

PITFALLS

1. The exposure provided with this technique is not as good as that obtained with an external approach. Moreover, it may be difficult to achieve fixation. If there is still some question of the reduction and fixation after application of the wire, the surgeon should proceed to plate fixation or an equally effective alternative.

2. The intraoral method should be avoided in patients with comminuted and multiple fractures. Other techniques, such as biphase, mesh, or reconstruction plate, provide much better stability and are more suited for these conditions (see later).

3. Splints or dentures should be avoided. These

INTRAORAL APPROACH FOR ANGLE FRACTURE

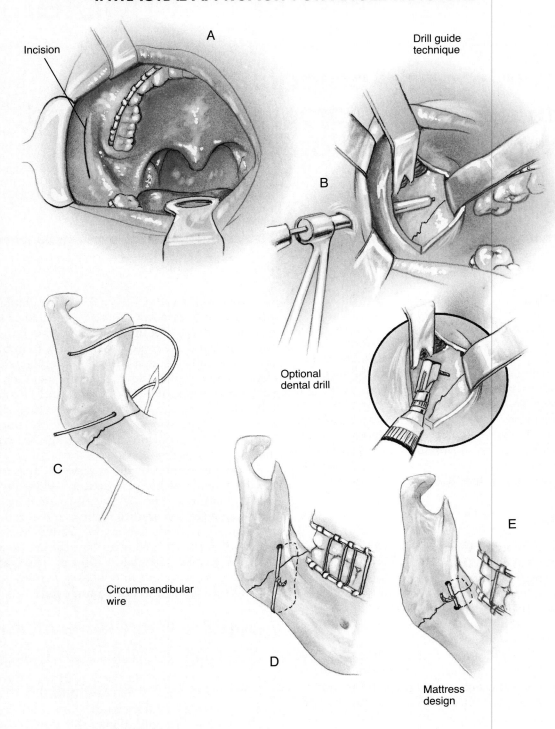

Incision

A

Drill guide technique

B

Optional dental drill

C

Circummandibular wire

D

E

Mattress design

can wear against the incision and cause subsequent chronic contamination and osteomyelitis. The technique thus becomes limited when it is applied to the edentulous patient.

COMPLICATIONS

1. Malunion can occur with the transoral approach, especially if there are inadequate reduction and fixation of the fracture. Treatment for malunion is described in Chapter 28.

2. Nonunion can occur following treatment of any mandible fracture. Once recognized, infection must be brought under control and devitalized bone removed from the fracture site. Usually another fixation method, such as a biphase apparatus, is required. Defects of the bone are corrected by the techniques described in Chapters 26 and 27.

3. Hypoesthesia and paresthesia are potential problems, especially if a wire is passed too close to the inferior alveolar nerve. By keeping the wire near the alveolus or near the lower border of the mandible, these complications can be avoided.

ALTERNATIVE TECHNIQUES USING COMPRESSION AND NONCOMPRESSION PLATE FIXATION

The intraoral approach can also be used for the application of internal rigid plate fixation. This technique is important when mobility is still present after interosseous wire fixation, when the patient is edentulous, or when it is desirable to avoid splints or dentures.

If teeth are available, they should be used for temporary occlusal relationships. The approach will require a larger incision than that used for the interosseous wire technique. The plates should be placed as close as possible to the inferior border of the mandible to avoid injury to the alveolar nerve.

a–c The Luhr or Arbeitsgemeinschaft fur Osteosynthesefragen (AO) plate can be used. Drill holes are placed with a speculum or through drill guides as described previously. The screws can be placed intraorally and the driver manipulated through the soft tissues to turn the screws. A dynamic compression plate may suffice, but if the alveolar ridge separates, an eccentric dynamic compression plate or a dynamic compression plate and tension bar should be applied. Closure of the wound and postoperative care are similar to those described earlier for the interosseous wiring technique.

d Another alternative is the noncompression plate. This plate utilizes a different principle, reinforcing lines of tension and distraction along the mandible. For this technique, a plate is applied subapically and medially to the oblique line of the mandible. This position provides a biomechanical advantage and prevents diastasis of the alveolus. The monocortical screws can be placed over the alveolar canal without injuring the nerve. The plates are usually 0.9 mm thick and 6 mm wide, with screw holes of 2.1-mm diameter. The core of the self-tapping screw is 1.6 mm. Usually one plate is sufficient; however, if stability is not sufficient, another plate can be applied more laterally and inferiorly to provide additional support.

INTRAORAL APPROACH FOR ANGLE FRACTURE *(Continued)*

ALTERNATIVE TECHNIQUES OF PLATING

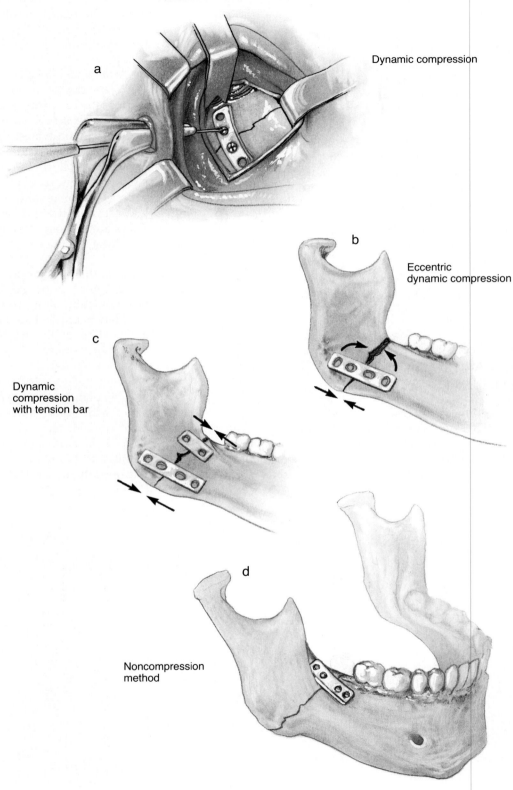

a

Dynamic compression

b

Eccentric
dynamic compression

c

Dynamic
compression
with tension bar

d

Noncompression
method

section VI

Body Fractures

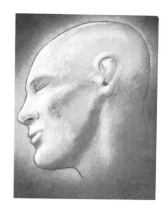

chapter 16

Open Reduction of Body Fractures With Interosseous Wiring and Intermaxillary Fixation
Alternative Techniques Using Figure-of-Eight and Parallel Wiring

INDICATIONS

Direct wiring of fragments and intermaxillary fixation with arch bars constitute a traditional method for managing mandibular fractures. The technique is easy to perform and often provides excellent reduction and fixation with minimal complications. The ideal patient for this technique is one who requires open reduction (i.e., who has an unfavorable fracture) and has a sufficiently healthy set of teeth. The technique is applicable to a mandibular body fracture when there is a marked displacement of the proximal and distal segments and/or multiple fractures involving the mandible. When the patient has atrophy of the mandibular body, as is often seen in the edentulous patient, then other techniques are probably more suitable (see Chapter 17).

PROCEDURE

A Anesthesia is best obtained through a nasotracheal intubation, as this will provide an excellent opportunity to establish occlusal relationships. The fracture is reduced manually, and arch bars are secured to the upper and lower dentition (see Chapter 8). The maxillary-mandibular relationships are subsequently established by applying several elastic bands to the loops of the arch bars.

The face and neck are prepared and draped as a sterile field. A curvilinear incision approximately 5 cm long is made in a neck crease two finger breadths below the body of the mandible. The area is infiltrated with 1% lidocaine containing epinephrine; the surgeon should then wait 5 to 10 minutes for vasoconstrictive effects.

B,C An incision is made through the skin and subcutaneous tissues. The plastysma is incised to the level of the superficial layer of fascia. The marginal mandibular branch of the facial nerve is identified by carefully spreading the fascia. A useful landmark is the anterior facial vein, which can be ligated at the inferior portion of the submandibular gland and safely lifted upward with the fascia. The nerve is thus protected by this maneuver. The dissection should extend to the inferior border of the mandible. If the facial artery crosses the field, the vessel should be ligated with a 2–0 silk suture.

D,E At the inferior border of the mandible near the fracture site, the periosteum is lifted off the lateral and inferior aspects. The fragments are reduced and stabilized with Dingman clamps. Drill holes are then placed 0.5 to 2 cm away from the fracture on a line perpendicular to the fracture, using a 0.045-inch K-wire and copious irrigation. A 25- or 26-gauge stainless steel wire is then introduced through one of the holes, grasped on the medial surface of the mandible with a small mosquito clamp, and pulled through. A loop of 30-gauge wire is inserted through the hole in the other fragment and passed in a similar fashion (see Chapter 13). The 26-gauge wire is threaded through the loop of the 30-gauge wire and back on itself. The 30-gauge wire is pulled forcefully, carrying the 26-gauge wire through the thickness of the jaw. The wires are disconnected, and the 26-gauge wire is pulled and twisted to reduce and secure the fracture. The wire is then cut and either bent into one of the holes or on itself to lie close to the surface of the mandible.

The wound is closed in layers. The periosteum is attached with 3–0 chromic sutures, and the platysma and subcutaneous tissues are repaired with either 3–0 or 4–0 chromic sutures. Excellent hemostasis should preclude use of drains. The skin is approximated with 5–0 nylon sutures.

At the conclusion of the procedure, the occlusion is checked and stability is further secured with application of elastic bands. The patient should be treated with prophylactic penicillin (or erythromycin) for 5 days, and radiographs should be obtained to verify completeness of the reduction and fixation. Healing of the jaw should be checked clinically and dental health maintained with frequent brushings and/or use of a water irrigation system. The strength of the jaw is tested at 6 weeks by having the patient bite on a tongue blade. If there is no movement at the fracture site or pain, the bands are left off, and the patient is then placed on a soft diet. One week later, the arch bars can be removed.

PITFALLS

1. Problems can develop from the use of arch bars; these are discussed in Chapter 8.

2. Accurate placement of the holes and interosseous wiring will ensure desirable force on the fracture line. If one of the holes is too low (or too high), there will be a tendency for sliding to occur. This can be corrected by better placement of the holes or by making additional holes in a figure-of-eight or double wire configuration as described later.

3. Remember to have the holes go through both cortices. This can be a problem in the oblique fracture, and failure to do so can lead to instability.

4. Postoperative radiographs are important to verify accurate fixation and reduction. Occasionally the wire will break, and if this occurs, the wound should be opened and the wire refixed. Radiographic evidence of inadequate reduction should also prompt reexploration and surgical correction.

5. In patients with multiple fractures, it is possible for intervening segments to rotate away from or into the floor of mouth. The disadvantage of wire fixation is that it does poorly in preventing medial and lateral rotation. To compensate for this deficiency, intermaxillary fixation should be in effect. If the segment continues to be unstable, the use of internal or external rigid fixation must be considered (see Chapter 18).

6. Avoid the interosseous wire technique in severely comminuted injuries. For such patients, it is better to achieve "normal" occlusal relationships and then stabilize the fracture with an internal or external fixation method (see Chapters 15 and 18). Open reduction and elevation of the periosteum may cause devitalization of the small fragments and should be avoided.

7. In patients with contamination (e.g., following gunshot wounds), it is better to first treat the patient conservatively with some type of intermaxillary fixation. At a later time, wires or plate fixation can be applied.

8. If the interosseous wire technique is to be used in children, the surgeon must make sure that the wires are placed close to the inferior margin of the mandible. This maneuver will avoid injury to the developing tooth buds. Intermaxillary fixation need be carried out for only 4 weeks; an alternative is the lingual splint described in Chapter 20.

COMPLICATIONS

1. Malunion is possible, especially if the patient has an unstable occlusal relationship. If this should

INTERMAXILLARY FIXATION OF BODY FRACTURE

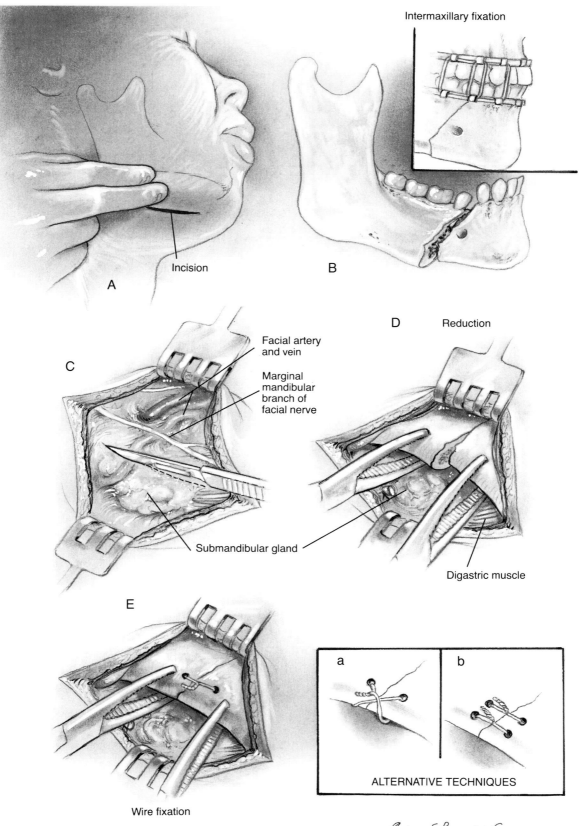

Intermaxillary fixation

Incision

A

B

C

Facial artery
and vein

Marginal
mandibular
branch of
facial nerve

Submandibular gland

D   Reduction

Digastric muscle

E

Wire fixation

a   b

ALTERNATIVE TECHNIQUES

Wm. Loechel

occur and healing has taken place, occlusal adjustments may be necessary. For more serious conditions, osteotomy and refixation must be considered (see Chapter 28).

2. Nonunion of the body fracture is rare except in patients with an edentulous atrophic mandible and in those who have comminution and contamination of the wound. Proper application of intermaxillary fixation and interosseous wiring will help prevent this complication from occurring. If delayed union or nonunion develops, the appropriate management is described in Chapters 25 through 27.

ALTERNATIVE TECHNIQUE OF FIGURE-OF-EIGHT WIRING

a The figure-of-eight wire is useful if the fracture fragments tend to slide or rock. The holes should be drilled accurately. A 26-gauge wire should be inserted through one of the holes, pulled through with a clamp from under the mandible, and then grasped and rotated through the other hole. The wire is again pulled through, and both ends are pulled and twisted on each other. The design of the figure-of-eight should be adjusted so that the wires do not cut into the fracture line.

ALTERNATIVE TECHNIQUE OF PARALLEL WIRING

b Another alternative for consideration is to use two sets of holes placed at right angles to the fracture. If the physician chooses this technique, the holes should be placed sufficiently low to avoid the inferior alveolar nerve.

chapter 17

Open Reduction of Body Fractures With Interosseous Wiring and Circummandibular and Circumzygomatic Splint Fixation
Alternative Technique Using an Onlay Rib Graft

INDICATIONS

Although the rigid plate technique is one of the more popular methods of treating the edentulous patient, occasionally there may be a need to apply splints or dentures with or without interosseous wires. Usually the interosseous wires are added if reduction of the fragment cannot be maintained with the splint or denture. The method is a conservative, proven approach to mandibular fractures and is equally applicable to isolated or multiple fractures of other parts of the mandible (i.e., condyle, angle, and parasymphysis).

PROCEDURE

The manufacture of splints and the adjustments necessary for dentures are discussed in detail in the chapter on condylar fractures (Chapter 9). For the body injury, the circummandibular wire must be placed away from the fracture site, and for most patients, one circummandibular wire is placed to each side of the injury. One wire is thus wrapped around the proximal segment and the other wrapped around the distal segment. Circumzygomatic wires are applied in a standard fashion.

A–D Before the splints or dentures are tightened and secured to each other, it is important to check the position of the fracture. The incision and the approach to the fracture are described in Chapter 16. The displaced fragments are identified, and when they are stable and in optimal position, interosseous wires can be applied. The periosteum is first elevated off a small area adjoining the fracture. Holes are then placed with a 0.045-inch K-wire using a minidriver in such a way that the pull will be at 90° across the fracture site. The deeper tissues are protected with a

malleable retractor. A 26-gauge wire is first passed from the outside to the inside. The wire is picked up with a loop of 30-gauge wire through the other hole and brought externally. The interosseous wire is twisted tightly down on the mandible. If the ends of the wire can be twisted into a drill hole, this is desirable.

The wound is closed in layers. The dentures (or splints) are secured and held together with elastic bands. A postoperative radiograph is obtained to evaluate the reduction. The patient is treated with prophylactic antibiotics for 5 to 7 days and evaluated weekly for healing and complications. Healing should be evident in 4 to 6 weeks, at which time the splints can be taken out of intermaxillary fixation and tested for removal.

PITFALLS

1. This technique should be avoided in patients with an atrophic, pencil-thin mandible. The anterior segment will not be sufficiently stabilized and will tend to pull downward, away from the posterior segment of the jaw. In such situations, the surgeon should probably use a plate or a rib onlay technique (see later).

2. Interosseous wires combined with splints or dentures can cause problems with respiration and nutrition. For these reasons, this technique is to be avoided in individuals who are elderly and/or debilitated. For such patients, the surgeon should seek an alternative method that provides early and rapid mobilization (e.g., rigid plate fixation or biphase fixation; see Chapters 10 and 18).

3. The body fracture can be associated with a laceration of the alveolar ridge. If this is the case, the denture or prosthesis can retard healing, and there

INTEROSSEOUS WIRING AND SPLINT FIXATION

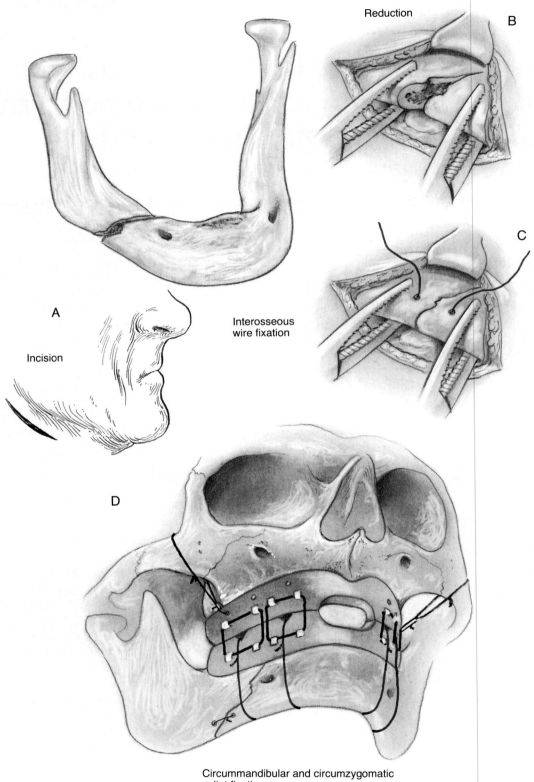

A

Incision

Reduction

B

Interosseous
wire fixation

C

D

Circummandibular and circumzygomatic
splint fixation

Wm. Loechel

can be a continuous contamination of the region by saliva. Should this complication develop, a rigid plate or external fixation technique should be applied.

4. The use of loose-fitting dentures or splints should be avoided. The fixation should be checked weekly and adjustments made to the circummandibular-circumzygomatic wires and intermaxillary bands.

5. The manufacturing of splints and adjustments of dentures can be costly and time consuming. The surgeon must consider the resources available and the cost of this method before selecting this technique.

COMPLICATIONS

1. Nonunion of the mandible is a rare complication. Postoperatively the patient should be evaluated for pain and inflammation around the denture (or splint). The fracture should also be evaluated radiographically for accurate reduction and fixation. Healing problems should prompt immediate evaluation and possibly a revision of the technique. The treatment for nonunion is described in Chapters 25 through 27.

2. If the patient develops osteomyelitis at the fracture site, the technique should be abandoned. The area of infection should be drained and devitalized bone removed. New cultures should be obtained. When such a situation develops, a biphase apparatus is an excellent alternative to hold the fragments in appropriate position and avoid the effects of a foreign body (see Chapter 10).

ALTERNATIVE TECHNIQUE USING AN ONLAY RIB GRAFT

A displaced fracture of an atrophic, pencil-thin mandible in a debilitated and elderly patient presents a formidable problem. In such a situation, the surgeon should avoid denture fixation and apply more stability directly to the mandible. Compression or reconstruction plates can be used, but occasionally the plate is too large for the area to be fixed, and application will cause severe damage to the perios-

teum and inferior alveolar nerve. If this possibility is a concern, the fracture site should be reinforced with a fresh bone autograft.

a–c Although a variety of donor sites can be considered, rib grafts are ideal because of their length, contour, and ease of harvest. For this procedure, the patient is placed in a lateral thoracoplasty position; the seventh rib is palpated, and a curvilinear incision is made over the angle of the scapula to the anterior axillary line. The latissimus dorsi muscle, the lower edge of the trapezius muscle, and the serratus anterior muscle are cut, and the periosteum is incised and elevated off the lateral aspect of the rib. Using Freer and Doyen elevators, the periosteum is elevated off the surface of the rib and then off the deep portion, carefully avoiding injury to the pleura.

d A side-cutting forceps is used to resect the appropriate length of rib. The periosteum is closed with 3–0 chromic sutures and the other soft tissues are closed in layers. If the pleura has been punctured, a chest tube must be used.

e The rib is held by an assistant. Using a sharp osteotome and mallet, the rib is split down the center. After the split has started, further splitting can be accomplished with heavy scissors or a knife.

f The mandible is approached as described in Chapter 16. In addition to the usual elevation of the periosteum near the fracture site, additional elevation is used to relax the periosteum that covers the alveolar ridge. The fragments are wired together as described previously, and the rib is placed into a subperiosteal pocket below the alveolus. The rib is held in position by two subperiosteal circummandibular 28-gauge wires. The wires are passed with awls as described in Chapter 9. The wound is closed in layers. Usually the graft provides sufficient support so that splints and dentures are not necessary. Moreover, if a splint or denture is applied, it may cause an erosion on the surface of the graft, creating the potential for contamination and breakdown of the wound. The patient should be maintained on a liquid nutrient diet during the 6 to 8 weeks of postoperative care. Prophylactic antibiotics should be administered for 10 to 14 days following the procedure.

ALTERNATIVE TECHNIQUE USING ONLAY RIB GRAFT

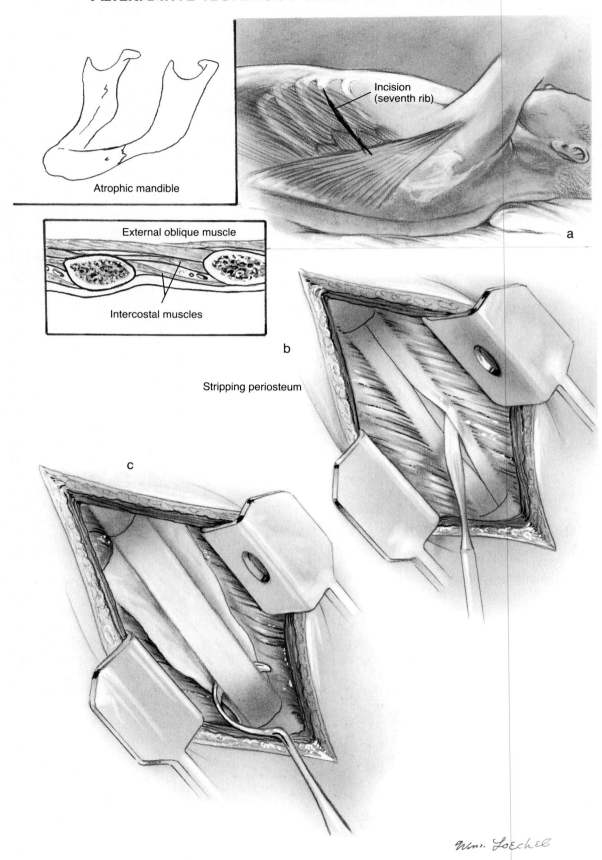

Atrophic mandible

Incision
(seventh rib)

External oblique muscle

Intercostal muscles

Stripping periosteum

a

b

c

Wm. Loechel

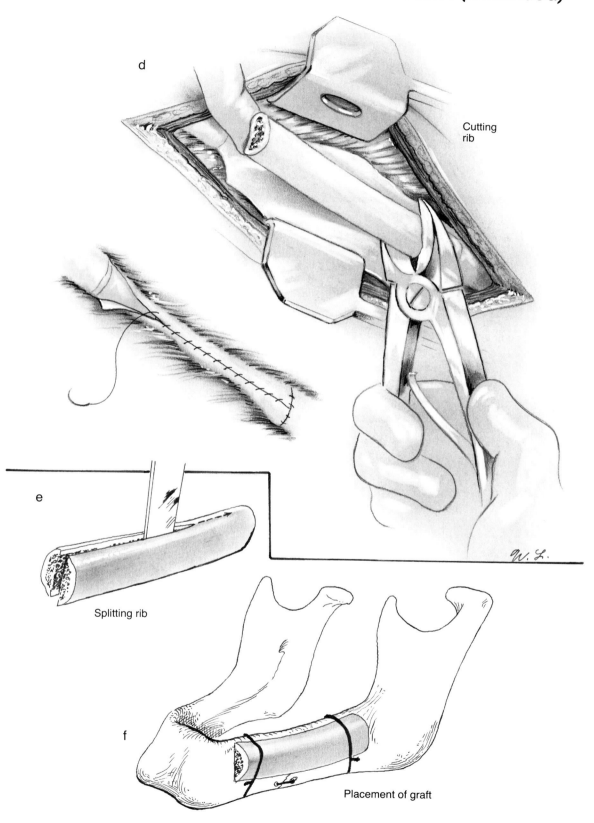

d

Cutting rib

e

Splitting rib

f

Placement of graft

chapter 18

Open Reduction of Body Fractures With AO Internal Rigid Plate Fixation
Alternative Technique Using Intraoral Reduction and Fixation

INDICATIONS

Internal rigid fixation is one of the most popular methods to treat unstable fractures of the body of the mandible, particularly when there are edentulous segments and/or multiple fractures. The technique is suitable for the edentulous patient with bilateral mandibular body fractures or body and parasymphyseal fractures of the contralateral or ipsilateral side. The rigid plate can also be used to cross over and stabilize small defects. An important advantage of this method is that it achieves early mobilization of the jaw, which is important for rapid restoration of masticatory, swallowing, and speech functions.

TECHNIQUE

Anesthesia is usually obtained with nasotracheal intubation. Ideally a temporary occlusal relationship is achieved by bringing opposing pairs of teeth together with Ivy loops or intermaxillary arch bar fixation. If the jaws are edentulous, occlusion can be approximated by a manipulation of the fractures into appropriate intermaxillary relationships.

The mandibular body fracture is approached by a curvilinear incision of approximately 8 to 9 cm in a neck crease two to three finger breadths below the middle of the jaw. The incision should be centered approximately at the level of the inferior border of the submaxillary gland. The area is infiltrated with 1% lidocaine containing 1:100,000 epinephrine. The surgeon should wait 10 minutes to achieve maximal vasoconstrictive effects.

The incision is carried through the skin, subcuticular tissues, and platysma to the superficial layer of fascia. While spreading the fascia with a hemostat, the surgeon should try to define the marginal mandibular branch of the facial nerve. At this level the nerve is near the inferior border of the mandible but can be retracted into the upper neck if the neck is overextended. Because the nerve often lies lateral to the anterior facial artery and vein (at the inferior border of the mandible), it is possible to ligate these vessels external to the submaxillary gland and, by lifting the fascia associated with these vessels, safely retract the nerve upward.

The dissection should be just external to the fascia covering the submaxillary gland. Working cephalad, the surgeon should identify the inferior border of the mandible and its periosteal covering. The periosteum is then incised and elevated to show the fracture site and the area that will be covered by the plate.

A–C If applying "strict" Arbeitsgemeinschaft fur Osteosynthesefragen (AO) techniques, the fracture is reduced and the fragments are immobilized at the inferior border of the mandible with a special reduction forceps. Two 8- to 10-mm holes are drilled with a 2-mm drill bit, 1 cm to each side of the fracture. The holes are then tapped with a 2.7-mm tap, and the sleeves of a reduction forceps are fixed with 8-mm screws. The forceps are then connected to the sleeves; the fragments are brought together and the forceps locked. Additional compression is achieved by pushing the screws up against the inferior border of the mandible. As an alternative, fairly good immobilization can also be obtained with an assistant holding bone clamps. Using this method, the surgeon can often forego the reduction forceps technique.

D With the fracture now reduced, a four-hole eccentric dynamic compression plate is fitted. The plate is bent with a curvature slightly greater than that of the outer cortex of the mandible.

E,F With a holding forceps the plate is placed over the area of fracture. A malleable retractor is then

COMPRESSION PLATING OF BODY FRACTURE

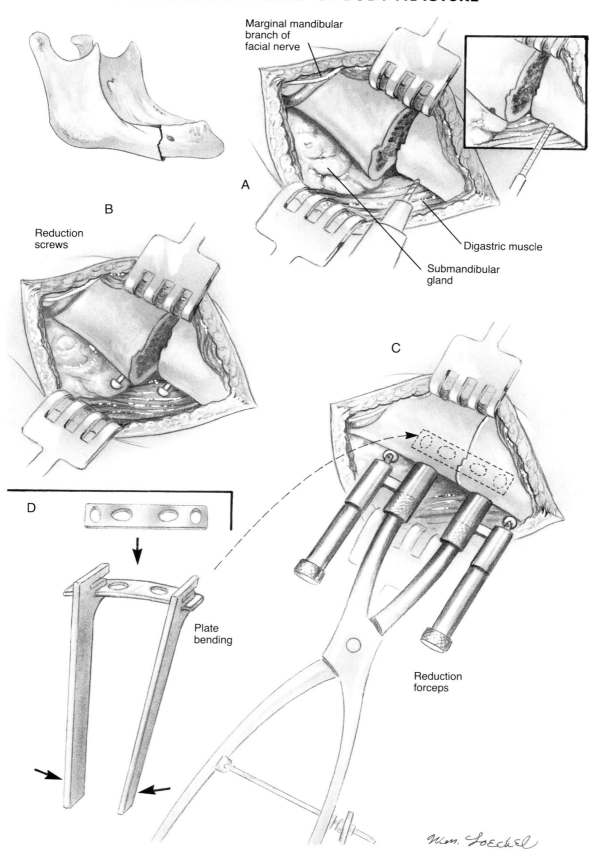

Marginal mandibular branch of facial nerve

Digastric muscle

Submandibular gland

A

B

Reduction screws

C

Reduction forceps

D

Plate bending

Wm. Loechel

slipped beneath the mandible for protection of soft tissues. One of the holes next to the fracture site is selected, and a 2-mm drill bit is used, with a drill guide, to create a hole. The drill guide arrow should be pointed toward the fracture site. A hole in the bone is then tapped with a 2.7-mm tap.

G,H A depth gauge will determine the appropriate length of screw needed so that the screw will engage both lateral and medial cortices. The screw is then loosely applied. A second drill hole is drilled on the opposite side of the fracture, and again, a screw is loosely placed into position. The plate holder can be removed and the screws tightened down to compress the fracture fragments. The outermost screw holes are then drilled with a guide, this time with the arrows pointing upward toward the alveolus. Two outer screws are placed and secured. Reduction compression forceps (or bone-holding clamps) are removed.

The wound over the plate is closed in layers. First the periosteum is closed with interrupted 2–0 or 3–0 chromic sutures. The platysma is approximated with 4–0 chromic sutures. Excellent hemostasis should preclude the use of drains. The skin is coapted with a running 5–0 nylon suture. The patient is placed on a 5- to 7-day course of penicillin (or erythromycin) and advanced to a soft diet. A radiograph is obtained to check reduction. The patient should be followed weekly for 6 to 8 weeks.

PITFALLS

1. Do not use the AO internal rigid fixation plate if a simpler method is more suitable. For example, in the patient with satisfactory dentition and a fairly favorable fracture, intermaxillary fixation using arch bars or Ivy loops must be considered. The plate technique should be avoided in children, in whom there is a potential for injury to the developing dentition. If the patient has an atrophic jaw and the plate occupies the height of the fragment, a smaller compression plate must be considered.

2. Plate bending must be exact. If the plate is not bent enough, the inner cortex will be retracted as the screws engage the bone. Overbending will have the effect of compressing the opposite cortex.

3. Screw holes that are stripped present a problem. One option is to remove the plate and drill new holes at a different level. Another alternative is to employ a self-tapping 3.2-mm emergency screw. This screw, placed in the same hole, will usually provide sufficient stability to the plate.

4. If a four-hole eccentric dynamic compression plate does not provide rigid fixation, the surgeon

should consider a plain dynamic compression plate and a tension band (see Chapter 15).

5. Do not injure the inferior alveolar nerve or unerupted teeth. This complication can be avoided by placing the plate within 1 to 2 cm of the inferior border of the mandible.

6. Often the screws of the compression plate will not fix small fragments. If there are areas of extensive comminution, it is better to use a reconstruction plate, titanium mesh, or a biphase apparatus (see Chapter 14).

COMPLICATIONS

1. Malunion can occur if the plate is improperly placed and the jaw heals in an abnormal position. This complication can be avoided by bringing the jaws into the proper occlusal relationships prior to fixation. In the edentulous patient, minor discrepancies can be corrected by modifications in denture fabrication. In the dentulous patient, the surgeon can consider occlusal adjustment at the surface of the teeth. Last, there is always the possibility of osteotomy and reconstruction of the mandible (see Chapter 28).

2. Osteomyelitis can occur at the site of the fracture and must be recognized and managed appropriately. The area of infection must be debrided of foreign bodies, and the offending pathogens should be identified and treated with intravenous antibiotics. Plate fixation can continue, but if the infection does not come under control, the plate should be removed and the fracture immobilized with an occlusal splint or external biphase apparatus.

3. Nonunion is uncommon (incidence less than 2%), but if it occurs, the plate should be removed, the edges of the fragments debrided, and the plate reapplied for rigid fixation. Defects of the mandible must be treated with a bone-grafting technique (see Chapters 26 and 27).

4. The plate may be palpable and noticeable in the thin-skinned individual. It may also project intraorally, affecting the fit of the denture. If this occurs, the plate can be removed through the original exposure several months later. Some patients complain of pain in the area, and if there are no other causes for the pain (e.g., infection, nonunion), the plate should also be removed.

5. Injury to the marginal mandibular nerve is possible and can be avoided by knowledge of the anatomy of the area and an atraumatic dissection technique. Considering that repair of the nerve is difficult and often unsuccessful, conservative management is a more prudent course.

COMPRESSION PLATING OF BODY FRACTURE *(Continued)*

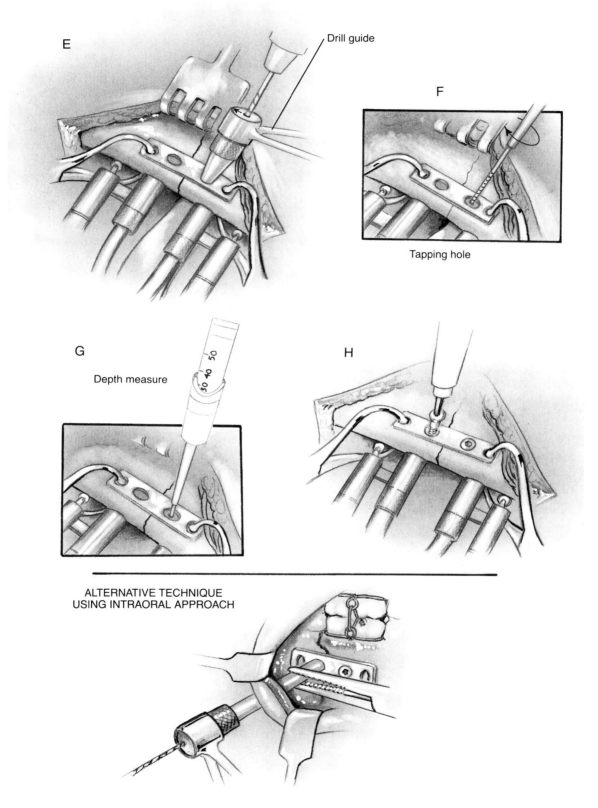

E

Drill guide

F

Tapping hole

G

Depth measure

H

ALTERNATIVE TECHNIQUE
USING INTRAORAL APPROACH

ALTERNATIVE TECHNIQUE USING INTRAORAL REDUCTION AND FIXATION

A rigid fixation plate can also be applied intraorally. This technique requires adjustment of the jaw into occlusal relationships and manual reduction of the fragments. The intraoral approach precludes the use of reduction forceps. Similar methods are described in Chapter 15 for the treatment of the mandibular angle fracture.

An incision is made 5 to 7 mm below the gingiva through the gingivobuccal sulcus, and the periosteum is elevated toward the inferior border of the mandible. The plate is then bent into an appropriate position and drill holes are placed. For this portion of the technique, the surgeon can use offset drills or small stab incisions made over the approximate area of the hole. The tissues can then be spread in the direction of the marginal mandibular nerve and a drill inserted through a guide or speculum. The screws can also be placed and twisted by a driver applied through the same hole. The mucosa is closed with chromic sutures and the patient treated as discussed earlier.

section VII

Parasymphyseal Fractures

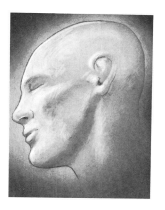

chapter 19

Open Reduction of Parasymphyseal Fractures With Interosseous Wiring and Intermaxillary Fixation
Alternative Techniques Using Rigid Internal Plate and External Pin Fixation

INDICATIONS

Because of the distracting forces of the suprahyoid musculature, the parasymphyseal fracture is relatively unstable, and the surgeon should be prepared for open reduction and fixation. The fracture becomes even more unstable when it is combined with other fractures of the mandible, and under these conditions, the mylohyoid, geniohyoid, and genioglossus muscles tend to rotate and pull the intervening fragment medially, posteriorly, and inferiorly. Stability in the dentulous patient can often be obtained with interosseous wires and intermaxillary fixation. In the edentulous patient, the surgeon has the options of interosseous wires and intermaxillary fixation

with dentures, internal rigid plate fixation, or external pin fixation. For the severely comminuted fracture, as seen with gunshot wounds, the external pin fixation technique is preferred.

PROCEDURE

A General anesthesia with nasotracheal intubation provides for evaluation of intraoperative occlusion and an excellent approach to the submental area. If the dentition is adequate, distraction of the alveolar ridge can be corrected temporarily with the application of a loop of 26-gauge wire around the incisor teeth. The surgeon should then establish intermaxillary fixation with arch bars, which will bring the fragments into appropriate position.

B The incision (4 to 5 cm) should be hidden beneath the chin. If the fracture lies to one side or the other, the incision can be made from the midline to a point just anterior to the submaxillary gland. The area should be infiltrated with 1% lidocaine containing 1:100,000 epinephrine, and the surgeon should wait 10 minutes to obtain maximal vasoconstriction for hemostasis.

C The subcutaneous tissues and platysma should be incised and the outer surface of the mandible exposed. The periosteum should be elevated, which in turn will release the insertion of the digastric muscle and show the fracture site. Injury to the mental nerve as it exits just inferior to the apices of the first and second premolars should be avoided. If the fragments are distracted, the fracture should be placed into an exact, interlocking position with Dingman or Lane bone-holding forceps.

D,E For interosseous wiring, holes are drilled to the side of the fracture with a 0.045-inch K wire and minidriver. Soft tissues are protected with a malleable retractor. A 25- or 26-gauge wire is then inserted through the holes from the external to the internal surface. The ends of the wires are grasped below the mandible, twisted tightly, and then bent beneath the projection of the mentum. The periosteum is closed with 3–0 chromic sutures. The platysma and subcutaneous tissues are approximated with 3–0 and 4–0 chromic sutures and the skin with a nonabsorbable suture. Drains should be avoided.

For most adults, healing will take place in 6 to 8 weeks, at which time the intermaxillary fixation can be removed. The patient should be kept on antibiotics (i.e., penicillin or erythromycin) for 5 to 7 days and evaluated weekly for displacement of the elastic bands and/or of fragments of the mandible. A postoperative radiograph should be obtained to verify adequate reduction and fixation. Oral hygiene is maintained with a toothbrush and/or water irrigation device.

PITFALLS

1. The fracture site can be misleading on radiographs. Triangular lines can suggest either a fracture extending through both cortices or a triangular free fragment. Failure to recognize the free fragment will cause instability and failure to heal. In such a case, the surgeon must ensure interosseous wiring and stabilization on both sides of the fragment. A maxi-

mum blood supply should be retained and periosteal elevation limited to the area of fracture.

2. Accurate placement of the interosseous wire is necessary to obtain a stable fixation. If the traction exerted by the wire is not perpendicular to the fracture site, the wire will loosen and break.

3. Solid fixation is very important. If the interosseous wire fails to achieve the objectives, the surgeon should consider rigid plate fixation.

4. Overtightening of the inferior edge of the symphysis can cause distraction of the alveolar ridge. To avoid this problem, make sure that the arch bar is tightened to the lower dentition. A loop of wire (a bridle) temporarily applied to the incisors will often keep the fracture tight at the alveolar ridge while the wire (or plate) is adjusted below.

COMPLICATIONS

1. Malunion of the parasymphyseal fracture can present as an over-, under-, or crossbite. Malposition of the front teeth can affect the biting of food and the general appearance of the lips. If such malocclusion or deformity develops in the early postoperative period, the fracture should be reduced and fixed again. After healing has taken place, the surgeon must consider orthodontic and/or orthognathic surgery (see Chapter 28).

2. Because the parasymphyseal fracture is relatively unstable and is probably the most distant from the inferior alveolar blood supply, it is prone to the unfortunate sequela of nonunion. This complication is often associated with infection, which must be identified and treated with appropriate antibiotics. Devitalized fragments of bone should be removed and major portions of the mandible stabilized with intermaxillary and/or external rigid fixation. If there is a defect, this should be treated as discussed in Chapters 26 and 27.

3. Hypoesthesia or paresthesia secondary to injury to the mental nerve is usually managed conservatively. Because this is a terminal nerve, sensation often returns. Injury to the nerve is avoided by understanding its location (below the apices of the first and second molars) and by applying atraumatic techniques during the surgery.

ALTERNATIVE TECHNIQUE OF INTERNAL RIGID PLATE FIXATION

a Parasymphyseal fractures can also be adequately treated with plate techniques that are described elsewhere (see Chapters 13, 15, and 18). Prior to the

REPAIR OF PARASYMPHYSEAL FRACTURE USING INTEROSSEOUS WIRING AND INTERMAXILLARY FIXATION

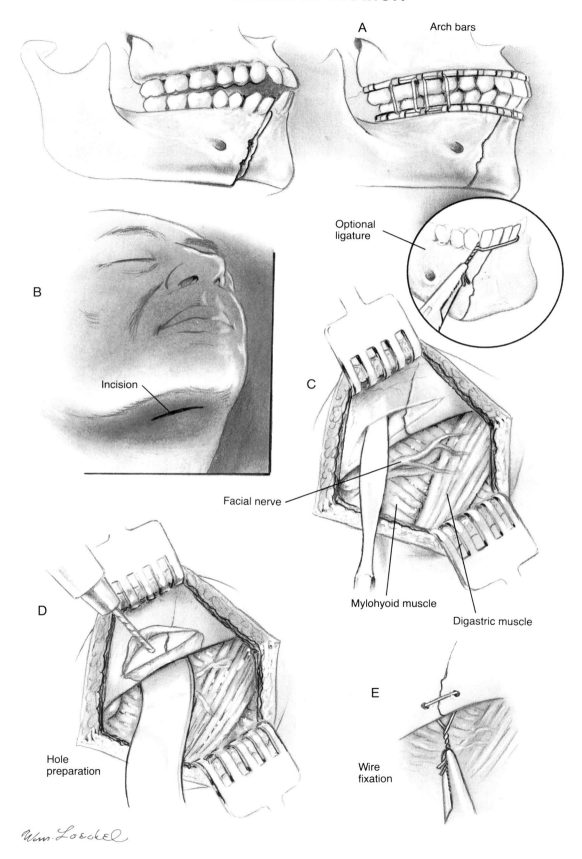

A

Arch bars

Optional ligature

B

Incision

C

Facial nerve

Mylohyoid muscle

Digastric muscle

D

Hole preparation

E

Wire fixation

application of plates, temporary occlusion should be achieved with either arch bars or Ivy loops. In the edentulous patient, manual approximation of occlusion can be performed. If the patient has a lower anterior dentition, loops of wires placed around the incisors will help to align the alveolus and prevent distraction.

b–d The submental incision is longer than the one used for interosseous wiring and requires a greater amount of periosteal stripping to accommodate the length of the plate. The contours of the mentum are complex, and sufficient time and attention should be allocated to bend the plate. In the edentulous patient, an additional tension bar is often necessary to prevent distraction at the alveolar ridge. Alternatively, eccentric dynamic compression plates can be applied. Patients may later complain about the prominence and feel of plates. Paresthesia and pain can occur if the plate is applied too closely to the mental nerve.

ALTERNATIVE TECHNIQUE USING EXTERNAL PIN FIXATION

External pin fixation is preferred over interosseous wiring in patients who are edentulous and/or who have comminuted fractures (see Chapter 14). The technique is useful when the surgeon wants to avoid using splints or dentures.

The biphase pins should be placed on each side of the area of fracture. Stab incisions should be made in the direction of the facial nerve and the pins applied so that they are perpendicular to the plane of the mandible. Several comminuted pieces of bone can be compressed between the more solid pieces of bone. If there is any question about the reduction of the intervening bone fragments, the pin method can be combined with the interosseous wiring technique described previously.

REPAIR OF PARASYMPHYSEAL FRACTURE USING INTEROSSEOUS WIRING AND INTERMAXILLARY FIXATION *(Continued)*

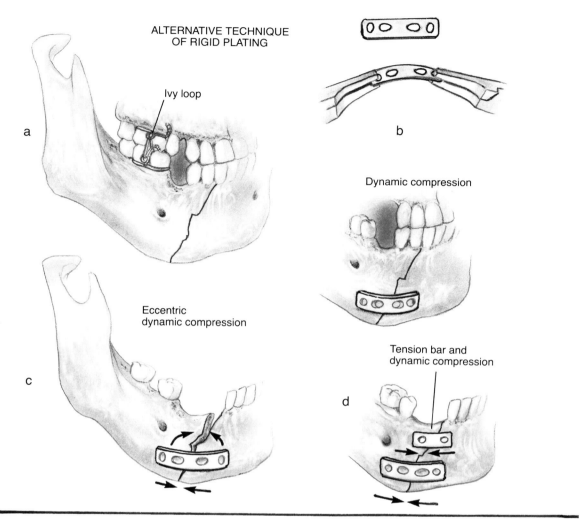

ALTERNATIVE TECHNIQUE OF RIGID PLATING

Ivy loop

a

b

Dynamic compression

Eccentric dynamic compression

c

Tension bar and dynamic compression

d

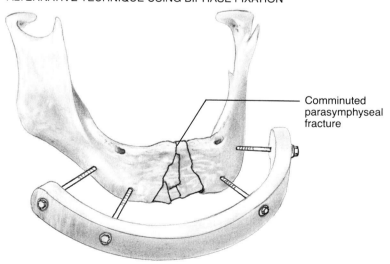

ALTERNATIVE TECHNIQUE USING BIPHASE FIXATION

Comminuted parasymphyseal fracture

Wm. Loechel

Closed Reduction of Parasymphyseal Fractures in Children Using Prefabricated Lingual Splints

Alternative Technique of Fabricating the Splint on the Patient's Dental Arch

In Consultation With Mark T. Marunick, DDS

INDICATIONS

Parasymphyseal fractures in children, unlike similar injuries in adults, need not be treated by open techniques. Pediatric fractures tend to heal rapidly, and even if the segments are not perfectly aligned, bone remodeling can bring about normal anatomic relationships. Furthermore, open reduction and fixation, either by interosseous wiring or fixation plates, put the developing teeth at risk and should only be applied very judiciously. For these reasons, the lingual splint method is an excellent method to use in small children. It is also well tolerated and easy to maintain.

PROCEDURE

A A lingual splint can be made with the techniques noted in Chapter 9. For this method, an impression of the lower jaw is obtained with alginate. The impression is then poured in plaster or stone to make a cast, and from this cast, a splint is fabricated.

B,C When displaced segments are encountered, cast surgery should be performed. For this procedure, the base of the involved cast should be trimmed with a divergent angle from bottom to top. The cast and entire base are duplicated. A flexible base former is lubricated and filled with a very watery mix of plaster. The base of the cast is lubricated and placed in the plaster. The lubricated tapered base will allow removal of the entire lower cast from the plaster boat.

D,E Cast surgery can then be performed in the area

of displacement. The cast is cut along the lines of the fracture and the segments are repositioned in the plaster boat. The segments are subsequently secured with wax.

F–H The stone cast is carefully removed from the plaster boat and a duplicate is made of the cast. The lingual splint is fabricated on the duplicate. To ensure the rigidity of the lingual splint, a heavy-gauge stainless steel wire is adapted to the lingual sulcus of the cast, 3 to 4 mm below the free gingival margin. The wire is luted to the cast with a few beads of wax. A separating medium (petrolatum) is carefully applied to the cast. Care is taken to keep the lubricant off the wire. Autopolymerizing acrylic resin is mixed, and when it thickens, it is adapted to the lingual aspect of the teeth and sulcus and around the wire. The acrylic should not extend over the occlusal surface of the teeth. After the acrylic is set, it is removed, trimmed, and polished. Small holes are directed through it to hold strategically placed circumdental wires. The splint should be 1.5 to 2 mm thick. If it is too thin, it can be reseated on the cast and additional acrylic added.

I The splint should be applied under general anesthesia. If sufficient teeth are available, the lips are retracted, and ligatures of 26-gauge wires are applied through the splint and between the adjacent teeth to be twisted at the buccal or lateral gingival surface. The wires are then tightened, cut, and bent toward the gum area. Usually four wires placed around "solid" molar teeth are sufficient to hold the splint to the teeth. The relationship of the upper and lower jaws is then evaluated for satisfactory occlusion.

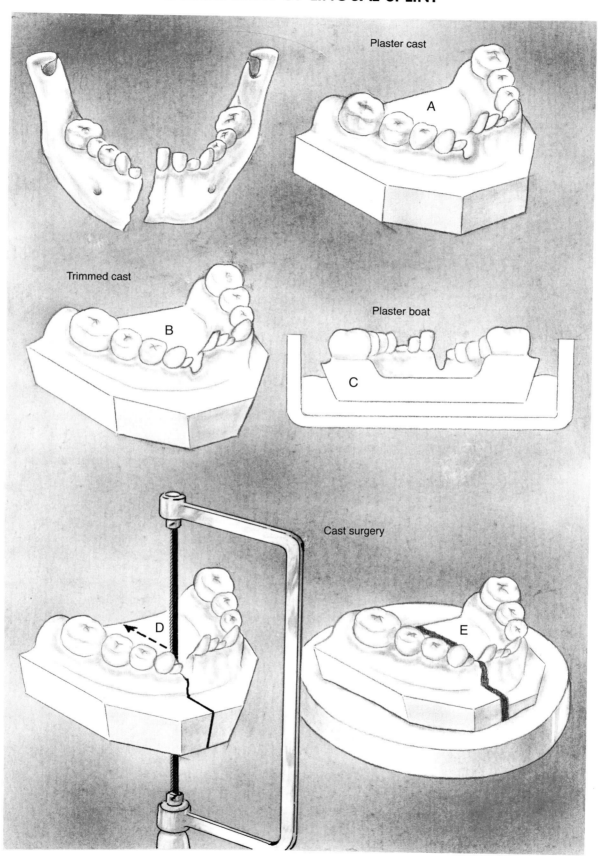

Plaster cast

A

Trimmed cast

B

Plaster boat

C

Cast surgery

D

E

Postoperatively the splint is checked daily to make sure that there is no loosening. The jaw is evaluated radiographically and clinically to verify reduction and fixation. Because healing is quite rapid, the splint can often be removed in 2 to 4 weeks. Antibiotics are provided for 5 to 7 days following the procedure.

PITFALLS

1. When treating symphyseal fractures, make sure there is not an associated condylar injury. If such a situation exists, the physician must check the state of the condyle every 2 weeks with radiographs to ensure that the condyle can be adequately mobilized. Short periods of intermaxillary fixation may be necessary to achieve adequate rehabilitation of the joint.

2. Because the deciduous teeth can be easily extirpated or loosened by the splint, the splint should be checked daily. If there is a loss of stability, new holes and wires must be applied. If there are no other teeth that can be ligated, the surgeon must consider new holes and circummandibular wires to hold the splint firmly to the alveolus (see Chapter 9).

COMPLICATIONS

1. Although nonunion and malunion are rare in children, the surgeon must be aware that they can occur and if they do, then treat with appropriate methods (see Chapters 25 through 28).

2. The most unrecognized complication of fracture in children is injury to the condyle with subsequent ankylosis and alterations in growth and development of the jaw. To avoid this problem, the surgeon should obtain radiographic analysis of the temporomandibular joint at the time of injury. If there is any suspicion of injury, the patient should be followed with appropriate radiographs every 2 weeks. In some condylar injuries, intermaxillary fixation may be necessary for short periods of time. As soon as intermaxillary fixation is completed, the child should be evaluated clinically and radiologically for healing.

3. Tooth injury can also occur in children. If the injury involves the deciduous teeth, it will probably not be a problem. On the other hand, if it involves the permanent dentition, consultation is advisable (see Chapters 22 and 23).

4. If the child has not developed teeth, the splint can be made to conform to the alveolar ridge. Grooves are made in the splint for the circummandibular wires.

5. If parasymphyseal and symphyseal fractures are associated with other fractures, there can be a marked displacement of intervening segments. In such a situation, the surgeon cannot be sure of the reduction or fixation, and an open method must be instituted. If this is necessary, then an interosseous wire can be placed as close as possible to the lower edge of the jaw. The interosseous wire method must be combined with intermaxillary fixation, arch bars, or with Ivy loops. If more stabilization is needed, it may be possible to combine the interosseous wiring technique with a lingual splint.

ALTERNATIVE TECHNIQUE OF FABRICATING THE SPLINT ON THE PATIENT'S DENTAL ARCH

If a prosthodontist is not available, there are "shortcuts" to making adequate splints. One way is to apply the autopolymerizing acrylic resin directly to the dentition or alveolar ridge. The technique is performed under general anesthesia. The teeth and/or alveolar ridge are reduced manually and treated with petrolatum. The acrylic is mixed, and when it becomes thick and can be handled, it is applied to the area while the jaw is held in a reduced position. As the acrylic is polymerizing, it must be removed, the tissues irrigated with cold water, and the acrylic readapted. Prior to final set, the splint is removed and placed in a bowl of water. These procedures will minimize heat transfer to the tissue and prevent the acrylic from getting locked into undercuts. The set acrylic is then carefully trimmed to remove overextensions into movable tissues. The peripheries of the splint are smoothed and holes are appropriately drilled for application of wires.

FABRICATION OF LINGUAL SPLINT *(Continued)*

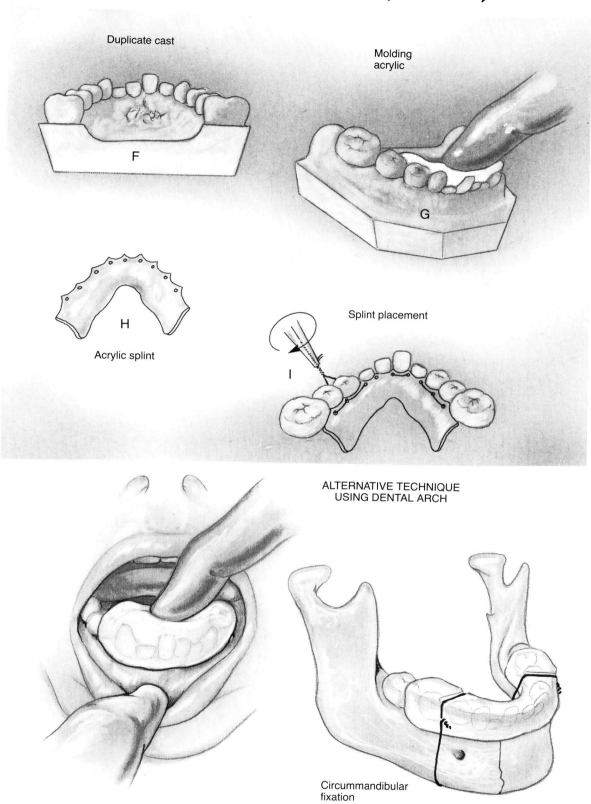

Duplicate cast

F

Molding acrylic

G

H

Acrylic splint

Splint placement

I

ALTERNATIVE TECHNIQUE
USING DENTAL ARCH

Circummandibular
fixation

Open Intraoral Reduction of Parasymphyseal Fractures With Interosseous Wiring and Intermaxillary Fixation
Alternative Technique Using Internal Rigid Plate Fixation

INDICATIONS

Because most parasymphyseal fractures are relatively unstable, open reduction and fixation must be considered. Usually an external approach is used, but if the surgeon wants to avoid external scars, the fracture can be approached directly through a gingivolabial sulcus incision. This technique provides a direct route to the fracture and an excellent exposure of the external cortex. One can then evaluate the contact of the fragments and the adequacy of the reduction from the lower border of the mandible to the alveolar ridge. Moreover, fractures involving the incisors and the alveolar ridge will not be missed and can be treated appropriately.

PROCEDURE

A Initially the surgeon should achieve normal occlusal relationships by loose application of intermaxillary fixation with arch bars to the upper and lower dentition. The arch bar (or, alternatively, a transdental loop of wire) across the incisors also tends to stabilize the parasymphyseal fracture so that when the inferior portion is reduced, there is no distraction of the fracture at the alveolar surface.

B–E Following infiltration with 1% lidocaine containing 1:100,000 epinephrine, an incision is made over the fracture site on the outer cortex of the mandible. This incision should be 5 to 7 mm below the gingival margin, but not so low that it injures the mental nerve. The periosteum is then elevated inferiorly and a periosteal flap held with Senn retractors. Care is again taken to avoid injury to the mental nerve, which exits between the apices of first and second premolars. The fracture is reduced manually and drill holes placed through the outer cortex and below the tooth apices on each side of the fracture. The drill holes are designed obliquely so that wires encompass only the outer cortex. A 26-gauge wire can be inserted through the hole on one side, and a loop of 30-gauge wire can be used through the other hole to pull the wire through it. The wire is tightened, and if reduction is accurate, the wire is cut and twisted down through one of the holes (or at least close to the surface of the mandible). The alveolar portion of the fracture is examined for distraction. The mucosa is closed with chromic sutures, and the arch bar is then tightened.

Postoperatively oral hygiene is maintained with frequent brushings and/or regular use of a water irrigation device. A radiograph should be taken to verify adequate fixation and reduction. Prophylactic penicillin (or erythromycin) is taken for 5 days and the jaw evaluated on a weekly basis. Following a test of jaw strength and stability at 6 to 8 weeks, the intermaxillary fixation can be removed.

PITFALLS

1. Because the interosseous wire secures the outer cortical portion of the mandible, it may not provide fixation as strong as that provided by other techniques. If there is instability following reduction and fixation, the surgeon must consider the possibility of applying a rigid plate to the area. This technique is described later in this chapter.

2. Avoid overreduction of the alveolar portion from an overtightening of the arch bar. If this occurs, the interosseous wire will not bring the fragments together, and the fracture will remain unstable. This problem can be avoided by loosely applying the arch bar and then tightening it after the interosseous wire has been applied.

INTRAORAL APPROACH TO PARASYMPHYSEAL FRACTURES

A   Intermaxillary fixation

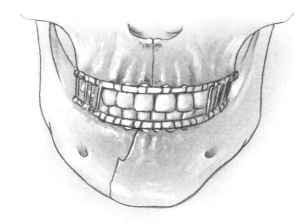

B   Gingivolabial incision

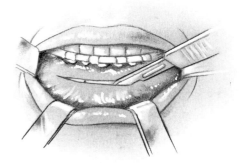

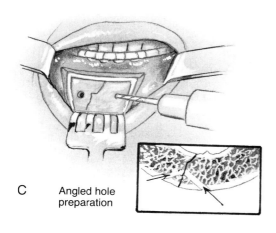

C   Angled hole preparation

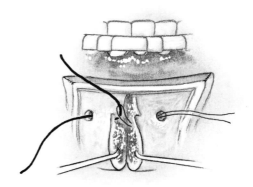

D   Pull-through technique

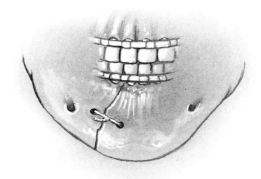

E   Wire fixation completed

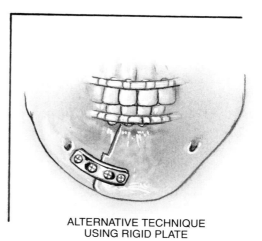

ALTERNATIVE TECHNIQUE
USING RIGID PLATE

Wm. LoechEl

3. Keep in mind that the mental foramen exits just beneath the apical portions of the first or second premolars. The incisions and/or periosteal elevation must be limited if injury to the nerve is to be avoided.

4. The drill bit has a tendency to overheat during the drilling of the oblique hole, and the area must be continuously irrigated to avoid burning of the bone. Excess heat can also cause breakage of the drill bit. Offset drills, if available, will more easily accommodate the required angle.

COMPLICATIONS

1. As with any mandible fracture, there is a potential for malunion. This complication can be avoided by accurate reduction and fixation and verification of preinjury occlusion. Treatment for this complication is described in Chapter 28.

2. Nonunion can occur and must be avoided. The physician must ensure that the fracture is accurately reduced and eventually shows signs of healing. The patient should be examined for evidence of infection, and if present, cultures should be obtained and appropriate antibiotics administered. Fragments that become devitalized must be removed. Further treatment for this complication is discussed in Chapters 25 through 27.

3. Paresthesias involving the lower anterior dentition and chin are possible from injury to the inferior alveolar and/or mental nerve. If this becomes a problem, the wire should be removed through the same intraoral incision.

4. Hypoesthesia resulting from injury to the mental nerve is usually transient; there is an excellent chance that sensation will return. This complication can be prevented by avoiding any direct trauma to the nerve.

ALTERNATIVE TECHNIQUE USING INTERNAL RIGID PLATE FIXATION

Internal rigid plate fixation is also possible using the intraoral approach. The incision is somewhat limited by the course of the mental nerve; this can become a problem when trying to obtain periosteal elevation for application of the plate. It is important to bend the plate to the exact contour of the bone. This can be assisted by using templates to test the curvature on the surface of the jaw. If the plate is bent too much or too little, there will be distraction at one of the cortical surfaces. The dynamic compression plate is preferred and is attached as described in Chapter 13. Postoperative care is similar to that used in intermaxillary fixation and interosseous wiring.

section VIII

Tooth and Alveolar Fractures

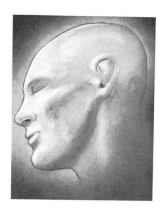

chapter 22

Repair of Tooth Injury
Alternative Technique of Orthodontic Brackets

In Consultation With Francis G. LeVeque, DDS

INDICATIONS

Injury to the dentition commonly occurs with mandible and/or maxillary fractures. Treatment of this injury depends on whether the tooth involved is deciduous or permanent, the severity of injury (including the number of teeth affected), the health of the injured tooth (or teeth), the overall condition of the noninjured dentition, the cost-effectiveness of the planned repair, and the need to retain affected teeth for a prosthesis or for the stabilization of a mandibular or maxillary fracture. If time permits, consultations with specialists such as dentists, endodontists, orthodontists, and oral surgeons are helpful.

In general, tooth fractures limited to the enamel should be managed electively; those injuries that penetrate the dentin may require dental dressings. When the injury involves the dental pulp and/or root, some form of endodontic therapy will need to be employed. Avulsed teeth require stabilization techniques, often in concert with endodontic procedures.

PROCEDURE
Incisal Edge Injuries Not Involving the Dentin

A For injuries involving the incisal edge but not the dentin, the teeth of the primary and permanent dentition are treated conservatively. The enamel can often be smoothed with an abrading disk. In cases of significant loss of tooth substance, a definitive dental restoration is indicated.

Incisal Edge Injuries Involving Enamel and Dentin

B Teeth with incisal edge injuries involving the enamel and dentin can generally be salvaged. First,

REPAIR OF TOOTH INJURY

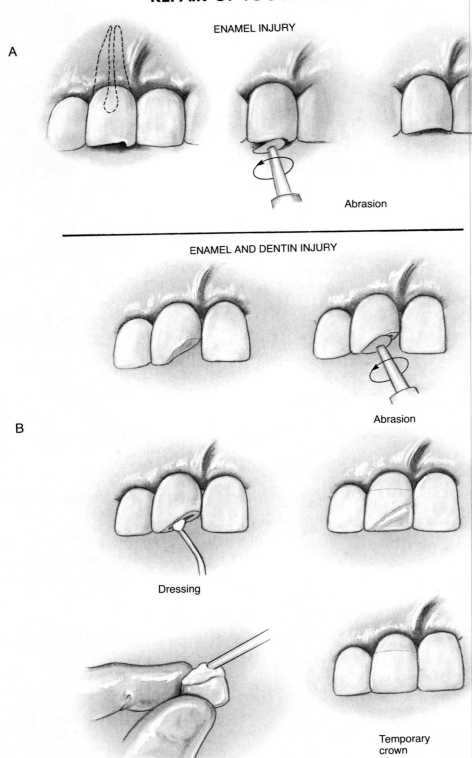

ENAMEL INJURY

A

Abrasion

ENAMEL AND DENTIN INJURY

B

Abrasion

Dressing

Cement

Temporary crown

unsupported enamel is removed by rotary instruments or dental chisels. The tooth is then pumiced, and if the injury is well within the dentin or is thermally sensitive, a dressing of calcium hydroxide or zinc oxide is placed over the exposed dentin. Then a temporary stainless steel or acrylic crown is cemented with any temporary dental cement. The definitive restoration can be placed sometime later.

Enamel, Dentin, and Pulp Injuries

C For complicated crown fractures involving the enamel, dentin, and pulp, much will depend on when the fracture is treated. Generally an uncomplicated fracture of the coronal portion of a tooth involving the pulp can be managed with direct pulp capping with calcium hydroxide and application of a temporary acrylic crown if performed within a few hours. If treatment occurs within 6 to 24 hours, extirpation of the coronal pulp should be completed (pulpotomy), a calcium hydroxide dressing placed on the root stump, and a temporary crown fabricated. After 24 hours, a complete endodontic procedure should be performed. For a deciduous tooth, a nonvital dressing should be placed after pulpotomy (formocresol).

Root Injuries

D For root fractures, the more apical the fracture, the better the patient prognosis. Root fractures in the apical third of the tooth are often stable, and conservative measures, such as fixation with acrylic or composite splints, can retain pulp viability. For these procedures, the tooth is coated with petrolatum; the acrylic is then molded and removed prior to curing. The acrylic should then be smoothed and replaced onto the tooth with a dental cement. If the tooth later becomes devital, appropriate endodontic therapy should be employed.

E Root fractures in the middle third and the coronal third carry a poorer patient prognosis. In most patients, if the fracture is close to the crown, the outlook is dismal, and extraction is usually the treatment of choice. The crown is removed, and the root is extracted through a small flap in the gingiva. The lateral alveolar bone is cut away, and the root is elevated with a downward (and/or upward) movement.

For fractures in the midportion of the root, rigid fixation with carefully fashioned acrylic splints should be employed. If pulpal death ensues, either endodontic therapy or extraction will have to be performed.

Displacement, Partial Avulsion, or Impaction Injuries

F In displacement, partial avulsion, or impaction injuries, the periodontal space, membrane, and pulp can be affected. A conservative approach is to regain the normal anatomic position of the tooth with careful manipulation and then to fix the tooth by means of a splint or orthodontic ligation.

Total Avulsion Injuries

G A permanent tooth that is completely avulsed is best reset within 2 hours. Replantation of an avulsed tooth more than 2 hours after injury can result in resorption, infraocclusion, and a variety of inflammatory responses that will require ultimate extraction. Briefly, the technique to be followed for replantation is as follows: the socket and tooth should be freely irrigated with normal saline. Using local anesthesia, the socket should be debrided. If the tooth is mature (i.e., with a closed apex), 2 mm should be amputated from the apex. In teeth with open apices, there should be no amputation. The tooth should then be stabilized by orthodontic appliances or an acrylic splint, and in approximately 2 weeks, endodontic therapy should be initiated.

PITFALLS

1. The diagnosis of tooth injury is very important in treatment planning. If the deciduous dentition is involved and the tooth is severely injured, it is probably more prudent to extract the tooth than to repair the injury.

2. If a tooth is severely carious or involved with significant periodontal disease, it should be considered for extraction. An exception may be a second or third molar that stabilizes the angle fracture and is not directly involved in the fracture. Extraction techniques are described in Chapter 23.

3. If the tooth is subluxated, displaced, or partially avulsed and is expected to exfoliate within 6 months, any efforts to retain it are not warranted, and the tooth should be extracted.

4. Patient attitudes are an important consideration. Many patients require revisional treatment, pulp testing, and delayed permanent restoration. If the patient is uncooperative and/or noncompliant, extraction may be the treatment of choice.

5. Avoid leaving nonvital teeth in fracture lines, as they are associated with portals of infection. Nonvital teeth can also act like foreign bodies and predispose the patient to osteomyelitis and, ultimately, nonunion of the fracture. The diagnosis can be made

REPAIR OF TOOTH INJURY *(Continued)*

ENAMEL, DENTIN, AND PULP INJURY

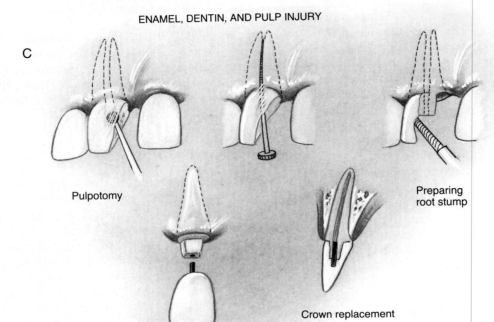

C

Pulpotomy

Preparing
root stump

Crown replacement

ROOT INJURY

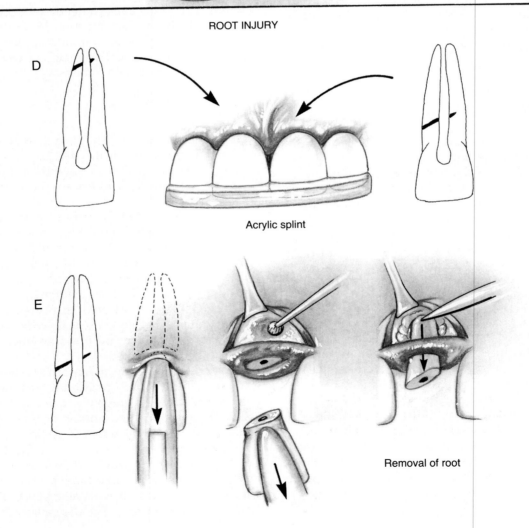

D

Acrylic splint

E

Removal of root

by dental radiographs and pulp testing. The tooth should also be evaluated for caries and periodontal disease. If the fracture line involves the tooth or is very close to the adjacent periodontal structures and the tooth is not necessary for stabilization, extraction must be considered.

COMPLICATIONS

1. Tooth injuries that are not successfully treated may cause the tooth to become nonvital and ultimately pose problems with resorption and/or infection. These teeth should be evaluated every few months with inspection and pulp testing. Radiographs should be obtained at least twice a year. Endodontic therapy can not only eliminate infectious processes, but also set the foundation for dental procedures to restore function and cosmesis.

2. Resorption of a tooth can occur following replantation. This process may be slow or accelerated. If there is no inflammation or infection accompanying the resorption, the tooth should be retained until function or appearance is compromised.

ALTERNATIVE TECHNIQUE OF ORTHODONTIC BRACKETS

Avulsed or displaced teeth can alternatively be stabilized by application of arch bars or orthodontic brackets. The arch bar is sufficient in teeth that are displaced laterally or lingually, but it will not give sufficient holding strength to a tooth that is being extracted; the orthodontic band is ideal for this condition.

For use of the band, the surgeon first applies dental etching acid to a 5-mm^2 area in the center of the tooth and to the two teeth on either side. An arch wire–accepting bracket is then attached with orthodontic bonding cement. Care should be taken to ensure that the brackets are aligned for easy placement of the arch wire. The arch wire is subsequently shaped and placed into the cemented brackets and the ends of the arch wire ligated to their appropriate brackets. The splint is retained for a minimum of 2 months. A radiograph should be obtained at the time of splint placement and then every month until the tooth is stable.

REPAIR OF TOOTH INJURY *(Continued)*

F   DISPLACEMENT

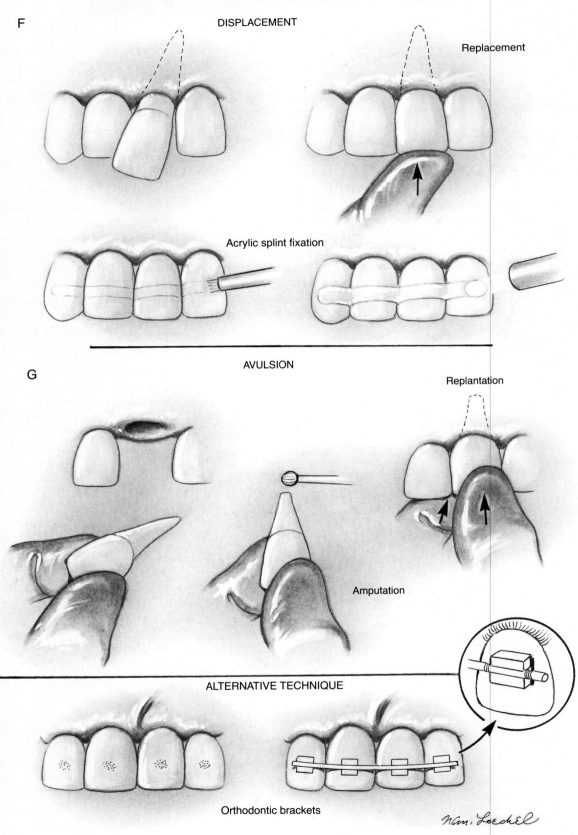

Replacement

Acrylic splint fixation

AVULSION

G

Replantation

Amputation

ALTERNATIVE TECHNIQUE

Orthodontic brackets

Wm. Loechel

chapter 23

Tooth Extraction

In Consultation With Francis G. LeVeque, DDS

INDICATIONS

Teeth that will compromise reduction and fixation of fractures should be considered for extraction. Usually these teeth have been assessed as nonsalvageable and are considered potential foreign bodies. If they are in or near a fracture line of the supporting jaw, they should be extracted before fixation. Otherwise they can be treated electively in the posttrauma period. Extraction should be considered on (1) those teeth that sustained sufficient injury to the tooth, periodontium, and alveolus to preclude a reasonable prognosis for retention (see Chapter 22) or (2) teeth with significant preexisting periodontal disease, periapical pathoses, and/or invasive caries; if left in place, such teeth could later become septic and may compromise the healing of soft tissue lacerations, alveolar fractures, and fractures of the jaws themselves.

Occasionally there is a question of salvageability. If this question arises in teeth that are on or very proximal to a fracture line, they should be removed. The caveats relating to jaw fracture stabilization and prosthetic retention must be carefully considered when planning these extractions.

The successful removal of a tooth or teeth depends on the skill of the operator, the availability of a proper armamentarium, and the presentation of the teeth slated for extraction. When possible, a referral to a dentist for the extractions is suggested.

PROCEDURES

Employing an atraumatic technique when removing teeth is of paramount importance. The retrieval of a retained, fractured cuspid root from dense alveolar bone will most often require significantly more force (and concomitant trauma) than the rather simple exercise of removing multiple periodontally compromised, mobile teeth. Before attempting dental extractions, a presurgical radiograph of the extraction site should be available. The radiograph will disclose the height and character of the supporting alveolar bone and root morphology, the knowledge of which should materially aid in the extraction. In cases of embedded molars or large or hypercementosed roots, or when the alveolar bone is dense or without appreciable loss of height, the use of rotary (drill) instruments should be seriously considered.

Elevation

A The judicious use of tooth elevation prior to application of an extraction forceps will usually facilitate luxation from the socket and prevent mucosal tearing. A periosteal elevator should first be used to separate the attached gingiva from the root surface of the tooth. Then a pointed straight-grooved elevator should be interposed between (1) the tooth and the alveolar bone (when a defect is present) and (2) the tooth to be removed and the teeth immediately adjacent. Careful instrumentation allows levering of the offending tooth without harming the adjacent one. This type of instrumentation can also prevent unwanted root fractures at the time of forceps delivery. In cases where repeated attempts at elevation fail to produce tooth movement, reduction of the investing alveolar bone should be considered. Also, teeth with multiple roots that exhibit compound angles to the crown should be removed with longitudinal sectioning. A dental drill or a roto-osteotome is necessary for these maneuvers, and the bone should be irrigated with physiologic solution during the use of one of these instruments.

Forceps Removal

Once the teeth are mobilized as a result of the elevation or are loose from preexisting periodontal disease or trauma, a special forceps should be used for the extraction. The application of the beaks of the forceps and the vectors of force applied to the forceps are important considerations.

UPPER ANTERIOR EXTRACTION

B The forceps used for the removal of maxillary incisors, canines, and premolars are all essentially the same. The beaks are straight projections of the handles without angulation. The beaks should be placed buccolingually. The forces employed should be apical, and for the removal of incisors and canines, an evenly applied rotational component will usually safely luxate the tooth. Sharp or jerky motions should be avoided, as these invite root fracture. For the premolars, the use of rotational forces should be discarded, as these teeth are often birooted. Once the beaks are securely placed, apical and controlled buccolingual forces should be steadily applied. Short buccolingual "rocking" excursions, rather than flamboyant movements, will reduce the incidence of unwanted fractures.

UPPER MOLAR EXTRACTION

C Maxillary molars usually have one lingual root and two buccal roots. In instances where the roots coalesce, are short, or are periodontally compromised, the use of a universal wide-beaked forceps is indicated. The forces for removal should be directed apically and buccolingually. Often the path of least resistance will be readily apparent (pulling coupled with rocking) and this is the path to follow for easy removal. If the roots are well formed and divergent, the use of an anatomic forceps is indicated. This type of forceps comes in both right- and left-sided models. The buccal beak is tapered and pointed and is designed to slide up between the two buccal roots. The lingual beak is wide and engages the lingual root at the neck of the tooth. Careful contraction of the handles of the forcep will expand the investing bone, and the buccolingual forces applied will usually luxate the tooth.

LOWER ANTERIOR EXTRACTION

D The forceps used for removing mandibular incisors, canines, and premolars are quite similar and can be readily interchanged. The beaks are moderately wide and bend down from the handles at about a 45° angle. The application of apical-rotatory forces will easily luxate a tooth with a nonangled root. For canines and premolars, the use of a buccolingual component along with the rotational force may be necessary.

LOWER MOLAR EXTRACTION

E,F The extraction of lower molars can pose significant problems. The root volume is impressive, and the tongue, floor of the mouth, and buccal tissues can obscure the field. The investing bone of the posterior mandible is unusually dense. The forceps used for removal of these teeth have both a buccal and a lingual beak of large proportion. These beaks are placed over the tooth so that their pointed tips engage the tooth at its root bifurcation. With the usual apical pressure, the forces are evenly and strongly applied in a buccolingual, rocking manner. In younger people, the use of a cow horn forceps can expand the alveolar bone to aid in the luxation of the tooth. In some adults, the tooth morphology often mandates sectioning of the crown to the root bifurcation before extraction.

Postextraction Care

Once the extractions are completed, hemostasis should be achieved by pressure and/or cauterization of small vessels. Thin interseptal bone should be removed and the socket periphery smoothed. The mucosa should be advanced and, if possible, loosely closed over the defect with 3–0 chromic sutures. Prophylactic antibiotics are administered for 5 days. Oral hygiene is maintained with daily chlorhexidine or 3% hydrogen peroxide mouthwashes.

PITFALLS

1. Inappropriate use of force can fracture the tooth, making it difficult to extract pieces of retained fragments. Such forces can also cause fractures of the alveolus and additional fractures to the bone of the jaw.

2. Remove all teeth that can adversely affect bone union. Retention of mobile, infected, or fractured nonsalvageable teeth in an area proximal to the jaw fracture may compromise the healing of the soft tissue and bone.

3. The need for dental extraction should have radiographic corroboration. Radiographs are essential for fully understanding tooth pathology, especially pathosis of the apex region and injuries that involve the alveolus, periodontium, and tooth proper.

COMPLICATIONS

1. Retained roots can be removed with careful use of angled elevators, root picks, and a variety of other specially designed instruments. In most instances, lateral pressure should be used to separate the tooth from the socket walls. Apical pressure should be avoided, as this vector of force could cause the loss of a root in the antrum, buccal pouch, or compartments inferior to the mandible. Careless instrumen-

TOOTH EXTRACTION

A

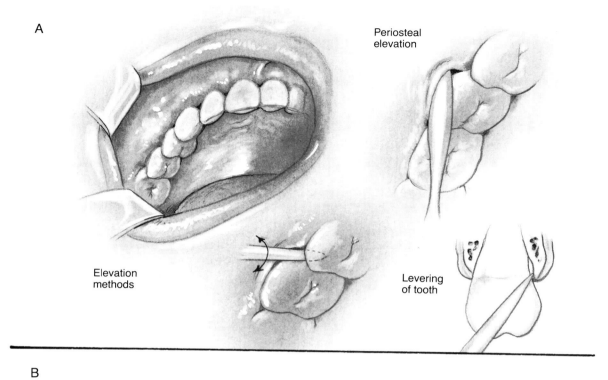

Periosteal elevation

Elevation methods

Levering of tooth

B

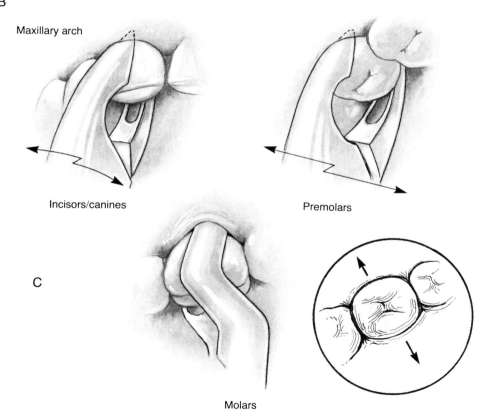

Maxillary arch

Incisors/canines

Premolars

C

Molars

Wm. Loechel

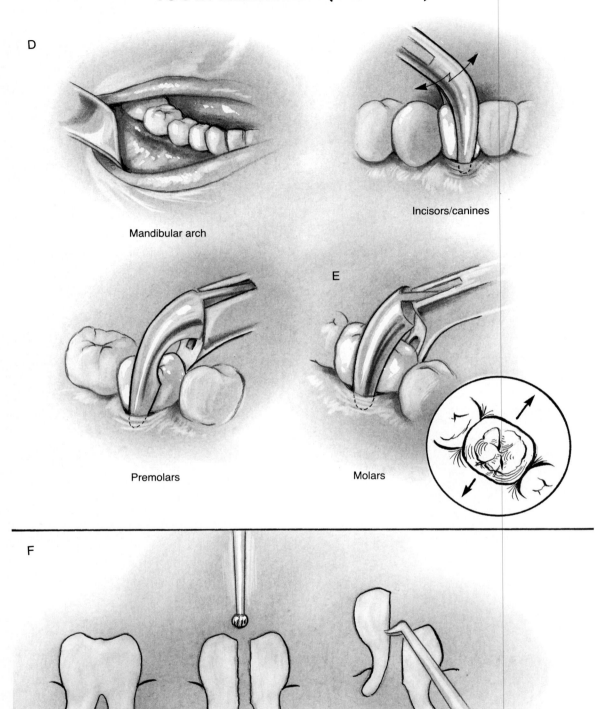

D

Mandibular arch

Incisors/canines

Premolars

E

Molars

F

Sectioning of crown

tation and loss of the root proximal to the inferior alveolar canal can cause injury to the nerve.

2. Dental or periodontal infection can spread and affect healing of the adjacent fracture. To avoid this problem, extraction should be as atraumatic as possible. All tooth fragments should be removed and the adjacent alveolus adequately debrided. Closure of the mucosa should be loose enough to provide for drainage and healing of the socket from below.

Prophylactic antibiotics and antiseptic mouthwashes are helpful adjuncts.

3. Extraction of the tooth (or teeth) can lead to instability of fixation. Postoperatively the patient should have radiographs taken to determine the position of the jaw fragments. If there is displacement of the fracture, an alternative fixation technique will have to be applied.

chapter 24

Closed Reduction of Alveolar Fractures

INDICATIONS

The alveolus is an important structure, and fractures of this area should not be taken lightly. The alveolus provides a neurovascular supply and structural support that are necessary for the health of the dentition, and in the edentulous patient, it produces a prominent ridge for stabilization of the denture.

Although many facial fractures are associated with fractures extending through the alveolar process, fractures confined to this process are relatively uncommon. Injury to the alveolus often takes place when there are abnormal forces exerted on the dentition, and thus the fracture is frequently seen with a dental injury; rarely is it observed in the edentulous patient. Decisions regarding treatment of the alveolar fracture must be coupled with management strategy for the dental injury.

PROCEDURES

For fractures of the alveolus in which the supported teeth are severely injured, the teeth should be extracted with a limited disruption of the alveolar periosteum attachments. This maneuver can best be achieved by stabilizing the alveolus with finger pressure and gently probing and elevating tooth fragments from their sockets with thin probes and elevators. Sharp edges should be trimmed with bone rongeurs, and soft tissues should be loosely closed over the defect.

For alveolar fractures associated with injured teeth that are important and will be retained, the teeth should be repaired according to procedures described in Chapter 22. These teeth probably should be treated after the alveolus has been reduced and fixed to the rest of the mandible.

A In patients with retained, restored, or even healthy teeth in the displaced alveolar segment, these teeth can be used for stabilization. The simplest approach is a manual reduction of the alveolar fragment, coupled with application of arch bars to the upper and lower dentition. The interdigitation of the teeth and rigidity of the bar will stabilize the fragment in a position that should be optimal for healing. The arch bar techniques are described in Chapter 8.

B,C In patients who have severe tooth injuries requiring extraction or in patients who are essentially edentulous, other methods must be considered. Often, small fragments of bone can be debrided and the orogingival mucosa closed over the area of injury. Alternatively, dentures, an acrylic covering, or a lingual acrylic splint with a soft liner can be used in combination with circummandibular wires. If the patient has an incomplete dentition, then a combination of arch bars and acrylic splints attached to the bars can be used to stabilize the intervening fragments.

Alveolar ridge fractures should be immobilized for at least 6 weeks. Oral health should be maintained with periodic brushings and irrigations. Antibiotics (i.e., erythromycin or penicillin) should be provided for 5 to 6 days.

PITFALLS

1. For the most part, treatment of the alveolus should consist of debridement, closure of the mucous membranes, and closed reduction with or without fixation. Attempts to open the fracture will further devitalize the fragments and potentially predispose them to infection.

2. Every attempt should be made to retain the alveolus. However, there are situations in which it may be better to remove the involved ridge of the mandible. This condition often develops following gunshot wounds in which there are multiple pieces of foreign material and devitalized bone. When this occurs, the alveolar mucosa is loosely closed over the area of resection.

3. Interosseous wires and plates applied to the alveolus should be avoided, as these materials often become exposed and act as foreign bodies. Moreover, an application of poorly fitting dentures can cause delayed complications of erosion and osteomyelitis.

4. Alveolar fractures require meticulous oral care.

TREATMENT OF ALVEOLAR FRACTURES

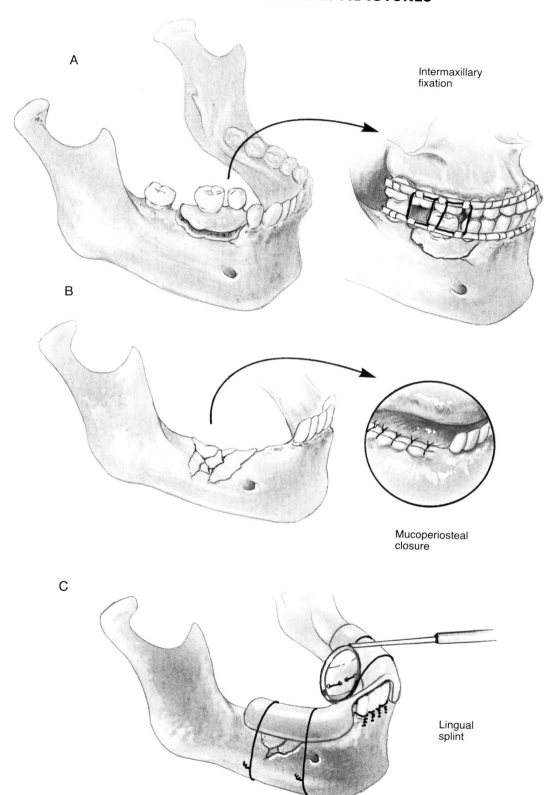

A

Intermaxillary
fixation

B

Mucoperiosteal
closure

C

Lingual
splint

Wm. Loechel

Lacerations and exposed sockets tend to harbor bacteria and debris. If the crevices are not kept clean, infection can develop in the underlying bone.

COMPLICATIONS

1. If infection should develop in the alveolar ridge, cultures should be obtained and the extent of the infection determined by radiographic analysis. Devitalized tissues should be removed; this may include the entire alveolar segment. Appropriate antibiotics should be administered for at least 10 days.

2. Displacement of the alveolus, especially in the patient who has teeth, can cause problems with occlusion. If the malocclusion is mild, a simple correction can be obtained by adjusting the crown surface with abrading disks. If displacement of the alveolar segment is severe and there is a need to retain the dentition, then the surgeon should consider orthodontic treatment. If this approach is not productive, refracture and restabilization can be implemented. When it is not necessary to retain the dentition of the alveolar segment, extraction may be the most prudent course of action.

3. Injury to the alveolus can ultimately cause devitalized teeth. In addition to direct trauma, the tooth is often subjected to indirect injury caused by disruption of the neurovascular supply to the alveolar segment. Evaluation by pulp testing may be indicated. If the tooth should lose viability, it may be possible to salvage it with endodontic therapy. If the dentition is associated with severe caries or periodontal disease, extraction should be performed.

Nonunion of the Mandible

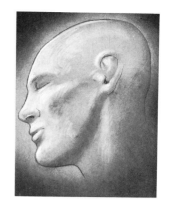

chapter 25

Early Treatment of Nonunion of the Mandible With External Pin Fixation (Biphase) Technique

INDICATIONS

Nonunion of the mandible is often the result of infection and is usually associated with pain and abnormal mobility of the jaw. The infection can be caused by contamination, retained foreign bodies, or failure to immobilize and reduce the fracture. Other contributing factors include an impaired blood supply and malnourishment, conditions that ultimately affect the healing of bone. All, or at least some, of the factors should be considered preliminarily before proceeding with the repair processes.

A stepwise progression of medical and surgical treatment is necessary. The goal is to obtain a clean, vascularized, and immobilized jaw. The biphase technique is ideal, as bicortical pins can be placed away from the fracture site and provide for an opportunity to treat the wound locally with debridement and irrigation. Moreover, the mandible can be completely immobilized during the "cleanup" period, which may allow for new bone to bridge the gap. The biphase is also an excellent method to stabilize the jaw during a bone graft procedure.

PROCEDURE

If the patient has a severely carious tooth, a fractured tooth, or a partially erupted molar in the fracture line, the tooth must be extracted (see Chapter 23). Osteomyelitis involving the periapical region of the tooth and/or the alveolar ridge must be treated with appropriate curettage. The mucosa can then be loosely approximated with 3–0 chromic sutures.

A,B The area of infection involving the mandible must be opened, drained, and debrided. Usually the surgeon can proceed through the original incision and open pockets of infection with a probing motion of the finger. Any devitalized bone noted previously on radiographs or on palpation should be removed. Large fixation plates can be left in place, but if there are small pieces of wire, mesh, or small plates directly involved with the infection, they should be removed. The bone edges should be freshened back to bleeding points with a bone rongeur.

C,D The biphase is then applied. If possible, occlusal relationships should be first obtained with arch bars or Ivy loops. In the edentulous patient, the fragments should be placed in approximate position and held with bone clamps. Two drill holes are then placed into each fragment on a line perpendicular to the fracture and at least several centimeters removed from the site of infection. The jaw is fixed in position with universal joints and bars and subsequently with a permanent acrylic bar (see Chapter 14). The wound is either drained with two to three Penrose drains sutured at the edge of the skin or packed several times a day with antiseptic-treated gauze (i.e., povidone-iodine). If the Penrose drain method is chosen, the drains are left in place for the long term, at least until drainage has stopped and the wound closes around the drains. For the packing technique, the packing must be changed several times a day, and entrapment of purulent material must be avoided. The wound is allowed to granulate from the deep surface, and when wound care becomes minimal, the patient can be discharged on oral antibiotics. Healing of the bone is monitored by inspection of the wound and serial radiographs. If formation of callous and bridging of the gap is suspected, then the biphase is maintained for at least 8 to 10 weeks. The acrylic can then be cut and the jaw tested for mobility. If the jaw is still mobile, the surgeon must suspect that fibrous tissue has grown between the fragments and that there is a need for more definitive surgical treatment.

If there is evidence that the mandible has not or will not heal, then the biphase must be maintained for 4 to 6 months and the patient considered for reconstructive surgery. Before proceeding, radiographs and clinical evaluations should verify no evidence of infection. The specific techniques for reconstruction are discussed in Chapters 26 and 27.

PITFALLS

1. It is often difficult to differentiate devitalized bone from healing bone. Because there is a tendency to try to retain as much bone as possible, there is also a tendency to keep any questionable bone, and if this bone is devitalized, infection will persist. Thus if drainage does not cease, the physician should be alerted to the possibility of reexploration and further debridement.

2. Remember that infections will delay healing for 2 to 4 weeks, and this time must be added to the healing process. Thus the patient should be in fixation for at least 6 to 8 weeks after infection has been controlled.

COMPLICATIONS

1. Failure to control infection usually indicates that there is insufficient debridement and/or drainage or there are underlying causes preventing bone healing. The patient should be thoroughly evaluated for immunologic and hematologic status. Vitamin and mineral deficiencies should be investigated. New cultures should be obtained and appropriate antibiotics (usually intravenous) administered.

2. Complications for the biphase procedure are described in Chapter 14 and are similar to those that would appear in the biphase treatment of a nonunion.

EARLY TREATMENT OF NONUNION

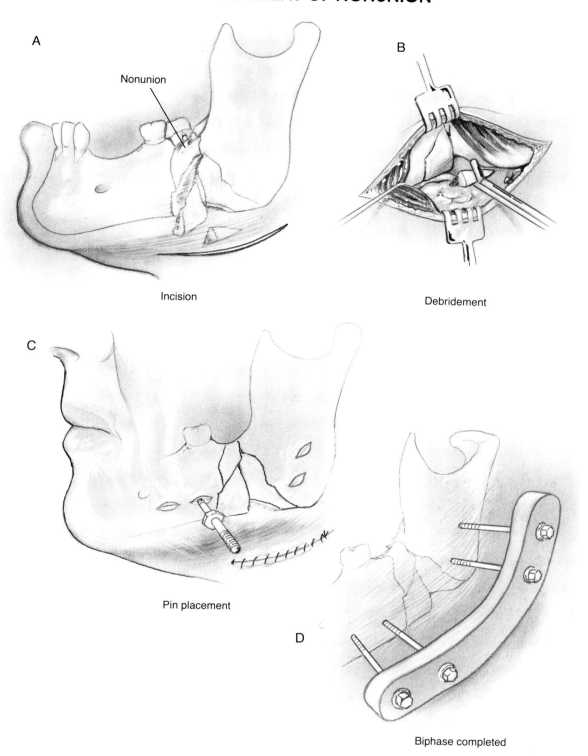

A

Nonunion

Incision

B

Debridement

C

Pin placement

D

Biphase completed

Repair of Nonunion of the Mandible With Reconstruction Plates and Iliac Crest Grafts
Alternative Technique Using External Pin Fixation (Biphase)

INDICATIONS

Nonunion of the mandible can occur in a variety of locations but is often found in an unfavorable angle or parasymphyseal fracture or in a fracture of an area of an edentulous atrophic body. Nonunion of the ramus, condyle, or coronoid process can also develop, but in these locations it does not usually pose a functional problem.

Jaw instability associated with a defect usually requires correction with a bone graft technique. To optimize conditions for surgery, the infection should be brought under control, and there should be a period of 4 to 6 months in which there is no evidence of soft tissue infection or osteomyelitis.

There are many methods for bone grafting and stabilization, but the reconstruction plate has become the most popular. This technique has the advantage of rigid fixation with early mobility and function of the jaw. Bone grafts can be harvested from a variety of sites, but the ileum is preferred. Iliac bone is easy to obtain and easy to shape and fit into the nonunion defect.

PROCEDURE

Harvest of Iliac Crest

To avoid confusion with an appendectomy scar, the left iliac crest should be selected as the donor site. Exposure is obtained by propping the left buttock with rolled towels or sandbags. The skin is prepared and draped as a sterile field. The incision is planned lateral to the crest to avoid a scar on the prominent part of the crest. This helps reduce discomfort that can be caused by pressure of a belt or waistband in this area.

A,B While pulling the skin medially, a 6- to 8-cm incision is made through the skin and subcutaneous fat. The anterior superior iliac spine is identified, and a cut is made through the periosteum from the spine to the flare of the ileum. Using heavy elevators, the periosteum is elevated off the crest. Laterally the elevation is more difficult because of the attachment of gluteus muscles, and these tendons must be incised with scissors or knife. Bleeding will be brisk, and hemostasis should be controlled with an electrocautery. The degree of elevation of the periosteum will depend on the amount of bone required for grafting, but a laterally directed subperiosteal pocket of about 6 × 10 cm can be safely developed without adversely affecting the hip joint.

C,D The graft is harvested with sharp, straight and curved 8- to 10-mm osteotomes. Using a straight osteotome, the bone is cut in a plane parallel to the outer table, taking a thickness of from several millimeters to almost the entire crest. The medial cortex should preferably be left intact. Inferiorly, the cut is developed along the anterior superior iliac spine. Superiorly, the limit is defined by the size of the bone required for the graft. The posterior cuts require a heavy retractor on the muscles, and usually a curved osteotome is necessary to obtain the appropriate direction and force. All bone cuts are then deepened, and when the osteotome tends to bind, it should be freed with a rocking action. Eventually the lateral plate bone becomes loose, and additional pieces of cancellous bone can then be removed with an osteotome and saved for the filling of small defects. The graft should be placed in a basin of blood until it is ready for implantation.

Hemostasis is achieved by applying bone wax to the external surface of the freshly cut ileum. Excess wax should be removed by forcefully wiping the wax with a sponge. Two medium-sized suction drains are placed through stab incisions and secured with 2–0 silk pursestring sutures. The periosteum is closed with 2–0 chromic sutures. The fat and subcutaneous tissues are brought together with 3–0 chromic su-

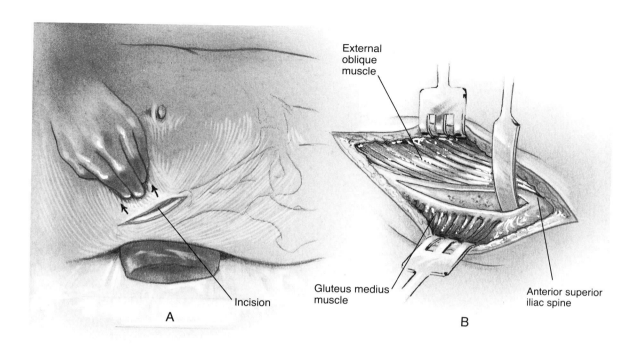

Incision

A

External
oblique
muscle

Gluteus medius
muscle

Anterior superior
iliac spine

B

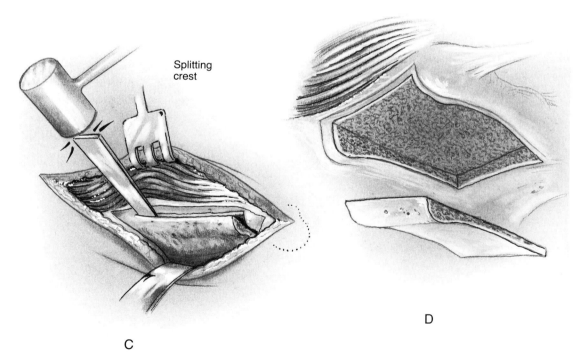

Splitting
crest

C

D

tures, and the skin is approximated with 5–0 nylon sutures.

REPAIR OF DEFECT

Occlusal relationships must be obtained. If there are sets of opposing teeth, they can be aligned with several Ivy loops. In the edentulous patient, stents or splints can be applied, but because the maxillary mandibular relationships can be readjusted at a later time with dentures, simple manipulations to approximate relationships of the jaws are all that are necessary. If the patient has a biphase apparatus in position, this can be quite helpful in stabilizing the fragments.

E Exposure of the mandibular defect will depend on the site of nonunion. Standard approaches are described in Chapters 13, 16, and 19. Longer incisions should be planned to accommodate the reconstruction plate.

F Periosteum should be elevated from all surfaces of the involved mandible, carefully avoiding entry into the oral cavity. If torn, the oral mucosa should be repaired immediately and the wound irrigated copiously with normal saline. The bone edges are often quite smooth and relatively avascular, and these edges must be freshened with bone rongeurs to at least a point at which fresh bleeding occurs.

G After adequate exposure of the outer surface of the mandible and approximation of the position of the mandibular fragments with bone forceps, the bone graft should be cut and placed into the defect. A wedging of the bone into position is desirable. Interosseous wires can be used temporarily to hold the graft in place.

H In planning for the reconstruction plate, the surgeon should place the plate so that at least two screws (but preferably three or four) can be placed into each segment of the mandible and at least one screw hole through the graft. A K-wire cutter should be available to cut the plate to the desired length. Special bending forceps are used to bend the plate to the contour of the recipient site.

I,J If an Arbeitsgemeinschaft fur Osteosynthesefragen (AO) reconstruction plate is chosen, then holes must be drilled, tapped, and measured for appropriate-sized screws. The first holes are placed in the mandible proximal and distal to the defect. The holes are drilled with a 2-mm bit and then tapped and measured so that the tip of the screw penetrates the inner cortex of the mandible. One 2.7-mm screw is loosely applied to just hold the plate in position. Another screw is then placed with a similar technique

to the other segment of the mandible. A hole is then drilled through the graft and a third screw used to secure it. Additional screws are added to provide rigid fixation. If there are any defects at the ends where the graft and mandible joint, these can be filled with pieces of cancellous bone. Additional pieces of bone can be used to adjust levels of the graft. If wires were used to temporarily hold the graft in position, they should be removed at this time.

The wound is closed by pulling the periosteum over the graft site with 2–0 chromic sutures. Dead space must be obliterated. This can be accomplished by freeing up the platysma and subcutaneous layers and inverting these soft tissues into the wound with 2–0 or 3–0 chromic vertical mattress sutures. Penrose drains may be used for 24 to 48 hours, but if the wound is dry, they should be avoided. The skin is approximated with 5–0 nylon sutures.

Extra pieces of iliac crest can be stored in a hospital bone bank, but if this is not available, the use of a "belly bank" should be considered. Usually the preparation of the hip includes the lower abdomen, which can be used for the bank. A small horizontal incision is then made just beneath the belt or waistline. A subcutaneous pocket is developed and the remainder of the graft inserted. The wound is then closed with subcuticular 4–0 chromic sutures and skin sutures of 5–0 nylon.

Postoperatively the patient is maintained on intravenous antibiotics for at least 5 days and continued on oral antibiotics for an additional 10 days. The patient can be started and maintained on a full liquid diet; chewing of food should be avoided for at least 2 weeks. The mouth should be washed several times a day with 3% hydrogen peroxide. The wound should be inspected weekly and radiographs obtained after surgery and at 6 to 8 weeks to evaluate adequacy of healing.

With regard to the hip, ambulation should begin as soon as possible. Drains are removed when the drainage is less than 20 to 25 mL per day. Sutures are removed at 7 days.

PITFALLS

1. Underestimating the amount of bone necessary to fill the defect is occasionally a problem. To avoid this situation, remove 25% to 50% more bone than is thought necessary to fill the defect.

2. Avoid hematomas of the hip, as they can lead to infection and pain. Hematoma can be prevented by fastidious hemostasis and also by checking for obstruction of the drainage tubes. The drains should not be removed until drainage is less than 25 mL per day.

ILIAC CREST RECONSTRUCTION FOR NONUNION *(Continued)*

E

Repair of defect

F

Nonunion

Incision

Debridement

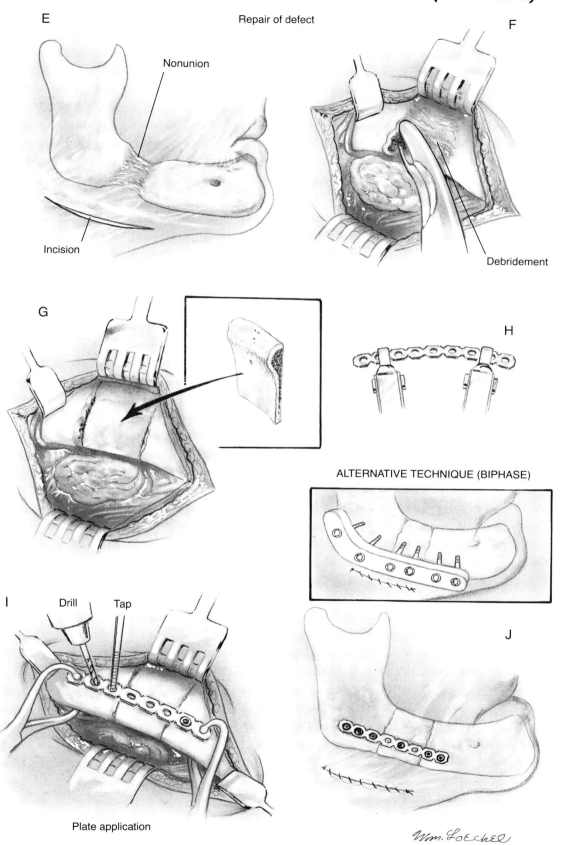

G

H

ALTERNATIVE TECHNIQUE (BIPHASE)

I

Drill   Tap

J

Plate application

Wm. Loechel

3. Sponges can inadvertently be left in the depths of the hip wound. A sponge count while closing can be extremely helpful.

4. In preparing the graft, it is necessary to try to provide a physiologic environment. Keep the graft bathed in a basin layered with blood. The surgeon should irrigate with lactated Ringer's solution while cutting and contouring the bone.

5. Do not reconstruct the jaw if there is any evidence of infection. The mandible must be treated and prepared with appropriate antibiotics and a period of immobilization for at least 4 to 6 months prior to bone grafting (see Chapter 25).

6. Pretrauma occlusal relationships should be obtained prior to grafting and fixation. Excessive bite forces can distract the fragments from the fracture site; these forces must be minimized by ensuring normal occlusion in the postoperative period.

7. Intraoral exposure will contaminate the wound. Lacerations created during the elevation of the periosteum should be closed immediately with 3–0 chromic sutures and the wound washed copiously with normal saline.

8. Dead space should be avoided and/or obliterated. Proper use of drains, rotation and/or advancement of subcutaneous tissues, and pressure dressings will help close the space and provide some prophylaxis against hematoma and infection.

9. The reconstruction plate must be rigidly fixed. Screws must be tight fitting, and this can only be achieved by placing the screw in a hole that is slightly smaller than the screw. Also remember that at least two screws, and preferably three, are required to stabilize the proximal and distal mandibular segments.

COMPLICATIONS

1. Iliac crest grafts are often associated with hip pain. Early mobilization of the joint is helpful and will prevent guarding and stiffness. Active rehabilitation is advisable.

2. Infection can be prevented by avoiding intraoral contamination, dead space within the wound, and less than optimal fixation. If the wound becomes infected, the infection should be drained and cultures obtained for the selection of appropriate intravenous antibiotics. Dead pieces of bone should be debrided. Sometimes the infection will come under control and the graft can be saved. However, if the amount of purulent drainage does not cease, the graft will have to be removed. If the plate is involved (i.e., the screw holes show evidence of osteomyelitis), then it should also be removed. Further immobilization can be achieved with other previously described techniques

(i.e., intermaxillary fixation, splints, stents, and biphase). A period of 4 to 6 months is again necessary before proceeding with reconstruction.

3. Oral rehabilitation is often a problem following a bone graft procedure. Obliteration of the gingivolabial or gingivobuccal sulcus will require a vestibuloplasty. If a large bone graft is used, the osseous integrated implant technique may be necessary for stability of the denture.

4. Facial deformity is common following an iliac crest implant. The bone plate and screws often show through the skin and must be removed. Resorption of the graft may be spotty, and irregularities of the bone will require a smoothing with cutting burs.

5. Bone grafting of the mandible is almost always associated with loss of sensation of the inferior alveolar nerve and loss of motion of those muscles innervated by the marginal mandibular nerve. Attempts at nerve graft are usually not successful and probably should not be attempted. Other methods for minimizing the cosmetic effects are neurotomy of the opposite side and/or muscle transposition to the involved site.

ALTERNATIVE TECHNIQUE USING EXTERNAL PIN FIXATION (BIPHASE)

External pin fixation has the advantage of immobilizing the mandible while treating the nonunion with debridement and antibiotics. The same method used for immobilization is employed for stabilizing the grafts that are used in the repair of the mandibular defect. The disadvantages of the technique are that the fixation apparatus must be taken apart to perform the surgery, it does not provide a fixation as rigid as that obtained with the plate, and it is clumsy to wear in the postoperative period.

The procedure requires setting the jaws into occlusal relationships. The biphase pins are then applied and held in position with universal joints and external bars (see Chapter 14). The hip graft is harvested and the recipient bed prepared as discussed previously. The hip graft is then fitted into place and held with two 26-gauge stainless steel interosseous wires. The acrylic is applied across the pins, the wires optionally removed, and the wound closed in layers.

Postoperative care requires intravenous antibiotics (5 to 7 days), followed by oral antibiotics for another week. Periodic radiographs should be obtained to ensure adequate healing. Pin holes must be kept clean with 3% hydrogen peroxide and daily applications of an antibiotic ointment. The acrylic bar is cut at about 8 weeks and the wound tested for stability. If there is any motion, the acrylic is reapplied; otherwise, the pins can be removed.

chapter 27

Repair of Nonunion of the Mandible With Titanium Mesh and Cancellous Iliac Crest Bone

INDICATIONS

Defects of the mandible resulting from infection and/or resorption of bone must be treated with a bone graft. The reconstruction plate and iliac crest graft technique is one of the more popular methods (see Chapter 26). However, this method becomes difficult to apply in patients who have comminuted or severely atrophic proximal or distal segments of the mandible. For these individuals, the mesh technique with cancellous bone grafts is preferred. The mesh is also strong enough to provide rigid fixation and early mobility of the jaw joint.

PROCEDURE

Cancellous bone is harvested from the iliac crest using the same exposure as that described for the removal of the solid cortical/cancellous block (see Chapter 26). After the lateral portion of the ileum is excised, the surgeon then removes 3 to 4-mm² pieces of bone with rongeurs from the deeper surfaces of the donor site and the graft. These small pieces of bone are placed in a blood-layered basin and the wound closed in a routine fashion.

A–D Surgical exposure of the jaw is the same as that used in the reconstruction plate technique (see Chapter 26). Bone should be cut back to healthy bleeding sites, and the periosteum should be elevated sufficiently to provide room for the mesh.

E With the proximal and distal segments held in anatomic relationships, a section of titanium mesh "crib" is cut to appropriate size and molded onto the inferior and lateral aspects of the recipient sites. Wire cutters and benders are needed, and if the mesh has to be bent more than 10° to 20°, it is probably better to cut the mesh and rotate its free edges over one another. Ideally, the lateral part of the crib should extend to the height of the mandible, whereas the

medial part should be lower and beneath the level of the alveolar ridge.

F The mesh is secured to the proximal and distal segments of the mandible by drilling small holes with a fine K wire and minidriver through the slots of the mesh. These holes should extend from the outer cortex of the mandible into the inner cancellous areas. Titanium screws are then selected, and using a special screw driver, these screws are applied to the holes. Multiple screws placed several centimeters apart should be sufficient to secure the mesh to each segment. Additional screws placed on the inferior portion of the jaw are helpful in bringing the mesh snug to the surface of the mandible.

When the lower jaw is stabilized with the mesh, small pieces of cancellous bone previously harvested from the hip are placed into the crib. The pieces are tightly packed to fill the entire mesh.

The periosteum is closed tightly around the mesh with 2–0 chromic sutures. The wound is then closed in layers, carefully obliterating the dead space. The wound should be dry, but if there is a need for it to be drained, the drains should be removed in 24 to 48 hours. A light compression dressing helps to keep the soft tissues tight against the graft.

The patient is treated with intravenous antibiotics for 5 days and oral antibiotics for an additional 10 days. The wound is evaluated weekly, and radiographs are obtained postoperatively and at 8 weeks. A full liquid diet will provide nutrition and avoid stress to the jaw. Care of the hip is described in Chapter 26.

PITFALLS

1. Precautionary measures and highlights of hip grafting are described in Chapter 26. Cancellous bone must be treated with the same care as in the cancellous/cortical block.

2. Because of the three-dimensional aspects of the titanium mesh crib, it is difficult to mold this to the contour of the jaw. The cutting and overlapping technique and multiple screw fixations help in achieving an optimal fit.

3. Avoid making the edges of the crib higher than the level of the reconstructed jaw. If this occurs, the edges can cut through the mucosa and can also cause problems with the fit of bridges and plates.

4. Do not use a filter paper lining, as was originally described with this technique. The paper interferes with wound drainage and revascularization of the graft.

5. Avoid binding on insertion of the screws. Titanium screws are fragile and will break if there is too much resistance. If tension should build, unwind the screw and redrill the hole. If the screw should break, ignore the broken part and start a new screw in another strategic area.

COMPLICATIONS

1. Infection in and around the graft postoperatively is associated with a grave prognosis. The wound should be immediately opened, cultures obtained, and the wound irrigated with 3% hydrogen peroxide. Infected cancellous bone is difficult to remove, but if the infection does not respond, there is no choice but to remove the mesh and graft material. The surgeon can then return to the original treatment plan of immobilizing the proximal and distal segments and selecting a method for correction of the nonunion.

2. Resorption of the bone graft can occur and should be identified in the posttreatment radiograph. If the jaw should remain stable, the complication can be treated expectantly. However, the surgeon should be aware that without bone, the mesh is susceptible to undue stress and may fracture. If this occurs, the mesh will have to be removed and a new form of reconstruction will have to be considered.

3. Occasionally a free edge of the mesh breaks through the oral mucosa or interferes with the proper fit of a denture or bridge. If either of these conditions occurs, the mesh must be removed. This process of removing the mesh is not easy, as the bone often heals over the mesh and must be removed with cutting burs. The screws do not come out easily, and if they break, parts of the screw will have to be left in bone.

REPAIR USING TITANIUM MESH

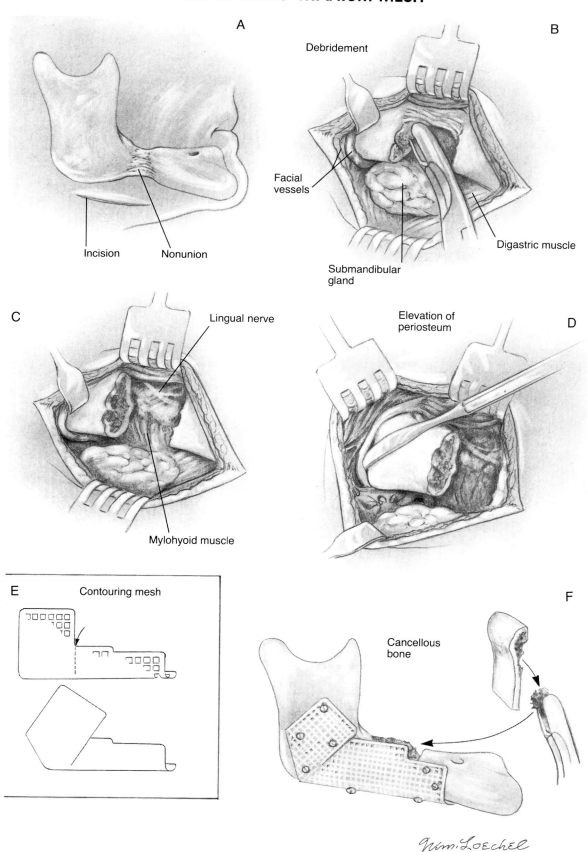

A

Incision   Nonunion

B

Debridement

Facial
vessels

Submandibular
gland

Digastric muscle

C

Lingual nerve

Mylohyoid muscle

D

Elevation of
periosteum

E   Contouring mesh

F

Cancellous
bone

Wm. Loechel

section X

Malunion of the Mandible

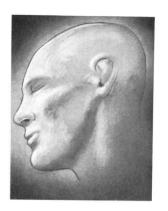

chapter 28

Osteotomy Techniques for Malunion of the Mandible
Alternative Technique Using Onlay Grafts
In Consultation With Mark T. Marunick, DDS

INDICATIONS

Malunion of the mandible can occur following a mandible fracture when there is imperfect reduction, inadequate fixation and stabilization, and periods of infection and resorption of the bone. The degree of malalignment usually dictates the degree of deformity and dysfunction. Correction should be considered for patients with malocclusion, temporomandibular joint disorders, and facial asymmetry. However, tolerances are variable, and the physician must evaluate the patient for individualized plans of management.

If the patient is edentulous, it is possible to correct many discrepancies of the mandible by denture modification. To some extent, dentures can be fabricated so that differences in the anteroposterior or horizontal plane can be adjusted. Compensation can also be carried out for open bite problems. However, severe interarch distance relationships that preclude denture fabrication may require osteotomies.

In patients with teeth, different techniques must be considered. For minor premature contacts, a conservative occlusal adjustment of the involved teeth may be needed. For moderate occlusal discrepancies, tooth reduction or endodontic therapy with crown fabrication and/or orthodontic treatment will generally resolve the problem. When a single tooth or several teeth provide a major discrepancy, extraction may be a simple and effective approach, especially when prosthodontic treatment will restore the dental arches and function.

For more serious malunions, the physician must consider strategic osteotomies to correct the maxillary and mandibular relationships. If the deformity is caused by malalignment of the fracture, an osteotomy is preferred, either in the fracture line or in a strategic site that will compensate for the problem. If the patient has a deformity and a dysfunction associated with a preexisting malocclusion, then it is more prudent to refer the patient for classic orthognathic surgery. If deformity is the only problem and function is adequate, onlay grafts can be performed over the area of deficiency.

PROCEDURE

Presurgical Considerations

To plan for osteotomy sites and methods of stabilization, it is important to study the fractures (i.e., their effects on malocclusion and/or deformity and the cause of the malunion). For this purpose, the surgeon should obtain the patient's previous records (including operative reports and radiographs), and a new set of radiographs and dental casts. Impressions, casts, face-bow registrations, jaw relationships, and surgical modification of casts are described in Chapters 9 and 20. Once the plaster boat is fabricated, it is indexed, a registration taken, and the cast placed back into the plaster boat and mounted on the articulator. The lines of fracture are marked out, and cuts are made through these lines. The fractured segments are then placed into anatomic and functional relationships with each other and with the opposing dental arch on the articulator and are held together with dental wax. Bone defects that would occur with repositioning of the fragments will have to be corrected with sliding osteotomies or with autogenous bone grafts. The operative dental casts are also useful in developing a lingual or interocclusal splint, which serves as a guide during the surgical procedure for the correct placement of the fragments (see Chapter 20).

Surgery

The incision and approach will depend on the site of the fracture. In general, the exposure is identical to that used for the external and open treatment of a mandible fracture. To obtain accurate relationships of the intermaxillary occlusion, nasotracheal intubation is preferred.

A–C After exposure of the osteotomy site, the periosteum should be stripped from the bone. Care must be taken not to open into the mouth, but if this does occur, the mucosa should be repaired immediately with 3–0 chromic sutures. Malleable retractors can be placed between the bone and periosteum so that the cuts will not injure the adjoining soft tissues.

The osteotomy can be performed with Lindeman burs, oscillating saws, or with fine, sharp osteotomes. However, the surgeon should recognize that the thicker the osteotomy line, the more chance there is for instability and the need for bone grafting. If the bone has healed completely, a stepwise cut or an oblique sagittal split will provide more surface area for postoperative stability. If the neurovascular bundle is intact, the surgeon should avoid injury to this structure.

D–F The site of osteotomy and the need for stability will determine the appropriate fixation technique. The lingual or interocclusal splint should be applied and will provide the relationships for the approximation of the segments (see Chapter 21). If the bones are in good contact, the surgeon can proceed with simple interosseous wiring and intermaxillary fixation with arch bars or Ivy loops or, alternatively, with temporary Ivy loops and rigid fixation plates (see Chapters 8, 15, and 18). If there is a deficiency, then a bone graft technique with plate or mesh fixation must be used (see Chapter 14).

Postoperatively the patient should be held in fixation for at least 6 to 8 weeks. Prophylactic antibiotics (i.e., penicillin or erythromycin) should be administered for 5 to 7 days, or longer if bone grafts are used. Oral hygiene should be maintained with gentle brushings and/or the use of a water irrigation device.

PITFALLS

1. An understanding of the pathophysiology is essential for obtaining good results. Occlusion can be observed on the casts, and additionally, one surgical hypothesis can be checked against another. An inadequate diagnostic workup is an invitation for problems.

2. Do not overoperate. If the patient's malocclusion can be corrected by occlusal adjustments or other dental treatment, then this is preferred to osteotomy and refixation. Moreover, most edentulous patients can be better treated with adjustments of their denture. If the problem is purely cosmetic, then the physician can even consider onlay grafts (see later). Consultation with appropriate dental colleagues is important in making these management decisions.

3. Avoid unnecessary contamination of the operative site. If a dental extraction is necessary, it is probably more prudent to delay a week or two before the definitive surgery. Try to avoid intraoral exposure, but if there is a tear, close the mucosa immediately with sutures.

4. Malunion of the condyle can be associated with temporomandibular joint ankylosis. If this occurs,

TREATMENT OF MALUNION WITH OSTEOTOMIES

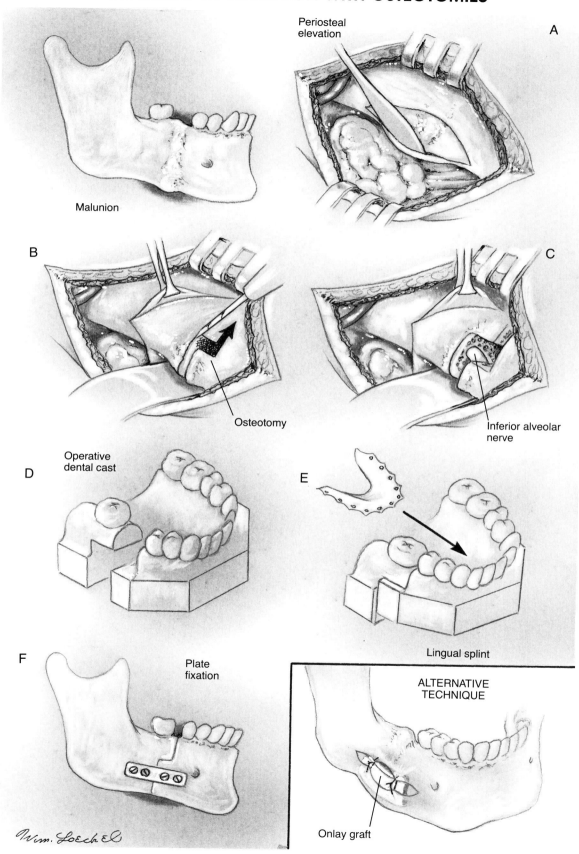

Malunion

Periosteal elevation

A

B

Osteotomy

C

Inferior alveolar nerve

D

Operative dental cast

E

Lingual splint

F

Plate fixation

ALTERNATIVE TECHNIQUE

Onlay graft

Wm. Loechel

the surgeon should consider creating a pseudarthrosis or even a condylectomy. Condylar reconstruction following condylectomy can also be considered as an option (see Chapter 29).

5. If malunion of the condyle is associated with satisfactory joint movement (as in subcondylar injuries), but also with shortening of the mandible and premature contact of the molars, it is probably better treated with a ramus osteotomy or a lower sagittal split osteotomy. In such cases, operative intervention of the condyle can cause more damage and should be avoided.

COMPLICATIONS

1. As in all mandibular injuries, infection and nonunion are possible sequelae. To prevent these problems, the surgeon should avoid intraoral contamination, drain hematomas and dead space, obtain exact reduction, and maintain a solid fixation during the healing process. Prophylactic antibiotics are also used, and if infection occurs, appropriate specific antibiotic treatment should be applied. Surgical management is discussed in Chapters 25 through 27.

2. Recurrence of malunion should be prevented by proper planning and execution of the surgical technique. If malunion should again develop, then the surgeon will again have to decide on the severity and significance of the malalignment of the fragments and on the appropriate measures for rehabilitation.

ALTERNATIVE TECHNIQUE USING ONLAY GRAFTS

Occasionally the malunion does not cause dysfunction and is only associated with deformity. If this is the case, the malunion can be corrected with onlay grafting techniques, rather than with an osteotomy. Using the onlay graft does not subject the patient to potential nonunion or dysfunction. However, morbidity will be associated with the donor site, and there may be subsequent irregularities of the graft that will require revisional surgery.

Adequate exposure for the repair will depend on the site of the deficiency. Care must be taken to avoid additional injury to the soft tissues—especially the muscles of mastication and the cranial nerves that supply these regions. The periosteum of the mandible should be elevated to create a pocket over the defect, and bone harvested from the hip or cranium is then contoured and placed into the pocket. The periosteum is tied snug around the graft with 2–0 chromic sutures. Postoperative care is similar to that described for other grafting techniques (see Chapter 26).

section XI

Temporomandibular Ankylosis

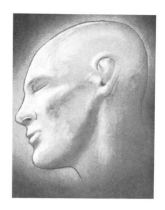

chapter 29

Treatment of Temporomandibular Ankylosis With Resection and Autogenous Rib Graft
Alternative Technique of Prosthetic Replacement

INDICATIONS

Immobility and consolidation of the temporomandibular joint are infrequent sequelae following injury to the head of the condyle and/or joint area. From a diagnostic standpoint, it is important to determine whether the patient's inability to open the mouth is secondary to scarring and contraction of soft tissues surrounding the joint or to a true fibro-osseous union between the condyle and glenoid fossa. Dynamic radiographs, in addition to computed tomographic (CT) scans, are important adjunctive diagnostic measures.

The diagnosis and condition of the patient will dictate therapeutic options. If the dysfunction is primarily caused by scarring, steroid injections and jaw opening exercises are warranted. If, on the other hand, there is bone formation and fusion, a more aggressive approach consisting of osteotomy or resection coupled with reconstruction should be considered.

What procedure to choose will depend on the location and degree of injury and the age of the individual. For the elderly person with complete ankylosis, osteotomy with a soft tissue interposition is all that is necessary. In the middle-aged individual, resection of the condyle and reconstruction with an alloplastic implant or autogenous bone can be considered. In most adults, however, rib graft is ideal, as it provides homologous, nonreactive tissues, a cartilage end for mobility, and bone-to-bone union for restoration of strength of the mandible. Growth is also possible as a result of the transfer of rib growth centers within the graft.

PROCEDURE

The patient's occlusion should be approximated by a loose intermaxillary fixation with arch bars or Ivy loops. Elastic bands will have to be removed during the procedure to check the mobility of the jaw. Preparations also require that the preauricular area be shaved and the face and neck established as a sterile field.

A–E The incision and approach to the temporomandibular joint is similar to that described in Chapter 10. The joint capsule and soft tissues should be incised and elevated off the bony structures to expose the affected area. The articular eminence, glenoid fossa (root of the zygoma), and condylar neck should be identified, but if this anatomy is obscured by fused pieces of bone, the surgeon should at least appreciate the relationships of the level of the middle fossa, the external auditory canal, and the articular eminence. Malleable retractors should then be inserted beneath the condylar head and neck to protect against injury to branches of the internal maxillary artery. The condylar head can be removed with cutting burs and rongeurs. An osteotomy can then be made along the neck of the condyle and intervening pieces of bone removed with rongeurs. Mobility of the jaw should be checked by passive opening and closing of the mouth. A new glenoid fossa is subsequently created by carving a concavity within the root of the zygoma.

F,G Another incision is made below the angle of the mandible to expose the angle and ramus region. This technique is similar to the one described in Chapter 13. The periosteum and masseter insertions are elevated to the neck of the condyle. A subperiosteal pocket is thus created close to the jaw and deep to the facial nerve structures. The ascending ramus of the mandible is grooved to receive the attachment of a rib graft.

H The seventh rib is harvested using the technique described in Chapter 17. The cartilage portion of the rib should be retained. This means that the rib must be handled gently, or the junction between the cartilage and bone will be broken. The length of the rib is designed according to the needs for reconstruction. The cartilage portion is rounded with a knife and the total length of the rib adjusted to accommodate firm contact to the new glenoid fossa and ramus of the mandible. The rib is then inserted from below into the newly formed glenoid fossa, and the bony portion of the rib is secured to the mandible

with several 25-gauge wires. No attempt is made to reattach the muscles of mastication, as they will attach to the grafted area during the healing process. The wounds are closed in layers.

Intermaxillary fixation should be maintained for 4 weeks (or 2 weeks in children). Intravenous antibiotics are administered for 5 days and oral antibiotics for another 10 days. Opening and closing exercises are initiated as soon as the intermaxillary wires or elastic bands are removed.

PITFALLS

1. The diagnosis of ankylosis must be accurate if the surgeon is to choose the appropriate procedure. Soft tissue scarring can be treated by conservative measures, whereas fibro-osseous union requires a more aggressive surgical approach. Beware, however, of extracapsular ankylosis caused by fusion of the coronoid to the zygoma (usually following zygomatic fractures) or fusion of the lateral pterygoid plate to the ramus of the mandible (occasionally following Le Fort III fractures), as these conditions require alternative methods for correction.

2. Ankylosis in the child is a serious problem, as the jaw will not develop normally and a significant facial deformity can result. Early diagnosis and treatment are important to minimize these effects. Rib grafting, with its potential for growth, is a preferred method of reconstruction.

3. Occasionally ankylosis is associated with infection of the mandible, infratemporal space, and external auditory canal. If this occurs, the infection must be brought under control before planning reconstructive surgery. Intravenous antibiotics must be administered, foreign bodies removed, and the area adequately debrided and drained. Reconstructive surgery should not be started until all signs of infection have been absent for several months.

4. Dental rehabilitation is an important part of the treatment process. As soon as the intermaxillary fixation is removed, an active exercise program should be begun. Occasionally these maneuvers must be combined with steroid injections to obtain relaxation of the adjoining tissues.

COMPLICATIONS

1. Bleeding from branches of the internal maxillary artery can be troublesome during the surgical procedure. To avoid this intraoperative complication,

RECONSTRUCTION AFTER ANKYLOSIS USING RIB GRAFT

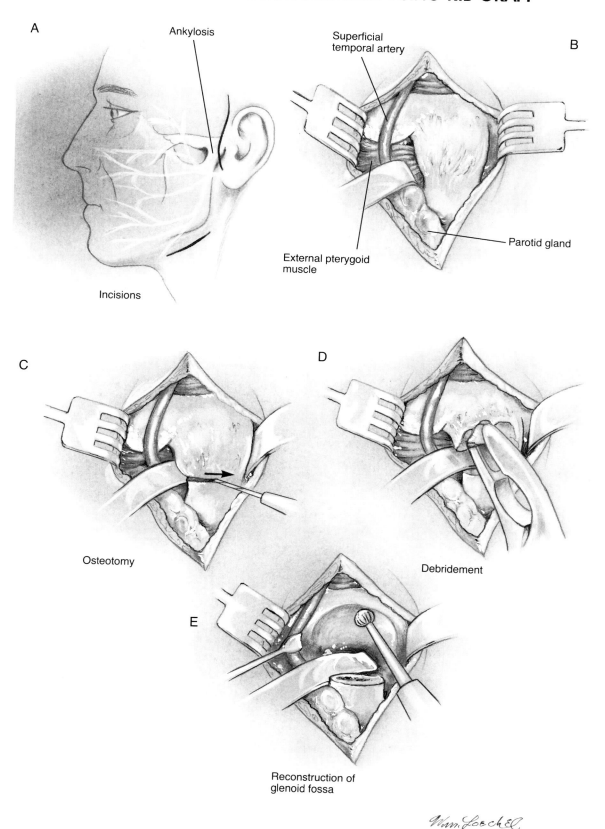

A

Ankylosis

Incisions

B

Superficial
temporal artery

Parotid gland

External pterygoid
muscle

C

Osteotomy

D

Debridement

E

Reconstruction of
glenoid fossa

Wm. Loechel

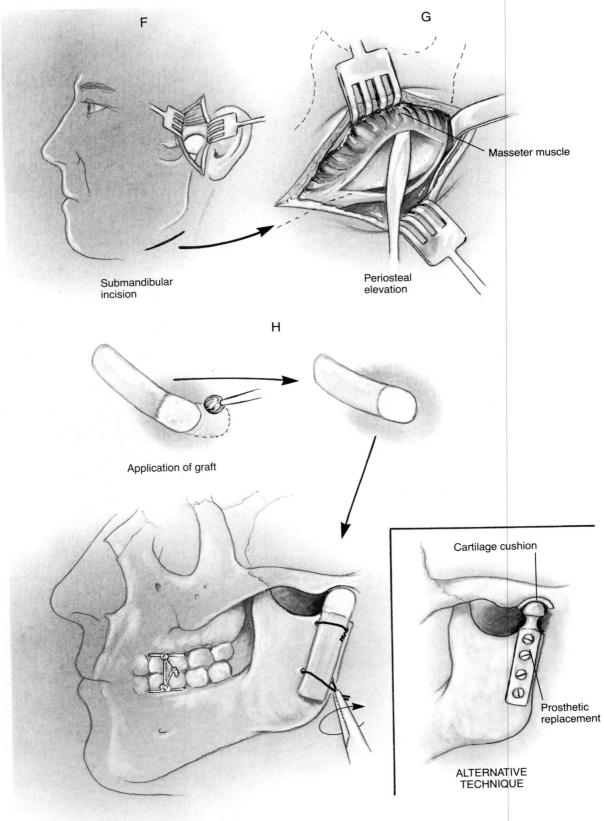

F

Submandibular
incision

G

Masseter muscle

Periosteal
elevation

H

Application of graft

Cartilage cushion

Prosthetic
replacement

ALTERNATIVE
TECHNIQUE

Wm. Loechel

the dissection should be close to the surface of the bone and carried out with blunt elevation and spreading clamp techniques. The deep tissues should be protected with a malleable retractor.

2. The seventh nerve root or one or several of its branches can be injured. This complication can be avoided by keeping the dissection close to the surface of the mandible. Also, retractors should be used judiciously on the soft tissues that cover the parotid and facial nerve area. Cauterization of the vessels should be avoided and bleeders clamped and tied. Any injury to the nerve should be recognized immediately and the condition of this injury determined by appropriate electrodiagnostic tests. If there are indications of anatomic interruption of the nerve, exploration and repair should be performed immediately (see Chapter 107).

3. Reankylosis is possible and can occur from infection, failure to remove bone spicules from the operative site, inadequate bone removal, or loss of grafts. Early function is encouraged to prevent the development of fusion at the temporomandibular joint. Steroid injections may help in the treatment of contracting scar tissues.

ALTERNATIVE TECHNIQUE OF PROSTHETIC REPLACEMENT

Following condylectomy, the condyle can be reconstructed with alloplastic materials. Many types of prostheses are available, but experience is limited, and follow-up data are not necessarily available. The advantages of the condylar prosthesis are its relative ease of insertion and avoidance of a donor site. On the other hand, there is a risk of infection and loosening and displacement of the implant.

The prosthesis is placed through the same exposure as that used in positioning the rib graft. The prosthesis should never be applied to a ''bare'' glenoid fossa, unless there is healthy intervening soft tissue. A cartilage cushion should be considered. The ramus is then grooved to receive the shank of the prosthesis, and to secure the implant, three or four screws are placed through the inner and outer cortices of the ramus. The periosteum is closed over the prosthesis with 2–0 chromic sutures, and the wound is closed in layers. Intravenous antibiotics are used for 5 days and oral antibiotics for at least 2 weeks following the procedure. Rehabilitation is similar to that discussed for the rib graft.

part three

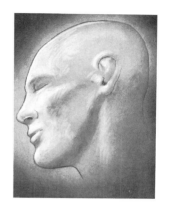

Maxillary Fractures

section I

Classification and Pathophysiology of Maxillary Fractures

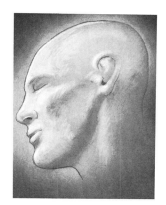

chapter 30

General Considerations

Maxillary fractures account for approximately 10% to 20% of all facial fractures. These midfacial injuries can be isolated or can occur in combination with fractures of adjacent structures such as the mandible, nasofrontoethmoid complex, orbit, or zygoma.

Many maxillary fractures are the result of violent blunt force to the facial skeleton. The displacement of the fracture will depend upon the degree and direction, and point of impact of the external force. Muscles that insert into the facial skeleton are believed to play only a minor role in the final position of the fragments.

A–D If the impact occurs primarily at the nasal bridge, the maxilla will be displaced downward along the sloping base of the skull, resulting in a lengthening of the face, retrognathia, and an open bite deformity. The maxilla may become impacted or hang loosely, floating from the cranium. Lateral blows to the facial skeleton can cause a lateral displacement associated with a crossbite dysfunction. Forces directed to the lower front of the midface can

produce a pyramidal fracture involving just the anterior maxilla and nasoethmoid complex. This same type of fracture can also occur in patients receiving a blow from beneath the chin, in which case the maxilla is often shortened and the fracture associated with zygomatic and hemipalatal fractures.

E–G Other forces to the maxilla can cause different types of injuries. Blows directed anteroposteriorly to the upper alveolus (or lower portion of the maxilla) can also separate the premaxilla and the alveolus from the nose and floor of the maxillary sinus. Limited sharp blows, usually from small objects, can produce isolated segmental fractures.

H For the most part, maxillary fractures are complex and difficult to define. A traditional classification, originally described by Le Fort, is useful, and most fractures fall into one of the Le Fort types. According to this system, a Le Fort III fracture (or craniofacial dysjunction) starts at the nasofrontal suture line and extends along the medial wall and floor of the orbit to pass through the inferior orbital fissure, lateral orbital wall, and zygomaticofrontal suture. The fracture line extends across the temporal surface of the zygoma and zygomatic arch, while a branch continues across the maxilla to separate the pterygoid plates from the basisphenoid. The Le Fort II (or pyramidal) fracture starts out at about the same level as a Le Fort III injury but passes more anteriorly to involve the lacrimal bones, the inferior orbital rim, and the anterolateral wall of the maxilla. The pterygoid plates may or may not be fractured. The Le Fort I fracture (Guerin type) crosses the nasal septum, the lower portion of the piriform apertures, the canine fossae, and the zygomaticomaxillary buttresses. The fracture then passes above the maxillary tuberosity to separate the maxilla from the pterygoid plates or, alternatively, to disrupt the lower from the upper two thirds of the plates. In most Le Fort fractures, the bony and cartilaginous portions of the nasal septum are also injured.

Other variations of the maxillary fracture are the medial maxillary, the split palate, and the segmental (partial maxillary or alveolar) fracture. These can occur alone or in combination with other midfacial injuries. The medial maxillary fractures commonly present with a skeletal depression between the nose and maxilla. A split palate often occurs with Le Fort II or III fractures or with fractures involving the malar bone. Alveolar or segmental maxillary fractures commonly are associated with Le Fort I fractures.

There can also be many combinations of injury. Le Fort I, II, and III fractures can occur on one side of the face (hemi–Le Fort), or there can be mixed fractures in which there are different fracture patterns appearing on opposite sides. Le Fort fractures can also be combined with medial maxillary, split palate, and segmental injuries.

The most important clinical aspect of the Le Fort classification is that these fractures involve buttresses and pillars that maintain the height, width, and projection of the face. The main vertical supports are paired and are called *nasomaxillary*, *zygomaticomaxillary*, and *pterygomaxillary* buttresses. There is also an unpaired frontoethmoid-vomerine buttress. The medially positioned nasomaxillary buttress extends upward along the frontal process of the maxilla (nasofrontal section of buttress) to attach to the base of the skull. The lateral zygomaticomaxillary buttress has two cranially directed components (zygomaticofrontal and zygomaticotemporal) that extend along the frontal and temporal processes of the zygomatic bone. The posterior pterygomaxillary buttress essentially attaches the maxilla to the pterygoid plates and the sphenoid bone. The median frontoethmoid-vomerine buttress connects the frontal bone to the surface of the palate.

There are also two main horizontal buttresses. One has two components, the superior and inferior orbital rims, and extends laterally across the zygomatic arch. The other traverses the maxillary alveolus to stabilize the palate and upper dental arch.

The goals in treatment of maxillary fractures are to (1) secure pretraumatic occlusion and (2) stabilize one of several buttresses that will restore the three dimensions of the face. In general, mandibular fractures occurring with the maxillary fracture should be treated first. The Le Fort III fracture should be stabilized at the zygomaticofrontal extension of the zygomaticomaxillary buttress and/or at the nasofrontal extension of the nasomaxillary buttress. The Le Fort II fracture needs fixation across the nasomaxillary, zygomaticomaxillary, and/or horizontal buttresses of the orbital rims. The Le Fort I fracture requires some type of stabilization across the lower part of the zygomaticomaxillary buttress and/or nasomaxillary buttress.

Treatment in children must be modified to account for more rapid healing and remodeling of the facial skeleton. The usual approach is conservative, and intermaxillary fixation with Ivy loops is often satisfactory. Fabrication of palatal splints with suspension can also be considered. For the high maxillary fractures, management generally parallels that in adults.

MAXILLARY FRACTURES

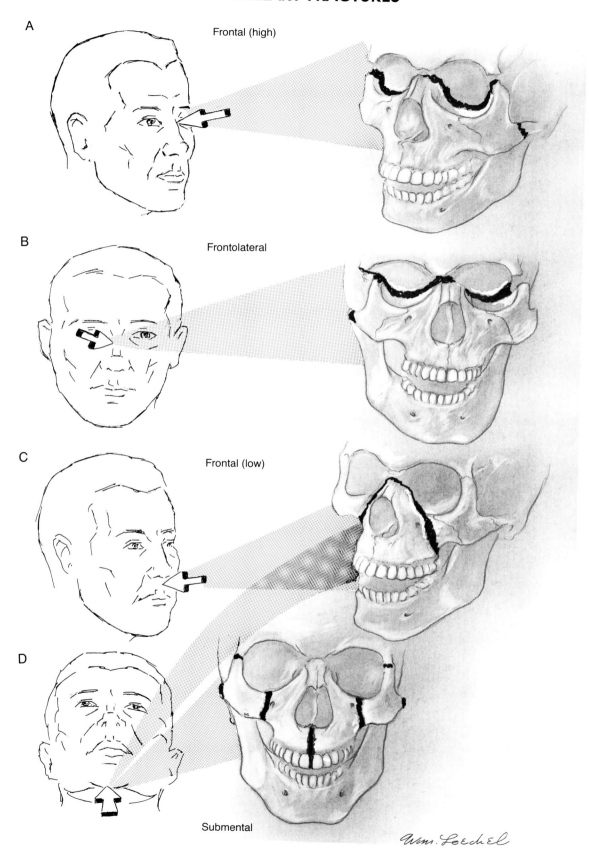

A   Frontal (high)

B   Frontolateral

C   Frontal (low)

D

Submental

Wm. Loechel

MAXILLARY FRACTURES *(Continued)*

E   Frontoalveolar

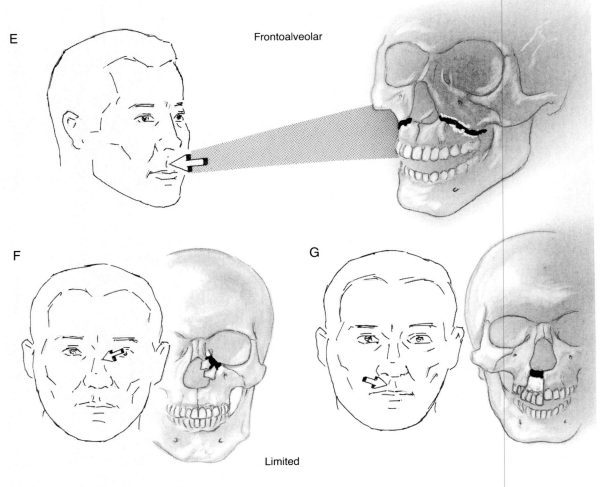

F   G

Limited

H   LE FORT CLASSIFICATION AND MAJOR BUTTRESSES

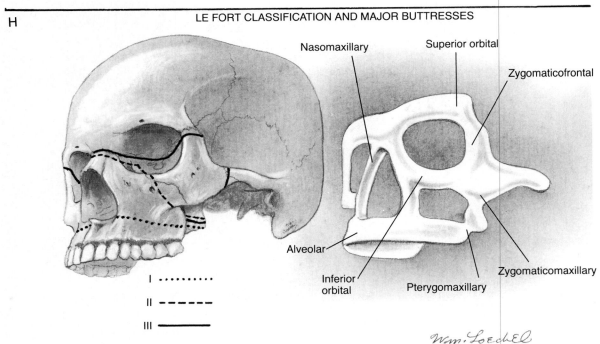

Nasomaxillary · Superior orbital · Zygomaticofrontal · Alveolar · Inferior orbital · Pterygomaxillary · Zygomaticomaxillary

I ··········
II ------
III ——

Wm. Loechel

section II

Le Fort I Fractures

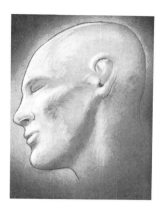

chapter 31

Repair of Maxillary Segmental Fractures

INDICATIONS

Sharp objects striking the midface can cause abrasions, lacerations, or partial avulsions involving the cheeks, lips, or adjacent gum tissues. Sufficient force, however, will also result in punched-out segmental fractures involving the dentition, alveolus, and lower portion of the maxilla.

Segmental fractures in patients with teeth generally can be reduced with digital pressure and stabilized with either a single arch bar or upper and lower arch bars and intermaxillary fixation. In the edentulous patient, dentures (or splints) suspended from stable portions of the skeleton can be fitted with arch bars, which are then secured to each other with wires or elastic bands (see Chapter 33). In some edentulous patients, direct interosseous wiring or plating may be a more expedient form of management.

PROCEDURE

Most segmental fractures can be treated with local anesthesia and sedation. If a general anesthetic is to be employed, nasotracheal intubation is preferred, as this will provide an opportunity to reduce and stabilize the fracture and immediately check for appropriate occlusal relationships.

To help control hemostasis and provide local anesthesia, the area of fracture is first infiltrated with 1% lidocaine containing 1:100,000 epinephrine. The fracture can then be simply reduced with digital pressure. If lacerations are present, the surgeon should use them to evaluate the adequacy of the reduction and then close the wounds with a 3–0 chromic sutures. Teeth should always be inspected, and any injuries to the crown portion should be treated accordingly (see Chapter 22). Loose or extirpated teeth should be repositioned and wired to an arch bar, which is subsequently stabilized by the adjacent uninvolved dentition.

Arch bar placement is described in Chapter 8. Wiring of the incisors may be necessary to obtain optimal stability. The surgeon should start with the upper arch, and if the fragments can be held with a rigid bar (i.e., Jelenko), then one arch bar will suffice for the fixation. However, if the fragments tend to move, additional rigidity using a lower arch bar and intermaxillary fixation should be employed.

Postoperatively the patient is treated with prophylactic antibiotics (i.e., penicillin or erythromycin) and chlorhexidine mouthwashes. The teeth should be

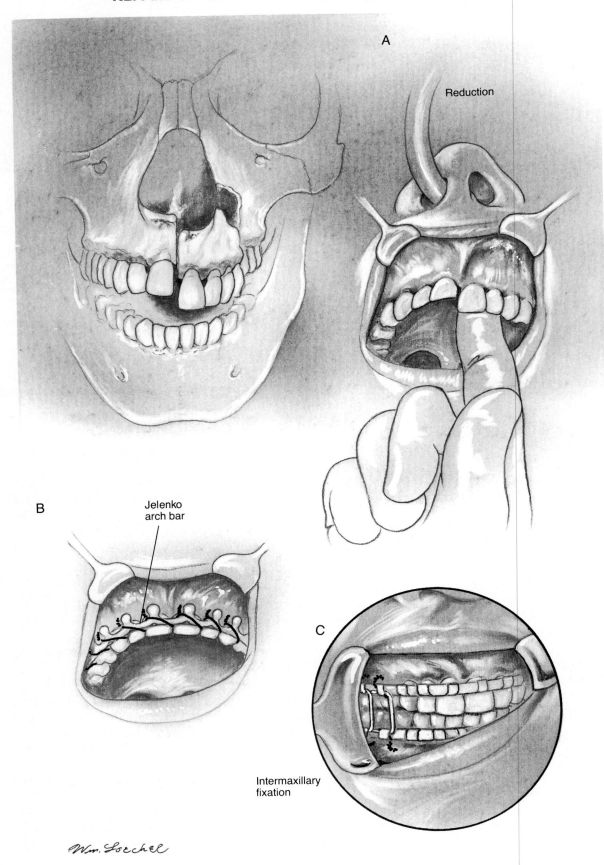

A

Reduction

B

Jelenko
arch bar

C

Intermaxillary
fixation

Wm. Loechel

gently brushed or treated with a water irrigation device daily. Most fractures will heal in 4 to 6 weeks, and at that time, the arch bars can be removed. Radiographic evaluation may be helpful, and the patient should be checked for several months thereafter to assure adequacy of healing.

PITFALLS

1. Fixation of segmental fractures often requires a stepwise approach. First, horizontal wiring of the teeth should be attempted. If this does not stabilize the fracture, the surgeon should proceed to arch bar fixation. Alternatively, orthodontic brackets can be applied (see Chapter 22). If instability is still present, intermaxillary fixation should be employed.

2. Careful evaluation of the teeth is important if permanent damage is to be avoided and infection of the alveolar fragments prevented. When there is concern regarding dental injury, dentistry consultation should be obtained.

COMPLICATIONS

1. The segmental fragment can become nonviable if its blood supply is severely compromised and/or infection develops in the area of fracture. This complication can be avoided by applying atraumatic techniques to the soft tissues and by ensuring accurate reduction and fixation. Additionally, the surgeon must be certain that the teeth are viable and will not act as portals of infection or as foreign bodies.

2. If malaligned segments have healed and are causing no deformity or difficulty, then no treatment is necessary. However, if malalignment is affecting appearance or masticatory function, then the complication must be treated. What option to choose will be dictated by the degree and extent of displacement and the need for natural dentition. Orthodontia and/or orthognathic surgery may have to be considered (see Chapter 42).

chapter 32

Reduction of Le Fort I Fracture With Disimpaction Forceps and Miniplate Fixation
Alternative Technique Using Intermaxillary Fixation

INDICATIONS

Le Fort I fractures are characterized by a retrodisplacement of the lower portion of the maxilla. Frequently the bone fragments are impacted, and there is premature contact of the molars with an open bite deformity. The maxilla may be shortened or lengthened. The patient may also present with epistaxis, ecchymoses along the gingivobuccal sulcus, and tenderness and crepitus along the fracture line.

The objectives of treatment are threefold: (1) to restore centric occlusion, (2) to reduce and stabilize the palatal segment to the closest rigid maxillary segment, and (3) to replace any septal dislocations. The classic fracture often requires a forceful reduction before the fragments can be manipulated into pretraumatic occlusal relationships. The method of fixation used depends on the postreduction stability of the fracture and the status of the dentition. If the fracture appears reduced and ''seems to fit,'' intermaxillary fixation with either arch bars or Ivy loops alone can be utilized. If instability is still present or the surgeon prefers not to use intermaxillary fixation, then miniplates can be applied along the medial and/or lateral buttresses. For those Le Fort I fractures associated with higher Le Fort injuries, additional miniplate fixation is the procedure of choice.

Other associated conditions will dictate alternative approaches. If the patient has comminuted fractures and is edentulous, the surgeon can simply treat with application of dentures, suspension wires, and intermaxillary fixation (see Chapter 33). In patients with associated alveolar segmental fractures, an arch bar with or without intermaxillary fixation should be considered (see Chapter 31). With a split palate fracture, the surgeon can use a special rigid arch bar (Jelenko) that is placed across the lower transverse buttress (see Chapters 31 and 40).

PROCEDURE

Reduction of Le Fort I Fracture

A General anesthesia is usually obtained with nasotracheal intubation or a tracheostomy. The surgeon should then reduce the maxillary fracture with digital pressure or with judicious traction of a tongue retractor or a bone hook behind the palate. If these techniques are not successful, a forceps reduction should be applied.

B The Rowe disimpaction forceps is designed to grasp and rock the lower maxilla symmetrically and to bring it forward. The right- and left-handed forceps have handles that are offset from each other. The straight blade of the forceps is first inserted into the floor of the nose; the curved portion, with its flat end, then fits around the alveolus and hard palate. Standing at the head of the patient, the surgeon grasps the forceps and applies constant pressure in a posterior-to-anterior direction. The forceps are simultaneously squeezed and rotated vertically and then horizontally to free and mobilize the segment. The maxillary fracture, when loosened, can then be molded back into a normal position. The patient's nose will bleed profusely during the reduction, but bleeding should stop in approximately 5 minutes.

Miniplate Fixation

C Several strategically placed Ivy loops should be used to secure adequate occlusal relationships. If the fracture extends to areas near the maxillary sinus ostea, the surgeon should consider an intranasal antrostomy to better aerate the sinuses in the postoperative period. This small opening can be made by incising the caudal end of the inferior turbinate,

DISIMPACTION TECHNIQUES

Le Fort I fracture

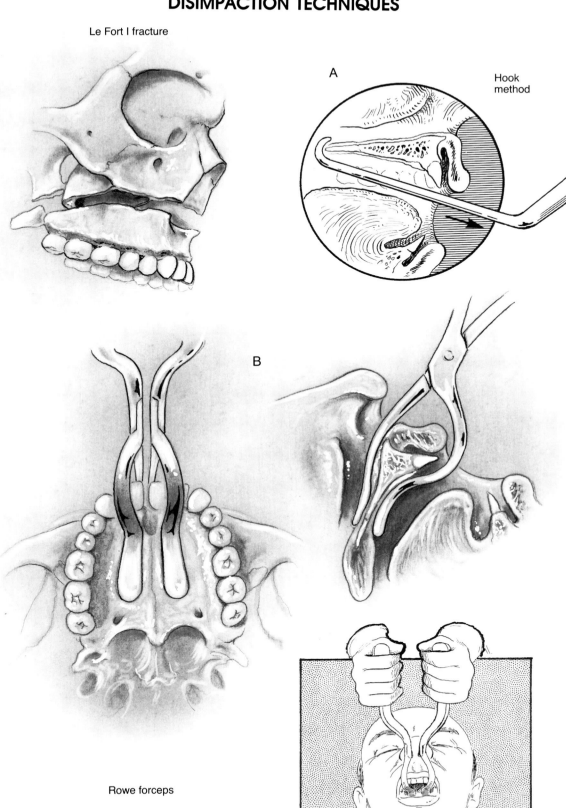

A

Hook method

B

Rowe forceps

Wm. Loechel

infracturing the turbinate, and then, with a Kelly clamp, puncturing through the inferior meatus. The opening is enlarged with Kerrison rongeurs. Preferably the antrostomy should be taken down to the floor of the nose so that there will be a continuity between the nose and antrum. A hole about the size of a dime is desirable. The inferior turbinate is then pushed back into a normal position.

D,E Exposure for application of plates is best achieved through a gingivolabial sulcus incision about 5 to 7 mm above the gingival margin from molar to molar region. The periosteum is elevated along the anterior wall of the maxilla, exposing the zygomaticomaxillary buttresses, canine fossae, nasomaxillary buttresses, piriform apertures, and anterior nasal spine. Care must be taken not to injure the infraorbital nerve and to keep as many fragments as possible attached to their periosteum.

Usually one plate across the zygomaticomaxillary or nasomaxillary buttress provides adequate fixation. The buttress should be stripped of periosteum to expose the area to receive the plate. The fragments should fit together, and any depressed fragments should be elevated into appropriate position.

F,G Compression or noncompression plates can be used to fit the area of fracture; this can be facilitated with a malleable template. A rigid plate is then selected so that there are at least two holes on each side of the fracture, and with the template as a guide, the rigid plate is bent to an appropriate fit. Holes through the buttress should then be drilled with a drill diameter that is slightly less than the screw diameter.

H,I Drill holes should be measured and screws selected that will penetrate just beyond the bone. Self-tapping screws are then applied to the holes on each side of the fracture and subsequently to the outer holes for additional support. If the maxilla is still unstable, another plate should be applied to the contralateral side. The incision is closed with interrupted 4–0 chromic sutures.

Postoperatively the patient is maintained for 5 days on penicillin (or erythromycin). As soon as optimal occlusion is ensured, the intermaxillary fixation can be removed and the bite checked for dynamic relationships. Postoperative radiographs should be obtained to confirm the adequacy of reduction and aeration of the sinuses. Clinical evaluation should be continued for at least 6 months to follow adequacy of treatment.

PITFALLS

1. Reduction of the fracture is probably the most important part of the procedure. Remember that plates are "unforgiving," and the patient will heal in the position in which the maxilla is fixed.

2. Beware of associated alveolar and palatal fractures, as these conditions will complicate the repair. Often the alveolar injury can be stabilized with an arch bar (see Chapter 31). Palatal splits require a plate across the premaxilla and/or placement of a heavy (Jelenko) arch bar (see Chapter 40).

3. The edentulous patient should be treated with the same concern for adequate reduction and immobilization given to the patient with teeth. Although the physician has the option of plate and/or wire fixation, there is also the traditional technique of using dentures with circumzygomatic suspension and intermaxillary fixation (see Chapter 33). The suspension method, however, can shorten the maxilla, and the surgeon must be careful not to overtighten the drop wires.

4. Occasionally reduction alone of a low maxillary fracture will bring about satisfactory stability. If such a situation develops, it is probably more prudent to place the patient into a short period of intermaxillary fixation and forego an open method.

5. Comminuted fractures of the lower midface can present formidable problems. If the bone fragments are displaced into the adjacent soft tissues, the surgeon should find these fragments and replace them into anatomic position. Stabilization can often be achieved with plate fixation and/or interosseous wiring. Sufficient portions of buttress are usually available, and bone grafting techniques should not be necessary.

6. Because the plate has the potential to be palpable or exposed, use only the minimum number of plates required to obtain fixation. Also, avoid plates that are too long, as these will often project beyond the alveolar ridge.

7. Make sure that screw placement does not affect the viability of tooth roots. If there is insufficient room between the plate and the tooth root, the surgeon should then consider interosseous wire fixation. A rule of thumb is that the screw should be placed no closer than the distance described by two times the height of the crown.

8. Treatment in children should be conservative. Remodeling of the maxilla can be expected, and the upper and lower jaws often will adapt to the occlusal plane. Intermaxillary fixation with Ivy loops or arch bars can be used in the mixed dentition; in the younger child, acrylic splints can be fit and secured to the piriform aperture and/or zygomatic arch.

COMPLICATIONS

1. Malunion of the maxilla from a Le Fort I fracture is a complication that can affect appearance and/or

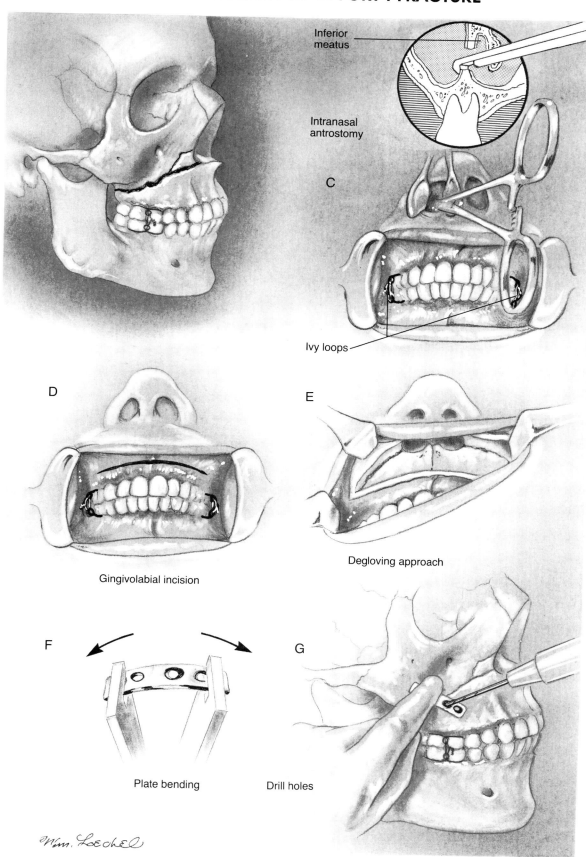

Inferior meatus

Intranasal antrostomy

C

Ivy loops

D

Gingivolabial incision

E

Degloving approach

F

Plate bending

G

Drill holes

Wm. Loechel

function. Generally the patient presents with a retrusion of the upper lip and columella. There is often an open bite and crossbite malocclusion. This problem can be avoided by accurate reduction and appropriate methods of fixation. If retrusion should develop in the early postoperative period, reduction should again be carried out and another method of fixation applied. At a later time, osteotomy and rigid plate fixation with or without bone grafts (see Chapter 42) must be considered. For those patients with minimal deformity and/or dysfunction, treatment may not be necessary.

2. Nonunion of the maxilla is extremely rare. Such a condition can develop from inaccurate reduction and/or poor fixation, but usually there is a history of infection or repeated trauma. The infection should be controlled with debridement and antibiotics. Loss of bone between fragments requires interposition bone grafts.

3. Sinusitis can also develop following midfacial trauma. This can often be avoided by an intranasal antrostomy and prophylactic antibiotic coverage. If the patient complains of pain and swelling of the face, then he or she should be evaluated radiographically. If sinusitis is present, appropriate antibiotics and drainage procedures should be administered.

ALTERNATIVE TECHNIQUE OF INTERMAXILLARY FIXATION WITH INTEROSSEOUS WIRES

a—c Intermaxillary fixation with either arch bars or Ivy loops is a proven method of treating low maxillary fractures. The technique is useful when reduction is not accurate or when the fracture is so minimal that the physician chooses to avoid an open method. The main disadvantage of intermaxillary fixation is that the patient cannot open his or her mouth, and nutrition and speech can be adversely affected for the duration of fixation. For those patients in whom instability is still present, plates (as described previously) or interosseous wires can be applied.

The method requires first the application of intermaxillary fixation with arch bars or Ivy loops (see Chapter 8). If the surgeon then decides that additional fixation is desirable, loose or malpositioned maxillary fragments are exposed through an incision of the gingivolabial sulcus. Elevation of the periosteum should be limited and displaced bone fragments reduced and placed into optimal position. The wiring should start at the most stable portion of the facial skeleton, working inferiorly until the buttress and alveolus are stabilized. Drill holes are made with a minidriver and a 0.035-inch K wire as a drill bit. A 28-gauge stainless steel wire is passed through the unstable fragment; a 30-gauge wire loop method is then used to pass the 28-gauge wire through the stable portion of the fracture. A 28-gauge wire is twisted down to hold the fragments in reduced position. The wound is closed with 4–0 chromic sutures, and prophylactic antibiotics (penicillin or erythromycin) are administered. The patient should be kept in fixation for approximately 4 to 6 weeks. Stability is determined at that time, and if it is adequate, the arch bars are removed. Postoperative radiographs are helpful in evaluating the reduction and aeration of the sinuses.

MINIPLATE FIXATION OF LE FORT I FRACTURE *(Continued)*

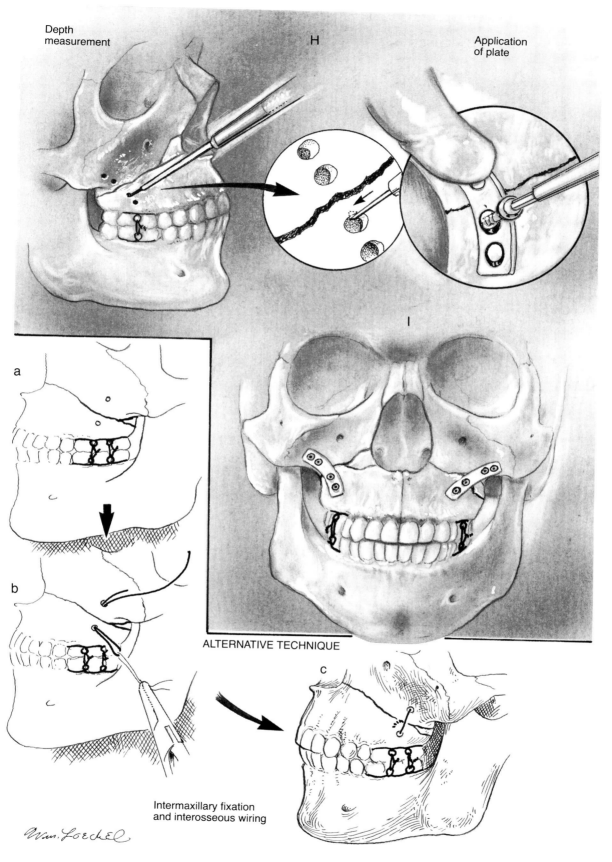

Depth measurement

H

Application of plate

I

a

b

ALTERNATIVE TECHNIQUE

c

Intermaxillary fixation and interosseous wiring

Repair of the Edentulous Le Fort I Fracture With Circummandibular and Circumzygomatic Denture Fixation

INDICATIONS

The edentulous patient, in contrast to the patient with teeth, will require special techniques for reduction and fixation of the Le Fort I fracture. The patient's denture provides an excellent opportunity to set the occlusion to the fit of the dentures and maintain the jaws in natural occlusion during the healing period. Miniplates (see Chapter 32) should be avoided, especially when the fracture involves comminution of the alveolus and when the plate will project over the edge of the gum line.

PROCEDURE

General anesthesia should be provided by way of a nasotracheal or tracheostomy tube. The surgeon should be able to open the mouth with freedom to attach and adjust the dentures.

Using digital pressure or traction from a bone hook behind the palate, the maxilla is reduced into anatomic position. If more force is necessary to achieve reduction, the surgeon should apply a Rowe disimpaction forceps (Chapter 32). The jaws are then placed so that the upper dental arch lies in correct relationship with the dental arch of the mandible.

A–D If necessary, the dentures should be repaired with acrylic cement (see Chapter 9). Arch bars or loops are attached to the dentures with cement or wires, and holes are drilled through the dentures for application of circummandibular, circumzygomatic and piriform aperture attachments. A soft lining is applied to those areas in which the denture will be in contact with injured soft tissues.

E,F The application of dentures is identical to that described in Chapter 9. However, care must be taken not to overtighten the wires, or the maxilla will be compressed and shortened. Drop wires from the zygomatic arch should be as vertical as possible. If there is still a rocking of the denture, an additional wire can be passed from the anterior nasal spine or piriform aperture to the midline of the denture. Intermaxillary fixation can be achieved with loops of 28-gauge wire or elastic bands.

Prophylactic antibiotics (penicillin or erythromycin) are desirable, and oral hygiene should be maintained postoperatively with chlorhexidine rinses. The tightness and position of the dentures and occlusal relationships should be checked daily, and adjustments should be made to correct traction from the vertical suspension wires. The patient should be started on liquids and advanced to a puréed diet. The period of fixation will vary from 4 to 8 weeks. Postoperative radiographs are helpful in evaluating the adequacy of reduction and aeration of the sinuses. The patient should be followed every 2 weeks during the first month and then monthly until the fracture has healed properly.

PITFALLS

1. Avoid loose-fitting dentures, as these will tend to cause erosion of the mucosa and displacement of the upper arch. The denture can usually be made to fit better by judicious application of a soft liner and periodic readjustment of the traction exerted by the circummandibular, circumzygomatic, and piriform aperture wires.

2. Do not overtighten the suspension wires, as too much traction can cause a shortening of the maxilla. The suspension wires will loosen as swelling of the soft tissue disappears, and the surgeon should be prepared to tighten the 28-gauge wire loop between the suspension wire and denture. The loop also serves conveniently as a safety factor, as overtightening will often break the loop before the maxilla is driven into the upper portion of the facial skeleton.

DENTURE FIXATION OF LE FORT I FRACTURE

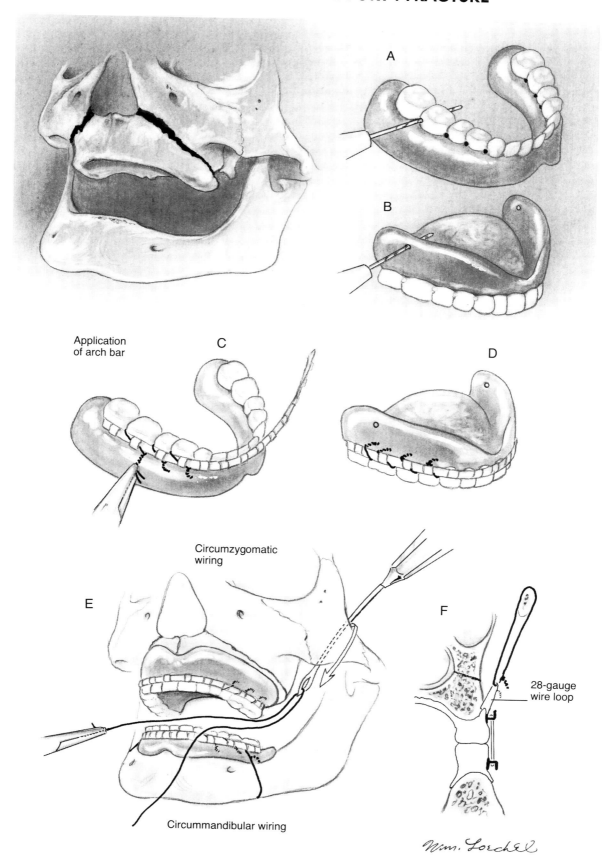

A

B

Application
of arch bar

C

D

Circumzygomatic
wiring

E

F

28-gauge
wire loop

Circummandibular wiring

COMPLICATIONS

1. Malunion, nonunion, and sinusitis are rare complications. These sequelae and methods of management are discussed in Chapter 32.

2. Specific to fixation with dentures is the potential problem of erosion of the mucosa beneath the denture and the possibility of osteomyelitis. This complication can usually be avoided by careful closure of lacerations and reduction of the bone fragments so that they do not cut through the mucosa. The surgeon must also avoid a loose-fitting denture, which tends to move and cause repeated trauma to the area. If an infection should develop, the dentures should be removed and the underlying soft tissues treated with local and parenteral antibiotics.

section III

Le Fort II Fractures

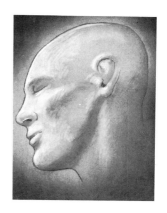

chapter 34

Noncompression Miniplate Fixation of Le Fort II Fractures
Alternative Technique Using Parietal Cortex Grafts

INDICATIONS

The pure Le Fort II injury is characterized by fracture of the nasal bones, the orbital rim (or rims), and the anterolateral walls of the maxilla. The maxilla is usually pushed backward and downward, causing a lengthened scaphoid deformity of the face. Premature contact of the molar teeth causes an open bite malocclusion. Fractures extending into the nasoethmoid complex can be associated with anosmia, cerebrospinal fluid leaks, and loss of consciousness.

An understanding of fracture lines and buttresses is essential to the planning and repair. Usually the Le Fort II fracture will pass high along the nasomaxillary (frontal) buttresses, through the horizontal buttresses of the infraorbital rim, and low across the zygomaticomaxillary buttresses. The degloving approach provides an excellent opportunity to evaluate and accomplish the repair. Stabilization of one or several zygomaticomaxillary buttresses will usually provide sufficient fixation to allow healing to take place, but if instability is present, additional fixation across the nasofrontal processes and/or the inferior orbital rims must be considered.

Rigid miniplate fixation is an unforgiving method and should not be employed unless there is complete reduction of the fracture and a return to pretraumatic occlusion. The plates should always be applied to areas of naturally thickened bone. Acute bone grafting is necessary only in rare instances in which the fragments are lost. Suspension techniques (see Chapter 33) generally are to be avoided, because they are inaccurate and can cause compression of the midfacial fragments.

PROCEDURE

General anesthesia is desirable and is preferably administered through a tracheostomy. Nasotracheal intubation makes it difficult to reduce the nasal fractures, and orotracheal intubation interferes with occlusal relationships.

The nose should be anesthetized with 4% cocaine

containing epinephrine, and the nose and gingivolabial sulcus should be blocked with 1% lidocaine containing 1:100,000 epinephrine (see Chapter 46). Usually the face and neck are prepared and draped as sterile fields.

The first portion of the procedure requires an application of arch bars and/or Ivy loops. The methods are described in Chapter 8. Generally, Ivy loops can be applied, but when many teeth are missing or loose, arch bars are indicated.

A,B To expose the lower maxillary fractures, an incision should be made in the gingivolabial sulcus, about 5 mm above the gingiva, from molar to molar region. The incision should be carried through the periosteum, and the periosteum should be elevated off the alveolus superiorly to expose the zygomaticomaxillary buttresses, canine fossae, and piriform apertures. A through-and-through septal-columella incision will facilitate the degloving and provide improved exposure to elevate the periosteum off the lateral walls of the piriform apertures. The surgeon can then also expose the infraorbital nerve and the frontal process of the maxilla.

C With the fracture lines visualized, the maxilla is reduced with digital or hook traction or with a Rowe disimpaction forceps (see Chapter 32). The lower maxillary fragments should be loosened and placed into an accurate position in relationship to the more stable upper portions. The nasal fractures, if present, are reduced at this time (see Chapter 46). Intermaxillary fixation is then applied with fine loops of 28-gauge wire or elastic bands.

D,E Once assured that reduction and occlusion are accurate, plates are applied. Noncompression plates with self-tapping screws are desirable. The plates should be contoured to the buttresses and secured with at least two holes placed over the more stable portions of bone. The initial drill holes are made close to the fracture with a drill bit just smaller than the diameter of the screws. The drilling should be irrigated copiously to prevent heat damage. Hole depths are then measured, and a screw slightly larger than the screw hole is selected and secured to the plate. Other holes are drilled and screws applied to give additional strength. Small fragments of buttress can be skewered with one or two screws. All fragments, however, should be elevated and reduced so that they are stable and in contact with the plate.

The zygomaticomaxillary buttresses are ideal places to achieve fixation, but if the maxilla is not stable, additional plates or wires must be applied to other buttresses. For the Le Fort II fracture, the surgeon has the option of exposing the inferior orbital rim through an infraciliary incision or the nasofrontal

process through a medial canthal incision and securing the fragments with interosseous wires. If the fracture line extends near the ostea of the maxillary sinuses, an intranasal antrostomy should be performed (see Chapter 32).

The mucosal incision is closed with interrupted 3–0 chromic sutures. The nose is packed for 24 to 48 hours with gauze or tampons treated with bacitracin ointment. The patient is given prophylactic antibiotics for 5 days. Intermaxillary fixation can be removed in 24 to 48 hours or, alternatively, it can be maintained for a variable period of time. Postoperative radiographs should be obtained to verify adequate reduction and aeration of the sinuses. Healing should be evaluated weekly for 4 to 6 weeks and then monthly for at least 6 months.

PITFALLS

1. Achieving an accurate reduction and ensuring pretraumatic occlusion are prerequisites for miniplate fixation. Rigid plates are unforgiving, and once they are applied, it is difficult, if not impossible, to change the relationship of the bone fragments.

2. Screws should be applied only through the thicker vertical and/or horizontal buttresses. The length of the screws should be controlled so that they do not penetrate the sinus and act as foreign bodies.

3. Avoid placing screws near or through the roots of teeth. This complication can be avoided by using L, T, or curved plates. If there is no room for the plate and screw, interosseous wires should be considered.

4. Additional stabilization of the Le Fort II fracture may be required at the infraorbital rim and/or nasofrontal processes. Although plates can be used, in thin-skinned individuals they will often be palpable and seen through the skin. In such situations, we prefer interosseous wires. The techniques are similar to those used for repair of nasal fractures (see Chapter 48) or malar fractures (see Chapter 52).

5. Le Fort II fractures rarely occur alone, and the surgeon must be prepared to reduce and fix other fractures associated with the injury. If the nose is fractured, the nasal fracture is reduced and treated as described in Chapter 46. Malar, orbital, and alveolar fractures must also be treated with appropriate techniques. Mandible fractures can complicate occlusal relationships and for this reason should probably be repaired before the reduction and fixation of the maxillary fracture.

6. Occasionally the midface is so comminuted that there are few, if any, bones of sufficient size to hold the plate, or the fragments of bone are so scattered

MINIPLATE FIXATION OF LE FORT II FRACTURE

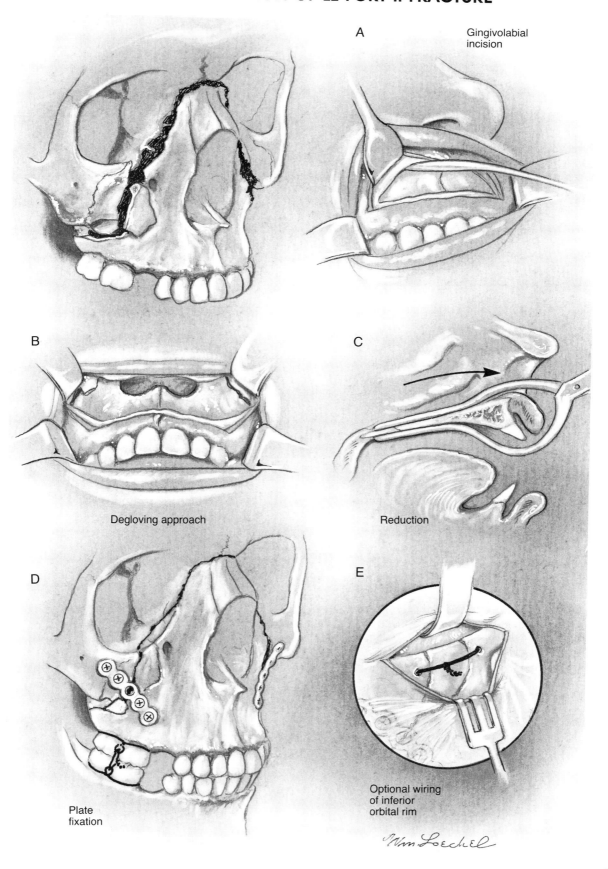

A — Gingivolabial incision

B — Degloving approach

C — Reduction

D — Plate fixation

E — Optional wiring of inferior orbital rim

Wm Loechel

163

that they are not readily available. In such a situation, the surgeon should consider harvesting a split parietal cranial bone graft and applying this graft across the remnants of the zygomaticomaxillary and nasomaxillary buttresses. Wires or plates can be used to hold the grafts in place (see later).

COMPLICATIONS

1. Malocclusion can occur following miniplate fixation, especially if the plates are applied when there is an imperfect reduction. To avoid this complication, the fractures should be aligned in exact interdigitation; the maxillary fragments must fit like a puzzle. The plates should be bent and applied in such a way that tightening of the screws does not distract the fragments. However, if malocclusion develops, the surgeon has the option of orthodontia, extraction of involved teeth, and/or osteotomies with refixation of the fragments (see Chapter 43).

2. Facial deformity associated with malunion of the maxilla is unlikely, especially if the reduction and occlusion are accurate. Also, plate fixation is rigid and there should be no postoperative slippage. However, if a deformity develops, orthognathic osteotomy techniques should be considered (see Chapter 43). For minimal deformity and/or dysfunction, no treatment may be necessary.

3. Infection of the maxilla and/or sinuses is a rare complication. Rigid and accurate fixation, intranasal antrostomy, and prophylactic antibiotics will usually prevent infection from occurring. If an infection develops, sequestered bone and foreign bodies will have to be removed. The infection should be cultured and appropriate intravenous antibiotics applied. The physician should also ensure that the antrostomy is open and aerating the sinuses.

4. Plate exposure can be a problem, but when it is properly treated, healing of the fractures should still occur. Usually the exposed plate area is treated with 3% hydrogen peroxide and local application of antibiotic ointment. Prophylactic antibiotics are administered. If the mucosa does not close over the plate, the plate should be retained as long as possible. If the wound is kept clean, the plate can be removed at the completion of healing.

5. Palpable or observable plates will eventually require removal. However, the plate should be left in place until all fractures have healed. Usually it can be removed through the original incision. The newer low profile miniplates may obviate this type of complication.

6. Tooth injury is possible, especially if a screw is placed too low and strikes the apex of the tooth. One way to avoid this complication is to make sure that the drill hole is placed in a position on the maxilla at least twice the height of the exposed crown of the tooth. If a tooth becomes injured, the plate will have to be removed and the tooth extracted or treated with appropriate endodontic therapy.

ALTERNATIVE TECHNIQUE USING PARIETAL CORTEX GRAFTS

a Split cranial grafts are indicated when the buttresses are comminuted and there is little, if any, bone left to secure the plate. Sometimes small pieces of bone are difficult to find, and even when found, they are too small to secure to a screw or wire.

b,c Bone is preferably harvested from the outer cortex of the parietal skull (see Chapter 60). The graft is applied through a degloving, infraciliary, or frontoethmoid approach. The graft should be contoured to the zygomaticomaxillary buttress and/or nasofrontal process and secured superiorly and inferiorly to the remaining fragments with fine 28-gauge stainless steel wires, plates, or lag screws. We prefer wire fixation, because the plates are difficult to contour to the different levels of the bone. Lag screws are also an excellent method of fixation, and a technique similar to that used in the mandible can be applied (see Chapter 13). Postoperative care requires a combination of intravenous and oral antibiotic treatment for at least 2 weeks.

MINIPLATE FIXATION OF LE FORT II FRACTURE *(Continued)*

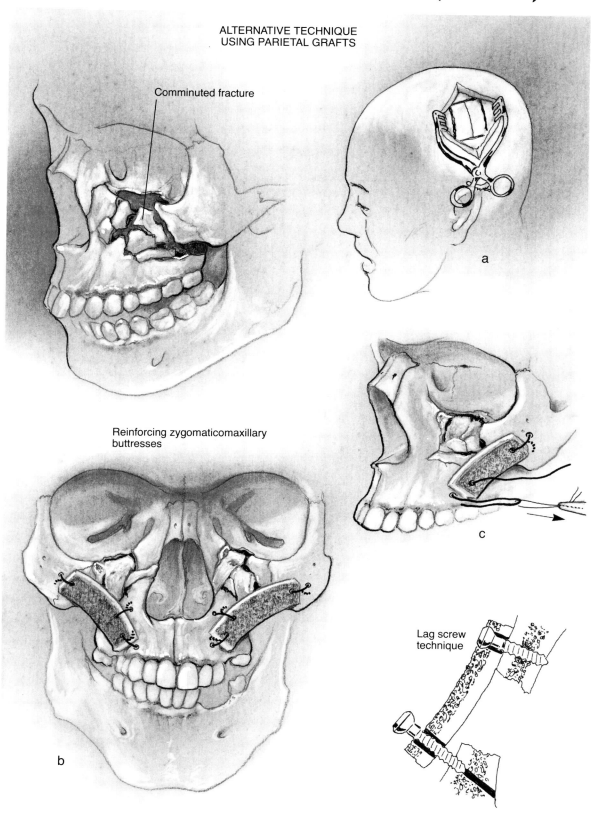

ALTERNATIVE TECHNIQUE
USING PARIETAL GRAFTS

Comminuted fracture

a

Reinforcing zygomaticomaxillary
buttresses

c

Lag screw
technique

b

Repair of Le Fort II Fractures With Intermaxillary Fixation and Interosseous Wiring

INDICATIONS

Most Le Fort II fractures should be treated by reduction and miniplate fixation (see Chapter 34). This rigid fixation plate technique provides early rehabilitation (i.e., oral intake and mastication) and improved stability during the healing process. Occasionally, however, an exact reduction of the fracture cannot be achieved, and when this occurs, semirigid methods should be employed. Intermaxillary fixation will usually bring the fragments into proper relationships. Interosseous wire fixation provides additional stability, allowing the fragments to unite and heal satisfactorily. If the adequacy of fixation is questionable, suspension wires can be used to augment stabilization, and in patients in whom there are comminuted buttresses, bone grafts should be considered.

PROCEDURE

Anesthesia is obtained by way of nasotracheal intubation or tracheostomy. This provides an opportunity to, at the same time, reduce the fracture, set the occlusion to pretraumatic relationships, and repair the injury. The patient's face should be prepared and draped as a sterile field. A solution of 1% lidocaine containing 1:100,000 epinephrine, injected into the incision lines, will help with hemostasis.

A The fractures are first reduced using digital or hook traction, but if this is not successful, Rowe disimpaction forceps should be applied (see Chapter 32). Arch bars are affixed to the teeth, and the jaws set into occlusal relationships with intermaxillary wires or elastic bands (see Chapter 8).

B The main maxillary fracture lines are exposed through a molar-to-molar incision about 5 mm above the gingiva proper. The periosteum is elevated off the maxilla to expose the piriform apertures and the zygomaticomaxillary buttresses. Displaced fragments are then reduced and placed into anatomic position.

To expose the orbital rims, infraciliary incisions are used. The dissection is carried out as in the blowout and malar fractures, carefully exposing the orbital rim, maxilla, and infraorbital nerve (see Chapter 52). Small fragments are reduced appropriately.

C,D Once the teeth and segments of the maxilla are in proper relationships, the bones are stabilized. Interosseous wires are placed along the inferior orbital rim using a minidriver with 0.035-inch K wire to drill the holes and a 28-gauge stainless steel wire to secure the fragments. A 30-gauge stainless steel wire loop can be used to pull out the deep end of the 28-gauge wire. The zygomaticomaxillary fragments are repaired in a similar way. The eyelid incision is closed with a single 3–0 chromic periosteal suture and a subcuticular suture of 5–0 nylon; the mucosal incision is closed with 3–0 chromic sutures.

The patient should be treated for at least 5 days with prophylactic antibiotics (penicillin or erythromycin). Dental hygiene is maintained with a water irrigation device or frequent brushings. Postoperative radiographs should be obtained to verify appropriate reduction and subsequent aeration of the sinuses. Intermaxillary fixation is maintained for 4 to 6 weeks. The patient should be evaluated monthly until there is assurance that the injury has healed properly.

PITFALLS

1. If reduction and occlusal relationships are accurate, the use of plate fixation should be considered (see Chapter 34). Rigid plate techniques provide for rapid healing and an opportunity for early mastication and oral intake.

INTERMAXILLARY FIXATION AND INTEROSSEOUS WIRING

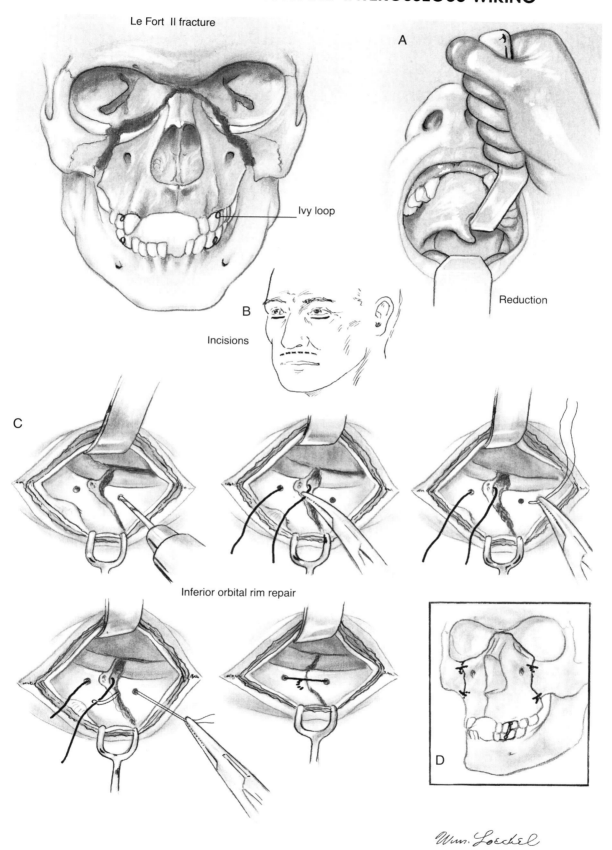

Le Fort II fracture

Ivy loop

A

Reduction

B

Incisions

C

Inferior orbital rim repair

D

Wm. Loechel

2. For the Le Fort II fractures, the occlusal relationships are important in maintaining reduction and fixation. Although Ivy loops can be used, the arch bar method provides more stability during the 4 to 6 weeks necessary for bone healing.

3. Interosseous wires should be applied from stable to unstable fragments, working from the superior portion of the facial skeleton to the inferior maxilla. Other sequences can distract the surgeon from proper orientation and cause malunion and deformity.

4. To avoid postoperative infection, the surgeon should remove the blood from the maxillary sinuses, and if the lines of fracture involve the sinus ostea, subsequent aeration of the sinuses should be provided by intranasal antrostomies. For these purposes, the inferior turbinates are infractured, 2- to 3-cm-diameter holes are made in the inferior meatus, and after the turbinates are placed back into anatomic position, the nose is lightly packed with antibiotic-soaked tampons (see Chapter 32).

5. For the severely comminuted Le Fort II fracture, the surgeon should consider rigid plates or bone grafts. These techniques can reinforce the buttresses, especially when the bone fragments are small and cannot be stabilized with wires and when the elevation of the periosteum threatens viability of the fractured segments. The rigid plate requires areas of buttress that are sufficiently strong and intact to hold the bone screws. The bone grafts can be fixed to small fragments of remaining buttress with either screws or interosseous wires.

COMPLICATIONS

1. Malocclusion and malunion are discussed in Chapter 34. If, in the early postoperative period, the maxillary bones are not satisfactorily reduced, intermaxillary fixation should be loosened and the tensions adjusted to compensate for the deficit. If reduction is still inadequate, the interosseous wires should also be loosened and the bone fragments reduced again and stabilized appropriately. If the bones have healed in malposition, the deformity and/or occlusal problems should be treated with orthognathic and/or orthodontic methods (see Chapter 43). Occasionally the surgeon can expose the healed fracture through the original incision, osteotomize the fragments and reposition them with plates or wires. If there is resorption of bone, interposition or onlay grafts will be required.

2. Infections following the repair of Le Fort II fractures have to be treated by debridement, drainage, removal of wires, and administration of antibiotics dictated by cultures and sensitivities of the micro-organisms. Adequate aeration and drainage of the sinuses must be ensured, and if this does not become apparent on subsequent evaluations, an antrostomy should be considered.

3. Nonunion of the maxilla following a Le Fort II fracture is uncommon and often responds to a longer period of fixation. If the fragments do not heal, the fracture lines will need to be freshened and bone deficits between the fragments stabilized with bone grafts and/or plates.

section IV

Le Fort III Fractures

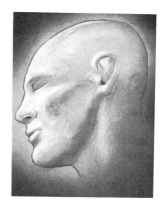

chapter 36

Repair of Le Fort III Fractures With Coronal Flap, Miniplate Fixation, Interosseous Wires, and Ivy Loops

INDICATIONS

Le Fort III fracture lines classically cross a series of horizontal and vertical buttresses of the face, separating the face from the base of the skull. The main fracture line extends from the bridge of the nose through the nasofrontal processes, the floor of the orbits, the zygomaticofrontal processes, and zygomatic arches. The nasal septum is also fractured, and the maxilla is separated from the pterygoid plates.

Exposure from above, coupled with additional incisions from below, provides an excellent opportunity to explore, evaluate, and repair the fractures. The coronal incision and approach expose the upper part of the vertical buttresses, and if the forehead flap is extended, the zygomatic arches can be repaired. Infraciliary and gingivolabial sulcus incisions can be used to expose fractures of both the orbital rim and floor and the lower maxilla, respectively.

A relative contraindication to the coronal flap is a balding hairline. An absolute contraindication is a need to retain soft tissue flaps that are based on the posterior branches of the superficial temporal arteries. Alternatively, traditional periorbital approaches can be used (see Chapters 52 and 58 through 60).

For Le Fort III injuries that are complicated by additional fractures through the cranium, orbit, lower maxilla, and/or mandible, certain precautions must be considered. Cranial and orbital damage requires a consultation with a neurosurgeon and ophthalmologist. As a general rule, mandibular repair should be performed first. In the case of a condylar fracture, the surgeon may have to consider open reduction and fixation.

Most Le Fort III fractures can be reduced and placed into occlusion with Ivy loops and then stabilized with rigid miniplates across major buttresses. Small fragments of bone can be molded into position and held with a basketing effect from the plate. If comminution of bone is extensive, bone grafts may be required. Rarely is there a need for an internal or external suspension, as these techniques can create abnormal forces that effect a shortening and retrusion of the midface.

PROCEDURE

Le Fort III fractures are best managed with a tracheostomy and general anesthesia. This method provides an excellent field for the surgeon, a separate field for the anesthesiologist, and an opportunity to check occlusion during and after the procedure. Nasal fractures can also be reduced without interference from the anesthetic tube.

A–C The coronal incision should extend from the preauricular creases above the pinnae and across the temples to form a gentle curve behind the hairline. A small area of hair should be shaved and the tissues injected with 1% lidocaine containing 1:100,000 epinephrine to help control bleeding.

The face is prepared and draped as a sterile field. Hair is held out of the way with elastic bands covered with towels and attached to the scalp. The incision is beveled along hair follicles and carried through the subcuticular and galeal tissues. Branches of the superficial temporal artery are clamped and ligated with 3–0 silk. A plane is then developed between the galea and periosteum, and the forehead tissues are elevated and rolled over the projection of the superior orbital rims. The periosteum should not be incised until the surgeon is close to the orbital rims, and the surgeon should attempt to preserve the supratrochlea and supraorbital vessels that enter the flap. Laterally the dissection should be in a plane just superficial to the temporalis fascia. Gentle retraction should avoid injury to the frontal branch of the facial nerve.

D–F With the flap rotated and held with fish hooks, the periosteum is incised along the zygomaticofrontal buttress. If the zygomatic arch needs to be exposed, the supraorbital arteries and nerves are released from their foramina with a small, sharp osteotome and the temporalis fascia incised and elevated off the arch. The nasal bridge fracture can be exposed by retraction and additional periosteal elevation off the frontal process of the maxilla and nasal bones. Incisions can be made along the lower eyelid (infraciliary) and the gingivolabial sulcus to expose the infraorbital rims and lower maxilla, respectively (see Chapters 32 and 52).

G Once all fracture lines are exposed, the maxillary fractures should be reduced with a Rowe disimpaction forceps (see Chapter 32). The fracture sites should be reevaluated, and the surgeon should ensure that the fragments are aligned. The relationships of the jaws should be examined and pretraumatic occlusion obtained with strategically placed Ivy loops (see Chapter 8).

H–K Miniplates are selected so that they will fit across the zygomaticofrontal fractures. Two screw holes should be available for solid bone fixation on each side of the fracture. The plates should be bent to the exact contour of the reduced fragments, and as the screws are placed, the surgeon should ensure that the bone fragments are retained in a reduced position. Screw holes are made with a drill bit that comes with the plating set. The depth of the drill should be controlled with a malleable retractor or, alternatively, the drill bit can be recessed so that it will not penetrate beyond the bone. Constant irrigation with saline should reduce the heat caused by the drilling and prevent further injury to the bone and soft tissues of the area. Drill holes should be measured so that the screws will pass through the bone but not project into the sinus (or soft tissues). The screws are applied first to holes located directly to the sides of the fracture and then to the outer holes for additional fixation.

For the classic Le Fort III fracture, zygomaticofrontal fixation should suffice. If the arch is severely comminuted and depressed, even after elevation, it may require direct wire or plate fixation. If the nasofrontal process is unstable, the surgeon can place 28-gauge wires or fine plates to approximate the fragments. If the inferior orbital rim needs repair, a separate eyelid exposure and wire fixation are indicated (see Chapter 52). As a general rule, the surgeon should use a minimum number of plates to obtain stability.

The coronal flap is returned to its original position and closed in layers. We prefer 3–0 chromic sutures to approximate the galea and several additional 3–0 chromic sutures in the subcuticular/subcutaneous tissues to coapt the skin edges. The skin is then closed with a running 5–0 nylon suture. Other incisions are treated with a layered closure.

To prevent swelling in the postoperative period, a light compression dressing of fluffs and expandable bandages is applied to the forehead, scalp, and ear areas. The patient should be treated with prophylactic antibiotics (i.e., ampicillin or cefazolin) for at least 5 days. Dressings are changed as needed and maintained for at least 5 to 7 days. Sutures are removed on the seventh day. Dental hygiene is achieved with a water irrigation device. Intermaxillary elastic bands or wires are removed when correct intermaxillary relationships are ensured. Postoperative radiographs should be used to verify the relationship of the bone fragments and subsequent aeration of sinuses. The patient should be evaluated every 2 weeks during the first month and then monthly until there is assurance that the injury has healed properly.

PITFALLS

1. Reduction of the Le Fort III fracture may require a forceful disimpaction. If there is a question of

CORONAL FLAP APPROACH FOR LE FORT III FRACTURES

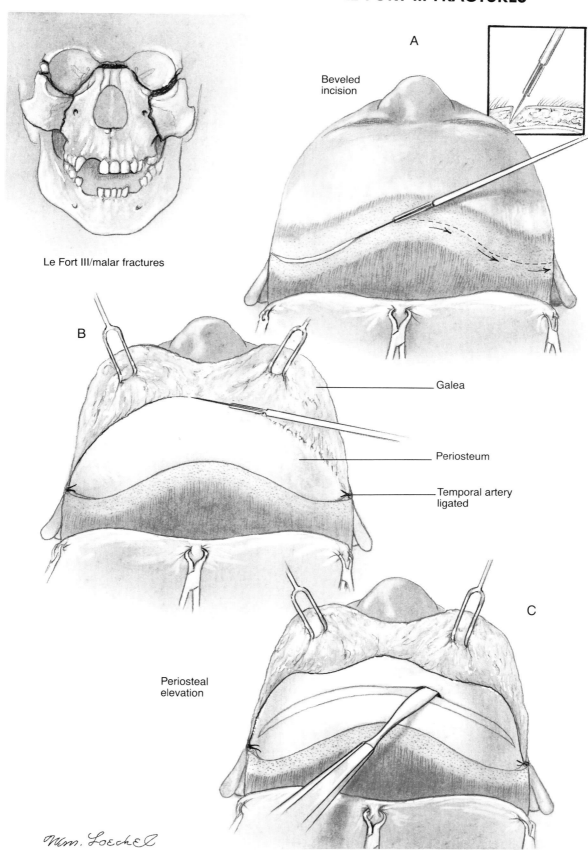

Le Fort III/malar fractures

A

Beveled incision

B

Galea

Periosteum

Temporal artery ligated

C

Periosteal elevation

Wm. Loechel

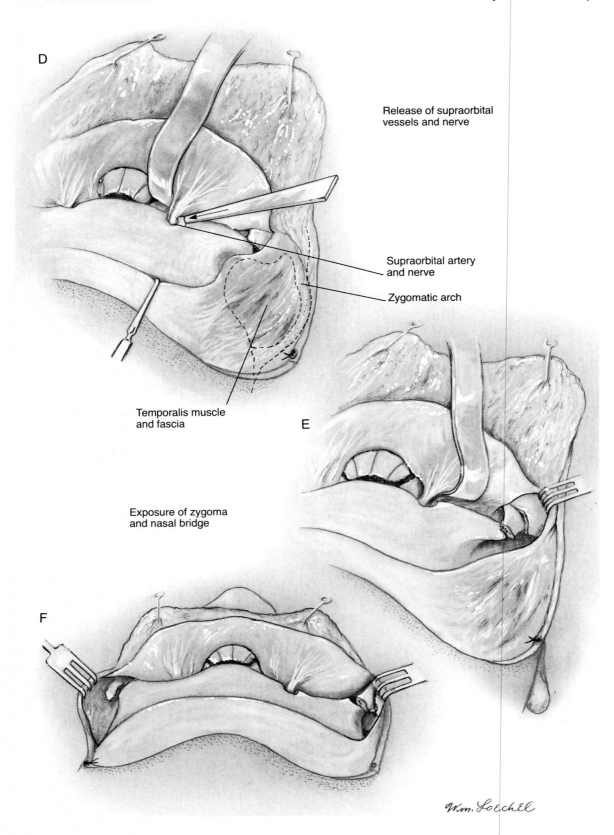

D

Release of supraorbital vessels and nerve

Supraorbital artery and nerve

Zygomatic arch

Temporalis muscle and fascia

E

Exposure of zygoma and nasal bridge

F

Wm. Loechel

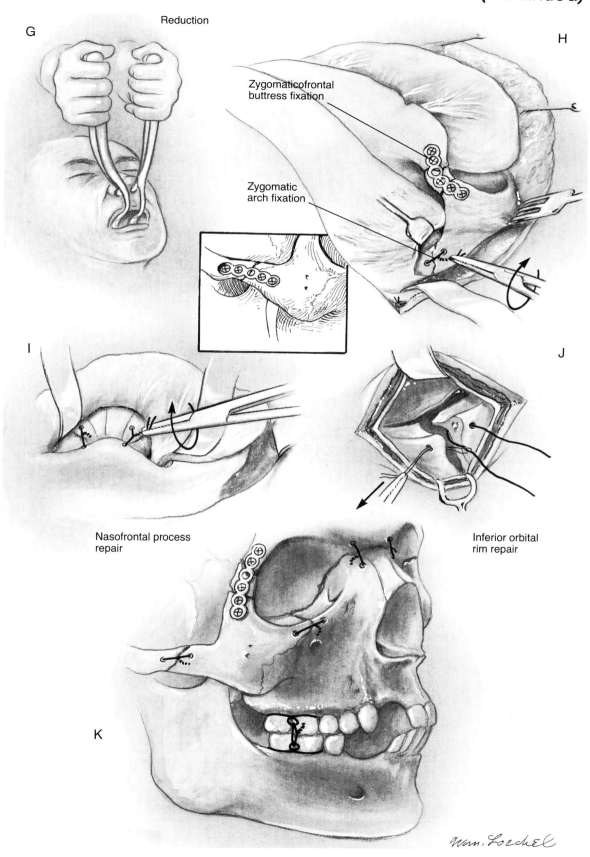

Reduction

G

H

Zygomaticofrontal
buttress fixation

Zygomatic
arch fixation

I

J

Nasofrontal process
repair

Inferior orbital
rim repair

K

Wm. Loechel

impending visual loss, the surgeon must carefully evaluate the site and the extent of the fractures in relationship to the orbit and retrobulbar tissues. Ophthalmologic consultation is advised. In experienced hands, a judicious application of force will reduce the fracture without untoward sequelae.

2. The coronal incision is ideal for exposure but should probably not be used in the patient who is bald (or balding) or in one who will need flaps based on the posterior branch of the superficial temporal vessel. Other alternatives are to use the infraciliary, eyebrow, and medial canthal incisions. The extended sub-brow incision can also be employed (see Chapter 71).

3. An accurate reduction of fragments to pretraumatic occlusion must be obtained prior to placement of the miniplates. The rigid plates are unforgiving, and healing will occur in the positions dictated by the plates.

4. Use gentle retraction on the flaps. Excessive pressure can cause injury to the supraorbital and frontal branch of the facial nerve, resulting in paresthesias and weakness of the forehead.

5. The supraorbital artery and nerve should be preserved, but if there is an orbital rim fracture that requires reduction and/or stabilization and the nerve and artery are in the way, then the vessel and/or nerve may have to be sacrificed. The patient should be warned prior to surgery that he or she may have some numbness of the forehead and periorbital region.

6. Although the zygomatic arch can be plated, the procedure can cause potential problems. The retraction necessary for plating places the facial nerve at risk. Moreover, the skin over the arch is very thin and the plate will often be palpable or observable and require later removal. The plate also is not easily removed without again performing a coronal incision. For these reasons, we prefer either a closed reduction or interosseous wire fixation.

7. Use only a sufficient number of plates to achieve fixation. One or two plates applied across the zygomaticofrontal buttresses often provide sufficient stability. If the maxilla is still unstable, additional plates can be added to other fracture sites. There is also the option of intermaxillary fixation for an extended period of time.

8. Plating should go from stable to unstable parts and thus in the direction of the frontal bone to the lower maxilla. In complicated cases in which fractures occur across the lower maxilla and mandible, the surgeon will have to first set the height of the mandible (i.e., repair condyle, ramus, and angle fractures), reduce the maxilla, and establish pretraumatic occlusion before aligning fragments with rigid plate fixation.

9. Avoid suspension wire techniques. Internal "drop-wire" suspension can cause a compression of the maxilla between the upper dentition and cranium. Retrusion can also occur. External suspension with a halo tends to pull the fragments up and out and can potentially create an overprojection of the midface. Although suspension techniques are fraught with untoward sequelae, they may be necessary when there is severe comminution and the surgeon is not sure of the adequacy of the reduction (see Chapters 37 and 38).

10. Comminuted bone fragments can often be treated by basketing techniques using plates (or wires). Most fragments can be found and manipulated into appropriate position. However, when there is an avulsion of tissue, as is often found with gunshot wounds, the bone deficit may require additional methods of support. Split cranial or rib grafts for either stabilization or reinforcement should be considered.

COMPLICATIONS

1. Infections are prone to develop in patients who have soft tissue injuries and/or contaminated wounds. Bone grafts are at risk, and plate exposure can occur. Most infections can be treated with appropriate antibiotics, debridement, and drainage; if necessary, the plate and/or grafts will have to be removed.

2. Sinusitis is rare following Le Fort III fixation. Most fractures pass above the maxillary ostea and below the nasofrontal duct ostea and do not affect drainage of the sinuses. Intranasal antrostomies are not necessary, but if sinusitis develops, the patient should be started on decongestants and antibiotics. Persistent sinusitis may require a surgical drainage procedure.

3. Weakness of the forehead can occur as a result of injury to the frontal branch of the facial nerve. To avoid this complication, the surgeon should apply gentle traction to the forehead flap. Extensive flaps should be avoided, especially if the zygomatic arch need not be repaired.

4. If there is injury to the supraorbital nerve, the patient can expect anesthesia and/or paresthesia of the forehead. The nerve is particularly at risk during maximal retraction of orbital tissues and with reduction and fixation of the superior and medial orbital rims. Loss of sensation is often transient, and some return of function is expected.

5. Nonunion of the maxilla is very rare. Some looseness of the maxilla can be tolerated, and with time, the maxilla will "tighten up" and require no additional surgical intervention. However, if maxil-

lary movement continues to be a problem, the fracture site will need to be explored, the bone edges freshened, and the fractures treated with interposition bone grafts. Plate fixation can also be applied.

6. Malunion and malocclusion will develop if the reduction is not accurate or there is a slippage of the fragments following the procedure. Occasionally there is a resorption of bone and, in children, the possibility of impaired growth of the maxilla. Malunion, resulting in deformity and/or dysfunction, will require osteotomy and/or bone graft techniques as described in Chapter 44.

7. Plates can be visible or palpable, especially in thin-skinned individuals or when the plates are placed over the frontozygomatic buttress, the nasofrontal process, or zygomatic arch. The complication can be avoided by using low-profile microplates or applying interosseous wires. If the plate causes a deformity, removal may be required.

chapter 37

Repair of Le Fort III Fracture With Intermaxillary Fixation and Interosseous Wiring
Alternative Technique of Denture Suspension Wiring for the Edentulous Patient

INDICATIONS

Although Le Fort III fractures are often managed with miniplate fixation, there are occasions in which miniplates are not advised and the more traditional interosseous wire methods should be employed. Miniplate fixation should only be used if the surgeon can obtain anatomic reduction of fragments and pretraumatic occlusal relationships. If these conditions cannot be met, then a less rigid technique, such as interosseous wiring, is preferred. Moreover, interosseous wires are easily concealed and generally will not cause the palpable and frequently observed irregularities found with plates.

PROCEDURE

A,B Essentially the patient is prepared for surgery as in the miniplate fixation technique (see Chapter 36). General anesthesia should be provided through nasotracheal intubation or a tracheostomy, but if the nose must be reduced or stabilized, tracheostomy is preferred. The maxilla is reduced with digital or hook traction or with a Rowe disimpaction forceps. The teeth are placed into optimal occlusal relationships with Ivy loops or arch bars, and the jaws are held together with fine wire loops or elastic bands.

C The fracture is exposed through a coronal incision (see Chapter 36) or, alternatively, through medial canthal, eyebrow, and infraciliary approaches (see Chapters 52, 59, and 60). A degloving gingivolabial sulcus incision is useful for complicated fractures that enter the lower maxilla and dental arch (see Chapter 34).

D,E Our preference is to apply 28-gauge stainless steel wires across the fractures of the horizontal and vertical buttresses. Drill holes are placed with a 0.035-inch K wire and a minidriver. The depth of the drill is controlled by the length of the K wire. Soft tissues are generally protected with a malleable retractor.

The first holes are placed on the cranial side of the fracture. Other holes are then made strategically on a line drawn at right angles to the fracture on the unstable segment (or segments). A 28-gauge wire is inserted through the drill hole on the unstable segment and pulled through the second drill hole with a loop of 30-gauge wire. The 28-gauge wire is then twisted with a heavy needle holder to abut the fragments. Only when the buttresses are completely reduced are the wires tightened down and bent flat against the bone or into one of the drill holes. Generally the frontozygomatic buttress and inferior orbital rim provide sufficient stability; additional support, however, can be obtained by wiring other fracture sites (i.e., zygomaticomaxillary).

All incisions are closed in layers using periosteal 3–0 or 4–0 chromic, subcuticular 5–0 colorless, or white nonabsorbable and cutaneous 5–0 or 6–0 nylon sutures. The wounds are dressed with antibiotic ointment, and the patient is maintained on prophylactic antibiotics (i.e., ampicillin or cefazolin) for at least 5 to 7 days. Intermaxillary fixation must be maintained for 4 to 6 weeks. Postoperative radiographs should be obtained to verify reduction of fragments and aeration of the sinuses. Occlusion

INTEROSSEOUS WIRING OF LE FORT III/MALAR FRACTURES

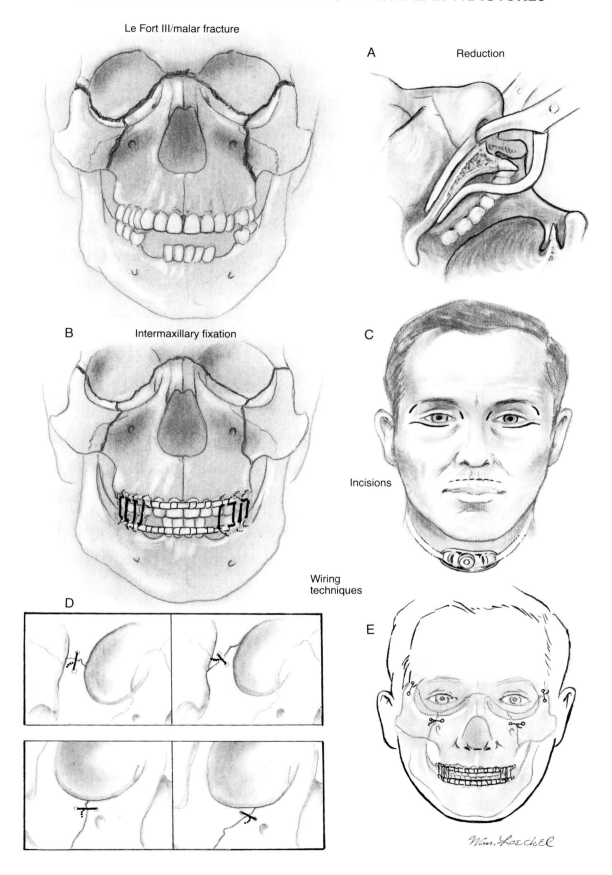

Le Fort III/malar fracture

A   Reduction

B   Intermaxillary fixation

C

Incisions

Wiring techniques

D

E

Wm. Loechel

should be checked on a regular basis and intermaxillary adjustments performed as necessary.

PITFALLS

1. Vertical and horizontal buttresses should be stabilized with wires and pretraumatic occlusion maintained with intermaxillary fixation. The technical aspects of the procedure (i.e., reduction of the fracture, incisions, retraction, and exposure) have the potential for the same complications discussed in Chapter 36.

2. Suspension wires should be avoided, as this technique can sometimes shorten the midface and drive the maxilla posteriorly and inferiorly along the base of the skull. However, in the edentulous patient, dentures may have to be used, and to hold the dentures, the surgeon may have to employ suspension techniques. In patients with Le Fort III fractures, the suspension wires have to be stabilized to the frontal bone (see later).

3. Comminuted fractures of the maxilla may be difficult to treat with interosseous wires, and in such cases, the surgeon should consider additional support with plates, bone grafts, or external fixation. If plates cannot be applied (i.e., there is insufficient stable bone for the ends of the plate), then the surgeon should consider rib or split parietal bone, either as onlay or interposition grafts. If there is uncertainty regarding the occlusal relationships and reduction, a halo should be used with planned postoperative evaluations and adjustments of tension on the apparatus (see Chapter 38).

COMPLICATIONS

1. Infection in the presence of interosseous wires requires drainage, local care, and appropriate antibiotics. If the infection persists, the wires should be removed. The surgeon should also ensure that adjacent sinuses are aerated and functionally drained.

2. Malreduction should be recognized early and treated appropriately. The interosseous wire technique is semirigid, and early malposition of fragments can be managed by a loosening, further adjustment, and tightening of the wires. If the bones have healed, orthodontia or osteotomy methods will have to be considered (see Chapter 44).

3. Nonunion of the maxilla is rare, and in most cases, longer periods of fixation will achieve healing. Persistent instability requires exploration, freshening of fracture sites, and reapplication of appropriate fixation methods.

4. Exposure or palpation of wires can be avoided by having the wire bent close to the maxilla or into a nearby drill hole. Projecting wires are usually managed with small incisions over the wire, a cutting of the wire, and a direct extraction of the wire loop.

ALTERNATIVE TECHNIQUE OF DENTURE SUSPENSION WIRING FOR THE EDENTULOUS PATIENT

Le Fort III fractures in the edentulous patient can usually be treated by reduction and rigid miniplate fixation, and in general, suspension techniques should be avoided. However, if the surgeon is not certain about the adequacy of the occlusion or reduction, then interosseous wires with dentures or splints (see Chapter 9) secured by a suspension method should be considered. This technique is also useful when there is a need for the suspension wires and denture to cradle small fragments of the alveolus and/or palate in anatomic position.

a,b The Le Fort III fracture is first reduced and the fractures approximated with wires (see earlier). A long (26 to 30 cm) 24-gauge wire is subsequently placed through the drill hole of the zygomatic process of the frontal bone, and the ends of the wire are passed with an awl or trocar behind the zygomatic arch into the gingivobuccal sulcus. The wire is pulled tightly and then twisted into a loop that is just exposed in the sulcus.

c To form a safety loop, a second loop of 28-gauge wire is applied between the 24-gauge wire loop and the denture near the region of the first molar. The denture is seated and secured into position by tightening the secondary loop. The lower denture is secured with a circummandibular wire.

d–f A pullout wire should also be fashioned. For this, a 26-gauge wire is passed through the first wire loop, just beneath its attachment to the frontal bone. The wire is bent back on itself and both ends passed with an awl or needle through the deep subcutaneous tissues to exit from the scalp at a point just beyond the hairline. The wire is secured to a button on the surface of the skin. When the fixation apparatus is to be removed, the long transmaxillary wire loop is cut, and the accessory scalp wire loop is used to pull it out. If there is difficulty in removing the suspension wire, a small incision can be made on the lateral orbital rim and the wire removed directly.

g The suspension procedure is usually performed bilaterally and the wires adjusted so that there is a vertical pull on the denture. If the upper denture

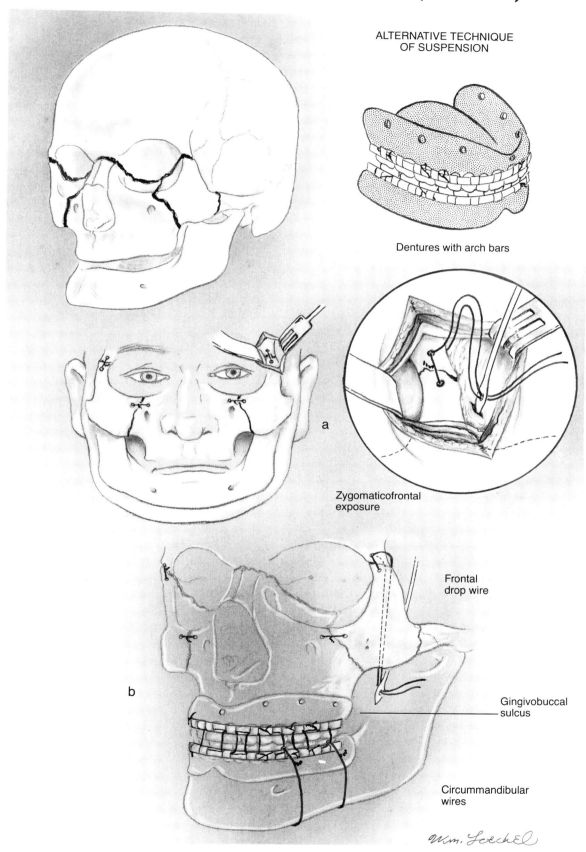

ALTERNATIVE TECHNIQUE
OF SUSPENSION

Dentures with arch bars

a

Zygomaticofrontal
exposure

b

Frontal
drop wire

Gingivobuccal
sulcus

Circummandibular
wires

Wm. Leechel

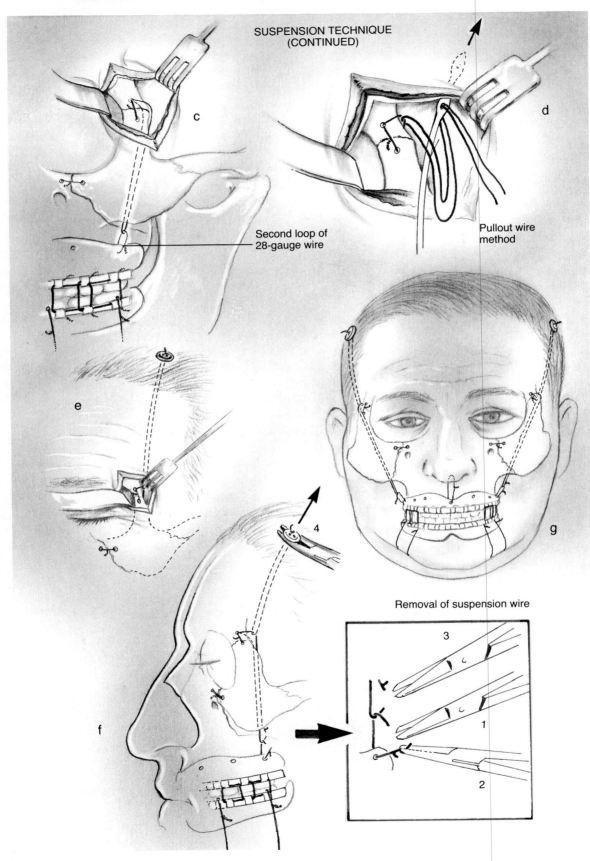

SUSPENSION TECHNIQUE
(CONTINUED)

c

Second loop of
28-gauge wire

d

Pullout wire
method

e

f

4

g

3

1

2

Removal of suspension wire

should rock, the surgeon should also consider a drop wire from the anterior nasal spine. Placement of this wire, the holes in the denture, and the intermaxillary fixation are described in Chapter 9.

Postoperatively the patient is treated as described in Chapter 36. In about 4 to 6 weeks, suspension wires and loops around the dentures are cut, and the suspension wires are removed with the pullout wire. The wire from the anterior nasal spine can be cut and removed directly.

chapter 38

External Fixation of Le Fort III Fracture With a Visor-Halo Frame

INDICATIONS

Almost all Le Fort III fractures can be treated with open reduction and interosseous fixation with wires and/or plates. However, in severely comminuted fractures, alone or in combination with other maxillary or mandible fractures, in which the reduction is in question and there is a tendency for retrusion, external traction and fixation, as provided by a halo frame, are indicated. The frame can also be used in patients with cranial bone injury in which the fracture of the frontal bone or anterior base of the skull precludes plate and/or wire fixation. The external halo device is helpful as an adjunctive method in support of other techniques of stabilization (i.e., interosseous wires and plates).

PROCEDURE

A The Le Fort III fracture is reduced and pretraumatic occlusion achieved by the methods described in Chapters 36 and 37. If wires or plates are to be applied, exposure is by way of coronal, periorbital, and/or gingivolabial sulcus incisions. The mandible should first be repaired, but the jaws should not be wired together (intermaxillary fixation) until the halo is fitted and adjusted into position.

B For the application of a Georgiade visor-halo, general anesthesia is preferred. Ideally the halo should be placed so that there is a 2-cm clearance between the halo headframe and the head. The halo is then secured in four quadrants along the skull with appropriate-sized pin-screws. The screws are inserted with a screwdriver so that the sharp pin penetrates the soft tissues and just engages the outer cortex of the cranium bone. The screws should be applied one or two turns at a time so that the halo does not shift from one side of the head to the other.

C Once the halo is in position, the visor portion is adjusted. Ideally the visor should be placed 2 to 3

cm above the brow. Offset outriggers are then secured along the visor so that the vertical bars lie directly in front of the malar prominences and upper incisors.

D–F For most fractures, only a few points of fixation are necessary for stabilization. The malar fixation points can be exposed through an infraciliary incision. Drill holes are then placed on the lateral maxillary border just below the body of the zygoma. A 26-gauge wire about 26 cm long is inserted through the hole and both ends are then brought out through a stab incision directly beneath the outrigger. The contralateral malar eminence is treated in a similar manner.

For stability to the lower maxilla, it is possible to attach a 26-gauge wire to the arch bar or to the anterior portion of a denture. This wire should lie just below the upper lip.

G After all wires are in position, they are attached to the turnbuckles, and the turnbuckles are tightened. Tension is adjusted so that there is just enough traction to pull the maxilla forward. This forward movement should accurately align the fragments in occlusal relationships. Once the surgeon has achieved optimal position of the fragments, the intermaxillary fixation can be tightened.

Postoperatively the position of the maxilla should be evaluated and the fixation apparatus adjusted accordingly. The cranial pins that hold the halo will become loose and will require tightening for several days. As the swelling disappears, the facial skeleton should be repositioned by adjusting the turnbuckles. The changes in tension of the wire can be used to pull or relax the attached bone fragments. Cephalometric analysis is often helpful in determining the skeletal relationships of the upper and lower jaws. Pin incisions should be treated daily with 3% hydrogen peroxide and antibiotic ointment. Otherwise, postoperative care should be similar to that used in wire and/or plate fixation (see Chapters 36 and 37).

HALO FRAME FIXATION OF LE FORT III FRACTURE

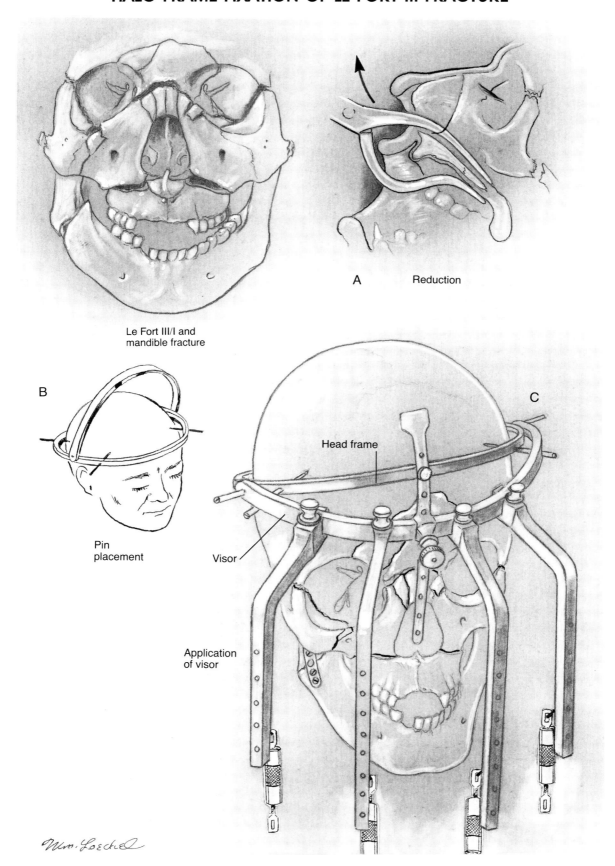

Le Fort III/I and
mandible fracture

A   Reduction

B

Pin
placement

C

Head frame

Visor

Application
of visor

D

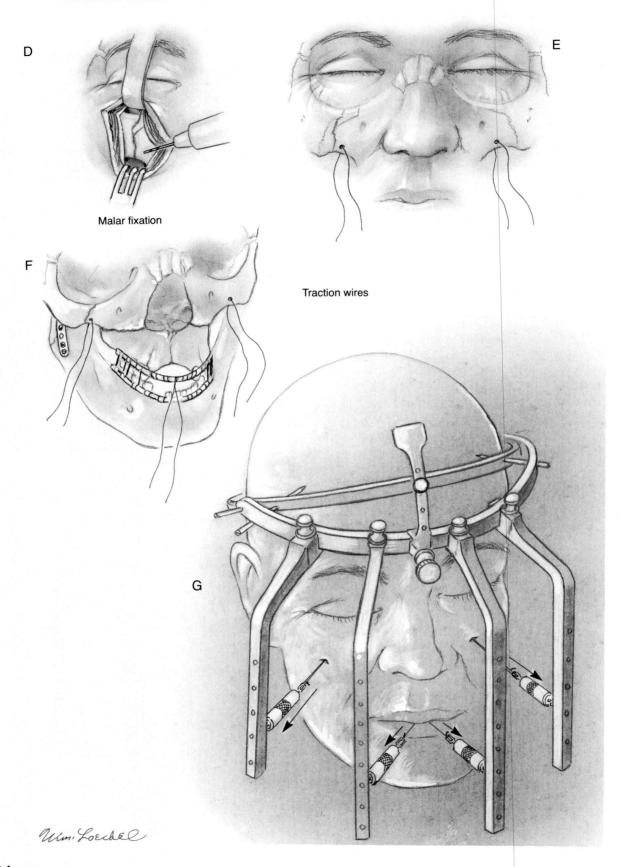

Malar fixation

E

F

Traction wires

G

Wm. Loechel

PITFALLS

1. The Georgiade halo is a complicated apparatus, and the surgeon should become familiar with its application by a preliminary take-down and replacement of its parts. Symmetric application of cranial screws is essential for the apparatus to fix tightly to the skull. However, the surgeon should avoid overtightening and penetration of the screw through the inner cortex.

2. A loosening of the screws in the postoperative period is common and can cause problems. The patient will complain of pain, and the apparatus may become dislodged. The screws should thus be tightened daily with a screwdriver (or the edge of a dime). The area around the screws should be kept clean with 3% hydrogen peroxide and antibiotic ointment.

3. Tension adjustments of the transcutaneous wires will be necessary for several days. Ideally traction should be at right angles to the plane of the face. As swelling disappears, changes in position and tension of the wires and outriggers will be required.

4. Shifts in occlusion can also occur, and thus the mouth and dental arch relationships should be evaluated daily. A cephalometric radiograph may be helpful.

5. The tighter the fit of the halo, the more comfortable it will be for the patient. Also, excessive weight on the halo can be avoided by using the minimum number of outriggers and wires necessary to achieve stability.

COMPLICATIONS

1. Infection of pin sites is prevented by keeping the skin clean with 3% hydrogen peroxide and antibiotic ointment. If an infection develops, the surgeon has the option of removing the pins and placing new pins in nearby holes. Antibiotics specific for the infection should be applied.

2. Penetration of the inner cortex of the cranium should not occur if the pin is screwed to the point at which the halo is tight to the skull. Each screw has a bevel, and this bevel should be used to evaluate the depth of the screw in relationship to the skull. If, on turning the screw, the screw appears to loosen as if it has penetrated through the inner cortex, the screw should be removed and placed in another site. The holes should be cleaned and treated with antibiotic dressings. A computed tomographic (CT) scan and neurosurgical consultation should be obtained.

3. Displacement of the apparatus can effect changes in the position of the fractures. Thus the screws and wires should be kept tight and the patient instructed to avoid additional trauma. If the halo becomes dislodged, it should be reapplied and secured in an ideal position.

4. Complications specific to the repair of Le Fort III fractures and prevention and management of these sequelae are described in Chapters 36 and 37.

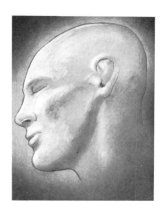

chapter 39

Repair of Medial Maxillary Fracture With Degloving Approach and Interosseous Wire Fixation
Alternative Techniques of Closed Reduction, Miniplate Fixation, and Late Reconstruction With Osteotomies and/or Onlay Bone Grafts

INDICATIONS

Medial maxillary fractures present with a characteristic deformity: a C-shaped deviation of the dorsum of the nose, with the tip and root of the nose maintained in a fairly normal position. The deformity can be confused with a simple nasal fracture, except the medial maxillary fracture is associated with an obvious depression of the medial maxillary wall and, in some cases, an extension of the depression to involve the frontal process of the maxilla and inferior orbital wall. The displacement of the medial maxillary wall usually causes nasal obstruction and potentially a disruption and twisting of the lacrimal collecting system. An accurate early diagnosis is essential, and once the injury is defined, reduction and fixation must be considered. Interosseous wires and miniplates are effective in stabilizing the repositioned bones.

PROCEDURE

Oral intubation is preferred. The face and neck are prepared with antiseptic solution and draped as a sterile field. The nasal mucous membranes are treated with pledgets soaked in 8 mL of 4% cocaine, to which is added five drops of 1:10,000 epinephrine.

187

The nose is then blocked in a standard fashion with 1% lidocaine containing 1:100,000 epinephrine (see Chapter 46). Additional amounts of anesthesia are infiltrated into the gingivolabial and gingivobuccal sulcus.

A–C An incision is made 5 mm above the gingival margin from the first molar on the side of exploration to the canine of the opposite side. Hemostasis is achieved with electric cautery. The periosteum is elevated off the alveolus and onto the anterior face of the maxilla. The dissection is continued upward, exposing the anterior nasal spine, piriform aperture, infraorbital canal, and neurovascular bundle. Additional exposure is obtained by making a through-and-through septal-columella incision and extending these cuts along the floor of the nose and the piriform aperture to expose the nasomaxillary buttresses.

D–G Further elevation of the periosteum will expose the frontal process of the maxilla, the nasal bones, and the inferior orbital rim. The thicker portions of the fracture are reduced with a Boies elevator and the smaller fragments with either a Cottle graduated elevator or single skin hooks. The fragments are secured with interosseous wires, which are applied through small drill holes made with a 0.035-inch K wire and minidriver. Usually a 28-gauge stainless steel wire is passed through the hole in the stable fragment and brought through the hole in the less stable fragment. A 30-gauge wire loop technique of passing the 28-gauge wire through the second hole is a valuable adjunct. Each wire is given a few turns, and in a planned rotation, wires are twisted to fix the fragments. The wires are then cut and the ends bent between the fragments.

Closure is accomplished by suturing the gingivolabial mucosa with 3–0 chromic sutures. The septum is secured to the columella with several 3–0 chromic mattress sutures, usually placed with a straight needle. The nose should be packed for 3 to 5 days with either a bacitracin-soaked nasal tampon or layered ½-inch, bacitracin-impregnated gauze. If the nasal bones are comminuted, a tape and plaster dressing is applied to the dorsum of the nose (see Chapter 46).

Antibiotics (i.e., erythromycin or penicillin) are prescribed for the duration of the packing. Following removal of the packing, the internal nose is kept moist and clean with sprays of normal saline several times a day. The patient should be evaluated every 2 weeks during the first month and then monthly until there is assurance that the injury has healed properly.

PITFALLS

1. The diagnosis is critical for an accurate and early treatment. The degloving approach is not necessary for simple nasal fractures, as these can be easily treated with a closed reduction technique (see Chapter 46). Moreover, the degloving exposure is not sufficient to treat a displaced inferior orbital rim or a fracture of the floor or medial wall of the orbit. These injuries require additional approaches (see Chapters 52 and 59).

2. Enophthalmos, hypophthalmos, and diplopia associated with the medial maxillary fracture suggest an orbital injury. When these signs and symptoms occur, an infraciliary incision and floor exposure are necessary (see Chapters 59 and 60).

3. Occasionally there will be cases in which it is more prudent to carry on a simple closed reduction of nasal bones and the medial maxilla (see later). This is indicated in a debilitated individual, especially one who cannot tolerate general anesthesia or the length of time required for the open procedure.

4. Although rare, the medial maxillary fracture can be associated with telecanthus and epiphora. If this occurs, a separate medial canthal incision should be carried out and the medial wall and rim of the orbit explored for injuries. The techniques for repair are discussed in Chapters 63 through 66.

5. Wire techniques are often satisfactory in fixing the nasomaxillary buttress. Miniplates are indicated when the interosseous wire is insufficient to maintain the desired anatomic position of the buttress and adjoining segments. They should also be employed when there is instability associated with injury of the other maxillary buttresses.

6. The medial maxillary fracture will heal rapidly, and if the diagnosis is not made early, there is a possibility of permanent deformity and dysfunction. If the bones are healed (and this usually occurs after 4 weeks), then the fracture must be reestablished with osteotomies and treated as in an early injury. To make the osteotomies, it is necessary to expose the orbit and nasal bones through a degloving, infraciliary and medial canthal approach. If there is resorption of bone, split parietal cranial grafts may be layered over the defect (see later).

COMPLICATIONS

1. Malunion of the maxillary and nasal bones can be corrected in the first few months with osteotomies, refracture of the segments, and reapproximation with wire or plates. At a later time, there is usually too much resorption of bone, and in such a case it is more prudent to employ split cranial grafts as an onlay to the area of deficit.

2. Early orbital complications such as enophthalmos, hypophthalmos, and diplopia can be treated early with reexploration, osteotomy (if necessary),

DEGLOVING APPROACH FOR MEDIAL MAXILLARY FRACTURE

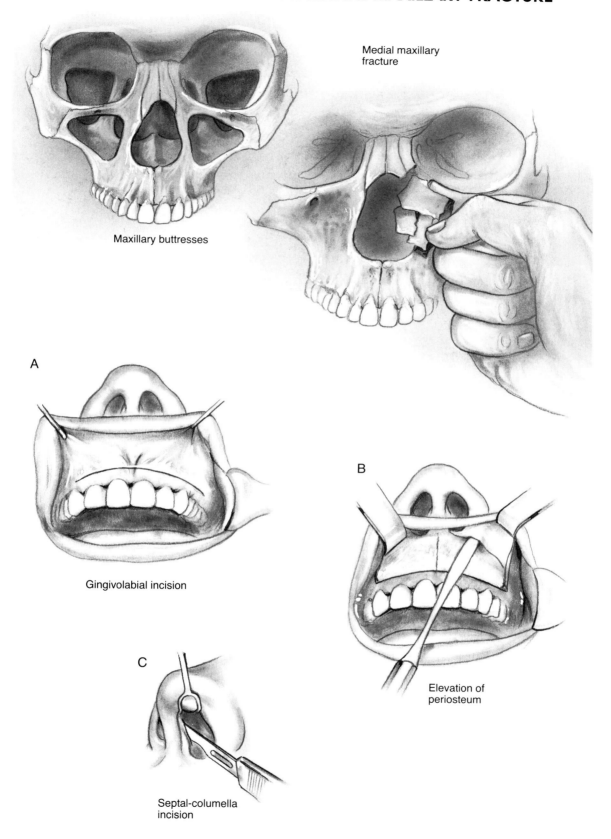

Maxillary buttresses

Medial maxillary fracture

A

Gingivolabial incision

B

Elevation of periosteum

C

Septal-columella incision

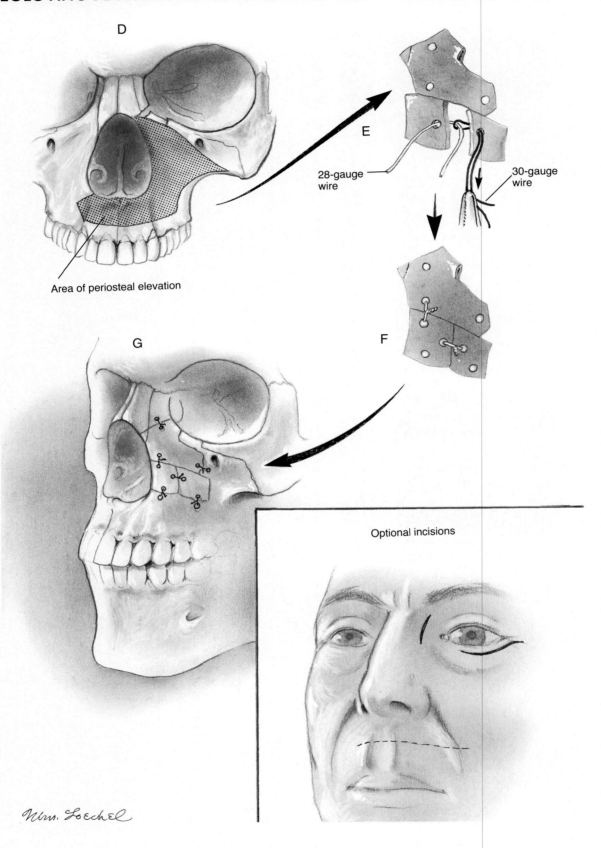

D

E

28-gauge wire

30-gauge wire

F

G

Area of periosteal elevation

Optional incisions

and repositioning of the fragments. For late complications, the patient must be evaluated for a complete reconstruction of the orbit (see Chapters 60 and 61).

3. Dacryocystitis is a potential problem, especially if the lacrimal drainage system is obstructed. The lacrimal system should be evaluated with appropriate dye tests. For obstruction at the outflow of the sac, dacryocystorhinostomy must be considered (see Chapter 68). However, the surgeon should make sure that a deviated septum or turbinate is not causing the obstruction, and if these conditions exist, they should be corrected before lacrimal collection system surgery.

4. Deformities confined to the nasal bones can be treated with standard rhinoplasty procedures (see Chapter 49). Usually the physician waits 4 to 6 months so that the bones become solid and the osteotomies can be controlled. If the bones are not healed, the osteotomies potentially can cause further instability of the nasal pyramid.

ALTERNATIVE TECHNIQUE OF CLOSED REDUCTION

A closed method of treatment is indicated for those individuals who are severely debilitated and cannot tolerate the general anesthetic usually given with an open procedure. For such a case, the nose is anesthesized with cocaine-soaked pledgets, and the nose is blocked with 2% lidocaine. Using a Boies elevator, the nasal bones and medial wall of the maxilla are elevated into position. The nose is then packed bilaterally with a tampon or gauze dressing (see Chapter 46). External tapes and plaster may be applied. The disadvantage of this particular procedure is that reduction may not be stable, and there can be a relapse of the fracture.

ALTERNATIVE TECHNIQUE OF MINIPLATE FIXATION

Complex or unstable fractures often require the stability of miniplate fixation. For this technique, the degloving approach is employed. The stable portions of the buttress should be exposed superiorly to the frontal process of the maxilla and inferiorly to the alveolus. After reduction of the fracture, a curved miniplate of appropriate length is placed across the stable portions. The plate is shaped and bent to accommodate the normal anatomic configuration. The plate is first secured to the stable portions of the buttress with drill holes and screws of optimal length and diameter. Additional screws are placed through

the plate into the underlying fragments, and the displaced fragments are drawn into anatomic position. After reduction and fixation, closure is accomplished as described with the interosseous wire technique.

ALTERNATIVE TECHNIQUE OF LATE RECONSTRUCTION WITH OSTEOTOMIES AND/OR ONLAY BONE GRAFTS

Osteotomy is a valuable adjunctive technique for the late deformity and dysfunction following medial maxillary fracture. The degloving approach provides exposure to the inferior portion of the fracture, but for the superior portion of the fracture that often extends to the frontal process of the maxilla and inferior orbital rim, additional periorbital incisions are necessary. The infraciliary incision, with a skin-muscle flap, provides excellent exposure of the inferior orbital rim. This direct approach also avoids injury to the infraorbital nerve. For the frontal process of the maxilla, a medial canthal incision one half the distance between the dorsum of the nose and inner caruncle is helpful. Elevation of the periosteum on the frontal process of the maxilla will demonstrate the fracture of the nasal bones and extension of the fracture toward the medial wall of the orbit.

a The osteotomies should be performed with a 3-mm osteotome (hand surgery type), directing the cuts along the fracture lines. With small elevators, the bones are reduced and repositioned into their anatomic relationships. If there happens to be some coexisting resorption, the surgeon can set small gaps and secure the bones with miniplates. Once significant resorption has occurred, interposed bone grafts will be required.

b,c In those cases of medial maxillary fracture in which resorption of bone is significant, the surgeon is advised to proceed directly with onlay grafts. Usually the objective is to fill the concavity caused by the depression of the medial maxillary buttress, but if these deformities extend to the frontal process of the maxilla or infraorbital rim, these areas also must be corrected.

Depending on the requirements to fill the defect, several pieces of split cranial bone graft are harvested from the ipsilateral parietal bone. The medial maxilla is exposed by a degloving, infraciliary and/or medial canthal approach, and the periosteum is elevated off the involved area. The cranial bones are carved to fit the defect and inserted beneath the periosteal pockets. The grafts are secured by closing the periosteum with 3–0 chromic sutures.

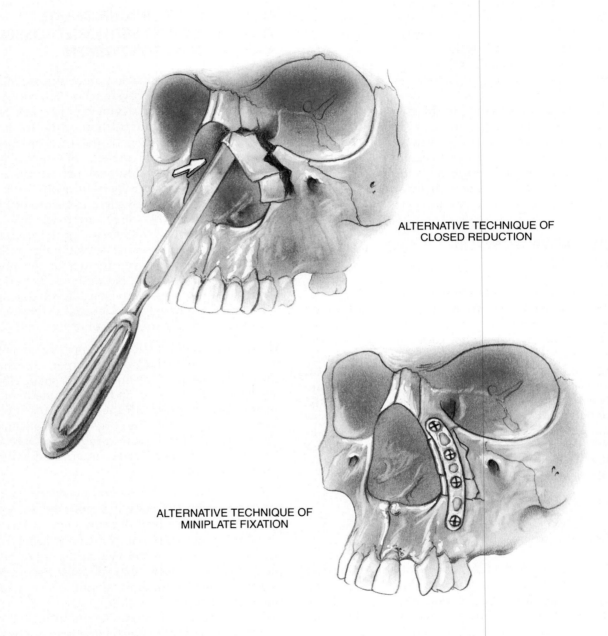

ALTERNATIVE TECHNIQUE OF
CLOSED REDUCTION

ALTERNATIVE TECHNIQUE OF
MINIPLATE FIXATION

ALTERNATIVE TECHNIQUES FOR MEDIAL MAXILLARY FRACTURE REPAIR
(Continued)

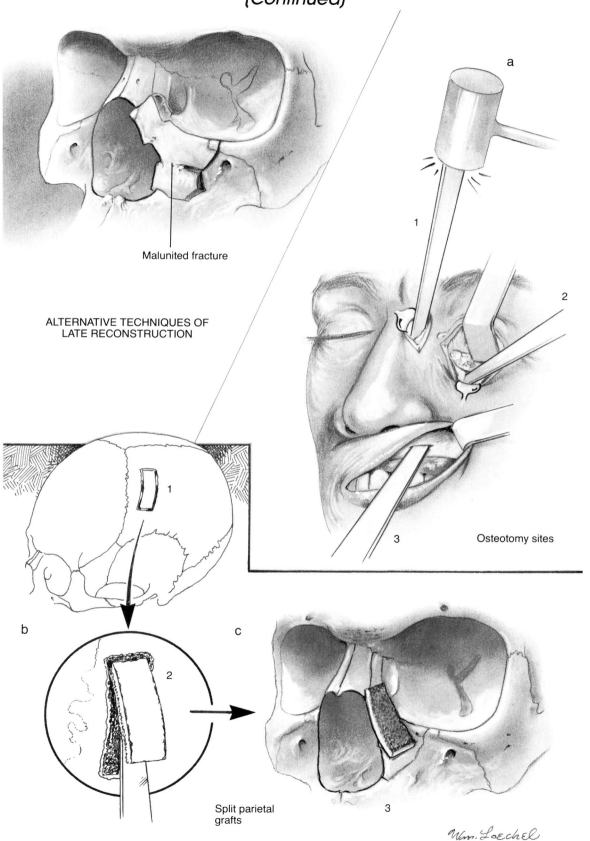

Malunited fracture

ALTERNATIVE TECHNIQUES OF
LATE RECONSTRUCTION

a

Osteotomy sites

b

c

Split parietal
grafts

Wm. Loechel

193

Palatal Split

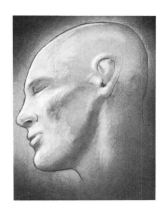

chapter 40

Repair of Palatal Split With Arch Bar Fixation
Alternative Techniques Using a Heavy Arch Bar (Jelenko) and Miniplate Fixation

INDICATIONS

A split palate in a patient with teeth is probably best treated with intermaxillary fixation. Setting the upper and lower jaws into occlusion and using the lower jaw to stabilize the upper jaw secures and stabilizes the dental arch. The teeth of the lower jaw also serve to stop inward and outward rotation of the hemipalates. The obvious disadvantage of intermaxillary fixation is that the patient's mouth is closed for 4 to 6 weeks and oral and masticatory functions are impaired for this period of time.

PROCEDURE

A Nasotracheal intubation or tracheostomy is performed. The maxillae should be mobilized as described in Chapter 32 so that the hemipalates are placed into anatomic position. Other facial fractures should also be reduced appropriately.

B,C An Erich arch bar is first attached to the lower dentition (see Chapter 8). The upper dental arch is then manipulated into approximate occlusion and the arch bar attached to the upper dentition to stabilize the midline split. If there is a large cleft, the surgeon can split the arch bar at the fracture and repair the arch bar later with horizontally placed 26-gauge wire loops. Alternatively, the surgeon can use a temporary 26-gauge transdental loop wire across the incisors. The upper and lower arch bars are subsequently secured to each other with elastic bands or 28-gauge wire loops. Reduction and fixation are evaluated, and occlusion is checked to ensure pretraumatic relationships. The associated facial fractures are wired or plated.

Postoperatively the patient is placed on oral antibiotics (i.e., penicillin or erythromycin). Reduction of fractures is confirmed by routine facial radiographs. Cleaning of the teeth and arch bars with chlorhexidine mouthwashes and a water irrigation device is important. Intermaxillary fixation is kept in place and adjusted when necessary for approximately 6 weeks. The patient should be followed monthly for at least 6 months. Puréed and soft diets are used to maintain nutritional status.

PITFALLS

1. Complete mobilization of the hemipalates is essential for the reduction and fixation. If the reduction is not accurate, the tension can be adjusted with the elastic bands or wires until the desired results are achieved. If this does not obtain pretraumatic relationships, then a formal open procedure with reduction should be performed.

2. In patients who are partially edentulous, Erich arch bars may not provide sufficient stability. For improved fixation, the surgeon should consider the heavier (Jelenko) arch bars, miniplates (see later), or palatal splints (see Chapter 41).

3. When approximating the fracture anteriorly, be careful not to distract the posterior segments of the palate. The arch bar should be tightened just until intermaxillary fixation and interdigitation of molars are complete. This sequence will prevent lateralization of the hemipalates.

COMPLICATIONS

1. Nonunion following a palatal split is frequently associated with malocclusion and problems with mastication. It usually becomes evident after removal of the arch bars, but if there is infection or soft tissue necrosis, it can be suspected at an earlier time. The complication can be avoided by accurate reduction and fixation, maintenance of local hygiene, and prophylactic antibiotics. Postoperative infection should be treated with cultures and specific antibiotic therapy. Initially the mobile maxilla can be treated as a delayed union with additional fixation, but if movement is still present after 8 to 10 weeks, the surgeon will have to consider alternative methods. As with other nonhealed fractures, it will be necessary to freshen the edges of the fracture, reduce the fragments, and apply rigid plates. Whether bone grafts are necessary will depend on the loss of bone and the malocclusion created by the loss of the bone fragments.

2. Malunion caused by a palatal split should be handled in the same way as malunion resulting from upper alveolar fractures. Occlusal readjustment, limited extractions, and orthognathic methods should be considered (see Chapter 42).

3. When the palatal fracture is associated with comminution and infection, it is possible for the patient to later develop an oroantral or oronasal fistula. Our preference is to first control the infection and then perform intranasal antrostomies (if the sinus is involved) and allow the wound to close by secondary intention. Contraction of the tissues will make for a smaller fistula and provide for an easier repair. We then consider a three-layer closure: (1) a trap door rotation of the superficial layers of palatal tissue; (2) insertion of a free piece of temporalis fascia between the palate and nasal flaps; and (3) a rotation of palatal flaps based on the greater palatine artery. Bilobed flaps can also be used.

ALTERNATIVE TECHNIQUE USING A HEAVY ARCH BAR (JELENKO)

If the reduction of the palatal split seems to proceed easily and the hemipalates seem to assume an anatomic position, the surgeon can employ the technique using a single heavy (Jelenko) bar. The heavy bar can act as a splint, and if it is applied accurately, it will immobilize the fragments in the desired position. The technique is particularly useful in patients with a partially edentulous jaw and in whom there is a need for stable support across the edentulous areas. However, the procedure should be abandoned if there is any instability and other methods of immobilization (i.e., intermaxillary, rigid plate, or prosthetic fixation) should be used.

For the heavy bar technique, the fractures should be reduced and occlusion ensured by an interdigitation of the teeth without premature contact. A Jelanko arch bar is then attached to the upper dentition with circumdental wires. If the occlusal relationships are questionable, the surgeon should apply an Erich arch bar to the lower dentition and use intermaxillary fixation as a guide.

Postoperatively the patient should maintain oral hygiene with chlorhexidine mouthwashes and water irrigation of the dentition. Prophylactic antibiotics should be used for 5 days and fixation maintained for approximately 6 weeks.

ALTERNATIVE TECHNIQUE OF MINIPLATE FIXATION

In many patients a single rigid miniplate across the premaxilla is sufficient for fixation. The technique is particularly suitable for the split palate in the edentulous patient, as the plate often provides sufficient immobilization for the fracture to heal. The disadvantage is that the anterior nasal spine and premaxillary crest can make it difficult to place the plate flat against the premaxilla; also, the plate can sometimes be felt, thus annoying the patient.

The rigid plate technique requires an accurate

REPAIR OF PALATAL SPLIT

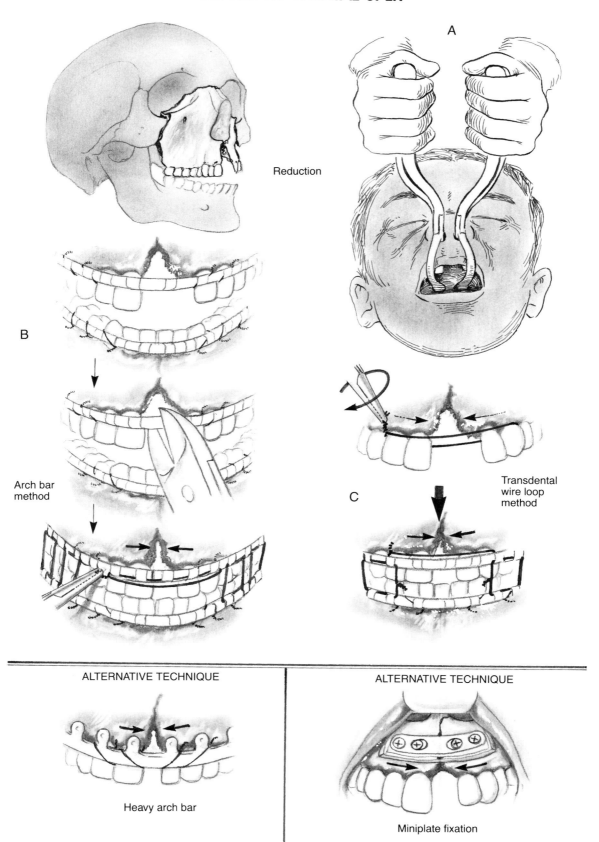

A

Reduction

B

Arch bar method

Transdental wire loop method

C

ALTERNATIVE TECHNIQUE

Heavy arch bar

ALTERNATIVE TECHNIQUE

Miniplate fixation

reduction of the dental arch to pretraumatic occlusion. The premaxilla is approached by a gingivolabial sulcus incision 5 mm above the margin of the gingiva. The periosteum is elevated to the level of the piriform apertures, and the fracture is exposed. If the fracture reduction and occlusal relationships are anatomic, the plate can be applied. If there is a pronounced ridge inferior to the anterior spine, this can be flattened with a cutting bur.

We prefer the minicompression plate with self-tapping screws. The procedure requires that the holes closest to the fracture be drilled first; other screws are then placed through the outer holes to give added support. Preliminary bending of the plate to an accurate contour prevents extraction of the fragments during application of the screws.

The incision is closed with interrupted 4–0 chromic sutures, and the patient is maintained on antibiotics for 5 days. A soft diet should be utilized throughout the fixation period (6 to 8 weeks).

chapter 41

Reduction and Fixation of Palatal Split With Prosthesis and Screws

INDICATIONS

In the edentulous patient who has dentures, the surgeon has the option of reducing the split palate and applying the patient's upper denture directly to the upper dental arch and palate. If there is some concern about the reduction, it is also possible to apply arch bars to the dentures, fix the dentures to the upper and lower jaws, and secure the dentures to each other with intermaxillary fixation. This technique provides the best opportunity to restore pretraumatic occlusion. Alternatively, if the surgeon does not want to use the patient's dentures or dentures are not available, a prefabricated splint can be used or occlusion can be approximated and a rigid fixation plate applied across the premaxilla (see Chapters 9, 20, and 40).

PROCEDURE

A–E Using general anesthesia administered through nasotracheal intubation or tracheostomy, the maxillary fractures are reduced as discussed in Chapter 32. Pretraumatic occlusion is approximated, and the upper denture is placed tightly against the reduced palate. Small holes are made with a bur on each side of the denture, and with appropriate drill bits (i.e., smaller than the screws), deeper holes are then drilled through the palate. Self-tapping screws, measured so that they just pass through the bone, are then used to secure the denture to the palate. If the maxilla is also unstable, drop wires with or without interosseous wires can be applied (see Chapter 33).

Postoperatively the reduction is assured by radiographic evaluation. The patient is treated with prophylactic antibiotics and oral hygiene maintained with chlorhexidine mouthwashes. Healing should occur by about 6 weeks, and at that time the denture can be removed.

PITFALLS

1. Although the prosthetic technique can be rapidly applied, it is a closed method and there can be problems with the reduction and fixation. Clinical and radiographic verification must be obtained in the postoperative period.

2. If there is any question regarding occlusion, the surgeon should apply arch bars to the upper and lower dentures and secure the upper denture to the zygoma with circumzygomatic wires and the lower denture to the mandible with circummandibular wires. The dentures are then placed into occlusal relationships and held with intermaxillary fixation.

COMPLICATIONS

1. Erosion beneath the denture is always a possibility. Unfortunately, until the denture is removed, there will be little evidence that this has occurred. Preventive measures are to secure a firm fit and cushion the denture on the alveolus with a soft liner. Prophylactic antibiotics and oral hygiene are helpful. Once erosion is noted, the denture should be removed and the area treated with ointment and local debridement and irrigations. If the damage is severe (i.e., oronasal or oroantral fistula) then flap closures may be necessary (see Chapter 40).

2. All of the complications associated with denture techniques can develop when using this method for repair of a palatal split. These conditions are discussed in Chapter 9.

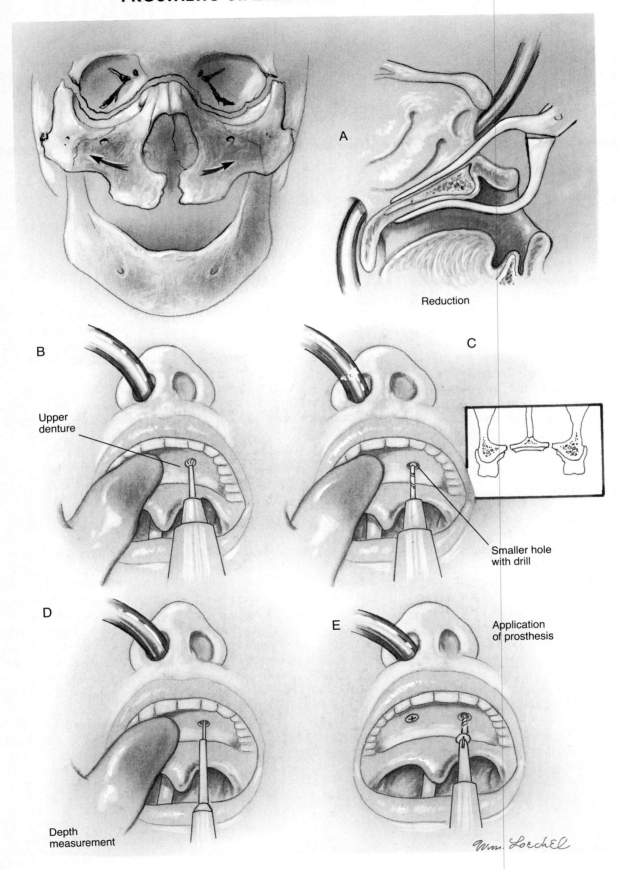

A

Reduction

B

Upper
denture

C

Smaller hole
with drill

D

Depth
measurement

E

Application
of prosthesis

Wm. Loechel

section VII

Malunion of the Maxilla

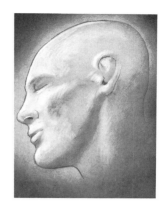

---

chapter 42

Correction of Low Maxillary Retrusion or Lengthening With Le Fort I Osteotomies
Alternative Technique Using Onlay Grafts

In Consultation With Robert Bruce MacIntosh, DDS

INDICATIONS

Malposition of maxillary fractures can impose functional and esthetic burdens on the trauma patient. Facial deformity and masticatory, temporomandibular joint, and speech dysfunctions are often presenting complaints. When they are severe, they evoke significant psychological changes. Malunion of the maxilla requires careful evaluation and application of modern craniofacial and orthognathic principles for appropriate therapy.

The objectives for surgical treatment are restoration of proper occlusion and a normal three-dimensional appearance of the face (i.e., in height, width, and projection) effected through strategic refracturing and stabilization of the bones. From an aesthetic standpoint, the surgeon should consider reconstruc-

tive surgery following malunion of Le Fort I fractures when there is retrusion of the upper lip, reduced projection of the nasal spine, or retraction of the columella. Additional indications are lengthening of the face and retrusion of the maxilla, particularly when there is a severe functional compromise of premature contact of the molars and an open bite deformity.

Pretreatment evaluation should include photographic, radiographic, and clinical assessment of the functional and aesthetic imbalance. For most Le Fort fractures, the surgeon should secure information regarding anosmia, cerebrospinal fluid leaks, loss of vision, diplopia, epistaxis, loss of facial sensation, and nasal obstruction. The surgeon should analyze the degree of flattening of the face in the anteroposterior direction, projection of the nose, and depression of the orbital rims and malar bones. Changes in the positions of the globes and intercanthal distances and in height and width of the palpebral fissures should be noted. Lateral and frontal cephalometric radiographs utilizing both bone and soft tissue densities will define the skeletal and soft tissue imbalances. Dental films, facial bone plain films, and computed tomographic (CT) scans (three-dimensional, when practicable) are also important parts of the evaluation. Dental occlusion should be recorded by standard nomenclature, wax bite registration, and dental models.

Careful review of all these diagnostic aids defines the indications for care and the particular procedures to be employed. Photographs taken in repose and in dynamic facial expression define the frontal, oblique, and lateral facial deformities; intraoral photographs record the functional imbalances of the dental occlusion. Radiographs show lines of fracture and aeration of the sinuses. Cephalometric films, particularly, define the skeletal deficiency and suggest the degree of movement necessary to establish skeletal norms and effect changes in soft tissue contour. Dental models should be appropriately sectioned and manipulated to define the movements necessary to restore proper occlusal relationships; interocclusal acrylic wafers made on the sectioned models often serve to guide and stabilize the occlusion during the surgical procedure. Orthodontic and prosthodontic consultations are helpful, and even mandatory, in determining the appropriate treatment plan.

PROCEDURE

Nasotracheal intubation is customary in the management of these problems, but if the patient has had a tracheostomy, this provides an ideal method of anesthesia. The face and neck are surgically scrubbed and draped as sterile fields. Arch bars or Ivy loops are applied to the dentition if the patient does not have the advantage of orthodontic appliances (see Chapter 8). The nasal mucous membranes are treated with 4% cocaine containing epinephrine, and the buccal sulci are infiltrated with 1% lidocaine containing 1:100,000 epinephrine. If palatal incisions are to be utilized, the same solution is deposited over the greater palatine and nasopalatine foramina.

A–E There are two commonly employed approaches through the soft tissue to the bone of the maxilla. One entails a horizontal incision made in the gingivolabial sulcus, 5 to 7 mm above the gingival margin, from one maxillary tuberosity region to the other. Through this incision, the periosteum is elevated off the anterior maxilla, exposing the anterior nasal spine, piriform apertures, infraorbital nerves,

and zygomas. Elevation of the periosteum should be extended along the floor and lateral walls of the nose with special Cottle elevators. Medially the mucoperichondrium and mucoperiosteum of the nasal septum are elevated in continuity with the mucosa of the floor of the nose (see Chapter 49). A subperiosteal dissection is also extended laterally and posteriorly around the maxillary tuberosities into the pterygomaxillary fossae, preserving the mucosa of these regions; exposure in this area is often somewhat limited.

F–H The second soft tissue approach is somewhat more difficult but often provides better mobility and freedom of the mobilized bone. Vertical incisions are made from the height of the gingivolabial sulcus inferiorly to the gingiva, at the midline (overlying the anterior nasal spine), in the bicuspid regions, and in the area of the terminal molars. A subperiosteal reflection through these incisions allows elevation of the tissues, as with the other approach. Additionally, however, the palatal soft tissues are reflected along a line of incision that extends in a horseshoe configuration from one greater palatine foramen to the other, coursing anteriorly in the trough between the alveolar arch and the horizontal palate, and across the midline in the area of the rugae. The elevation of the palatal tissues eliminates their restrictive influence on displacement of the maxilla, particularly advancement.

Osteotomies are performed with Lindeman burs, electric saws, or mallet and chisels. Horizontal cuts are initiated through the lateral rim of the piriform aperture at a level at least 5 mm above the apices of the dental roots. The appropriate level can be estimated by measuring the length of the canine crown and making the osteotomy at a point 5 mm higher than twice the crown length. Ideally, although not usually possible, the sinus mucosa can be protected by carrying the osteotomies just through the thickness of the maxillary bone. The nasal mucosa should be preserved by elevating it off the lateral wall and floor of the nose while the osteotomies are being made at these two sites with the osteotomes. Using subperiosteal tunnels, the cartilaginous septum, the vomer, and the perpendicular plate of the ethmoid are separated from the palate with the septal chisels. Posteriorly the maxilla is loosened from the pterygoid plates with a curved osteotome directed into the pterygomaxillary groove.

If the maxilla has been approached through the optional lateral vertical incisions and the soft tissues of the palate are reflected distally, additional mobility can be obtained by a posterior sectioning of the maxilla. This is accomplished with a vertical osteotomy made through the maxillary tuberosity anterior to the pterygomaxillary interface and onto the palate

LE FORT I OSTEOTOMIES

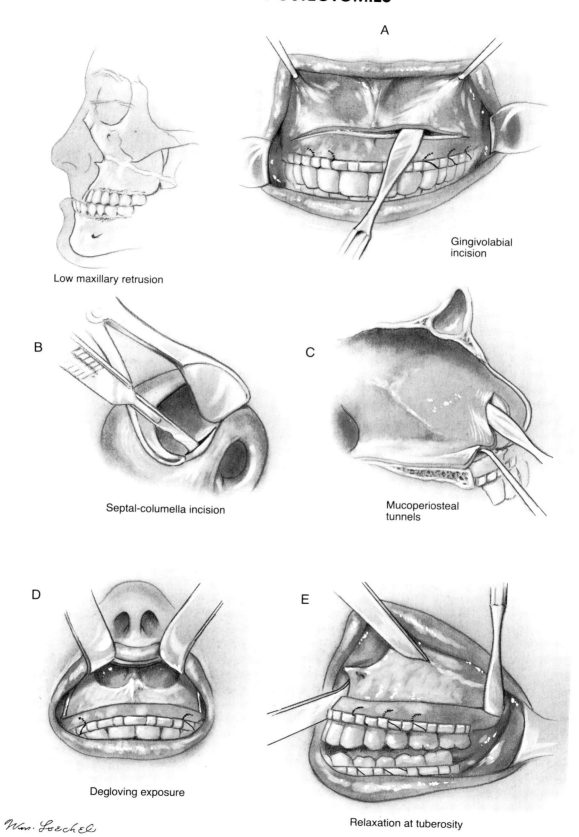

A

Gingivolabial
incision

Low maxillary retrusion

B

Septal-columella incision

C

Mucoperiosteal
tunnels

D

Degloving exposure

E

Relaxation at tuberosity

Wm. Loechel

203

LE FORT I OSTEOTOMIES *(Continued)*

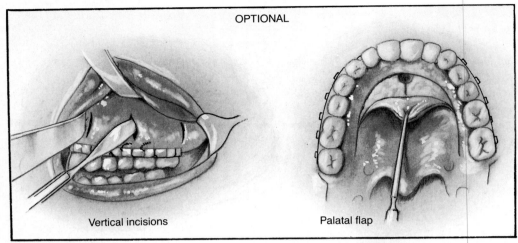

OPTIONAL

Vertical incisions

Palatal flap

F

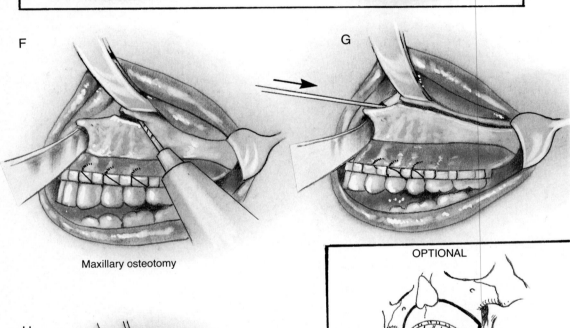

Maxillary osteotomy

G

H

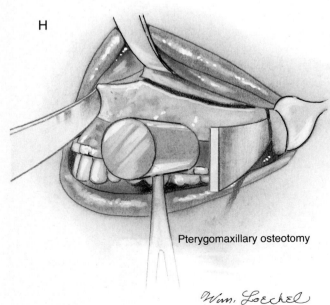

Pterygomaxillary osteotomy

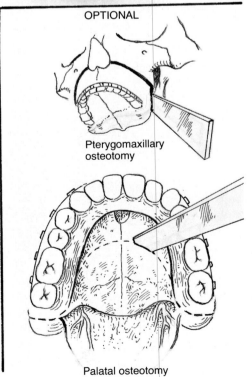

OPTIONAL

Pterygomaxillary
osteotomy

Palatal osteotomy

Wm. Loechel

204

to continue as a transverse bone cut across the palatal midline to the same region on the opposite side. Blood loss in the posterior aspect of the wound is quite often less with this approach.

I–K Following completion of the osteotomies, the maxilla is mobilized by applying torque to the bone along the fracture lines with osteotomes or elevators and applying traction to the maxilla with Rowe disimpaction forceps. The operator must be careful, in the down-fracture mobilization, to avoid injury to the descending palatine vessels, which should become visualized on the lateroposterior walls of the nose as the maxilla is drawn inferiorly; if the palatal tissues have been reflected and the posterior vertical osteotomies are made anterior to the pterygomaxillary interfaces, the descending palatine arteries will remain intact within the stable posterior bone and the reflected palatal soft tissues and will not be as affected by the mobilization of the maxilla.

L Once the maxilla is fully mobilized and the desired functional relationship with the lower dentition attained, it is next stabilized in this position. Miniplate fixation, as an option, offers the advantage of greater stability, at least in the short run, but has the disadvantage of inflexibility, thus allowing little margin of error in repositioning the mandible and the condyles and often requiring subsequent removal. The application of miniplates is described in Chapter 32. Intermaxillary fixation is applied to the previously placed arch bars or Ivy loops, usually with 26-gauge stainless steel wire. If teeth are missing or the occlusion is otherwise complex, an acrylic occlusal splint prepared preoperatively on the surgical models facilitates precise positioning of the dentition (see Chapter 8). If miniplate stabilization is not used in the edentulous patient, preoperatively prepared acrylic splints are mandatory to provide the appropriate functional relationships of the maxillae; such splints are first secured to the individual jaws and then to each other with intermaxillary wires. In intermaxillary fixation, elastic bands may be applied more quickly and replaced more easily than wires, but they have the disadvantage of applying continuous dynamic traction, which can loosen teeth and/or displace the fixation apparatus (see Chapter 33). Once fixation is applied, any significant deficits between the bone fragments should be obliterated, depending on size, with grafts from the outer parietal plate, the mandible, or the iliac crest.

Postoperative care parallels that utilized in primary management of the Le Fort I fracture. Prophylactic antibiotics are administered for 5 to 10 days. Strict adherence to oral hygiene is mandatory and is often best effected with an electric intraoral water spray device. Stabilization is maintained for 6 to 8 weeks.

Monitoring postoperative progress with standard radiographs, cephalometric films, and photographs is very helpful. The patient should be examined at regular intervals to intercept, and hopefully correct, developing problems and to obtain an objective evaluation of the final result of surgery.

PITFALLS

1. The tooth roots should be preserved. A point 5 mm above the apex of the canine root should be marked along the facial skeleton to ensure proper placement of the osteotomy.

2. Avoid unnecessary injury to the blood supply to the mobilized maxilla. When the transverse incision in the vestibule is used, most residual blood supply is derived from the palatine arteries, and they should be preserved. When the vertical vestibular incisions are used and the palatal soft tissues reflected, the palatal blood supply is obviated in the early postoperative stages, and the viability of the maxilla depends on the vessels coursing inferiorly through the lateral soft tissues. The nasal and antral mucosal supply can be important with either technique, and to whatever degree possible, this mucosa should be left intact.

3. Mobilization of the maxilla should be complete. Appropriate traction and torquing with the osteotomes along the lines of osteotomy and careful but firm application of the Rowe disimpaction forceps should be utilized.

4. It is important to stabilize the mobilized maxilla in the proper occlusal position. This is facilitated by careful preoperative analysis of the wear facets on the teeth, study of the preoperative dental models, and careful construction of acrylic splints to stabilize the maxillary and mandibular dentitions to one another, particularly in patients with missing teeth or otherwise confusing preexistent malocclusions.

5. To avoid instability caused by defects between the bone segments, bone grafts are necessary along the anterior and posterior buttresses of the maxilla and pterygoid plates. Miniplate or direct wiring fixation is often required to hold such grafts in their anatomic positions.

COMPLICATIONS

1. Brisk intraoperative bleeding may occur during the procedure but will usually stop within 5 to 10 minutes in patients with normal coagulation profiles. When a large vessel has been transected, gauze packing within the mouth and pharynx and nasal packing treated with 4% cocaine containing epinephrine will help to control the bleeding.

2. Postoperative respiratory problems can occur as a result of pharyngeal edema, excessive secretions within the posterior mouth or pharynx, or drowsiness resulting from fatigue, unusual blood loss, or overmedication with sedatives or analgesics. Extubation thus should not be carried out until the patient is alert and all bleeding has been brought under control. The patient with a tracheostomy has an obvious advantage with regard to this problem.

3. Infection and/or necrosis of the mobilized segment can best be avoided by careful handling of the soft tissues. The blood supply is essential, and the surgeon should attempt to preserve most nasal and sinus mucosa, as well as the mucosa of the posterior maxilla. Special attention to preservation of the palatine vessels during manipulation of the maxilla is important. Infection is usually managed with cultures and appropriate antibiotics. Healing will often be delayed, with a resultant need for a prolonged period of intermaxillary fixation. True necrosis may take weeks or even months to run its course, and the degree of debridement necessary will be determined by the extent of the tissue death; additional surgery of one type or another is almost always necessary in such cases.

4. The factors that cause a regression and/or relapse of the maxillary position are not clear, but stable fixation and maintenance of normal occlusal relationships during the healing period should help prevent this complication. Bone grafting across bony defects also is a deterrent to postoperative change. Miniplates probably offer the best chance of at least short-term stability. Significant regression mandates additional procedures such as orthodontic care, onlay grafts, or surgical repositioning of part or all of the maxilla.

ALTERNATIVE TECHNIQUES USING ONLAY GRAFTS

Upper lip retrusion or accentuation of the nasolabial fold can often be improved with onlay graft techniques. These procedures are useful in those instances in which the occlusion is satisfactory and corrective osteotomies to improve aesthetics would result in unacceptable shifts of the dentition. Onlay procedures are also indicated as small secondary improvements for those patients in whom orthognathic surgical procedures produce incomplete aesthetic change. Onlays provide simple, expedient improvements, and although early good results can be expected, the surgeon must be aware of the tendency for unpredictable healing and resorption when autogenous bone is used. Such grafts are harvested from the cranium (see Chapter 58), rib (see Chapter 17), or iliac crest (see Chapter 60) and are best immersed in blood or wrapped in antibiotic-soaked sponges until ready for implantation.

Autogenous or bank cartilage and alloplastic materials, most commonly silicone rubber or polytetrafluoroethylene, may also be employed as onlays. The latter have an advantage in that they do not undergo resorption, but their disadvantages include potential mobility and greater chance of infection. Alloplastic grafts have also been shown to evoke significant foreign body reactions.

The areas to be grafted are exposed through small gingivolabial sulcus incisions and subperiosteal dissections sufficient to create pockets just large enough for insertion of the grafts. The graft is appropriately trimmed and inserted and the periosteum closed tightly with chromic sutures. If the graft proves too mobile, it can be secured to the underlying bone with fine steel wires or lag screws; however, the screws can sometimes fracture the onlay, and quite often, because of palpability, they require subsequent removal.

The patient should be treated postoperatively with antibiotics and a light compression dressing. Strict oral hygiene is mandatory.

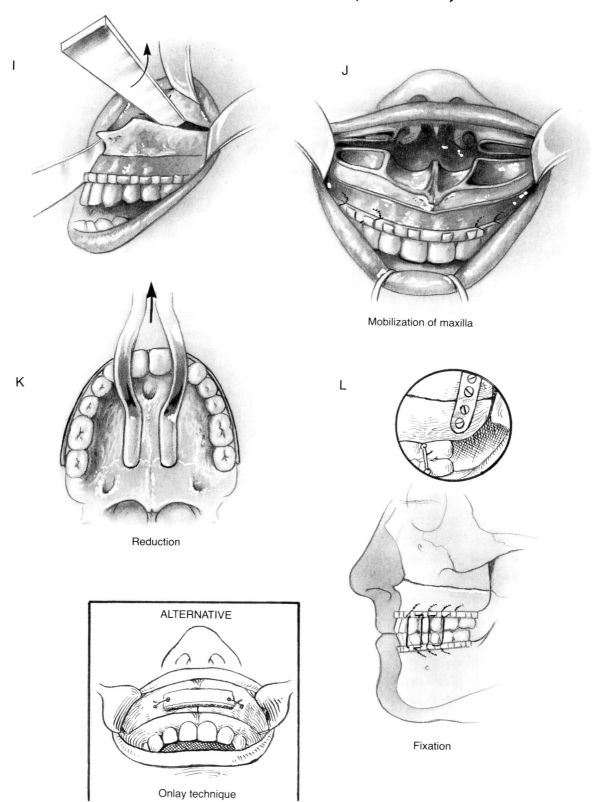

I

J

Mobilization of maxilla

K

Reduction

L

Fixation

ALTERNATIVE

Onlay technique

Wm. Loechel

chapter 43

Correction of Maxillary Retrusion or Lengthening With Le Fort II Osteotomies

In Consultation With Robert Bruce MacIntosh, DDS

INDICATIONS

Deformity and dysfunction following Le Fort II maxillary trauma can present a formidable problem to the reconstructive surgeon. The patient often has a retrusion of the midface and changes in the length of the face. Apertognathia (open bite) and other imbalances in the occlusion are common. In addition, the fracture is often associated with nasal obstruction, telecanthus, epiphora, and displacement of the medial wall of the maxilla. Like patients with malunions resulting from low maxillary fractures (see Chapter 42), these patients require a sophisticated evaluation of respiration, olfactory and masticatory functions, and aesthetic imbalance. Photographic records in both passive repose and dynamic facial muscle function, radiographic imaging (including cephalometry), wax bite registration, and dental models are all pertinent to proper evaluation.

Corrective Le Fort II osteotomies are best applied to those patients with symmetric midfacial retrusion in which there is symmetry of the nasal bones and normal maxillary height. Malunion resulting from unilateral Le Fort II fracture or from a bilateral but asymmetric fracture are more difficult to correct because of the complexity in planning asymmetric corrective procedures. In any case, corrective Le Fort II osteotomy should be considered when evaluations indicate that both reestablishment of functional dental occlusion and improvement in nasomaxillary aesthetics are required for effective rehabilitation. The preparations for orthognathic surgery of this type are described in Chapter 42.

PROCEDURE

A preexisting tracheostomy is ideal for providing anesthesia. Nasotracheal intubation can be used but makes any required nasal surgery difficult. Orotracheal intubation precludes the establishment of good dental occlusion and should be avoided. Tonometric values are recorded preoperatively.

A Exposure is obtained through the gingivolabial, medial canthal, infraciliary, or other infraorbital incisions. The gingivolabial incision exposes old fractures on the lateral aspect of the maxilla and provides access for lateral maxillary, retromaxillary, and lower nasal osteotomies. Medial canthal incisions allow exploration of the attachment of the nasal bones to the frontal process of the maxilla and the frontomaxillary buttresses. Infraciliary incisions provide access to the inferior orbital rim and floor of the orbit. These exposures, in combination, provide adequate access for the corrective osteotomies and allow the operator to avoid injury to the medial canthal ligament, the lacrimal sac, the soft tissues of the orbit, and the infraorbital nerve.

B The medial canthal incision is laid in a generally vertical curvilinear direction, one half the distance between the caruncle of the eye and the dorsum of the nose. After cautery or ligation of the angular vessels, the periosteum of the nasal bones and frontal process of the maxilla are elevated, and the trochlea is detached from the orbital rim. By avulsing or clipping the anterior ethmoidal vessel, the surgeon can explore the medial wall of the orbit superiorly and deep to the medial canthal ligament. For visualization of the bridge of the nose, the periosteum should be completely elevated off the nasal bones and lower portion of the frontal bone.

C The infraciliary incision is made about 2 to 3 mm below the cilia and lateral to the puncta of the lower eyelid. A cuff of periosteum is developed inferior to the orbital rim, and the periosteum is then elevated off the rim and floor of the orbit. The periosteal pocket should be connected with the one developed along the medial wall of the orbit.

D–G Using malleable retractors to protect the me-

Le Fort II Osteotomies

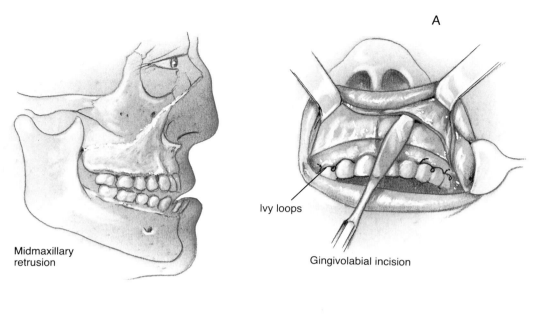

Midmaxillary retrusion

Gingivolabial incision

Ivy loops

A

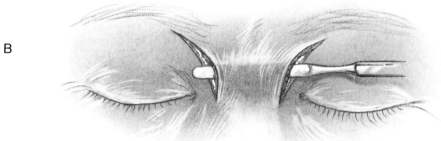

B

Medial canthal incisions

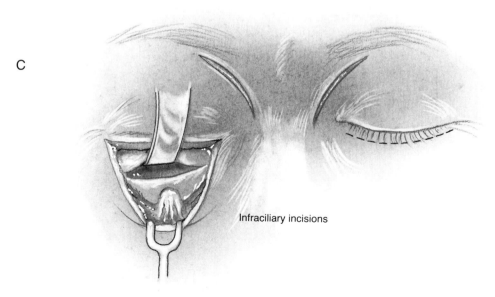

C

Infraciliary incisions

Wm. Loechel

Le Fort II Osteotomies *(Continued)*

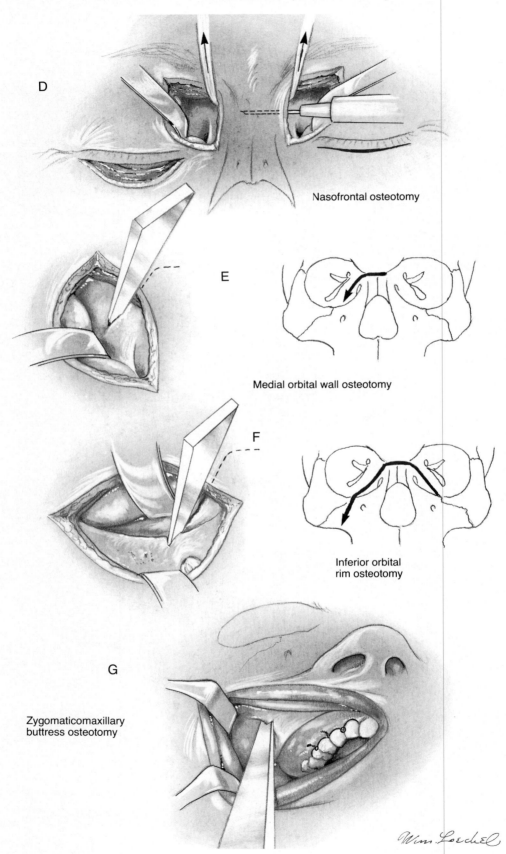

D

Nasofrontal osteotomy

E

Medial orbital wall osteotomy

F

Inferior orbital
rim osteotomy

G

Zygomaticomaxillary
buttress osteotomy

dial canthal ligament, the lacrimal sac, and orbital soft tissues, Lindeman or other fine burs are used to lay an osteotomy across the bridge of the nose, just below the nasofrontal suture line. Working on one side at a time, this cut is next extended inferolaterally across the frontal process of the maxilla and along the medial wall of the orbit. Through the medial canthal and/or infraciliary incision, the bone cut is extended across the floor of the orbit with small, sharp osteotomes or fine bone burs. The orbital floor osteotomy is carried laterally to the point for transection of the orbital rim. The bone cut is brought across and through the rim and onto the lateral face of the zygoma. The osteotomy, from this point inferiorly through the anterior wall of the maxilla, can be made at least partially from the superior approach or from below through the intraoral incisions.

Exposure of the maxilla intraorally need not be as extensive as that for the Le Fort I osteotomy. Horizontal incisions in the gingivolabial and gingivobuccal sulci to ensure full exposure of the zygomaticomaxillary buttresses need only extend from the maxillary tuberosity areas anteriorly to approximately the bicuspid regions. The same exposure can also be obtained through optional vertical incisions made from the height of the sulcus inferiorly to the attached gingiva at the bicuspid and tuberosity regions on either side, with the mucoperiosteal tissues between the incisions being elevated off the bone in a tunneling, subperiosteal fashion. Use of the vertical incisions allows reflection of the palatal soft tissues; this often eliminates any restrictive tendencies of those tissues to mobilization of the maxilla, while providing direct access to the bone of the palate for placement of an osteotomy (see Chapter 42). No subperiosteal reflection is necessary from the midline to the zygomaticomaxillary buttress, as no osteotomy will be placed in this area. The elevation of periosteum is restricted to the area from the anterior maxilla superiorly to the infraorbital rims, with care being taken to protect the infraorbital nerve with the retractors. The subperiosteal exposure is carried posteriorly to the pterygomaxillary interface.

G Using Lindeman burs and/or osteotomes, a bone cut is made inferiorly from the infraorbital rim, either vertically from the lateral aspect of the rim, so as to include the prominence of the zygoma, or obliquely from the rim further medially so as to traverse the anterior maxilla either superiorly or inferiorly to the infraorbital nerve. Again, this cut may be made in part through the infraorbital exposure. In any case, this facial osteotomy will cut through the base of the zygomaticomaxillary buttress at a variable point and then course directly posteriorly above the apices of the teeth to the maxillary tuberosity region.

H The pterygomaxillary osteotomy is carried out through the horizontal or vertical (optional) incisions. If the maxillary osteotomy is carried all the way to the pterygomaxillary junction, it is joined to a vertical separation between the plates and the tuberosity effected with a curved osteotome; if the horizontal osteotomy is terminated in the tuberosity itself, anterior to the pterygomaxillary junction (an optional procedure), it is joined to a vertical bone cut made with the bur vertically through the tuberosity and medially onto the palate. In this latter instance, a bone cut is made transversely across the palate to join the vertical osteotomy coming through the tuberosity on the opposite side. Separating the maxilla through the tuberosity sites avoids some of the bleeding encountered when the maxilla is separated from its junction with the pterygoid plates and provides a more stable posterior surface for support of any interpositional bone grafts.

I,J To complete the separation of the maxilla from the skull, the vomer and perpendicular plate of the ethmoid, as well as the lateral wall of the nose, must also be released. These bone cuts are effected first by directing a small, sharp osteotome through the osteotomy at the bridge of the nose diagonally downward and backward toward the posterior part of the palate and, second, slightly laterally through the osteotomy at the bridge to transect whatever portion of the lateral nasal wall may be still intact high in the superior portion of the nose. The surgeon can ensure the correct angle of the osteotome as it courses through the septum by placing a finger within the nasopharynx and palpating it as it penetrates the posterior nares. Final mobilization of the maxilla is effected through lifting and torquing with the osteotomes along the osteotomy sites and careful disimpaction with the Rowe forceps. Complete mobility of the sectioned midface is necessary to ensure proper adaptation to the mandibular dentition, correct adaptation and stabilization of any grafts, and a lessened tendency toward postsurgical regression.

Bleeding will be brisk as the osteotomes are placed, particularly following total mobilization. If the patient has normal coagulation profiles, however, the bleeding should stop in several minutes. The surgeon should wait until all significant bleeding has stopped before proceeding with the fixation portion of the procedure.

K There are several acceptable methods of establishing occlusal relationships and fixation. Usually the occlusion is stabilized with Ivy loops or, preferably, with arch bars, with or without an interocclusal wafer. The proper occlusal relationships will have been determined preoperatively through study of the dental models as described in Chapter 42. In the edentulous patient, proper functional relationships

Le Fort II Osteotomies (Continued)

H

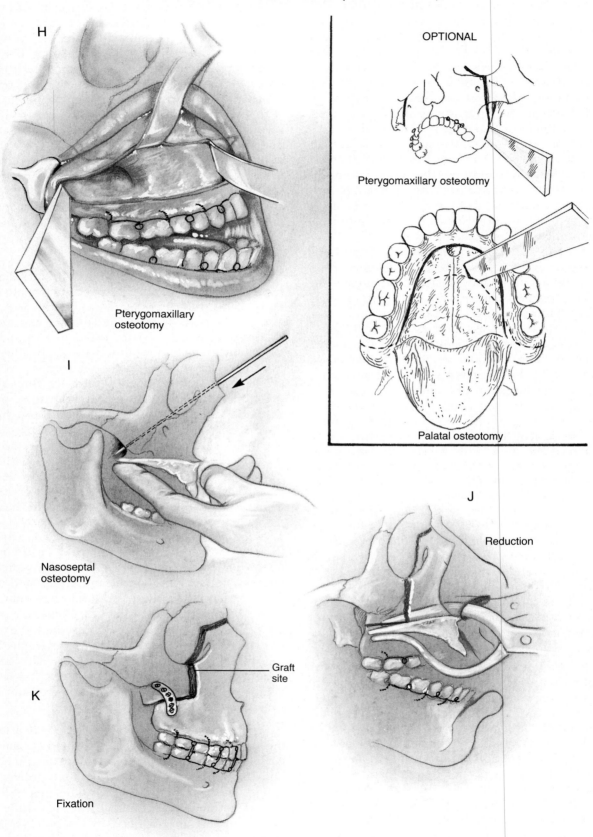

Pterygomaxillary
osteotomy

OPTIONAL

Pterygomaxillary osteotomy

Palatal osteotomy

I

Nasoseptal
osteotomy

J

Reduction

Graft
site

K

Fixation

of the maxilla and mandible are determined preoperatively and the mobilized maxilla stabilized with intermaxillary fixation of the patient's preexisting dentures or specially fabricated maxillary and mandibular acrylic splints. The latter are stabilized with either bone screws or wire fixation.

Following establishment of intermaxillary fixation, the fracture lines are inspected and the interosseous defects stabilized with autogenous grafts obtained from the cranium, rib, or iliac crest. Often the grafts can be appropriately morticed and wedged into position so that they themselves do not require fixation. Stabilization of the mobilized midface, however, is mandatory; miniplates offer the best stability, at least for the short term, but craniomandibular or craniofacial wiring offer greater adaptability and versatility.

Tonometric values are again recorded, and all facial incisions are closed in layers. The patient is treated for at least 5 days with intravenous antibiotics (i.e., cephalosporins or penicillins). Facial films obtained several days postoperatively are helpful in evaluating aeration of the sinuses, and cephalometry will demonstrate the revised skeletal relationships. Oral hygiene is best maintained with chlorhexidine or hydrogen peroxide washes, and the dentition is best cleaned with a water irrigation device. Intermaxillary fixation is maintained for a 6-week period.

PITFALLS

1. The Le Fort II osteotomy is best applied to the patient with a retrusion of the midface and a fairly normal architecture of the nose. The patient with a major nasal deformity is probably better treated with a Le Fort I correction and subsequent independent rhinoplasty, with or without implants to the nose.

2. Avoid injury to the soft tissues during osteotomy. The best insurance against this type of complication is adequate exposure of the bony surfaces and judicious use of retractors and sectioning instruments. If the medial canthal ligament or lacrimal sac are injured, they should be repaired during the procedure. Small tears of the periorbita can be left open to heal by secondary intention.

3. Assure proper dental occlusion. This requires a comprehensive preoperative evaluation and osteotomies that gain complete mobility of the maxilla. If instability is still present after occlusion is obtained, external halo fixation may be used. This will help stabilize the fractures during the entire course of the healing and provide an opportunity to adjust projection and length of the face. Changes in skeletal status can subsequently be checked with cephalometry (see Chapter 38).

COMPLICATIONS

1. Most of the complications related to corrective Le Fort II osteotomies are similar to those related to other midface corrections (see Chapters 42 and 44). Postoperative bleeding, breathing difficulties, infection, and malunion are all possible as a result of the Le Fort II procedure, and the surgeon should become familiar with the methods that are available to prevent and treat these difficulties.

2. Nasal obstruction and deformity is common with the Le Fort II injury and may not be adequately addressed with corrective Le Fort II osteotomies alone. Adjunctive septorhinoplasty procedures may be required. These considerations are discussed in Chapter 49.

3. Residual contour defects following healing of corrective Le Fort II osteotomy sometimes require additional care. Various materials can be used in these efforts, but probably cranial bone or alloplastic grafts offer the best assurance of success. These procedures are usually executed as subsequent revisional operations, but occasionally, when such deficits can be anticipated preoperatively, they can be carried out at the time of the Le Fort II osteotomy.

chapter 44

Correction of Midfacial Retrusion or Lengthening With Le Fort III Osteotomies

In Consultation With Robert Bruce MacIntosh, DDS

INDICATIONS

Le Fort III osteotomies are primarily used for midfacial retrusion associated with inadequate malar and infraorbital rim projection. Such patients usually present with concave facial profiles ("dishface" deformities) and lengthening of the face. A retruded maxillary dentition is characteristic, very often in association with the open bite malocclusion and multiple deformities and dysfunctions found with fractures of the orbits, nose, malar bones, and/or mandible.

Evaluation of the malunited Le Fort III injury mandates assessment of aesthetic compromises and functional imbalances, most particularly in the skeletal and dental relationships. As in malunion resulting from lower maxillary fractures, these patients require a sophisticated clinical evaluation, photographic records, radiographic imaging, bite registration, and dental models (see Chapter 42). Orthodontic and/or prosthetic consultation is often helpful in defining the dental and skeletal considerations. Orbital and nasal deformities are particularly important, and ophthalmologic consultation is often mandatory. A neurosurgical opinion is advisable whenever cranial injury is part of the original trauma.

Once all diagnostic criteria have been duly weighed, the surgeon must determine whether Le Fort III refracturing offers a significant advantage over less hazardous lower midfacial repositioning combined with onlay cosmetic procedures.

PROCEDURE

Tracheostomy is the preferred method of providing ventilation and anesthesia and should be carried out as a preliminary procedure either under local anesthesia or following a temporary oral intubation. Ivy loops or, preferably, arch bars are adapted to the teeth, and the entire face and neck are then surgically scrubbed and draped as sterile fields. Tonometric values are recorded.

A combination of incisions is necessary for adequate access to the skeleton. The more common combinations are coronal and maxillary gingivolabial incisions or frontoethmoid (medial canthal), infraorbital, and gingivolabial sulcus incisions.

A The coronal incision, made in an area shaved prior to the sterile scrubbing, should extend superiorly from just above the preauricular creases on one side to a point just posterior to the recesses of the temporal hairline. It is then placed anterosuperiorly several centimeters behind the hairline in a gentle curving configuration to a similar position on the opposite side. Infiltration of the scalp with a vasopressor containing local anesthetic assists hemostasis. The incision can be carried through the periosteum but is usually made just through the galea, with the soft tissues reflected anteriorly in a supraperiosteal fashion. The flap is progressively rotated anteriorly to a level just above the superior orbital rims, at which point the periosteum is incised throughout the width of the reflection. Branches of the superficial temporal artery are controlled with cautery or suture ligation.

B The dissection progresses subperiosteally along the superior orbital ridge and the bridge of the nose. The supraorbital neurovasculature is reflected with the flap; the supraorbital foramina, if present, are opened gently with fine osteotomes to facilitate the maneuver. Progressive subperiosteal reflection allows exposure of the superior and medial walls of the orbit and freeing of the trochlea. Additional relaxation and exposure are obtained by clipping the anterior ethmoidal artery.

Laterally the surgeon should elevate the attachment of the temporalis muscle at the frontozygomatic process. Continuation of the subperiosteal dissection allows release of the lacrimal gland from its fossa.

214

Le Fort III Osteotomies

A

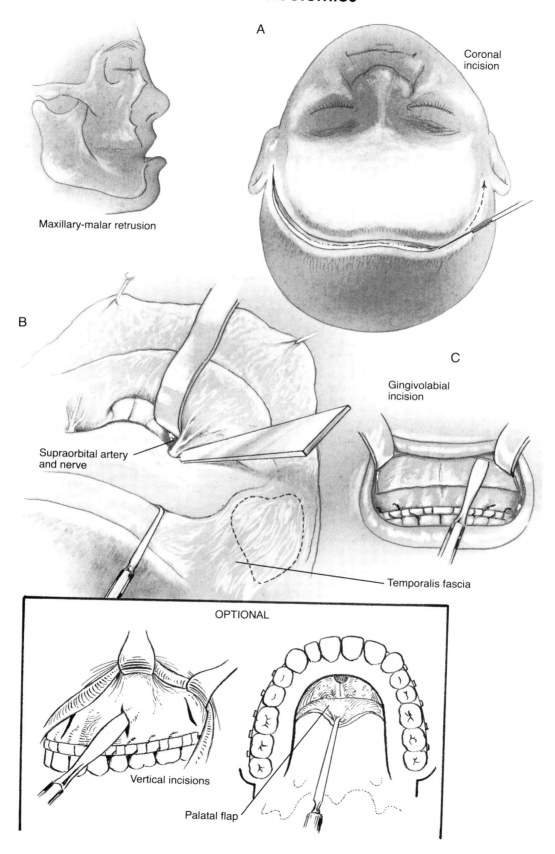

Maxillary-malar retrusion

Coronal incision

B

Supraorbital artery
and nerve

C

Gingivolabial
incision

Temporalis fascia

OPTIONAL

Vertical incisions

Palatal flap

The lateral canthal ligament is also relaxed with its periosteum, and the dissection is continued along the body and arch of the zygoma. To maintain function of the temporal branch of the facial nerve, long periods of forceful retraction on the soft tissues must be avoided.

C The options for exposure of the maxilla intraorally are those used for execution of the reparative Le Fort II osteotomy as described in Chapter 43. One of the approaches entails a horizontal incision in the height of the buccal sulcus, extending from the bicuspid area posteriorly to the pterygomaxillary interface; in this case vascularity of the posterior maxilla at the alveolar level is maintained through the palatal soft tissues. The second option utilizes vertical incisions made from the height of the sulcus inferiorly to the attached gingiva in the cuspid and third molar regions and a curvilinear reflection of the palatal soft tissues extending from one greater palatine foramen, forward across the rugae, and then posteriorly to the opposite foramen; in this case vascularity to the lower posterior maxilla is maintained through the vertical soft tissue drapes. Subperiosteal reflection through either of the lateral incisions allows exposure of the anterior and lateral walls of the maxilla, the zygomaticomaxillary buttresses, the infraorbital nerves, the nasomaxillary junctions, and the piriform aperture. When the palatal reflection is used, direct exposure of the bone of the palate is gained, and the resistance of the palatal tissues to maxillary displacement is obviated.

D Exposure of the orbital rims and floors is accomplished through infraciliary approaches. Access to the nasomaxillary interface through the intraoral exposure and to the orbital floor through the bicoronal flap is limited.

E–G The osteotomies begin at the bridge of the nose, and through the exposure from above, a horizontal cut is made just beneath the nasofrontal suture line. This cut is then brought laterally across the frontal processes of the maxillae and onto the medial walls of the orbit; with appropriate retraction, the osteotomy will not produce injury to the medial canthal ligament or lacrimal sac. With a fine osteotome or fine surgical bur, the osteotomy is carried inferiorly on the medial walls to the floors of the orbits, just behind the lacrimal collecting systems. Once these cuts are completed on both sides, the osteotome is placed into the bone cut at the bridge of the nose and directed inferoposteriorly toward the soft palate through the substance of the septum to free this structure from the base of the skull. The direction and depth of this osteotomy can be controlled by a finger placed in the nasopharynx.

H,I On the lateral walls of the orbits, osteotomies are made at a variable distance below the frontozygomatic suture line, either transversely through the full thickness of the lateral orbital rims or sagittally through the rims for a variable distance inferiorly; the latter cut results in a less abrupt interruption in lateral rim contour and broader contact of bony surfaces. The sagittal osteotomies of the rims should be made with very fine osteotomes or with the fine surgical bur. Through this same exposure, the zygoma (or arch) is osteotomized in a stepwise fashion.

On one side at a time, the orbital contents are retracted medially, and a bone cut is made through the lateral orbital wall inferiorly onto the floor of the orbit anterior to the inferior orbital fissure. The orbital contents are then gently elevated and this bone cut connected in the floor of the orbit to the osteotomy previously made on the medial wall. The bone cut across the floor of the orbit should be made approximately 1 cm proximal to the inferior orbital rim to avoid trauma to the orbit in the region of the apex. Access to the floor is often limited through the coronal approach, and it is in these instances that access through an infraorbital incision proves beneficial.

J The bodies of the zygomas are next sectioned free of the zygomatic arches. To complete these fractures, the maxilla must be separated at the alveolar arch levels in the region of the pterygoid plates. This may be achieved with an osteotome directed medially and slightly superiorly into the pterygomaxillary fissure or with an osteotomy extending from a point high on the maxillary tuberosity near its junction with the plates, inferiorly through the full thickness of the alveolar arch anterior to the pterygomaxillary junction, and across the hard palate to a similar position on the opposite side. This optional osteotomy requires reflection of the palatal soft tissues but lessens the chance of significant bleeding from the descending palatine artery and the pterygoid venous plexus.

K Even careful placement of all osteotomies does not guarantee mobility of the maxilla, and complete separation of the midface commonly requires forcible displacement with the Rowe disimpaction forceps and/or active elevation or torquing with osteotomes placed into the osteotomy sites. Complete mobility must be gained, however, if the surgeon is to ensure proper positioning of any grafts, establishment of correct dental occlusion, and a lessened chance of postoperative regression. Bleeding is usually brisk during these mobilization maneuvers but will come under control spontaneously as mobilization efforts are completed.

L Once complete mobilization is gained, preopera-

D

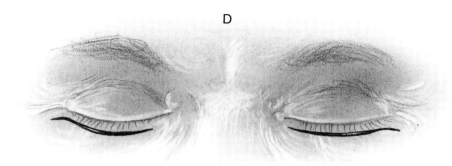

Infraciliary incisions

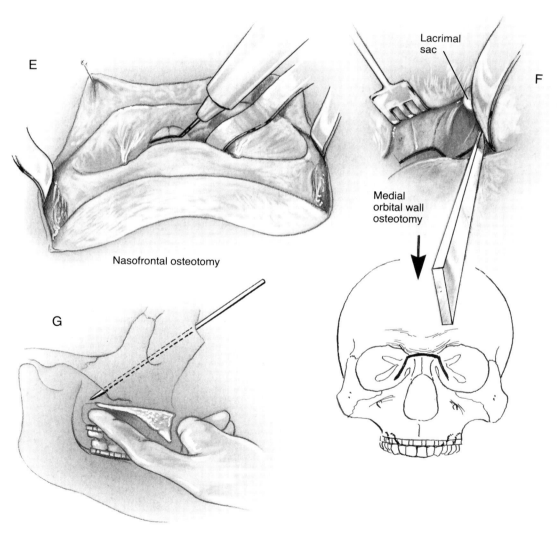

E

Nasofrontal osteotomy

F

Lacrimal sac

Medial orbital wall osteotomy

G

Nasoseptal osteotomy

Le Fort III Osteotomies *(Continued)*

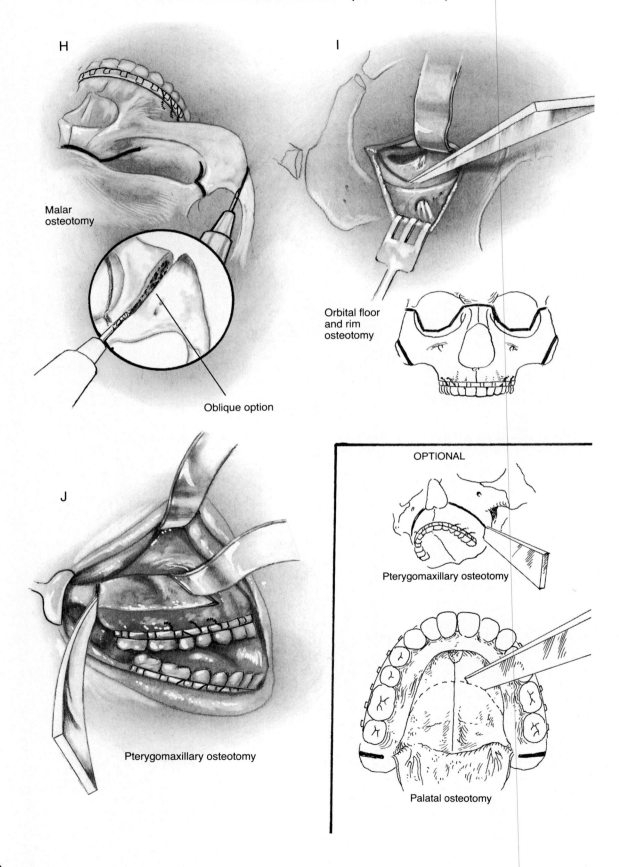

H

Malar
osteotomy

Oblique option

I

Orbital floor
and rim
osteotomy

J

Pterygomaxillary osteotomy

OPTIONAL

Pterygomaxillary osteotomy

Palatal osteotomy

Le Fort III Osteotomies *(Continued)*

K

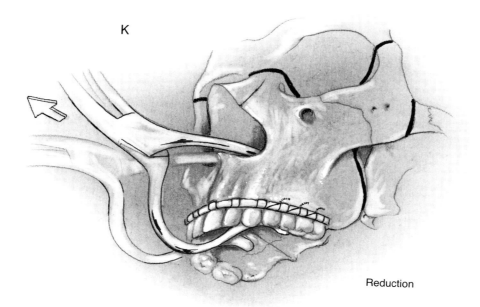

Reduction

L

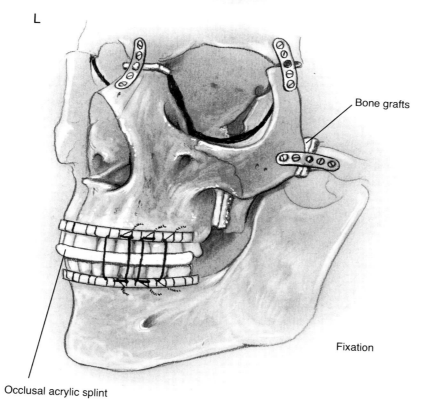

Bone grafts

Fixation

Occlusal acrylic splint

tively determined dental occlusion is established and stabilized with intermaxillary wiring, often with the use of an intermaxillary occlusal acrylic splint. Bone grafts, preferably autogenous and taken from the ileum, rib, or parietal cortex, are placed into the osteotomy defects. Careful contouring and wedging often precludes the need for assisted stabilization of these grafts, but the maxilla, especially if it is loose, requires stabilization with miniplates and/or craniofacial and/or craniomandibular wiring suspension. Fixation plates generally provide greater stability, at least initially, but suspension wiring is more versatile and adaptable. Head frame stabilization may offer the advantage of adjustment of the fixation in the postoperative period.

The incisions, with the exception of the intraoral, are closed in layers, though it is often impossible to reapproximate the periosteum at every osteotomy site. A light compression dressing is applied over the scalp flap. Tonometric readings are taken at the completion of the procedure.

Postoperatively the patient is carefully monitored for evidence of hematoma or changes in sensorium and vision; immediate drainage of recognized intraorbital hematomas is mandatory. Antibiotics (usually cephalosporins or penicillins, with or without aminoglycosides) are maintained intravenously for approximately 5 days following surgery. Stability of the dental occlusion is monitored clinically. Radiographs taken within the first few postoperative days allow evaluation of graft positions, aeration of the sinuses, and cephalometric change. The patient should be examined at regular intervals for at least 1 year postoperatively to intercept any tendencies toward skeletal regression.

PITFALLS

1. Ensure appropriate indications for the procedure. The Le Fort III osteotomy is a complex operation demanding intimate familiarity with the anatomy and objective evaluation of the gains to be anticipated. The technique should not be used when less extensive osteotomies and/or onlay grafts will suffice. It should be used cautiously in older patients and probably not at all in patients who have sensorium or vision instability.

2. Be prepared for profound bleeding. Brisk bleeding is to be expected during the osteotomy, especially following application of the disimpaction forceps and other final mobilization procedures. Pharyngeal and/or nasal packing may be helpful if blood loss is excessive. Blood transfusion may be necessary.

3. Do not attempt the procedure without a tracheostomy. All anesthetic techniques short of tracheostomy entail significant compromises in access and/or safety and should not be employed. Postoperative respiratory care is also facilitated with the tracheostomy.

4. Adequate mobility of the osteotomized segment must be gained. The pterygomaxillary area is a site of particular resistance, but additional mobility is sometimes achieved by cutting residual pterygoid muscle attachments. The surgeon can also place posterior vertical osteotomies through the tuberosities and anterior to the pterygomaxillary complex. Incomplete sectioning through the septum and through the orbital osteotomies can usually be eliminated with the final disimpaction maneuvers.

5. Appropriate advancement of the facial skeleton should be appreciated. In many patients, reestablishment of the occlusion automatically reestablishes the pretraumatic midfacial proportions. On the other hand, if the original trauma was asymmetric or otherwise erratic, reestablishment of the dental occlusion may not guarantee a satisfactory aesthetic result. If the patient is partially or completely edentulous, determining the proper dental relationships or stabilizing the occlusion intraoperatively can be difficult; in these cases, preoperatively designed interocclusal acrylic stabilization devices can be very helpful.

6. Care must be taken to avoid postsurgical regression. Intermaxillary dental fixation must be maintained for at least 6 weeks, and bone grafts placed at the site of osteotomy must be firmly fixed in position and held with either wedge force or direct plate or wiring fixation. The myriad of interfaces along the osteotomies generally aids in stabilization but does not obviate the need for careful stabilization of the mobilized midface with miniplates and/or wires. Halo frame application is an excellent option, not only for stability during the 6- to 8-week course of healing, but also to provide selective traction in the early postoperative days to allow minor correction in skeletal position.

COMPLICATIONS

1. Bleeding and airway obstruction can be life-threatening complications. Intraoperative bleeding generally does not occur as the result of severance of major vessels, and so it can usually be treated with hypotensive anesthesia, a vasopressor containing local anesthetic infiltration, gauze packing, and appropriately administered blood or blood product transfusion. A Le Fort III osteotomy should not be executed without a tracheostomy, as damage or kinking of the endotracheal tube, irritation of the vocal cords during the long procedure, or leakage of blood

around the cuff can all lead to significant ventilatory problems. The tracheostomy puts control of respiration both intraoperatively and postoperatively out of the surgical field, and the anesthesiologist and surgeon can work independently of one another. Postoperatively the tracheostomy affords easy assisted ventilation and tracheal hygiene.

2. Injury to the cribriform plate can result in cerebrospinal fluid leakage. This maloccurrence can generally be avoided by keeping the osteotome strictly in the midline, directing it downward toward the soft palate, and controlling its position with a finger in the nasopharynx. If a cerebrospinal fluid leak fails to stop, antibiotics should continue beyond the projected time, and the surgeon should consider repair of the dura using either a frontoethmoid or an intracranial approach (see Chapters 86 and 87).

3. Enophthalmos, hypophthalmos, and/or diplopia may also occur. Small diastases in the orbital floor can be managed with Gelfilm or Marlex mesh, but larger defects are best treated with autogenous bone grafts. Major displacements of an orbital wall are also best managed with appropriate grafting techniques (see Chapters 58 and 60).

4. Visual compromise, including blindness, is best avoided by placing the osteotomy in the floor of the orbit, no more than 1 cm proximal to the inferior orbital rim, and limiting the vigor of dissection and retraction. The dissection along the medial wall of the orbit should be restricted to the area anterior to the posterior ethmoidal artery. Retractors should be intermittently relaxed, and impingement of the retractors on the retrobulbar tissues must be avoided. Persistent bleeders in the area of orbital dissection should be treated with bipolar cautery or vascular clips. Any decrease in visual acuity should prompt an early ophthalmologic consultation, and hematoma of the orbit must be evacuated as soon as it is recognized. Tonometry at the completion of the procedure often provides an early indication of increasing intraorbital pressure. Other aspects of evaluation and treatment are described in Chapter 58.

5. Residual facial imbalances or occlusal disharmonies can occur following healing of the reparative Le Fort III osteotomy. Such imperfections can often be improved with onlay grafts, preferably of autogenous cranial bone or alloplastic material. Minor occlusal disharmonies can be accommodated with orthodontic or dental restorative measures, but major imbalances resulting from malposition or unacceptable regression may require additional osteotomies. Rarely is it necessary to recreate the entire Le Fort III sectioning.

part four

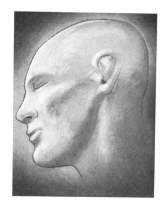

Nasal Fractures

section I

Classification and Pathophysiology of Nasal Fractures

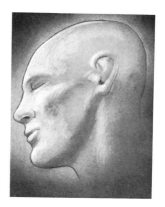

chapter 45

General Considerations

A Nasal fractures are the most common facial fractures. They occur frequently in children and are more often seen in men than in women. The projection of the nose from the face predisposes to injury; the midline septum offers little support, and there are additional weaknesses along the grooves created by the anterior ethmoidal veins. Because there is a greater cartilage-to-bone ratio in children compared with adults, fractures in children usually involve cartilage, whereas in adults the bone is usually broken and displaced, and the cartilage is involved secondarily.

A classification of nasal fractures is difficult because there are many variations. If the impact is from a frontal direction, the fracture will involve, in order, the nasal tip; the nasal dorsum, septum, and anterior nasal spine; and the frontal processes of the maxilla, lacrimal, and ethmoid bones. With a lateral oblique force, fractures will involve, in order, the ipsilateral nasal bone; the contralateral nasal bone and septum;

and the frontal processes of the maxilla and the lacrimal bone. On the basis of this pathophysiology, several syndromes can be defined; these are discussed in the text that follows.

TIP FRACTURE

B1 As a result of frontal impact, the nasal tip alone can be fractured and malpositioned. Usually the lower (caudal) portion of the fracture rotates inward and downward, while the upper (cephalic) portion rotates upward and outward. This rotation causes the development of a small hump and supertip depression.

FLATTENING OF THE NASAL DORSUM WITH SPLAYING OF NASAL BONES

B2 With more force from the anterior direction, the nasal bones are prone to fracture at a higher level

225

and will be pushed inward. The lateral part of the nasal bones at the same time will be splayed outward. The cartilaginous septum will buckle, the anterior nasal spine may fracture, and the nose will have a flattened appearance.

FLATTENING OF THE NASAL DORSUM WITH SPLAYING OF THE FRONTAL PROCESS OF THE MAXILLA

B3 In this condition, the anterior force is powerful enough to fracture the nasal bones, the frontal process of the maxilla, and the anterior nasal spine. Usually fractures are comminuted and tend to lateralize. The nose becomes markedly depressed, the columella becomes retracted, and the medial canthal ligaments are frequently relaxed, creating a telecanthus.

DEPRESSION OF THE LATERAL NASAL BONE

C1 A force from the lateral oblique direction often causes a depression of the nasal bone on one side of the nose. Simultaneously there is a raising of the nasal bone on the opposite side. The septum may buckle. Typically, the patient displays a C- or S-shaped deformity of dorsum of the nose.

DEPRESSION OF IPSILATERAL NASAL BONE AND FRONTAL PROCESS OF THE MAXILLA

C2,C3 If the lateral oblique forces are excessive, the fracture can extend to the frontal process of the maxilla. Usually the dorsum and septum are markedly displaced (more so than the ipsilateral nasal bone depression), and there is a depression of the medial wall of the maxilla. This fracture is a variant of a medial maxillary fracture and is described in Chapter 39.

NASAL FRACTURES

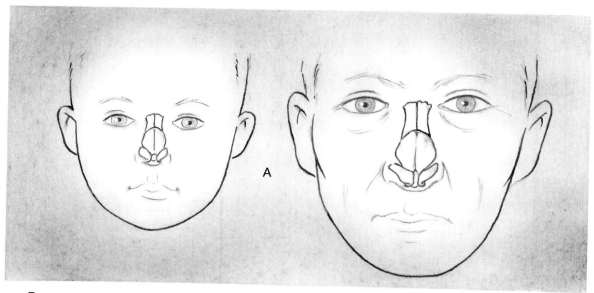

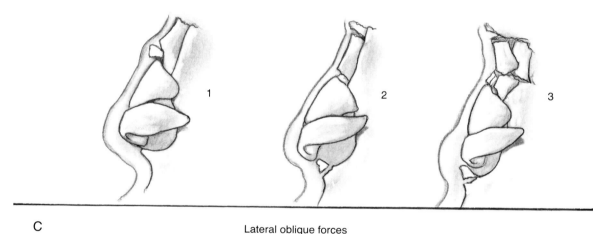

B   Frontal forces

1   2   3

C   Lateral oblique forces

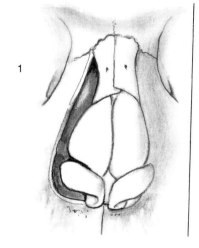
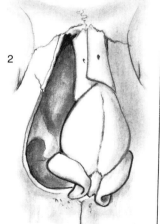
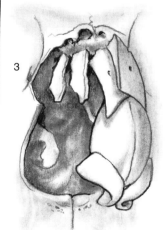

1   2   3

227

section II

Management Strategies

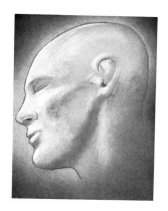

chapter 46

Closed Reduction of Nasal Fracture by Manipulation

INDICATIONS

Closed reduction usually provides satisfactory results in most types of nasal fractures. It should at least be given a trial, and if it is not successful, the surgeon can still treat the fracture by open reduction and/or elective rhinoplasty. The closed technique is also associated with minor morbidity. It is characterized by a short, easy-to-perform operation and rapid recovery.

The ideal patient for the closed technique is an individual who had a straight, nonobstructed nose prior to the injury and who sustained a tip or depressed ipsilateral nasal bone fracture. The technique is also effective in treating the acutely displaced septum and associated hematoma. The procedure will be limited if there is a frontal bone and/or lacrimal bone fracture or if the fracture also involves the medial wall of the maxilla. Nasal fractures associated with cribriform plate and cerebrospinal fluid leaks are probably better treated with techniques that avoid obstructive nasal packing. Timing of the surgery is

important. The procedure is best applied when most swelling has subsided (after about 5 days). After 10 to 14 days some healing will have occurred, and in these situations, other (open) methods should be considered.

PROCEDURE

A–C Sedation and anesthesia are an important part of the technique. If the surgeon chooses local anesthesia with sedation, the patient should be given sufficient medication for relaxation, cooperation, and amnesia. The nasal mucous membranes are then sprayed with ¼% oxymetazoline hydrochloride (Neo-Synephrine) followed by several sprays of 4% lidocaine. Additional levels of topical anesthesia should be obtained by strategic placement of cotton pledgets, moistened in a solution of 8 mL of 4% cocaine containing five drops of 1:10,000 epinephrine. This solution will provide sufficient vasoconstriction for the duration of the procedure. The pledgets are usually placed for about 10 minutes beneath the nasal dorsum, at the posterior edge of the middle turbinates, on the floors with extension into the inferior meati, and on the septum.

D,E After application of topical anesthesia, the surgeon should also block the nose with a local anesthetic. A 2% solution of lidocaine containing 1:100,000 epinephrine should be injected along the dorsum, the anterior maxilla, and the base of the septum to anesthesize the infratrochlear, infraorbital, and greater palatine nerves. Additional infiltration of the tip area should block the superior alveolar nerve and branches of sensory nerves to the skin.

If the patient chooses a general anesthetic, the same application of topical and local medications is advised, as these will provide for better visualization and control of bleeding. Moreover, in the postoperative period there will be less need for pain control and sedation.

F,G Manipulation should be carried out with the head slightly elevated so that the surgeon's light will illuminate most of the nasal cavity. Standard operating room lighting should be adjusted to minimize distortions and shadows. For the simple depressed unilateral nasal bone fracture, a Boies elevator can be used, but before elevation, the surgeon must make sure that the elevator is placed just beneath the depressed bone and not into the cribriform plate area. The depth of insertion is thus controlled by measuring externally the distance from the angle of the glabella to the tip of the nose and then applying the elevator just short of that depth. With a slowly increasing force, the nasal bone is elevated. The degree of elevation is controlled with external pressure exerted by the other hand, molding the fragments into appropriate position. Often the side opposite the depressed nasal fracture is also displaced laterally, and in such a situation, the contralateral bones should be pushed inward to develop the ideal pyramid.

For the nasal tip fracture, the elevation should be directed to the front part of the septum under the dorsum, and with the other hand, the dorsum should be molded into appropriate position. Bilateral comminuted fractures require bilateral elevation and a massaging of the fragments to achieve the desired effect.

H The septum should next be inspected. Often elevation of the dorsum will return the septum to the midline, but if this has not occurred, the surgeon can apply Ashe forceps to simultaneously elevate the dorsum and replace the septum to the midline. The septum should then be inspected to make sure there are no mucosal tears and a hematoma has not developed.

I,J Fractures of the nose and septum should be stabilized by external and internal splints. For a severely disrupted septum that has been repositioned in the midline, internal splints made of polyethylene can be trimmed and secured to the columella with a broadly based 3–0 nylon mattress suture. If the septum holds the midline and also has not been severely lacerated, the nasal openings can be packed with a light, bacitracin-treated gauze. Alternatively, a nasal tampon (with or without the polyethylene plates) can be used to control pressure and prevent bleeding.

K Splints to the external nose are easily made by an application of tape and plaster (see Chapter 47). The skin of the nose is first treated with an adhesive solution and the skin covered with pieces of tape applied to hold the nose in a normal anatomic position. About six to eight pieces of plaster are cut in the shape of a small shield; the plaster is then dipped into warm water and molded to the nose. The surgeon must be careful to keep the plaster from getting into the eyes. A drip pad over the nares is subsequently applied and secured to the cheeks.

The patient should be treated with antibiotics for the duration of the packing. Sufficient stability is usually obtained at 5 days, and at that time, internal and external splints can be removed. Crusts that subsequently develop on the mucous membrane should be actively and prophylactically treated with normal saline douches.

PITFALLS

1. Timing of the surgery is important. If the surgeon operates too early, the anatomy of the nasal structures can be obscured by swelling and ecchymoses. If operation occurs too late, the nasal bones will have united, and reduction will be difficult, if not impossible, to carry out. Ideally nasal fractures in children should be treated in 5 to 7 days. In adults, it is possible to obtain reduction up to 10 to 12 days after injury.

2. Results can be compromised by associated injuries. Radiographs of the nose can miss fractures of the facial bones, and the surgeon should not rely only on the patient's nasal appearance and examination of the nose. If there is any suspicion of additional injuries, the patient should be evaluated by computed tomographic (CT) scans in the horizontal and frontal planes. If additional fractures are found, appropriate techniques should be used to specifically address those fractures.

3. Adequate sedation and/or anesthesia is important to get good results. The uncooperative patient will often move about in the operating room and

CLOSED REDUCTION OF NASAL FRACTURE

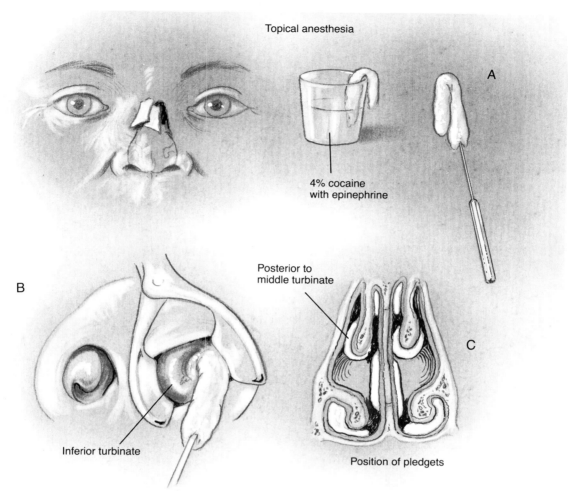

Topical anesthesia

A

4% cocaine
with epinephrine

B

Inferior turbinate

Posterior to
middle turbinate

C

Position of pledgets

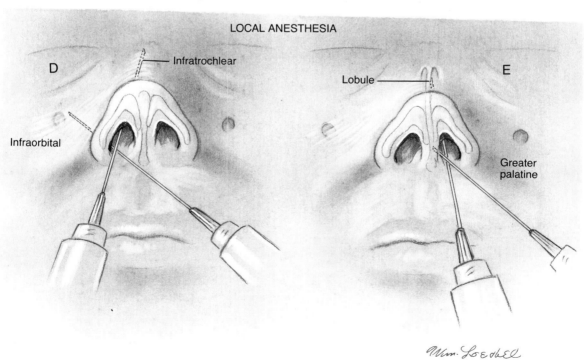

LOCAL ANESTHESIA

D

Infratrochlear

Infraorbital

Lobule

E

Greater
palatine

CLOSED REDUCTION OF NASAL FRACTURE *(Continued)*

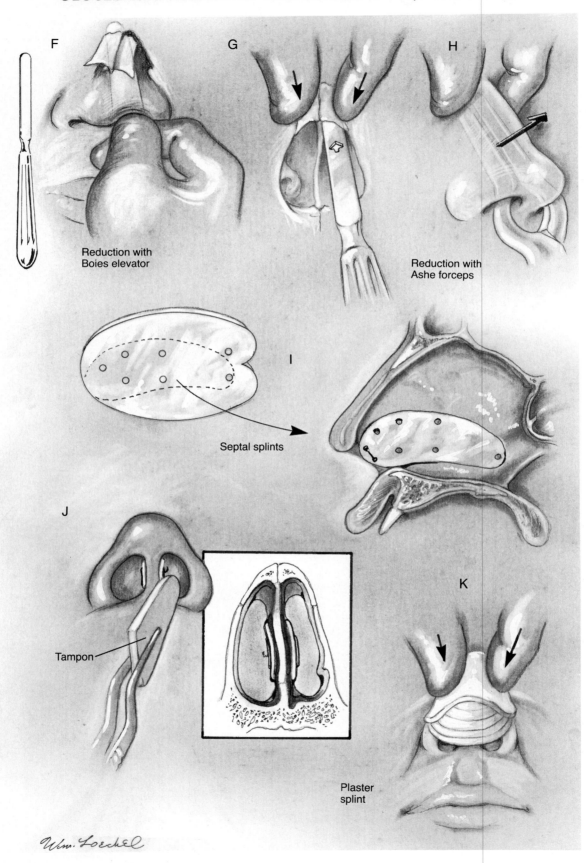

F

G

H

Reduction with
Boies elevator

Reduction with
Ashe forceps

Septal splints

I

J

Tampon

K

Plaster
splint

Wm. Loechel

cause bleeding. Moreover, postoperative restlessness and confusion can cause reinjury and should be avoided. Using the internal and external splints should at least prevent some of the postoperative traumatic sequelae from occurring.

4. Although the closed method is successful in most cases, the surgeon must be prepared for a semiclosed approach. Occasionally the septal fracture will leaf onto itself, or the nasal bones will not be reduced or held in the desired position. If such a situation develops, the septum can be exposed by a limited Killian incision and the fracture treated by removal of projecting bone and/or cartilage. The nasal bones can be reduced by making a cartilage-splitting or intercartilaginous incision and then manipulating the bones with small, needle-nosed rongeurs (see Chapter 48).

5. Packing should not be used for the reduction. It should be applied secondarily only after manipulation of bone and cartilage. The packing should support the structures in their anatomic position.

6. Improper application of septal splints can cause necrosis and perforation. To avoid this complication, the septum must have no evidence of hematoma. The suture that holds the splints must be placed into the fleshy part of the columella, not the intermembranous part, and the tie should be through a wide (3- to 4-mm) mattress suture. This approach will avoid excessive pressure and necrosis of intervening tissues.

COMPLICATIONS

1. Failure to reduce the fracture can lead to deformity and/or nasal obstruction. Although a rhinoplasty may be performed, the multiple relatively loose fragments will make control of the osteotomies difficult. Our preferred approach is to wait until the nose is healed (i.e., 3 to 6 months) and then proceed with a rhinoplasty to correct the specific postinjury deformities.

2. Septal hematoma must be recognized and treated appropriately. Failure to do so predisposes to necrosis of septal cartilage, saddle deformity, and retraction of the columella. If a septal hematoma develops, the area should be drained by a small vertical incision through the septal mucosa. The blood must be evacuated by suction. The mucosa should be placed back into normal position, which is then maintained by intranasal packing.

3. Infection following nasal injury is rare, but if it occurs, it can cause significant problems to the support of the nose. There can also be scarring of the overlying skin. Infection can be avoided, for the most part, with proper surgical techniques and prophylactic antibiotics.

chapter 47

Closed Treatment of Comminuted Nasal Fracture With Lead Plates
Alternative Technique Using Tape and Plaster

INDICATIONS

A forceful blow from the frontal or lateral oblique direction can often cause comminution and displacement of the nasal bones and septum with or without fractures of the adjoining ethmoid, lacrimal, and maxillary bones. When this injury occurs, the nasal bones and septum are usually reduced with a Boies elevator and/or Ashe forceps. The maxillary and nasoethmoid injuries are treated separately. If the nasal bones are unstable and tend to move laterally, the surgeon must consider retention plates made of lead or other suitable materials. The technique is also useful when there is a cerebrospinal fluid leak and the surgeon is trying to maintain reduction while avoiding an obstruction caused by nasal packs. If nasal obstruction is not going to be a problem, nasal packing and plaster splints can be considered.

PROCEDURE

A The lead plate technique is applied to the nasal fracture after reduction and fixation of other associated craniofacial injuries. Preparation should include vasoconstriction of the nasal mucous membranes with 4% cocaine containing epinephrine and an adjunctive block consisting of 1% lidocaine containing 1:100,000 epinephrine (see Chapter 46). If the vibrissae of the nose are blocking visualization of the internal nose, they should be trimmed accordingly. The nasal bones and septum are then reduced with the Boies elevator and Ashe forceps.

B–D The plates that will be molded to the outer surface of the nose are cut from malleable, thin lead sheets. The plates are designed in the shape of a rectangle, 1 to 1.5 cm × 2 to 3 cm; the corners should have a gentle curve. The plates are pressed and bent to fit over the nasal bones and a portion of the upper lateral cartilages. A soft Silastic sheeting is cut just slightly larger than the plates and placed under the plates as a protective cushion. The plates (with Silastic) are again adjusted to the nose, and two scratches are made on the outer surface of the plates in a line parallel to the long side of the plate and at least 1.5 cm apart.

E–G The plates and Silastic are placed together and a 1-mm drill hole is placed through the markings. The plates are then reapplied to the surface of the nose. A fine wire suture swaged onto a long needle is then passed through the more cephalic hole of the plate (and Silastic) and then directly through the marks on the skin, through the nasal bones and septum. The needle is passed through the opposite plate (and Silastic) and back through the caudal markings on the plate and nose. This mattress closure is then tightened to accurately secure the plate and compress the nasal bones.

The plates may require further adjustment, and if they cut into the skin, the edges should be bent appropriately. An antibiotic ointment is applied to the edges of the plate. If the septum requires stabilization and/or nasal bleeding is a concern, a light, antibiotic-soaked packing can be applied to the nasal passageways. The plates are removed in 7 to 10 days. Prophylactic antibiotics should be used for the duration of treatment.

PITFALLS

1. The plates should be applied to narrow the nasal bones. With swelling from the trauma, there will be a tendency for the nasal bones to splay, especially near their attachment to the frontal processes. This problem can be avoided by making sure the wire is placed posteriorly on the plates and the plate itself rests on and compresses the frontal process of the maxilla.

2. Avoid a closure that is too tight, or else the

REPAIR OF COMMINUTED NASAL FRACTURE

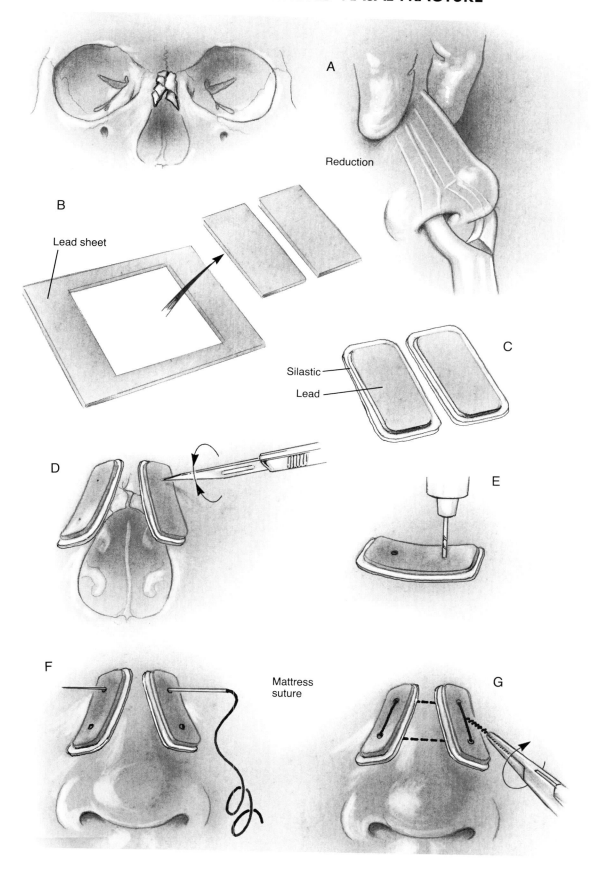

A

Reduction

B

Lead sheet

C

Silastic

Lead

D

E

F

Mattress
suture

G

plates will cause necrosis and scarring of the skin. The soft Silastic can serve as a cushion and should be used as a lining beneath the plates.

3. Note also that if the wire is applied too loosely, the plates will tend to shift out of position. A decrease in swelling following the repair is to be expected, and during the 24 to 48 hours following the procedure, the surgeon should reexamine the compression and tighten the wire accordingly.

COMPLICATIONS

1. Malunion of the nasal bones will occur if the initial fixation is not accurate or the plates slip out of position. The surgeon must make sure that the reduction is effective in loosening impacted fragments and that the plates are designed to hold the fragments into normal anatomic position. Because it is cosmetically desirable to have a narrow dorsum, the surgeon should attempt to achieve this effect. Plate position should be continuously monitored, and if there is a displacement of the plates and/or the nasal bones, the plates should be reapplied. If deformity occurs, corrective rhinoplastic surgery can later be considered (see Chapter 49).

2. Infection can occur around the plates, especially if there is a preexisting skin injury or a new injury created by undue pressure of the plate. This complication can be avoided by adjusting plate tension, applying local antibiotic ointments, and administering prophylactic parenteral antibiotics. If infection develops, the plates will have to be removed. The infection will require appropriate debridement and antibiotic therapy as determined by culture.

3. Scarring can occur from pressure necrosis and/or infection. These scars should be allowed to mature and then treated by revisional techniques. Wide areas of tissue loss may require local advancement and/or rotation flaps.

ALTERNATIVE TECHNIQUE USING TAPE AND PLASTER

Because of the potential pitfalls associated with application of lead plates, the surgeon can also choose to apply a plaster cast and fix the cast tightly to the skin of the nose. The obvious disadvantage of this technique is that the cast is "permanent," and as the swelling disappears, it cannot be adjusted to the new contour. Moreover, adhering the cast to the nasal skin does not provide fixation as secure as that obtained with a mattress wire. There will thus be a tendency for the cast to slip prior to the desirable 7- to 10-day period of fixation. Packing of the nose with a plaster cast may be indicated for control of bleeding and/or additional support of the nasal skeleton, but it is contraindicated in those patients with a cerebrospinal fluid leak.

a–c The plaster technique first requires reduction of the nasal bones and, if needed, internal splinting with antibiotic-treated gauze. A tape dressing is then applied. The skin must be clean and coated with appropriate adhesive. Quarter-inch strips of soft, pliable tape are then cut and placed over the entire tip and dorsum. Overlapping of the strips will prevent development of skin marks.

d–f The plaster cast is made in the shape of a shield from approximately six pieces cut from a four-inch roll. The narrow portion fits into the intercanthal space, and the wide part covers the upper lateral and cephalic portions of the lower lateral cartilages. The cast should reach the frontal processes of the maxilla so that the nasal bones can be kept medial to these processes. The plaster is then soaked quickly in hot water and applied immediately to the nose. A dry 4 × 4 sponge placed over the plaster will catch any excess plaster and prevent it from entering the eyes. The cast is then pressed against the taped nose, making sure that the dorsum is sufficiently narrowed. Pressure should be exerted symmetrically until the plaster has set. A small 2 × 2–inch drip pad is applied to the nostrils and secured to the cheek skin with a thin strip of adhesive.

ALTERNATIVE TECHNIQUE OF TAPE AND PLASTER

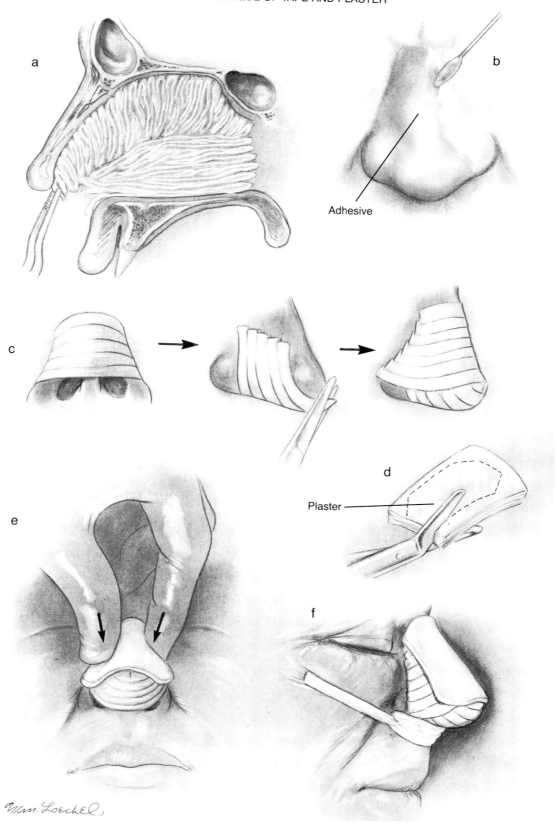

a

b

Adhesive

c

d

Plaster

e

f

Wm. Loechel,

chapter 48

Open Reduction and Fixation of Nasal Fractures
Alternative Technique Using Cantilevered Bone Grafts

INDICATIONS

Because most nasal fractures can be adequately treated with closed reduction techniques (see Chapters 46 and 47), the indications for open reduction are controversial. Most of the time, the nasal bones, including the septum, can be reduced and stabilized with internal nasal packs and external splints. However, a case can be made for opening and reducing (1) fractures that have started to heal in malposition and (2) fractures that extend to the frontal process of the maxilla and frontal bones. Alternatively, if any of the closed methods fail, one of the open techniques should be considered.

PROCEDURE

The nose is treated with local and topical vasoconstrictive agents as described in Chapter 46 and then prepared and draped as a sterile field. The design of incisions and approaches depends primarily on the pathologic condition that is to be corrected.

A,B For a *septal deflection,* the incision should be placed caudal to the area of leafing or deflection. This means either an intermembranous incision (between the columella and septum) or a Killian incision, 1.5 to 2.0 cm cephalad to the caudal border of the septum. If the deflection is associated with buckling and the buckling creates a spur at the junction of the septum with the maxillary crest, then the incision should be carried onto the ledge of the nostril and the floor of the nose approached simultaneously.

C,D Through these incisions, the surgeon should carefully raise the mucoperichondrium off the septum and, if indicated, the mucoperiosteum off the nasal floor. The correct subperichondrial plane can often be obtained by scraping along the side of the septum with a sharp elevator until the blue color of the cartilage becomes apparent. The surgeon can

then proceed cephalad with a subperiosteal dissection.

E,F The elevation should extend beyond the area of the fracture, but it should also cross over in front of the fracture and raise the mucoperichondrium of the opposite side. With mucoperichondrial flaps elevated off the area of deflection, the deflection can be removed, trimmed, and/or scored to fit into a relaxed anatomic position.

G,H Takahashi rongeurs should be used to cut off pieces of displaced cartilage and/or bone. A twisting action of the rongeurs will avoid inadvertent extraction of the fractured segment and injury to the cribriform plate. Scoring can be accomplished by making partial cuts through the curvature of the cartilage with a Beaver knife. Stability of the cartilage can be reinforced by through-and-through fine chromic sutures. If there is a tendency for leafing to occur, a figure-of-eight suture can be applied; this will prevent sliding of the fragments.

I,J For septal fractures involving the maxillary crest and for fractures in which there is a sharp spur, the surgeon must take special precautions not to tear the mucosa. Approaching the deviation with one of the tunnels described previously will relax the septal mucoperichondrial/mucoperiosteal tissues. The spur, however, may prevent safe elevation and should also be exposed by relaxation of the floor tissues from below. The combined approach will allow the surgeon to tease and cut away the attached mucoperichondrial flaps. The floor tunnel is developed with special Cottle elevators that are narrow, sharp, and curved to fit over the piriform aperture. The floor mucoperiosteum is raised and elevated toward the septum beneath the spur. A special speculum with a more pointed blade (Cottle) is then introduced into both tunnels. When the speculum is opened gently, the spur area will be exposed. The mucoperichon-

OPEN REDUCTION AND FIXATION OF NASAL FRACTURE

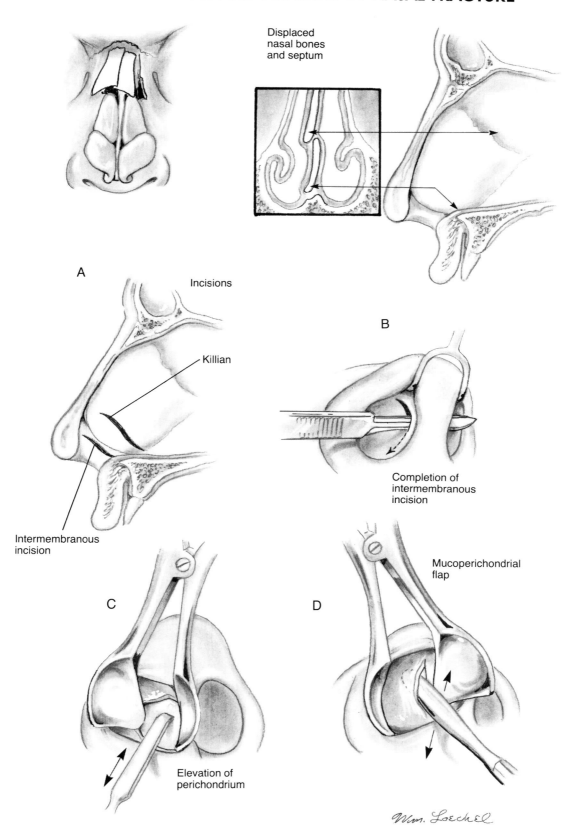

Displaced nasal bones and septum

A

Incisions

Killian

Intermembranous incision

B

Completion of intermembranous incision

C

Elevation of perichondrium

D

Mucoperichondrial flap

Wm. Loechel

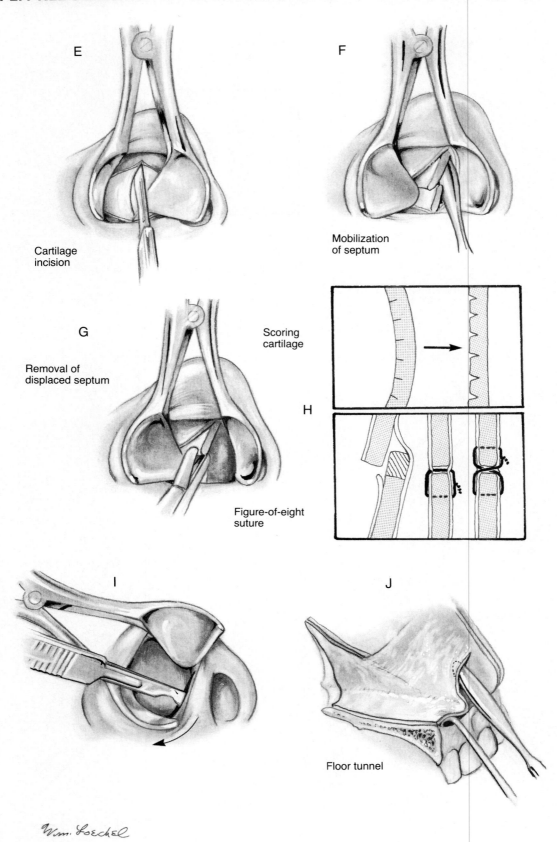

E

Cartilage incision

F

Mobilization of septum

G

Removal of displaced septum

Scoring cartilage

H

Figure-of-eight suture

I

J

Floor tunnel

Wm. Loechel

drium/periosteum can then be teased off of the projection.

K,L If the septum is displaced to the side of the crest, reduction will require removal of several millimeters of the cartilage inferiorly. This will allow the septum to swing like a door back into its normal position. A 4–0 chromic suture through the periosteum near the anterior nasal spine and the inferior portion of the cartilaginous septum can be helpful in maintaining the position of the septum. Sometimes a displaced maxillary crest can be repositioned, but if it is unstable, it is probably more prudent to remove it completely.

M Caudally placed incisions through the intramembranous septum can be closed with a 4–0 chromic mattress suture attaching the columella to the caudal septum. More cephalic incisions on the septum can simply be held closed with the nasal packing. Polyethylene splints should be applied to those septums in which instability remains. Nasal packing consisting of tampons or antibiotic-treated gauze is useful in controlling any residual bleeding. The packing also adds support to the septum. These methods and postoperative care are described in Chapter 46.

N For the *early malunited nasal bones* characterized by a limited depression, it is possible to make an intercartilaginous incision, expose the upper lateral cartilage and bone from below, and reduce the bone accordingly. Through this incision, the surgeon should first undermine the skin on the dorsum. A Lempert rongeur can then be inserted with one blade in the pocket and the other in the nasal passageway. The instrument is closed and the bone (including the upper lateral cartilage) rotated into position. The incision should be held closed with packing. An external cast is helpful.

O For *nasal fractures extending to the frontoethmoid region,* additional approaches are necessary for the reduction and fixation. A curvilinear medial canthal incision one half the distance between the dorsum of the nose and the caruncle of the eye will give satisfactory exposure of the frontal process of the maxilla and the nasal, lacrimal, and parts of the ethmoid bones. The same incision can be used bilaterally, and if additional exposure must be obtained toward the midline, the upper part of the incision can be connected with the horizontal limb (open sky approach). Another possibility is to use the coronal incision and forehead flap described in Chapter 36, but this technique is limited in exposing the medial wall of the orbit. It also requires extensive elevation of periosteum, which can jeopardize viability of comminuted fragments.

P,Q Depressed nasal bone fractures should be exposed by judicious elevation of the periosteum. The fragments should be elevated into position and maintained with strategic placement of fine wires. For this method, a minidriver with a 0.035-inch K wire is used to place holes across from each other in adjoining fragments. Irrigation with normal saline is necessary to avoid burning of the bone. Stainless steel wire (28-gauge) is then passed through the holes, and the fragments are secured by twisting down the wires appropriately.

The wounds are closed in layers. The periosteum is approximated with 3–0 chromic sutures, the subcutaneous tissues with 4–0 chromic, and the skin with 6–0 nylon. Intranasal packing is used if there is a need to stabilize the septum, but rarely is packing necessary to support the wire fixation. Prophylactic antibiotics are administered for 5 days.

PITFALLS

1. Maintain the supporting structures of the nose as much as possible (i.e., 1.5 cm of caudal septum and 3 to 5 mm of dorsal septum).

2. Splints and packing techniques should be applied in such a way as to prevent hematoma and necrosis of septal tissues. Polyethylene splints should be placed outside the mucosal flaps; pressure exerted by the splints should be appropriate to prevent accumulation of blood beneath the flaps, support the septum in the midline, and avoid necrosis of tissues.

3. Limit incisions and subperiosteal dissections, especially if there is significant comminution of the nasal bones. The open rhinoplasty approach (see Chapter 49) should be avoided, as this method requires an extensive dissection and undermining of tissues. The technique can cause additional trauma. It also will not give sufficient exposure to the lateral part of the nasal bones where they attach to the frontoethmoid region.

4. Interosseous wires should not be palpated through the skin. Fine wire should be used to secure the bones and the ends of the wire twisted through a hole or into the space between the fragments. Most rigid plates can be seen or felt and therefore should be avoided.

COMPLICATIONS

1. Potential infection can be minimized by atraumatic techniques and prophylactic antibiotics. If infection develops, packing and/or splints should be removed. Cultures should be obtained and the nose irrigated with saline douches.

2. Malunion of the nose with or without obstruc-

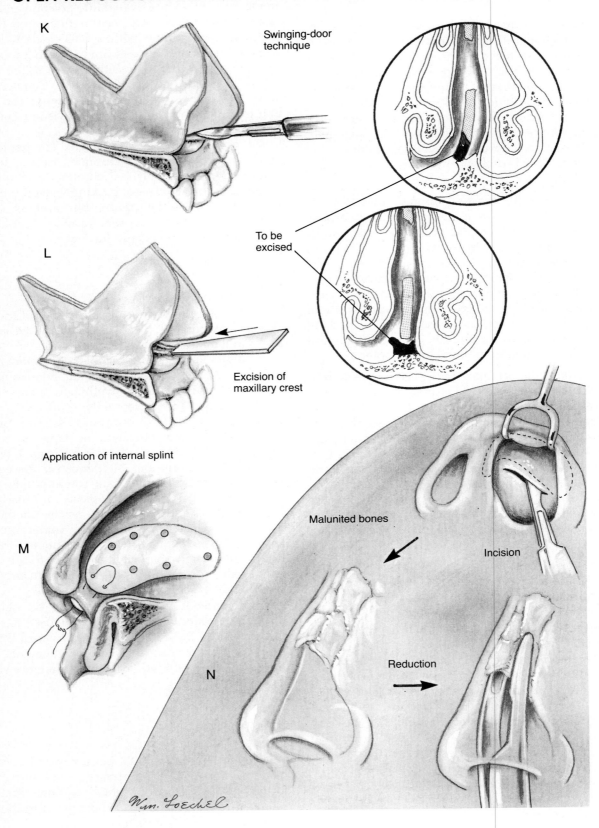

K

Swinging-door technique

To be excised

L

Excision of maxillary crest

Application of internal splint

M

N

Malunited bones

Incision

Reduction

Wm. Loechel

OPEN REDUCTION AND FIXATION OF NASAL FRACTURE *(Continued)*

Frontoethmoid
nasal fracture

"Open sky" incision

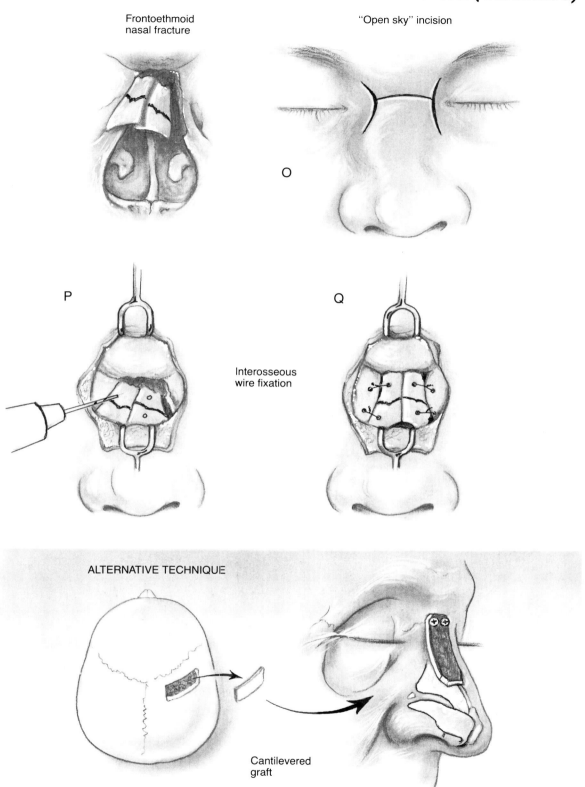

O

P

Q

Interosseous
wire fixation

ALTERNATIVE TECHNIQUE

Cantilevered
graft

Wm. Loechel

tion will require a septorhinoplasty. These techniques are described in Chapter 49.

ALTERNATIVE TECHNIQUE USING CANTILEVERED BONE GRAFTS

If comminuted fractures of the nasal bones and septum are associated with fractures of the adjoining buttresses, there may be insufficient support to maintain the projection of the nose. In such cases, interosseous wiring or lead plating methods will fail to establish nasal projection, and cantilever techniques must be considered.

Exposure through the coronal incision and forehead flap is desirable (see Chapter 36). The dissection should extend to the dorsum of the nose so that a subperiosteal and subcutaneous elevation can be achieved at least to the level of the lower lateral cartilages. A 1.5 × 4.5–cm graft is harvested from the outer cortex of the parietal bone. The graft is then rotated so that the cortical surface is placed along the frontoethmoid junction and the graft extended over the dorsum of the nasal bones. The graft is secured to the frontal bone by two small bone screws (self-tapping type) or by a 26-gauge wire passed through the frontal cortex and around the graft. The incisions are closed in the standard fashion. External casting is not necessary and probably should be avoided, as it can cause pressure and necrosis of those tissues caught between the graft and cast.

chapter 49

Septorhinoplasty for Nasal Deformity Following Trauma
Alternative Techniques Using Open Rhinoplasty and Cartilage Grafts

INDICATIONS

Probably the most common complication following nasal injury is malunion of the bony cartilaginous framework with or without obstruction. A variety of deformities can be described alone or in combination: dorsal hump; C- or S-shaped deviation of the septum; depression of the dorsum; saddle deformity; deviation of the tip; fallen tip; retracted columella; asymmetry of the nasal bones; asymmetry of the upper lateral cartilages; and asymmetry of the lower lateral cartilages. In addition, the septum can be displaced to one side or another; buckling can occur in the caudal-cephalic or superior-inferior directions. If any of these conditions develop, the patient can be considered for a septorhinoplasty.

Timing of the surgery is important. Ideally the procedure should be performed after the deformities have stabilized; this usually occurs 3 to 6 months after the injury. However, earlier repair can be contemplated if there is (1) obstruction, (2) a simple deformity requiring minimal correction, or (3) severe deformity affecting the patient's well-being.

Before embarking on septorhinoplasty, information should be obtained on the condition of the nose prior to injury and the nature of the new deformities. The patient should have the same expectations as the surgeon and be completely informed about results and complications. Sinus radiographs should verify that there is no sinusitis. Photographs are important to document the preoperative status.

PROCEDURE

The surgery can be performed under local anesthesia with sedation or under general anesthesia. Regardless of choice of anesthesia, the nose should be treated with topical 4% cocaine (containing five drops of 1:10,000 epinephrine) and local blocks of 1 or 2% lidocaine containing 1:100,000 epinephrine (see Chapter 46). The face is then prepared with an antiseptic solution and draped as a sterile field.

The surgeon has the option of several approaches. Some are more logical than others, depending on the location and severity of the deformity. The surgeon's experience and techniques will also be factors. For most deformities, a transfixion incision using either an intercartilaginous or intracartilaginous (cartilage-splitting) incision is satisfactory. For those patients requiring low dorsal implants and/or repair of the tip, delivery through a rim incision is helpful. The transfixion incision also provides an opportunity to do a septoplasty through the same incision.

A Intercartilaginous incisions are made bilaterally, one side at a time. The area to be incised is exposed by placing the blade of the nasal speculum (or double-ball retractor) under the lower lateral cartilage. The cephalic border of the lower lateral cartilage will tend to subluxate over the lower border of the upper lateral cartilage; a groove will develop, and it is this groove where the incision is made. The No. 15 blade should enter the subcutaneous space and not injure the overlying skin.

B As an alternative, the intracartilaginous (cartilage-splitting) incision can be made directly through the lower lateral cartilages. Exposure is obtained by holding the rim with a double-ball hook and pressing downward on the upper border of the lower lateral cartilages with a middle finger so that the cartilages evert into the nasal vestibule. An incision is then made parallel to the rim; the chosen distance from the rim will depend on the desired effect. If there is a need to retain most of the tip support, the incision should be 1 to 1.5 cm cephalad and parallel to the rim. If there is going to be more sculpting, the incision can be made closer to the rim. The incision, while carried through the lateral cartilages, should again avoid injury to the overlying skin.

C The incisions provide entry points for undermining the skin over the cartilaginous and bony dorsum of the nose. Both the cartilage-splitting incision and the intercartilaginous incision can then be extended into a transfixion incision. With the tip of the nose elevated with a double-ball hook and the columella pulled forward with a suture or columella forceps, a button knife is used to incise the tissues over the septum and between the septum and columella to the anterior nasal spine. This frees the lower lateral cartilages and the skin from the upper lateral cartilages and nasal bones.

D,E The rim incision, which is the third alternative, is well suited for cases in which small implants are to be inserted over the cartilages (and/or dorsum) and for tip projection techniques. The incision should be placed in a groove that usually separates the rim of the ala from the hair-bearing skin region. Initially the tips of the scissors are pointed away from the cartilage and then toward the rim. Once around the cartilage, the tips can be rotated and the cartilage separated from the overlying skin. The incision often has to be extended medially along the border of the columella to provide sufficient exposure.

F The septoplasty is usually performed at this stage; details of this procedure are illustrated in Chapter 48. Deviations of the septum often cause deviations to the external nose, and therefore straightening of the septum must take place before the external nose is repaired. The intramembranous incision, which is part of the transfixion incision, can be extended to the nostril sill to gain additional exposure for the floor region. The floor-septum approach is useful in managing sharp spurs and/or dislocation of the quadrilateral plate off the maxillary crest.

With the help of a focused light, a submucosal flap is started at the intramembranous septum. The dissection is continued at a level beneath the perichondrium, and to achieve the appropriate plane, the surgeon should scratch the perichondrial covering over the septum with a sharp elevator or small knife. The correct depth can be appreciated by the appearance of "blue" cartilage. Continued scraping should cause retraction of the edges of the perichondrium, and once this occurs, the dissection should proceed posteriorly with a Freer elevator. The flap should be created only on one side of the septum, as this will protect the soft tissues of the opposite side and prevent problems with necrosis and perforation.

Once the deviation (or leafing) is encountered, an incision can be made through the septal cartilage and

the dissection carried out subperichondrially and subperiosteally cephalad on the opposite side. This should expose portions of the remaining quadrilateral plate, perpendicular plate of the ethmoid, and vomer. Deviated parts of cartilage and/or bone can be removed with Takahashi rongeurs. Large segments of cartilage can be harvested with a swivel knife. Twisting motions of the rongeurs will avoid extension of fractures to the cribriform plate.

For spurs in the floor region, it is probably more prudent to use a floor approach in combination with the septal flap. The perichondrial fibers of the septum decussate beneath the septum, and a combined approach allows the fibers to be directly cut. Also, elevation of the septal mucosa over the spur can be made more easily when the surgeon elevates the mucosa from above and below the area of deflection.

Special instruments are usually needed for the floor dissection. First sharp elevators are used to expose the rim of the piriform aperture. Then using a curved Cottle elevator, the mucoperiosteum is elevated off the "blind side." Switching to a more gentle curve of the instrument allows elevation of the periosteum off the remainder of the floor. A thin-bladed Cottle speculum is introduced, with one blade into the floor tunnel and the other into the septal tunnel. The speculum is opened gently, and the junction between the tissues where the fibers decussate is cut with a sharp scissors or knife. The dissection continues cephalad until a complete floor and septal flap is developed. With this exposure, Takahashi rongeurs or a 3-mm chisel are used to resect bony and cartilaginous spurs. Dislocated septal cartilage can often be treated by taking off a 2- to 3-mm section inferiorly and scoring the main concavity. If the septum does not return to the midline, the mucosa on the opposite side may be preventing the rotation and should be elevated accordingly.

To retain sufficient support of the nose, the surgeon should maintain at least 1.5 to 2.0 cm of cartilage inferiorly and 0.3 to 0.4 cm of cartilage dorsally. Alternatively, if the surgeon does not want to remove any cartilage, it is possible to move the cartilage back to a midline position by a scoring method. For this technique, multiple parallel cuts should be made on the concave side. The convex surface should be left intact with periosteal attachments. When the deviations are complex, crosshatching may be necessary to achieve desired effects.

G The rhinoplasty part should now be carried out for the other deformities. Assuming that the tip of the nose needs to be rotated upward or made more narrow, the tip area should be exposed. Rotation usually is achieved by removing the cephalic border of the lower lateral cartilage. If the surgeon has chosen the cartilage-splitting incision, then the ce-

SEPTORHINOPLASTY

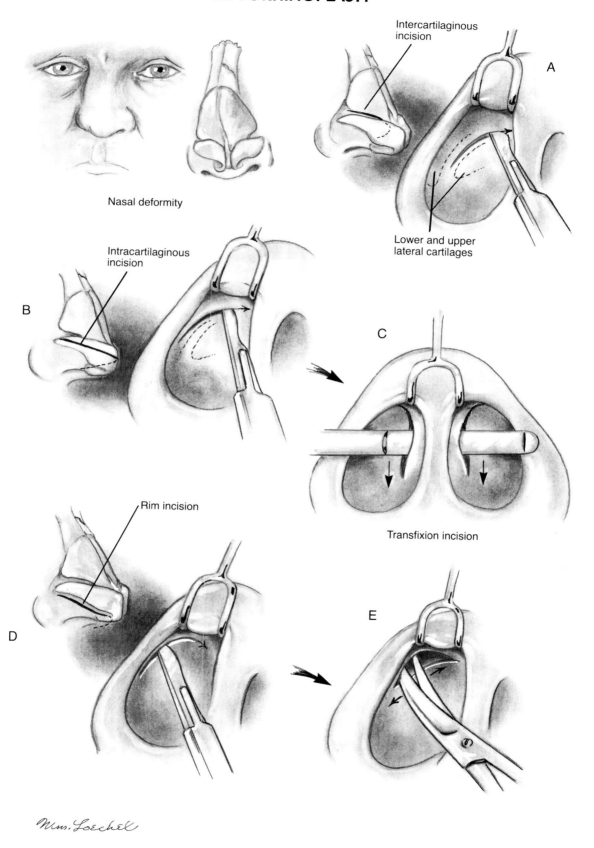

Nasal deformity

Intercartilaginous incision

Lower and upper lateral cartilages

A

Intracartilaginous incision

B

C

Transfixion incision

Rim incision

D

E

Wm. Loechel

phalic flap is pulled downward with a sharp hook and that portion of cartilage cephalad to the incision should be removed. This will leave a strip of lower lateral cartilage caudally. If the dome needs further narrowing, a small wedge of cartilage can be removed retrograde in the region of the dome. This can be accomplished by everting the rim, elevating the perichondrium on both sides of the strip for several millimeters, and making diamond-shaped cuts in the dome with a sharp scissors.

H For those patients requiring more tip work, the lower lateral cartilages should be delivered. Exposure is facilitated by combined rim and intercartilaginous incisions as described previously. The handle of the double-ball retractor is useful in rotating the mucosa and cartilage into view. The surgeon can then design the cephalic border resection and, if necessary, free up the domes for more narrowing, rotation, and projection with a direct suture technique. Usually the cephalic borders are trimmed, leaving a strip inferiorly. The medial crura are then freed up for several millimeters along the columella, and the dome is marked bilaterally with a marking pen. The mucosa beneath the domes is elevated, and the domes are delivered symmetrically into one or the other nostril. They are then held together with a thin-bladed forceps and secured with a 4-0 colorless or white nonabsorbable suture. The knot is buried between the projected domes.

I Tip definition can subsequently be enhanced by removal of the cartilaginous hump. The mucosa beneath the cartilages should be elevated. After exposing the upper lateral cartilages and their attachment to the septum with an Aufricht retractor, the perichondrium is excised. Variable amounts of cartilage from the lower dorsum are removed with a small sharp knife or corrugated nasal scissors.

J,K Following these maneuvers, the surgeon can then appreciate the degree of bony hump deformity that has to be resected. The periosteum should be first elevated. The hump can then be removed with straight saws, and irregularities can later be corrected with a bone rasp. The glabella is deepened, if necessary, with a small chisel and glabellar rasp. If the dorsum needs narrowing, a graduated 6- to 7-mm osteotome is inserted along the sides of the septum, and the bony septum is released (one side at a time) to the glabellar angle.

L–N Lateral osteotomies to narrow the nasal pyramid are performed with offset saws or a 4-mm osteotome. If the bones are thick, the saws can be used to start the cut. Completion of the osteotomy can be accurately accomplished with an osteotome. For the saw technique, incisions are made just in front of the inferior turbinates. The periosteum is elevated off the junction of the frontal process of the maxilla and nasal bones to create a pocket that extends just anterior to the medial canthal ligament. Sawing is facilitated by stabilization of the head by an assistant. Usually the saw cuts are directed along the junction of the nasal bones and frontal process of the maxilla. The cuts are completed with curved, guarded osteotomes. Superiorly the cuts are directed to the glabella angle. As an option, the surgeon can choose just the osteotome technique. For this, the osteotome is directed above the inferior turbinate, along the same path that would be used for the saw. However, the osteotomy ideally should only cut the periosteum and bone on the inner side of the nose, leaving the outer periosteum intact. This technique tends to be less traumatic but can be quite difficult if the nasal bones are thick and in a markedly abnormal position. Narrowing of the nose is completed by exerting finger pressure along the nasal bones and pushing the bones toward each other. A rocking motion often completes the fracture.

At this stage some refinements can be implemented. Additional dorsal irregularities can be removed with appropriate rasps or scissors. More rotation and projection can be achieved by removal of a wedge of the caudal septum.

O The intermembranous incision is closed by attaching the septum to the columella with 4-0 chromic mattress sutures. The rim and intracartilaginous incisions are closed with a single 4-0 chromic suture. The septum can be stabilized with thin polyethylene plates. The nose is packed gently with a tampon or antibiotic-treated gauze, and an external plaster dressing as described in Chapter 46 is applied. Antibiotics are prescribed for 5 to 6 days. The packing is removed at 2 days, septal splints are removed at 5 to 7 days, and the external dressings are removed at 7 to 14 days.

PITFALLS

1. Careful planning of each step is required for a successful correction of the deformity. Preoperative analysis with photographs and a set of sinus radiographs (to ensure that sinusitis is not present) should be part of the workup.

2. Many deviations of the external nose are caused by deviation of the septum. The septoplasty therefore becomes the foundation of the procedure. It should come first, and following the septoplasty, all deformities should be reevaluated.

3. Exposure and lighting of the septum is important. Avoid excision of septal tissues that cannot be

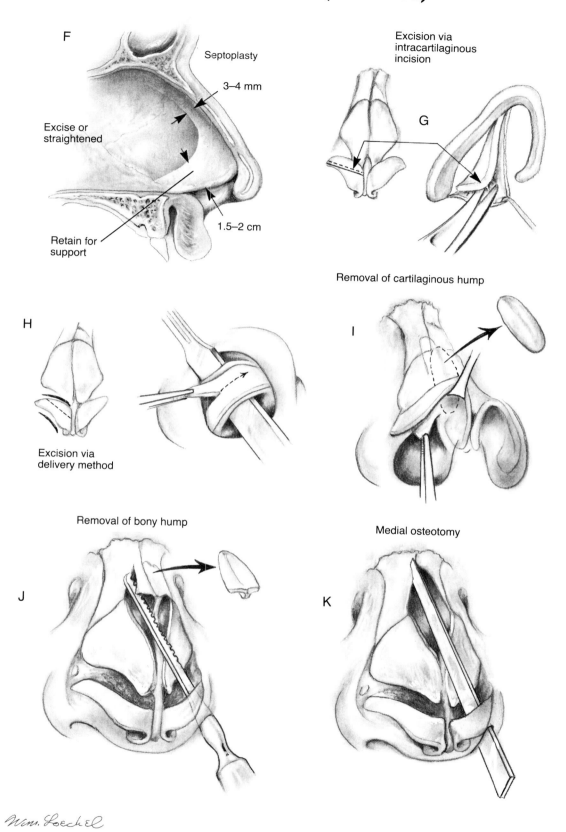

F

Septoplasty

3–4 mm

Excise or
straightened

Retain for
support

1.5–2 cm

Excision via
intracartilaginous
incision

G

H

Excision via
delivery method

Removal of cartilaginous hump

I

Removal of bony hump

J

Medial osteotomy

K

Wm. Loechel

Lateral osteotomy

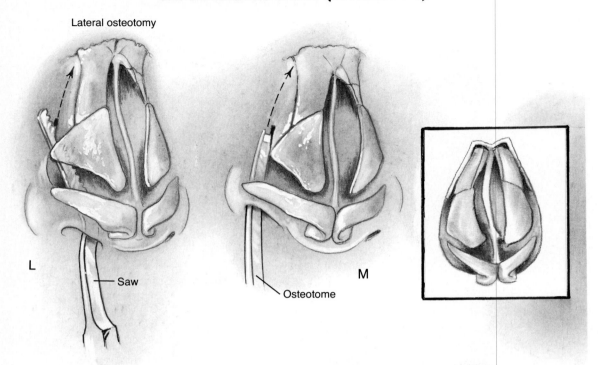

L

Saw

Osteotome

M

Infracture

N

Nasal splint

O

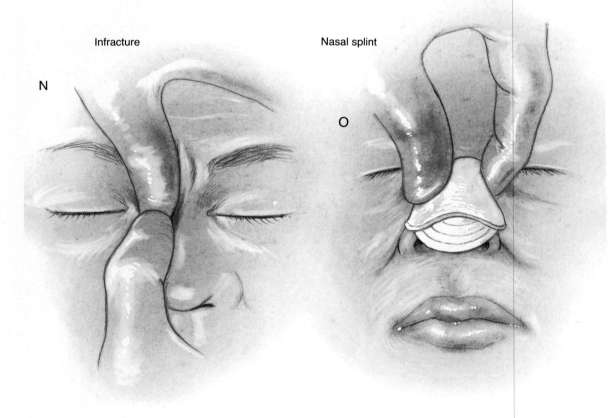

Wm. Loechel

visualized. Ensure that the mucosa has been elevated before removal of any of the fragments.

4. Although the surgeon has the choice of doing the cartilaginous tip before or after the bony skeleton, there are advantages to doing the cartilage work first. Often there is less bleeding than after an osteotomy, and considering that the tip is the "delicate" part of the procedure, optimal exposure is desirable. Moreover, tip projection can be a guide to the level of hump removal.

5. Always ensure symmetry of the procedure. A maneuver performed on one side should be followed immediately by the same maneuver on the opposite side. If pieces of tissue are being removed, they should be placed in front of the surgeon and compared directly to see if they are mirror images of each other.

6. It is always better to make an error in removing too little than in removing too much. Additional amounts of tissue can be removed at any time. However, it is difficult to add tissues and have them restored to normal anatomic contour.

7. Do not remove too much of the lateral portion of the cephalic border of the lower lateral cartilages. This lateral "tail" area is important for maintaining postoperative tip projection. It is also safer to keep the domes and rims intact, although incisions and some trimmings may be necessary in the more difficult cases.

8. When bringing the domes together, remember that it is possible to obliterate the tip highlights. To prevent this from occurring, place the mattress suture on the medial crura side of the dome. The higher placement certainly provides more projection, but the lower placement is better in creating the natural splaying that occurs in the tip region.

9. The level of the lateral osteotomy depends on the desired correction. If more projection of the dorsum is needed, the osteotomy should be placed close to the maxilla. For those patients who just need a narrowing of the dorsum, an osteotomy can be placed in a more intermediate position.

10. Postoperatively swelling can be reduced with elevation of the head and cold compresses. Another option is to administer steroids that will reduce the swelling and inflammatory response.

COMPLICATIONS

1. Epistaxis can occur in the immediate postoperative period. This can sometimes be avoided by making sure that all bleeding has stopped before terminating the procedure. However, if the patient bleeds following the surgery, the surgeon should (1) reduce the blood pressure with analgesics, sedation, and/or blood pressure–lowering agents; (2) apply cold compresses to the face; and (3) adjust and tighten packing. If these maneuvers are unsuccessful, the packing will have to be removed and the bleeding corrected with cauterization and/or repacking. Sometimes more pressure is needed on the bleeding sites.

2. Occasionally the nasal deformity cannot be completely corrected, or a new one may develop. Soft tissue swelling such as that seen with a "polybeak" can sometimes be treated with a direct injection of 20 mg/mL of triamcinolone. Cartilaginous depressions can later be filled with cartilage implants. Repeat septorhinoplasty, in part or as a whole, must sometimes be considered.

3. Nasal obstruction can occur as a result of the procedure. If the problem is caused by deformity (i.e., spurs, displacement of the septum, and/or deviated nasal bones), another septoplasty and/or rhinoplasty must be considered. Some of the more serious problems, such as a collapsing valve, are difficult to treat, and the reader is referred to a more appropriate text or journal.

4. Infections in the postoperative period are rare, but if they do occur, they can cause loss of skin with scarring and loss of skeletal support, later showing as a saddle deformity and retracted columella. These dreaded complications can sometimes be avoided by ensuring that there is no infection such as acne or sinusitis before starting surgery. The surgeon should also ensure that there is no intraoperative hematoma formation. Prophylactic antibiotics should be used throughout the period of packing or stabilization. If infection develops, cultures should be obtained and the appropriate antibiotic administered. Infectious disease consultation is desirable.

ALTERNATIVE TECHNIQUE USING OPEN RHINOPLASTY

The open rhinoplasty is another method for approaching nasal deformity following trauma. Exposure of the nasal architecture using this technique is far superior to that with any others, and this procedure is best used when the deformity is complex or there is any confusion as to what is causing the deformity. In performing the open procedure, the surgeon must be aware that there will be a small incision across the columella and that there can be more than the expected edema in dependent areas of the nose.

a,b The area is prepared and draped as in the standard septorhinoplasty. An incision is marked at the junction of the lower and middle thirds of the columella with a small V directed superiorly. The lateral portions of the incision are brought just beneath the rim and then along the rim superiorly to create the rim incision as described previously. The dissection proceeds through the skin, just in front of the medial crura and lower lateral cartilages. Curved scissors are directed away from the edge of the cartilages and then rotated on top of the cartilages to start the superiorly directed subcutaneous elevation. Skin flaps are developed to about the midlevel of the nasal bones.

The procedures that are used for correction of the nasal deformities and/or obstruction are the same as those described for a septorhinoplasty. The effects of trimming and/or removal can be appreciated by repeatedly placing the flaps into their original position. After completion of the procedure, the skin over the columella is closed with interrupted 6-0 nylon sutures. The dressings and postoperative care are the same as those for the standard rhinoplasty procedure.

ALTERNATIVE TECHNIQUE USING CARTILAGE GRAFTS

For those patients with a saddle deformity, retracted columella, or upper or lower lateral cartilage defects, implantation of cartilage can be a useful adjunctive procedure. Cartilage can be harvested using a septoplasty technique, but if there is insufficient material, either because of trauma or previous surgery, then the preferred donor site will be the conchal bowl of the ear.

The patient's face and neck should be prepared and draped in the standard fashion, exposing both the ears and the nose region. Vasoconstrictors are applied to the nose, and the ear is blocked with 1% lidocaine containing epinephrine.

a′,b′ An incision is then made at the lateral edge of the conchal bowl and a subperichondrial flap elevated to the external auditory meatus. Conchal cartilage of desired shape and size is elevated from the deep surface of the perichondrium. Bleeding is controlled with an electric cautery, and a small elastic band drain is secured to the skin. The skin is closed with interrupted 6-0 nylon sutures. A mastoid dressing of fluffs and stretch gauze (applied later) can be removed at 24 to 48 hours.

c′ Grafts harvested from the conchal bowl can be applied to the nose in a variety of techniques. For the saddle deformity, the surgeon can use a rim or intracartilagenous incision. The pocket should be just slightly larger than the desired implant. Contact of the implant with the cartilages and/or bone is encouraged. Implants that are too thin can be made larger by layering pieces of cartilage on each other and holding them together with 3-0 chromic ties. The cartilage can be trimmed to appropriate size and shape; a keel design is desirable for the saddle deformity. Closure and postoperative care are the same as those used for a rhinoplasty.

d′ For the columella retraction, incisions are made through the medial crura inferiorly and subcutaneous pockets created with a sharp scissors from the anterior nasal spine to the tip of the nose. Slivers of cartilage are then introduced into this pocket. Incisions are closed with a 3-0 nylon mattress suture.

e′ For small deformities involving the lower and upper lateral cartilages, isolated rim incisions can be used. The skin is dissected free from the lower and/ or upper lateral cartilages and the implant placed into this pocket. This incision should be closed with a single 4-0 nylon suture.

SEPTORHINOPLASTY *(Continued)*

ALTERNATIVE TECHNIQUE USING OPEN RHINOPLASTY

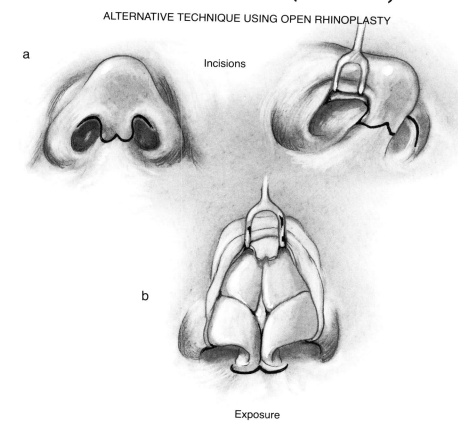

a

Incisions

b

Exposure

ALTERNATIVE TECHNIQUES USING CARTILAGE GRAFTS

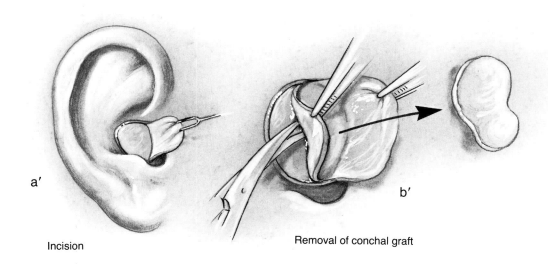

a'

Incision

b'

Removal of conchal graft

SEPTORHINOPLASTY (Continued)

ALTERNATIVE TECHNIQUES USING CARTILAGE GRAFTS (CONTINUED)

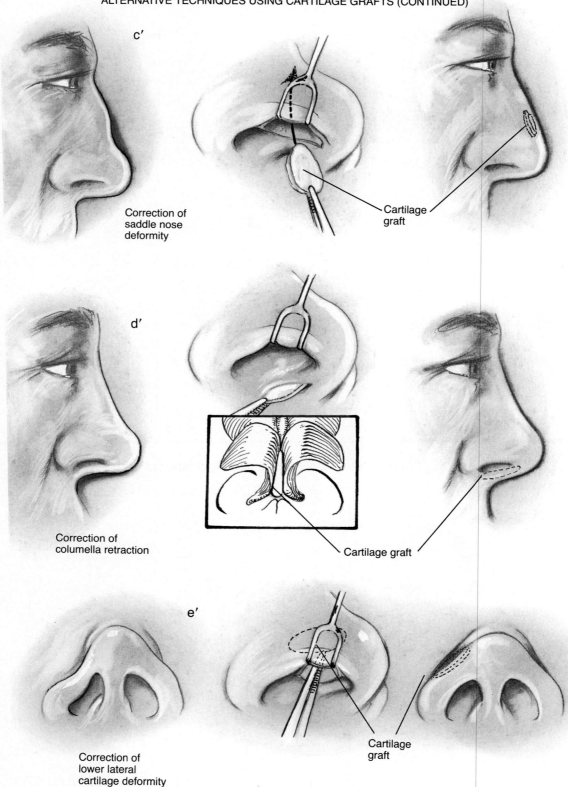

c′

Correction of
saddle nose
deformity

Cartilage
graft

d′

Correction of
columella retraction

Cartilage graft

e′

Correction of
lower lateral
cartilage deformity

Cartilage
graft

part
five

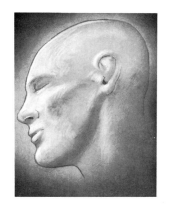

Malar
Fractures

section I

Classification and Pathophysiology of Malar Fractures

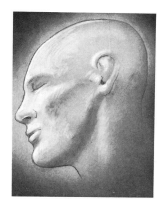

chapter 50

General Considerations

A–E The malar bone (zygoma) attaches to the craniofacial skeleton by frontal, maxillary, and temporal projections, forming a tripod, and by broad suture lines that connect the malar bone with the sphenoid and maxillary bones. The displacement of the bone depends on the direction and magnitude of external forces and the pull of the masseter muscle. The malar complex tends to move inward or outward and/or rotate along a vertical or anteroposterior (longitudinal) axis. Sometimes this block of bone is comminuted; at other times, part of the bone, such as the rim or arch, is displaced. There are many classification systems, but probably the most important factor is the relationship of the alteration in position of the bone to the development of clinical signs and symptoms.

F–H Rotation and depression of the malar fracture often causes abnormalities of the orbit. Typically, when the malar bone is depressed and rotated clockwise, the orbital walls will expand, resulting in enophthalmos and/or hypophthalmos; also, there will be a downward displacement of the lateral canthal ligament. The infraorbital nerve is frequently involved with the fracture, causing hypoesthesia of the cheek and upper dentition. If the bone rotates inward, the orbit is made smaller, and the patient presents with hyperophthalmos and some degree of exophthalmos. Displacement of the malar bone inward and downward can compromise the space occupied by the coronoid process, resulting in trismus and pain on mastication. Unilateral epistaxis, subconjunctival hemorrhage, and periorbital ecchymoses are additional common findings.

MALAR FRACTURES

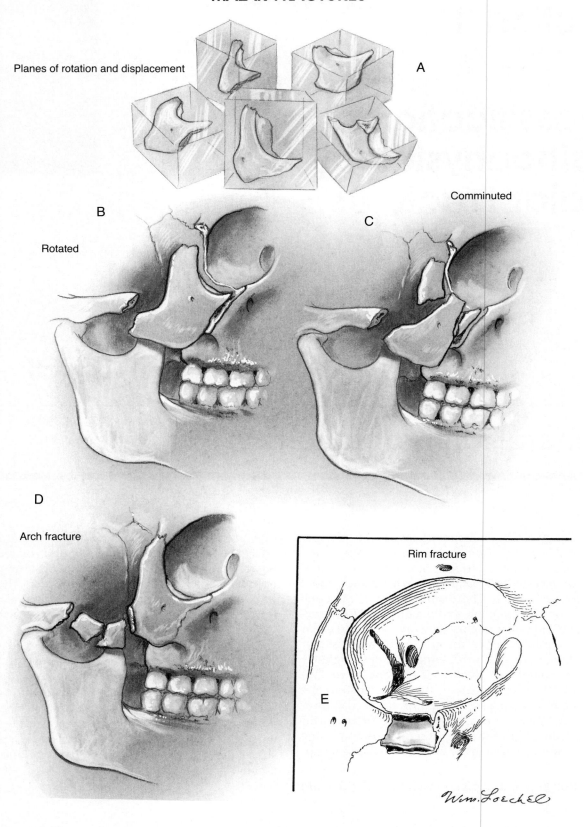

Planes of rotation and displacement

A

B

Rotated

C

Comminuted

D

Arch fracture

E

Rim fracture

Wm. Loechel

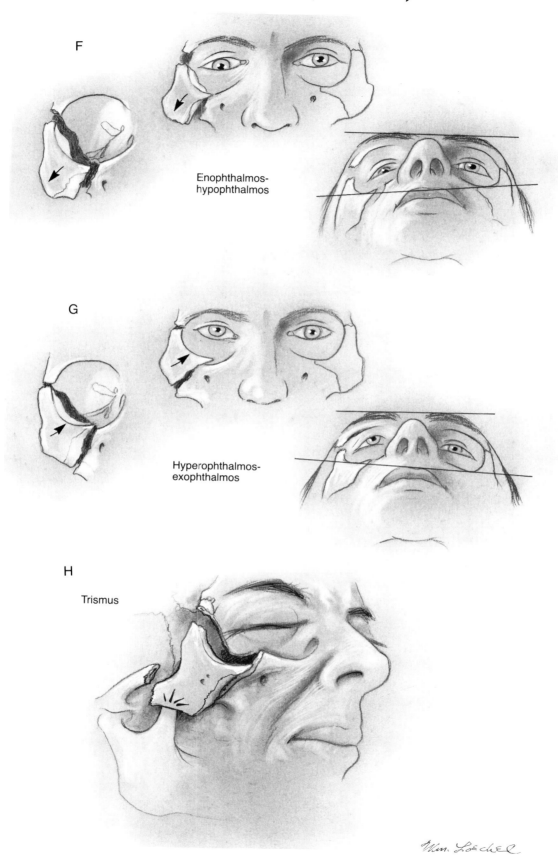

F

Enophthalmos-
hypophthalmos

G

Hyperophthalmos-
exophthalmos

H

Trismus

Management Strategies

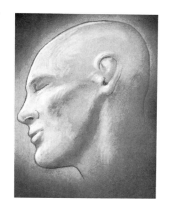

Semiclosed Reduction of Zygomatic Arch Fractures Using Eyebrow, Temporal Hairline, and Intraoral Approaches

INDICATIONS

Fracture and rotation of the zygomatic arch are often associated with a deformity of the lateral cheek. The area of depression may not be appreciated until all swelling has disappeared. Severe displacement of the arch can cause an impingement on the coronoid process and result in trismus and pain on mastication. Injury to the masseter may also cause trismus, but this effect should clear in several days; mechanical obstruction will persist longer. There are many surgical approaches to the arch fracture, but the most popular ones use incisions that are hidden intraorally or in the eyebrow or temporal hair line. Tunnels are then created beneath the arch that can then be used to elevate the arch into correct position. Direct open approaches are avoided because of the potential damage to the frontal branch of the facial nerve. Closed methods, such as reduction with a suture or

towel clip, can be used, but they have the disadvantage of being unable to control the rotation. Moreover, the surgeon loses the opportunity to stabilize the fragments by packing beneath the displaced arch.

PROCEDURE

Surgery should be planned when swelling has disappeared and the degree of deformity can be appreciated. The procedure usually is performed under orotracheal anesthesia. The face should be prepared and draped as a sterile field and the area of depression marked on the skin with a marking solution.

A The eyebrow approach uses an incision through the lateral eyebrow. Some hemostasis can be obtained by infiltration with 1% lidocaine containing epinephrine. The incision is made through the orbicularis oculi and periosteum, exposing the zygomaticofrontal suture line. The periosteum is then elevated laterally and the temporalis muscle retracted from the frontal process of the zygoma. A Joseph elevator is utilized to develop a tunnel along the lateral wall of the orbit beneath the temporalis muscle to the level of the arch. Once the elevator is at the arch, it can then be advanced to the lateral anterior aspect of the maxilla. The Joseph elevator is removed and replaced with a heavy, curved Kelly clamp. The clamp is levered on the prominence of the frontotemporal bone and the arch elevated laterally. The arch is then molded back into position with the other hand. Usually the arch is stable enough that no packing is necessary, but if the arch is unstable, the surgeon can pack beneath it with pieces of Gelfoam. Penrose drains can be used but will cause a widened scar.

B The popular Gillies approach uses an incision just behind the temporal hairline. Usually a small area is shaved, and the incision is made parallel to the hair follicles. The superficial temporal artery may be exposed and either retracted from the wound or ligated. The superficial temporalis fascia is then incised and the elevator used to develop a tunnel beneath the fascia and zygomatic arch. Reduction is carried out with a heavy, curved clamp or Boies elevator. As with the eyebrow approach, the arch is overcorrected and then molded back into position with the opposite hand. Gelfoam or Penrose (½-inch) drains can be used for packing and brought out through the incision. The temporalis fascia, subcuticular tissues, and skin are closed in layers.

C The buccal (Keen) approach requires an intraoral incision through the gingivobuccal sulcus mucosa. Using a blunt clamp, the tissues are spread and a tunnel developed just lateral to the maxilla and beneath the zygomatic arch. A heavy clamp is introduced through the opening, and the arch is elevated into position. If the arch is unstable, the surgeon can pack Gelfoam beneath the bone; Penrose drains should probably be avoided. The buccal mucosa should be loosely closed.

Postoperatively the patient is kept from putting pressure on the cheek area. Drains should be removed in 5 to 7 days. Prophylactic antibiotics (i.e., penicillin or erythromycin) are administered while the packing is in place. Postoperative radiographs should be obtained to ensure adequate reduction.

PITFALLS

1. Depression of the zygomatic arch is easily camouflaged by swelling of soft tissues. Thus patients should continue to be evaluated until the arch structure can be seen and palpated. Trismus or pain on mastication are clues that there is a substantial depression of the bone.

2. Make sure that the subtemporalis fascia tunnels lie beneath the arch. Remember that the temporalis fascia inserts into the arch, and for an instrument to achieve reduction, it must be placed deep to this fascial layer.

3. Avoid repeated attempts at reduction, as this will cause instability. One or two forceful attempts at elevation at the appropriate site with sufficient pressure should achieve the reduction. If the fracture becomes unstable, packing should be used to support the fragments.

4. Although packing can be safely used through the hairline incision, packing applied intraorally can potentially cause an infection, and packing through the brow sometimes causes a widened scar. High levels of antibiotics are suggested. Occasionally Gelfoam can suffice as a safe packing medium.

5. Closed techniques may be employed for those patients who are too unstable for anesthesia (see optional method). A towel clip strategically placed around the arch can be used to elevate the arch into approximate position. If the arch is still unstable, a suture can be placed around the arch and attached to a tongue blade, which is secured to the surface of the adjoining facial skeleton.

COMPLICATIONS

1. Unsatisfactory reduction is probably the most common complication of the procedure. Usually in these cases the surgeon has failed to insert the instrument beneath the arch, or the arch is too unstable and falls back to its posttraumatic position. The position of the arch is best evaluated by a postoperative submental vertex radiograph, and if the arch is in malposition, reduction and fixation should be repeated.

2. Infection should be avoided with proper postoperative care. Intraoral packing must be removed within several days; packs through the hairline and eyebrow may be left longer but should be inspected daily for evidence of infection. Antibiotic coverage is a very important adjunct. If signs of infection are present, the packing should be removed, cultures obtained, and appropriate antibiotics administered.

3. If the arch heals in malposition and the patient complains of trismus and/or deformity, other procedures must be considered. A coronoidectomy, described in Chapter 11, is a possibility. Deformity of the arch can also be treated with osteotomy and/or onlay grafts (see Chapters 54 and 55).

SEMICLOSED TECHNIQUE FOR ZYGOMATIC ARCH FRACTURES

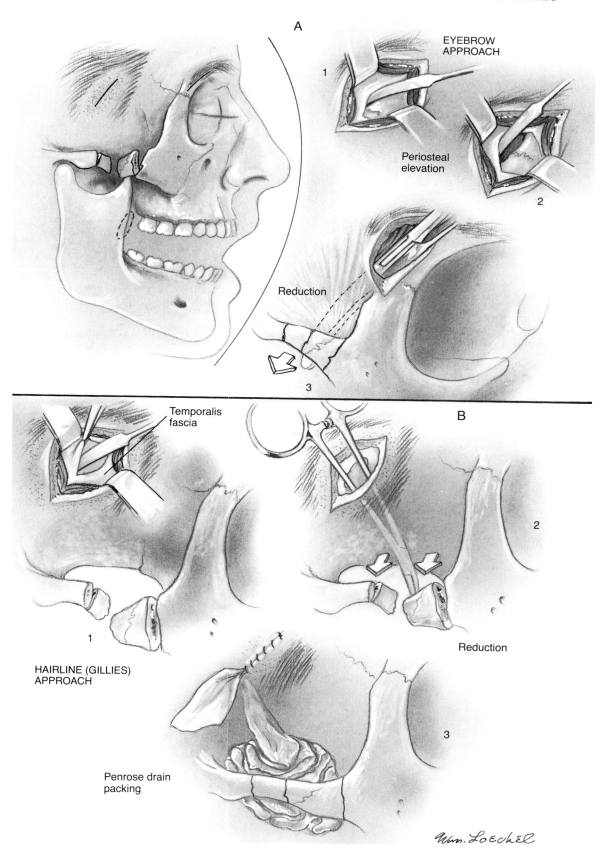

A

EYEBROW APPROACH

Periosteal elevation

1

2

Reduction

3

Temporalis fascia

B

2

Reduction

HAIRLINE (GILLIES) APPROACH

1

Penrose drain packing

3

Wm. Loechel

C

BUCCAL (KEENE) APPROACH

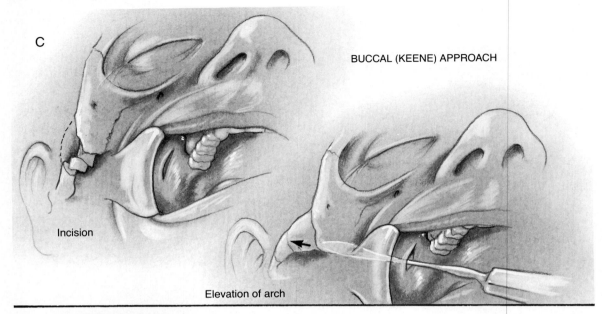

Incision

Elevation of arch

OPTIONAL METHOD
USING TOWEL CLIP

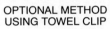

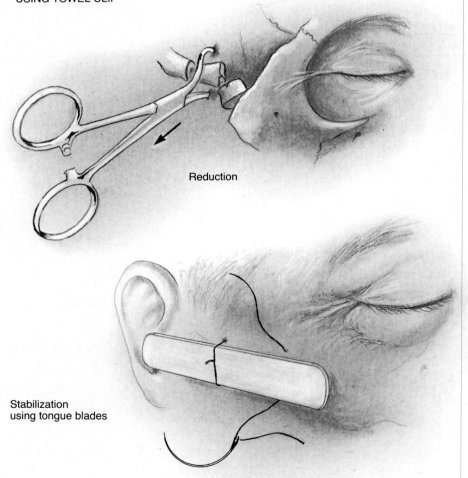

Reduction

Stabilization
using tongue blades

chapter 52

Open Reduction of the Malar Fracture With Interosseous Wire Fixation
Alternative Technique for Repair of Blow-in Fractures

INDICATIONS

Facial asymmetry and trismus, as consequences of a malar fracture, are probably the most common indications for open reduction and fixation. Usually the patient presents with a depression of the cheek and an inferior displacement of the lateral canthal ligament. The zygomatic arch can also be displaced laterally to give a widened appearance to the midfacial area. The patient may complain of an inability to open and close the mouth, pain on mastication, and no improvement in jaw function over time.

Other indications for surgery are those associated with the orbital floor component of the fracture (see Chapter 58). If the fracture rotates into the orbit, exophthalmos may be observed. Loss of tissues into the maxillary sinus and/or enlargement of the orbit can cause enophthalmos and/or hypophthalmos. Diplopia secondary to displacement of the inferior rectus muscle is also a concern.

Occasionally the malar fracture is only minimally displaced but is associated with a palpable defect of the orbital rim. As posttraumatic swelling disappears, the patient can develop a notable deformity. Surgical correction is desirable.

One controversial indication is hypoesthesia. There is no proof that reduction of the malar fracture improves the return of function of the infraorbital nerve, but it is logical to assume that this injury is caused by compression and that decompression with reduction should be effective in treating the sequela. Therefore it is reasonable to explore the canal and remove those fragments of bone that may project into the nerve (see Chapter 56).

PROCEDURE

A Under general orotracheal anesthesia, the face is prepared and draped as a sterile field. The entire face is exposed so that the surgeon can evaluate cheek projection in more than one plane. Infraciliary (or high eyelid) and eyebrow incisions are mapped out with marking solution. The infraciliary incision is made 2 to 3 mm below the cilia and lateral to the puncta; it can be extended into one of the "crow's feet" creases laterally. The high eyelid incision, which can be used as an alternative to the infraciliary incision, can be made in a high crease line below the puncta and lateral to a line drawn perpendicular to the pupil. The eyebrow incision, about 2.5 cm long, is made within the lateral eyebrow, carefully cutting the skin parallel to the orientation of the hairs.

B,C Using the infraciliary or high eyelid incision, the surgeon should separate the orbicularis oculi from the orbital septum and follow the septum to the anterior wall of the maxilla. As described in Chapter 58, the periosteum is incised and a cuff of tissue developed and elevated from the orbital rim. The fracture should be visualized, and if there is any comminution, the surgeon should attempt to keep the periosteum intact over the fragments. The infraorbital nerve should be identified and these soft tissues protected from further damage. The periosteum should also be elevated from the orbital floor, freeing up any tissues that are caught in the floor part of the fracture.

D,E Using the exposure of the eyebrow incision, the orbicularis oculi muscle fibers are spread, and the periosteum is incised at the level of the zygomaticofrontal suture line. A Joseph elevator is used to elevate the periosteum medially and laterally. With a Freer elevator, the periorbita and lacrimal gland are dissected free from the lacrimal fossa. The fracture line often entraps tissue near the inferior orbital fissure; these displaced tissues should be elevated and freed. The dissection should be continued laterally and posteriorly around the frontal process of the zygoma and then downward to create a pocket beneath the zygomatic arch. This pocket should be

WIRE FIXATION OF MALAR FRACTURE

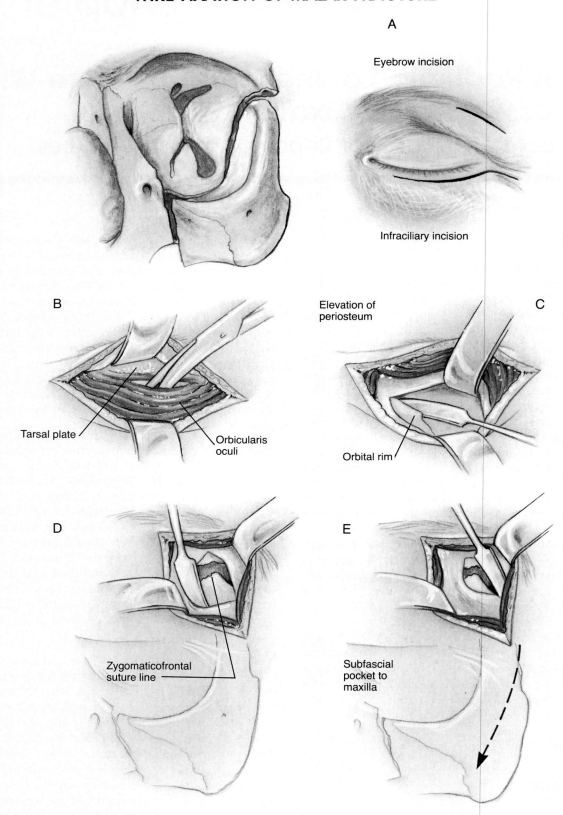

A

Eyebrow incision

Infraciliary incision

B

Tarsal plate

Orbicularis oculi

Elevation of periosteum

C

Orbital rim

D

Zygomaticofrontal suture line

E

Subfascial pocket to maxilla

extended to the anterior wall of the maxilla, as it will become useful in the reduction of the fracture.

F Reduction is carried out through both the eyebrow and infraciliary or high eyelid exposures. A large, curved clamp is inserted through the eyebrow incision and beneath the arch of the zygoma to the lateral wall of the maxilla. Through the infraciliary or high eyelid incision, a small elevator or osteotome is inserted between the fragments of the anterior wall of the maxilla. Both instruments are then raised simultaneously, and with steady pressure, the malar bone is elevated anteriorly and laterally. The bone is then manipulated into the desired position. The zygomaticofrontal and inferior rim fractures are evaluated for adequacy of reduction. Confirmation is obtained by palpation of the zygomaticomaxillary buttress and by ensuring that these fragments are correctly aligned. Cheek projection should be the same on both sides.

G,H Fixation is achieved with a 28-gauge stainless steel interosseous wire technique. A minidriver equipped with a 0.035-inch K wire is used to drill holes (with irrigation) on each side of the zygomaticofrontal fracture. The drill holes should be directed through the orbital wall or toward the infratemporal fossa. A 28-gauge wire is then passed through the drill holes and the wire twisted against the wall. Similar drill holes are placed on each side of the fracture at the inferior orbital rim or anterior maxilla. At these points the wire is placed through the hole on one side of the fracture and then pulled out with a 30-gauge wire loop on the other side. The 28-gauge wire can then be twisted firmly across the fragments and rotated downward along the face of the maxilla. The orbital floor should be inspected, and if there is a deficit, this condition should be treated with polyethylene mesh as in Chapter 58.

Single 4-0 chromic sutures are used to approximate the periosteum over the inferior and lateral orbital rims. The infraciliary or high eyelid incision is closed with a running 5-0 subcuticular nylon suture. The eyebrow incision is closed with a 4-0 chromic subcuticular suture, followed by a running or interrupted 5-0 nylon suture through the skin. The patient is maintained on antibiotics (i.e., penicillin or erythromycin) for 5 days and instructed to keep pressure off the cheek area. A soft diet is recommended for 24 to 48 hours. Radiographs are obtained in 2 to 3 days and the cheek projection evaluated at that time. Sutures are removed at 5 to 7 days.

PITFALLS

1. An accurate diagnosis is a prerequisite for appropriate treatment. Radiographs and computed tomographic (CT) scans should be obtained in several planes, carefully evaluating the rims of the orbit, floor of the orbit, zygoma and zygomatic arch, sphenoid attachments, and lateral wall of the maxilla. A clinical appraisal should also include palpation of the adjoining facial structures and an analysis of cheek projection. Waiting until all swelling has disappeared will improve the accuracy of the evaluation.

2. The repair process should employ the principle of three-point reduction and two-point fixation. Fractures at the zygomaticofrontal suture line and infraorbital rim should be directly evaluated; the zygomaticomaxillary buttress should be palpated. If there is any suspicion that the zygomaticomaxillary buttress is not in correct alignment or that instability continues, an incision should be placed in the gingivobuccal sulcus and this area exposed and evaluated directly. Additional wires can be placed at this fracture site (see **I**).

3. Be careful not to injure the tarsal plate, as trauma to this structure can later cause ectropion. Leaving some orbicularis oculi fibers attached to the plate will help avoid the development of this complication.

4. While the minidriver is being used to drill holes, the soft tissues should be protected with a malleable retractor. Also, to prevent heat damage, there should be a constant flow of irrigation solution (isotonic saline).

5. Because a malar fracture is often associated with injury to the floor of the orbit, the surgeon must ensure that the reduction of the malar bone does not cause additional damage to the floor. To avoid this problem, the floor of the orbit should be initially exposed and then reevaluated prior to closure. Occasionally the floor will need to be repaired, as in a blowout fracture (see Chapter 58).

6. Small fragments of bone that become loose at the inferior orbital rim can contribute to instability, and, if they are not retained, they can cause a step deformity. Every attempt should be made to keep the periosteum on these fragments. Occasionally the fragments can be stabilized with a "basket" formed by the interosseous wire (see **J**). Their position can also be maintained by a closure of the periosteum over the fragments.

7. Special techniques are required for fractures in which there is comminution of the malar bone (see Chapter 53). In general, these fractures are better treated with strategically placed miniplates (see **K**).

8. Delay in treatment can be associated with resorption and malunion of the malar bone. When 4 to 6 weeks have elapsed after injury, osteotomy, refracture, and use of the interosseous technique is satisfactory. If later treatment is required, the surgeon should consider osteotomy (and/or grafts) or onlay grafts alone (see Chapters 54 and 55).

WIRE FIXATION OF MALAR FRACTURE *(Continued)*

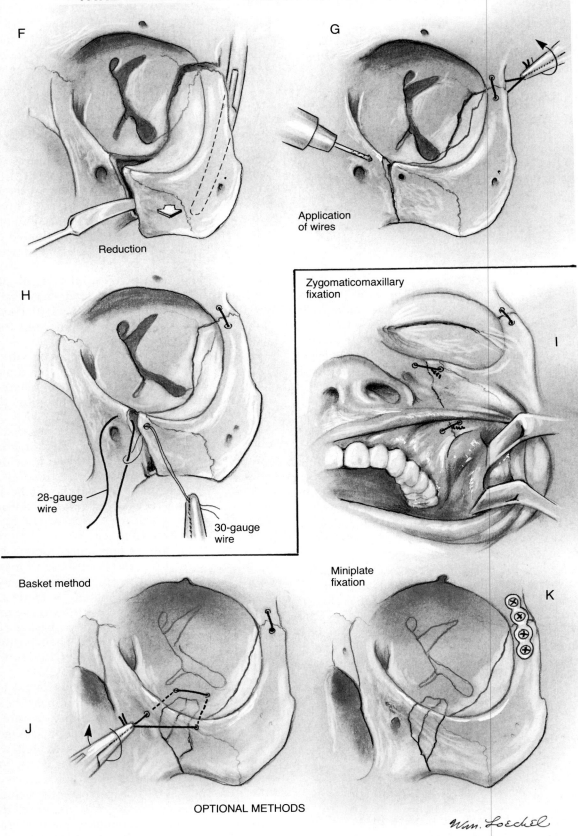

F

Reduction

G

Application
of wires

H

28-gauge
wire

30-gauge
wire

Zygomaticomaxillary
fixation

I

Basket method

J

Miniplate
fixation

K

OPTIONAL METHODS

Wm. Loechel

9. Blow-in fractures are an infrequent variant of malar fracture and can be also associated with orbital floor damage. The diagnosis and management of these fractures are discussed later.

COMPLICATIONS

1. Blindness is rare following treatment of the malar fracture. However, the surgeon must be aware of the possibility of an intraorbital hematoma, optic nerve compression, and retinal artery occlusion (see Chapter 58). Ophthalmologic evaluation should always be obtained before surgery. To avoid iatrogenic injury, the fracture sites should be exposed before manipulation, and the forces of reduction should be sufficient to reduce the fragments without causing new fracture lines.

2. Orbital deformity and dysfunction (e.g., enophthalmos, hypophthalmos, and/or diplopia) are common complications. These conditions and methods of treatment are discussed in Chapter 61.

3. Postoperative depression of the malar bone can be avoided by an accurate reduction and adequate fixation. Although it is unlikely that the masseter will pull the malar bone out of position, the patient should be placed on a soft diet for several days. We instruct the patient not to lie on that side and to avoid any activities in which there is potential physical contact. If the cheek becomes displaced, immediate exploration and correction should be considered. If malunion has occurred, osteotomy and onlay bone grafts may be necessary (see Chapters 54 and 55).

4. Trismus following repair of the malar fracture may indicate an inadequate reduction and continued impingement of the malar bone (or zygomatic arch) on the coronoid process of the mandible. The patient often complains of pain on opening and/or closing

the jaw, and some cheek depression is usually observed. In the early stages (i.e., up to 6 weeks), osteotomy of the malar bone should be considered. If there is no significant deformity, then a coronoidectomy is the preferred treatment (see Chapter 11). If the complication is seen later, then coronoidectomy with or without augmentation of the malar eminence should be considered.

ALTERNATIVE TECHNIQUE FOR REPAIR OF BLOW-IN FRACTURES

Downward and rotatory forces on the malar bone can cause the bone to be displaced into the orbit. Characteristic signs and symptoms are depression of the cheek, hyperophthalmos (elevation of the globe), and exophthalmos. The zygomatic arch may be displaced laterally. A step deformity can be observed or palpated along the inferior orbital rim. There may also be difficulty in opening and closing of the mouth and double vision on upward and downward gaze. A tent-shaped configuration of the floor of the orbit and a medial displacement of the lateral maxilla on radiographic examination confirm the diagnosis.

a The blow-in fracture should be explored through the infraciliary (or high eyelid) and lateral eyebrow incisions. Infiltration of the incision sites with 1% lidocaine containing 1:100,000 epinephrine should be considered for hemostasis.

b–d Blow-in fractures are explored as described for the laterally displaced malar bone (see earlier). Reduction is accomplished by elevation in an anterior and lateral direction. Interosseous wiring or placement of a single plate at the zygomaticofrontal suture can be used. Closure of the incision and postoperative care are identical to those used in other malar repairs.

ALTERNATIVE TECHNIQUE FOR BLOW-IN FRACTURE

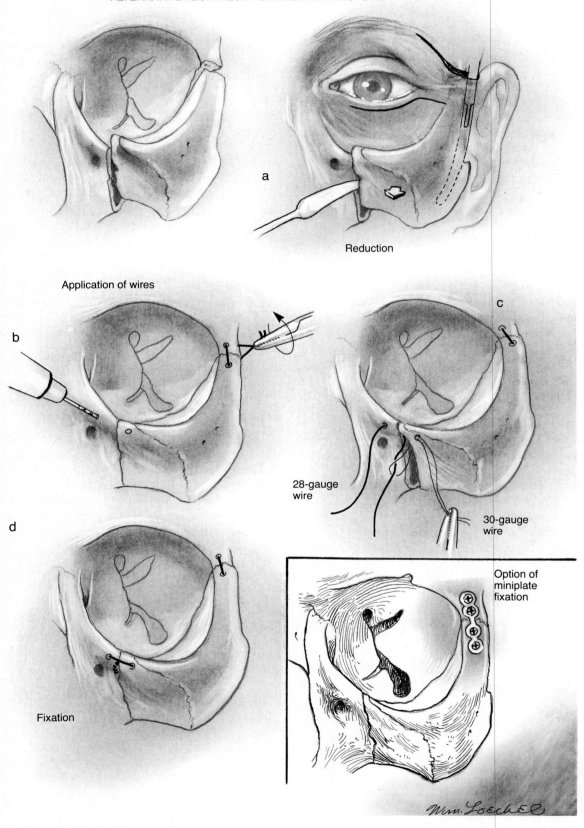

a

Reduction

Application of wires

b

c

28-gauge
wire

30-gauge
wire

d

Fixation

Option of
miniplate
fixation

Wm. Loechel

chapter 53

Open Reduction and Miniplate Fixation of Comminuted Malar Fractures

INDICATIONS

The more severe malar fractures are characterized by comminution of the body and processes of the bone. There is often marked swelling of the face and radiographic evidence of many small, displaced fragments. Orbital and cranial injury is common. Once the swelling has diminished, the physician can appreciate the depression of the cheek and changes in facial contour. It is not unusual to observe an alteration in eye position and, in some cases, a movement of the eye with mastication. These comminuted fractures can be managed with wire techniques, but a miniplate is preferred. The surgeon can choose either the compression or noncompression type, both in a variety of metal materials and thicknesses.

PROCEDURE

A–E Sufficient exposure can usually be obtained through the eyebrow and infraciliary incisions; occasionally a buccal incision is necessary to evaluate and treat the fractures of the vertical support buttress. The exposure and reduction of the fracture are as described in Chapter 52.

F–H The frontozygomatic separation can be treated with a variety of plates. If the compression type is chosen, the periosteum should be sufficiently elevated to allow placement of a four- or five-hole curved miniplate. The plate should be placed across the fracture so that at least one compression hole and one stabilization hole lie to the side of the fracture. As an option, a thin malleable template is then applied to the surface of the reduced fracture. A rigid plate is bent to the appropriate contour and shape of the template. The rigid plate is applied, and a drill hole is made through one of the compression holes and through the thickness of the orbital rim. The hole depth is measured, and a screw of appropriate length is applied to secure the plate to the bone. In preparing for the other compression hole,

the surgeon must understand that the plate will cause the underlying bone fragments to move toward each other, and the second drill hole must be strategically placed according to the status of the reduction. If the reduction is already tight, the drill hole should be made about midway through the oval compression plate hole. If more compression is needed, the drill hole should be placed farther away from the fracture line in the plate hole. The outer two stabilization holes can then be secured with appropriate drill and screw techniques.

I Alternatively, the surgeon can apply noncompression mini- or microplates, usually designed with self-tapping screws. The thickness of the plate may vary. The titanium plate is quite thin (0.5 to 0.6 mm), whereas the stainless steel and other alloy plates are slightly thicker.

J Usually the plate provides sufficient rigidity to stabilize the malar bone. If there is still some movement, the surgeon can place additional plates along the inferior orbital rim or zygomaticomaxillary buttress. If the malar bone is stable but a small piece of rim is unstable, interosseous wiring, as described in Chapter 52, can be utilized across the fracture site. Often small fragments of bone along the orbital rim can be stabilized by simple reduction and closure of the periosteum. Orbital floor exploration should be carried out before and after the reduction and fixation. If necessary, the orbital floor should be repaired with the appropriate autogenous or alloplastic implant.

For closure, the periosteum is approximated over the plate with 4-0 chromic sutures. The incisions and the skin edges are coapted as described in Chapter 52. Postoperative care is identical to that used with the interosseous wire technique.

PITFALLS

1. Because plating of a malar fracture provides rigid fixation, fractures must be accurately reduced

MINIPLATE FIXATION OF MALAR FRACTURE

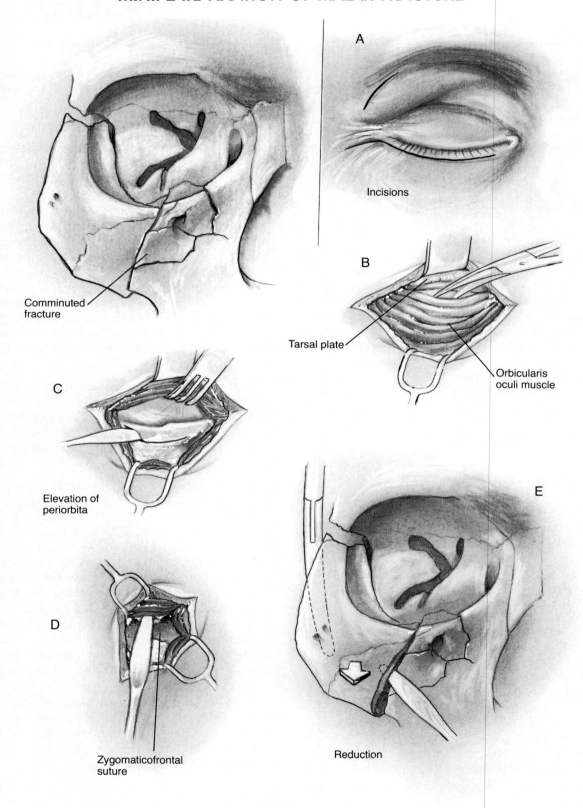

A

Incisions

Comminuted
fracture

B

Tarsal plate

Orbicularis
oculi muscle

C

Elevation of
periorbita

D

Zygomaticofrontal
suture

E

Reduction

F

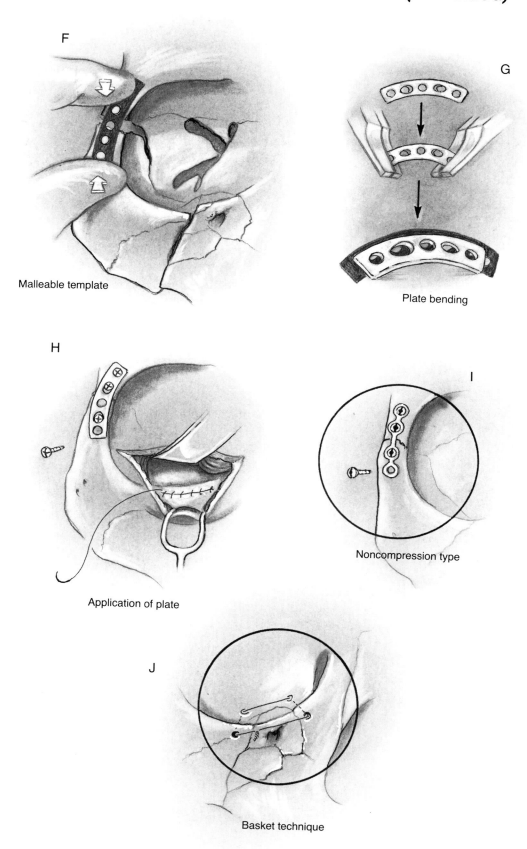

Malleable template

G

Plate bending

H

Application of plate

I

Noncompression type

J

Basket technique

and the plate bent and applied so that there is no displacement of the fragments. If the plating changes orientation of the fragments, it should be removed and a more optimal position obtained.

2. Plates may be palpated or observed through the skin, especially in those patients who have prominent orbital rims and thin skin. For this reason, the patient should be told that the plate may be temporary, and that after the bones have healed, the plate may have to be removed.

3. In applying the compression plate, the screws should first be placed through the compression holes and then through the stabilization holes. If the reduction is accurate, less compression is needed, and the drill holes can be placed in the center of the oval plate holes. However, if more compression is needed, the drill holes should be placed toward the outer edge of the plate holes. If this is not done, the screws will not be recessed and, as a result, will be seen or palpated through the skin. Noncompression plates are thinner, and although they are not as rigid as compression plates, they will provide satisfactory strength. Such plates have fewer problems with the screws and/or the plate being seen or palpated through the skin.

COMPLICATIONS

1. Deformity of the cheek and/or orbit are unfortunate sequelae of malar fractures. Such complications can be minimized by accurate reduction and fixation. Three-point reduction and complete immobilization with plating techniques are desirable. On the other hand, the surgeon must ensure that the plate does not change the orientation of the fragments. If this occurs, the plate should be removed and placed accurately. If the bone heals in a malposition, an osteotomy and/or onlay grafts must be considered (see Chapters 54 and 55).

2. The plate can sometimes be seen or felt through the skin. This occurs more often in thin-skinned individuals who have prominent orbital rims. These effects can be minimized with the new titanium plates and miniscrews, which have a very low profile. However, if the plate creates a deformity, then after healing has been completed, the incision should be opened and the plate should be removed.

3. Although rare, the plate can be associated with pain. If this occurs, healing should be ensured and the plate removed from the site.

chapter 54

Repair of Malunited Malar Fracture With Osteotomies
Alternative Technique Using a Coronal Approach

INDICATIONS

Residual deformity following malar fractures presents a formidable challenge. Depression of the cheek is often associated with enophthalmos, hypophthalmos, and limitations in mastication and conjugate gaze. If some healing has taken place, it is possible to osteotomize the fractured lines and reset the malar bone into proper position with interosseous wire and/or plating techniques. However, if the processes of the zygoma have undergone resorption, then the bone will be unstable following osteotomy and adjunctive bone grafts become important.

PROCEDURE

A Osteotomies can be performed through the standard eyelid, infraciliary, or high eyelid crease and eyebrow incisions (see Chapter 52). General anesthesia and infiltration of the incision with 1% lidocaine containing epinephrine are desirable to help control hemostasis.

B,C It is important in this procedure to strip the periosteum from the fracture lines. Through the eyebrow incision, the soft tissues of the orbit should be retracted medially and the periosteum elevated along the zygoma-sphenoid suture line to the inferior orbital fissure. The periosteum is also elevated off the posterior wall of the frontal process. A tunnel is developed beneath the zygomatic arch to the lateral maxillary wall. Using the lower eyelid approach, the floor of the orbit should be explored and the periosteum elevated posteriorly to the junction of the infraorbital canal and inferior orbital fissure. The periosteum should also be elevated laterally to connect with the dissection that was performed through the eyebrow incision. Additionally, periosteum should be released from the anterior wall of the maxilla and malar bone to expose the zygomaticomaxillary buttress.

D Following these maneuvers, the fractures (or suture lines) should be evaluated. The soft tissues of the cheek should be retracted and osteotomies carried out through the fracture lines with sharp-pointed 3- to 4-mm osteotomes. The initial cut is started at the zygomaticofrontal suture and follows the fracture or suture line to the inferior orbital fissure. The next cut starts at the inferior orbital rim and follows the fracture laterally to the inferior orbital fissure. The osteotome is then turned and directed downward along the lateral face of the maxilla through the zygomaticomaxillary buttress. A heavy clamp (Kelly) is then inserted underneath the zygomatic arch, and with an elevator directed through the inferior orbital rim osteotomy, the malar bone is rocked and lifted into the preferred position (see Chapter 52). The arch or any other parts of the malar bone that were not osteotomized will usually fracture along the natural suture lines.

E,F The malar bone should be fixed with wires or miniplates. Usually 28-gauge stainless steel interosseous wires applied to the zygomaticofrontal buttress and inferior orbital rim are sufficient. The more unstable fragments require multiple wires or a miniplate. Closure of the wounds and postoperative care are identical to those used in the repair of malar fractures (see Chapter 52).

PITFALLS

1. The osteotomy technique is best applied to fractures that have partially healed and can be opened with a "nudge" of the osteotome. If the bones have healed completely and the fracture sites have undergone resorption, the malar bone will not "fit." Bone grafts will have to be placed behind the osteotomy sites to secure a firm fixation.

2. To avoid entry into the intracranial cavity while performing the osteotomies, the osteotome should

275

OSTEOTOMIES FOR MALUNION OF THE MALAR BONE

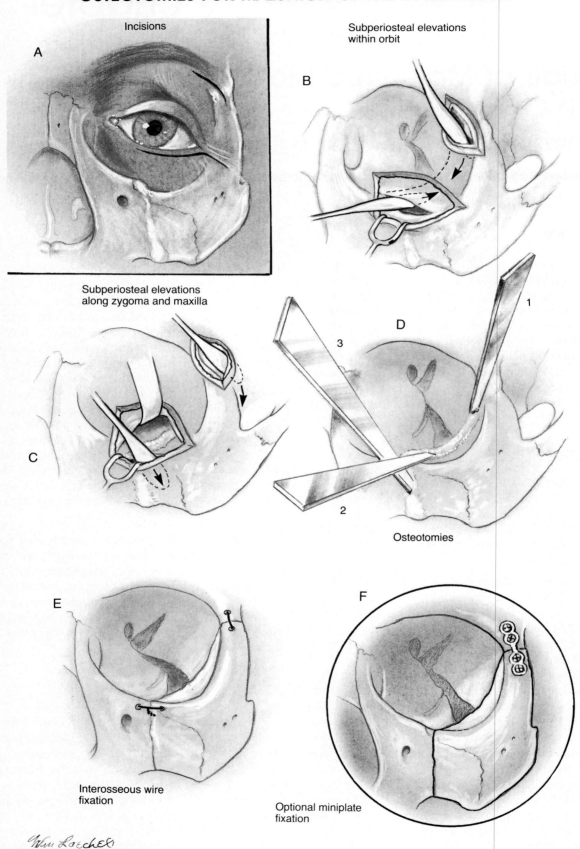

A Incisions

B Subperiosteal elevations within orbit

Subperiosteal elevations along zygoma and maxilla

C

D Osteotomies

E Interosseous wire fixation

F Optional miniplate fixation

be at or below the suture lines. The osteotome should also just penetrate the bone, so that if there is dura beneath the osteotomy site, it will not be cut. Postoperatively the patient should be observed closely for development of any intracranial signs or symptoms.

3. If the malar bone cannot be reduced following the osteotomies described previously, the surgeon should consider another osteotomy through the junction of the arch and the body of the zygoma. As an alternative to the eyebrow incision, the surgeon can use a coronal approach and expose even more of the arch for the osteotomy (see later and Chapter 44).

4. Avoid using oscillating saws for the osteotomy. The width of the saw determines the width of the cut, and removal of too much bone can affect the fixation. For these reasons, use of the sharp, thin osteotome is preferred. It also provides for irregularities in the bone that can be used to hold the malar bone in its natural position.

COMPLICATIONS

1. The most feared complication of the osteotomy technique is a dural tear, which can be associated with bleeding and cerebrospinal fluid leak. Usually the tear can be avoided by keeping the osteotome shallow and just below the cranium. Should the patient develop or experience any intracranial signs and symptoms, neurosurgical consultation should be immediately obtained.

2. Instability of the fragments following osteotomy can be a problem. This can be somewhat avoided by early diagnosis and narrow osteotomies. However, if the malar bone is unstable, it can be additionally secured at the zygomaticomaxillary buttress with a rigid plate. Deficits at the osteotomy site should be filled with free bone grafts from the parietal or hip region.

3. Blindness is a possibility, especially if the fracture extends into the retrobulbar and optic nerve regions. Direct compression of the optic nerve, retrobulbar hemorrhage, and retinal artery occlusion are all possible. These complications should be recognized and treated immediately (see Chapter 58); ophthalmologic consultation should be obtained.

4. Exposure of the zygomatic arch places the frontal branches of the facial nerve at risk. Injury can be avoided with judicious use of retraction and limitation of the dissection to a subperiosteal plane over the arch.

ALTERNATIVE TECHNIQUE USING A CORONAL APPROACH

a,b A malar osteotomy can also be carried out through a standard coronal approach. The incision is the same as that described in Chapter 36, except that the dissection is continued along the frontal process of the zygoma and superficial temporal fascia to the zygomatic arch (see Chapter 44). In carrying out the dissection, the surgeon should recognize that the deep temporal artery has a branch that comes through the fascia, and the frontal branch of the facial nerve lies in the soft tissues just superficial to the fascia. Also, the fascia becomes continuous at the superficial musculoaponeurotic layer just above and lateral to the arch. Exposure from above, however, will show most of the arch, the frontal process, and the lateral half of the body, but the floor of the orbit cannot be appreciated. To give this exposure, the surgeon should use a lower eyelid (infraciliary-subtarsal) approach.

c—e The subperiosteal elevation and osteotomy maneuvers are identical to those used for the direct exposure method described earlier. The surgeon can additionally osteotomize the zygomatic arch. Wire and/or plate fixation should be applied and the flap replaced and closed in a routine fashion. The patient is placed on prophylactic antibiotics for 5 to 7 days, and the malar bone is clinically and radiographically evaluated for adequacy of reduction and fixation.

ALTERNATIVE TECHNIQUE USING CORONAL APPROACH

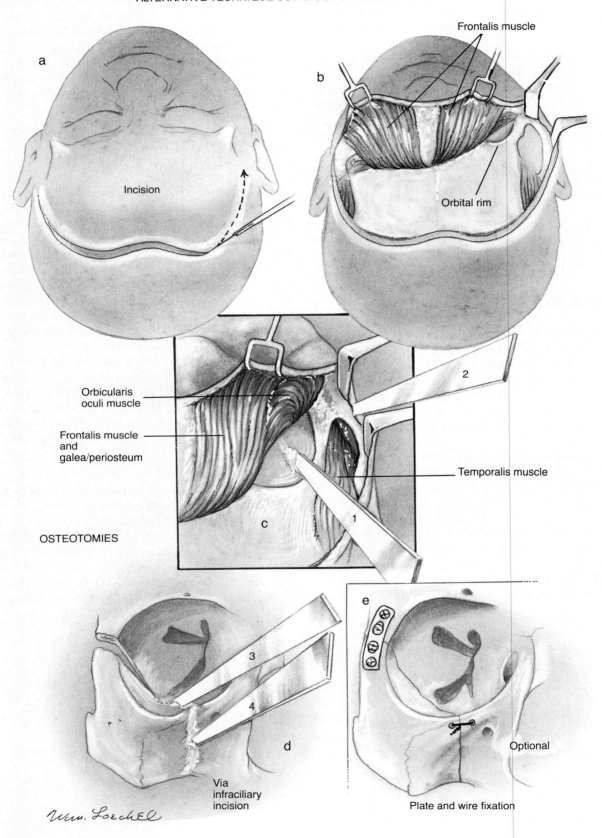

a

Incision

b

Frontalis muscle

Orbital rim

Orbicularis oculi muscle

Frontalis muscle and galea/periosteum

Temporalis muscle

c

OSTEOTOMIES

2

1

d

3

4

Via infraciliary incision

e

Optional

Plate and wire fixation

Wm. Loechel

chapter 55

Treatment of Malunited Malar Fracture With Onlay Hip Grafts
Alternative Techniques Using a Coronal Approach and Cranial or Rib Grafts

INDICATIONS

The malpositioned, completely healed malar fracture is probably best treated with onlay bone grafts. When the malar fracture heals, the bony processes are absorbed and sutures and fracture lines obliterated. Under such conditions, osteotomy is difficult to perform, and even with a freeing up of the bone, there will be marked instability and a probable need for adjunctive grafts. The malar onlay graft technique is also suitable for those patients in whom the orbit or other parts of the facial skeleton need grafting. The procedure will not help alleviate associated trismus or difficulty in mastication resulting from the malar bone impinging on the coronoid process. For the latter condition, osteotomy and/or intraoral coronoidectomy should be considered (see Chapters 11 and 54).

PROCEDURE

The face, neck, and hip should be prepared and draped as a sterile field. The hip graft is obtained as described in Chapter 60. Either hip can be used, as the graft can be contoured and bent into a variety of shapes. Ideally the graft should have a curvature that corresponds to the cheek, but if the graft needs to be bent further, this can be achieved by partial osteotomies with Lindeman burs through the outer cortical layers. The bone graft can then be bent to the contour of the anterior maxilla and zygomatic processes. Additional contouring can be obtained with cutting burs.

A,B Exposure for onlay grafting is accomplished through a subciliary incision extended through a "crow's foot" crease. To reduce bleeding, the area should be infiltrated with 1% lidocaine containing epinephrine. The proper plane is easily obtained by incising between the orbicularis oculi and the septum orbitale. The tarsal plate should be protected during these maneuvers by leaving a small strip of muscle on the plate. The dissection should continue to the inferior orbital rim. A periosteal incision is then made over the anterior wall of the maxilla just beneath the rim. A cuff of soft tissue is elevated superiorly, and the floor of the orbit is explored to the junction of the infraorbital canal and inferior orbital fissure. The subperiosteal dissection should continue laterally to free up the periosteal attachments along the frontal process of the zygoma and the outer wall of the orbit. This will relax the lateral canthal ligament. Additionally, periosteum is elevated off the anterior arch and the body of the malar bone. Medially the infraorbital nerve is exposed; if it is in the way of grafting, it should be sacrificed. To obtain appropriate contour the subperiosteal dissection may often have to be extended to the lateral aspect of the nasal bones.

C–E The bone graft is shaped to fit over the maxilla and malar bone and adjusted to the desired level in relation to the orbital rim. Several additional small pieces of bone are then placed on top of the frontal process of the zygoma and the anterior floor of the orbit. These additional pieces of bone are used to construct a smooth orbital wall. The bone is held firmly by 2-0 chromic sutures placed through the adjacent periosteum. The infraciliary incision is closed with a running 5-0 nylon subcuticular suture. A light compression dressing is applied to help stabilize the grafts and prevent swelling.

Postoperatively the patient is maintained on intravenous antibiotics. The reconstruction is inspected every 2 to 3 days with appropriate dressing changes. The dressings are maintained for approximately 10 days, and the sutures are removed at 5 to 7 days.

ONLAY HIP GRAFTS FOR MALUNION OF MALAR BONE

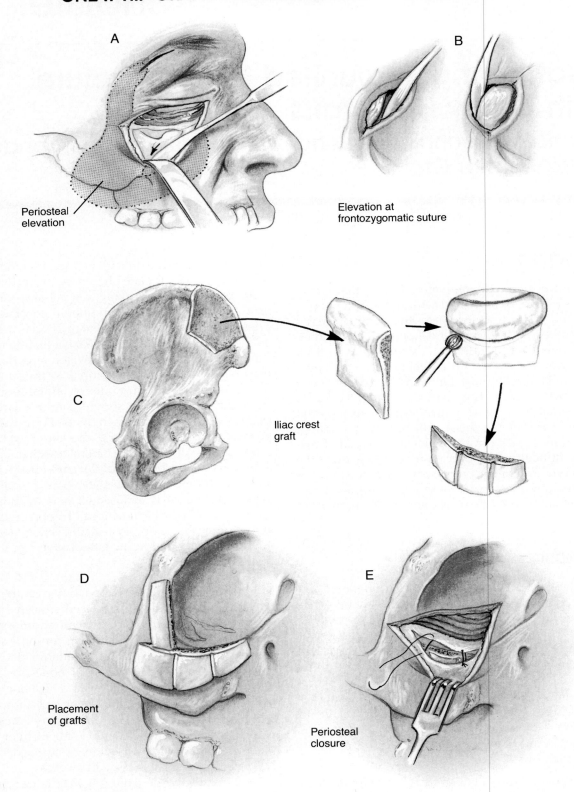

A

Periosteal
elevation

B

Elevation at
frontozygomatic suture

C

Iliac crest
graft

D

Placement
of grafts

E

Periosteal
closure

PITFALLS

1. Ideally the malar graft should be one piece of bone. This will ensure more stability and a smoother contour of the cheek. Fracture of the graft can be avoided by using sharp, cutting instruments and gentle handling of the bone. Osteotomies performed in preparation for bending of the graft should be strategically placed through the cortex, and bending should be done with just enough force to bend without breaking the bone. If the graft should fracture, each part can be applied to the malar and maxillary bones separately and immobilized with chromic sutures and periosteal closure.

2. Do not rely on remodeling to create a smooth cheek contour. Fill all defects and cracks with pieces of cancellous bone.

3. Dressings are important and must be properly placed if they are to assist in stabilization of the graft. The eye should be treated with an ophthalmic ointment and two eye pads placed over the closed eyelid. Fluff dressings are then built up over the cheek, around the ear, and over the eye and held with wraps of stretch type dressings. A figure-of-eight design around the upper neck and chin is helpful in keeping the dressing in a desired position.

COMPLICATIONS

1. Movement of the graft can result in an irregularity of the cheek and subsequent failure to correct the deformity. This complication can be avoided by securing the grafts with heavy chromic sutures through the periosteum and by the dressings described earlier. The patient also should be instructed to avoid any pressure and contact activities that could affect the grafted area.

2. Irregularity of the graft can develop with time. Resorption is unpredictable and occurs in a spotty fashion. A palpable and noticeable irregularity of the cheek can be corrected by exposing the graft through the same incision and smoothing it with cutting burs.

3. Infection can jeopardize the survival of the graft and can be avoided with the use of prophylactic antibiotics, atraumatic techniques, and optimal hemostasis. If infection develops, the wound should be debrided and cultures obtained. Failure to control the infection requires removal of the graft.

ALTERNATIVE TECHNIQUE USING A CORONAL APPROACH AND CRANIAL GRAFTS

The malar bone can also be approached by combining parietal onlay grafts with coronal and subciliary eyelid incisions. The coronal approach is described in Chapter 54. Harvest of the bone graft is discussed in Chapter 60. The grafts will have a natural curve, but unfortunately they are brittle, and there is little capability to bend the graft further without causing a fracture. Thicker grafts can be obtained by placing grafts on top of one another and securing them with heavy chromic sutures. Also, the sides can be beveled to the appropriate contour. Resorption is believed to be less with cranial grafts than with grafts from the rib or hip region.

ALTERNATIVE TECHNIQUE USING RIB GRAFTS

Rib grafts are ideal to use as onlay grafts for the malar deformity. When split, the grafts can be bent to exact curvature, and multiple grafts can be placed on top of each other for additional thickness. The grafts are beveled and secured beneath the periosteum with 2-0 chromic sutures. The major disadvantage of the rib graft is that absorption is very unpredictable and often exceeds that observed with other graft methods.

ALTERNATIVE TECHNIQUES FOR MALUNION OF MALAR BONE

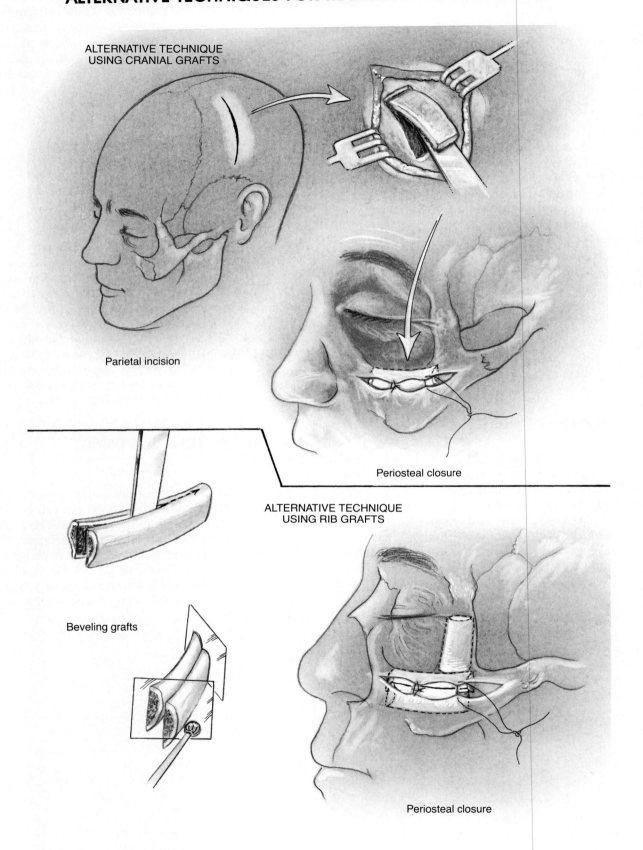

ALTERNATIVE TECHNIQUE
USING CRANIAL GRAFTS

Parietal incision

Periosteal closure

Beveling grafts

ALTERNATIVE TECHNIQUE
USING RIB GRAFTS

Periosteal closure

chapter 56

Decompression of the Infraorbital Nerve

INDICATIONS

Fracture of the malar bone is often associated with loss of sensation over the cheek and upper dentition. Return of sensation is variable, and occasionally the patient develops pain and paresthesias. If an injection of 2% lidocaine to the infraorbital foramen alleviates this pain, then the surgeon should consider a decompression of the infraorbital nerve.

PROCEDURE

A–D Under general anesthesia, the face is prepared and draped as a sterile field. Bleeding is partially controlled with a prior injection of 1% lidocaine containing 1:100,000 epinephrine. An infraciliary or high eyelid (subtarsal) incision will provide adequate exposure.

The skin-muscle flap, which is lifted between the orbicularis oculi fibers and the septum orbitale, should be used to gain access to the anterior wall of the maxilla (see Chapter 52). The orbicularis oculi and zygomaticus muscle attachments are cut and the periosteum incised just beneath the inferior orbital rim. The periosteum is elevated off the superior wall of the maxilla to expose the infraorbital nerve and foramen. Using a sharp elevator (Cottle), the nerve is dissected free from the foramen. The foramen can be enlarged with rongeurs; additional depressed fragments are elevated from the floor of the orbit and either removed or replaced into anatomic position. The wound is then closed in layers.

PITFALLS

1. The results of infraorbital nerve decompression are variable. If the patient does not obtain relief, there is always the option of reoperating and lysing the nerve. However, the surgeon must be aware of the neural supply carried by other branches of the infraorbital nerve through the maxilla and recognize that the decompression is aimed only at the anterior portion of the nerve that innervates the cheek tissues and the anterior upper dentition.

2. The patient must be warned that the procedure may also cause hypoesthesia. Scar tissue at the foramen can make the dissection difficult, and the nerve can be inadvertently injured.

3. Neuromas at the foramen are not easily treated. Decompression will not help in such cases, and it is more practical to lyse the nerve and remove the mass of neural tissues.

COMPLICATIONS

Probably the most common complication of the procedure is the return of hypoesthesia. The patient should be warned of this possibility, and the surgeon should take precautions to prevent it from happening. Scar tissues at the foramen should be gently teased from the nerve. The rongeurs should be directed away from neural tissues, and depressed fragments of bone in the infraorbital canal should be elevated or removed.

DECOMPRESSION OF INFRAORBITAL NERVE

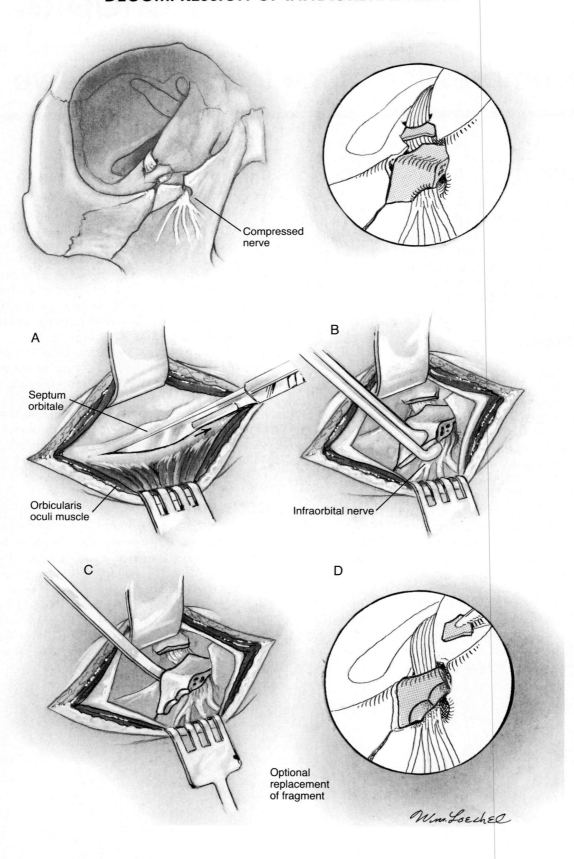

Compressed nerve

A

Septum orbitale

Orbicularis oculi muscle

B

Infraorbital nerve

C

D

Optional replacement of fragment

Wm. Loechel

part
six

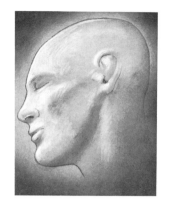

Orbital Wall
Fractures

section I

Classification and Pathophysiology of Orbital Wall Fractures

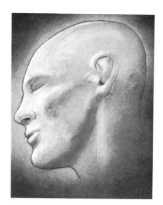

chapter 57

General Considerations

A–C The most common site of a blowout fracture is the orbital floor, but similar injuries can be noted, in order of prevalence, on the medial, lateral, and superior walls. The pure blowout fracture is generally understood as a trap-door rotation of bone fragments involving the central area of a wall. However, if the injury is associated with a fracture line extending to one of the orbital rims, it is then considered an impure type of fracture. The impure fractures are commonly found with malar, maxillary, naso-orbital, and frontal bone fractures.

D–F The defect created by the blowout fracture is variable in size and often filled with soft tissues of the orbit. If there is minimal edema formation, significant defects will translate into an increase in the orbital volume described by the walls and a reduction of intraorbital contents. These events can lead to the clinical appearance of hypophthalmos and/or enophthalmos.

The fat tissues that enter the blowout contain fibrous septae, which in turn support the position and mechanical activity of the extraocular muscles. In a small defect, the muscles may become trapped, but it is usually the septae that are displaced; it is this change in position of the septae that causes alterations in muscle performance. Changes in the globe position can also have an impact on the tension and contraction of the muscle. In addition, there is a possibility of direct neural and/or muscular damage. All of these factors, alone or together, can cause a failure in conjugate gaze and produce the symptom of diplopia.

Different sites and sizes of the wall defect produce different clinical pictures. Large defects on the floor often cause hypophthalmos and/or enophthalmos, but because the large opening does not usually trap muscle or fat, extraocular movements can be excellent, and diplopia should not occur. However, small defects of the floor can entrap the fat and/or muscle, restrict muscle activity, and cause diplopia on upward gaze; enophthalmos or hypophthalmos should be a minor complaint. Defects on the medial wall, depending on size, can be associated with enophthalmos; if a muscle is disturbed, it is usually the medial rectus, which in turn can affect medial and lateral gaze. Injuries affecting the junction of the medial and inferior walls are often relatively large, and enophthalmos will usually be apparent. Fractures of the other walls of the orbit can also affect volume/content relationships of the orbit and muscle activities; these effects are generally determined by the size of the wall defect and relationship of the muscle to the injured wall.

BLOWOUT FRACTURES

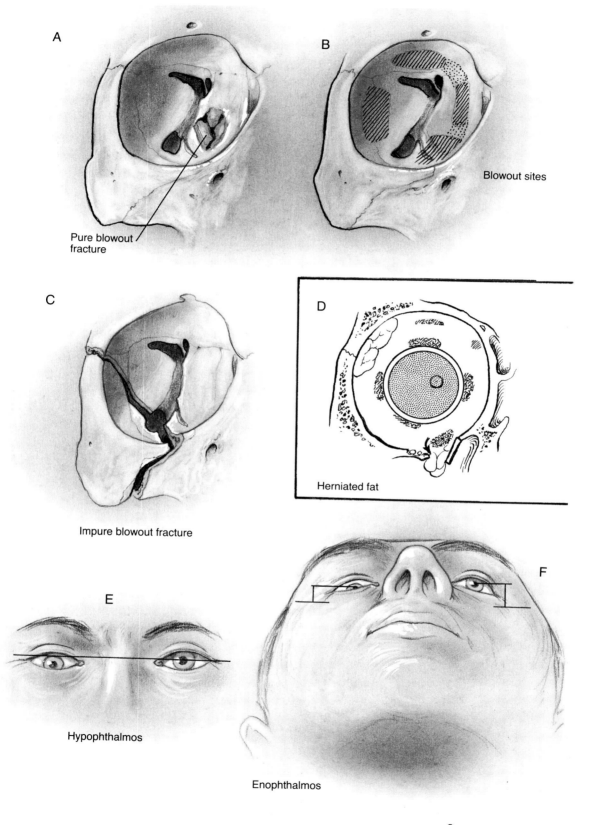

A

Pure blowout
fracture

B

Blowout sites

C

Impure blowout fracture

D

Herniated fat

E

Hypophthalmos

F

Enophthalmos

Wm. Loechel

section II

Management Strategies for Orbital Wall Fractures

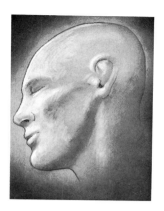

chapter 58

Repair of Orbital Floor Fractures With Polyethylene Mesh
Alternative Techniques Using Parietal Bone Grafts and the Caldwell-Luc Approach

INDICATIONS

Most blowout fractures need to be repaired surgically; some can be treated by conservative management. Usually the latter are associated with minimal displacement of an orbital wall and no diplopia. These conditions, however, must be substantiated radiographically and by repeated examinations; otherwise, what appears to be an unimportant injury becomes associated with a progressive malposition of the globe, neuromuscular imbalance, and persistent deformity and dysfunction. There are both absolute and relative indications for exploration and corrective surgery to avoid these sequelae.

Absolute Indications

1. Acute enophthalmos (>2 to 3 mm) and/or hypophthalmos (>2 to 3 mm).

2. Mechanical restriction of gaze associated with diplopia.

Relative Indications

1. Conditions that can later cause enophthalmos and/or hypophthalmos; theoretically, 2 to 3 mm of a 1.5- to 2-cm^2 area of displaced wall or soft tissue can cause these deformities. These changes generally can be recognized on horizontal and coronal computed tomographic (CT) scans.
2. Persistence of diplopia, presumably caused by small defects and mechanical changes that are not perceptable by forced duction tests; such cases should have no evidence of neural injury.

The timing of surgery is important. Surgery performed too early can be associated with an inaccurate diagnosis, swelling that obscures surgical planes and anatomic landmarks, and excessive bleeding that accompanies the inflammatory phase of healing, whereas exploration performed too late may reveal malunion and resorption of bone with contraction of soft tissues by scar. Therefore surgery is best performed at 7 to 10 days. If associated craniofacial fractures are also to be treated, the procedures should be coordinated so that they can be carried out at the same time. In general, children will heal early and should be done early. Adults can be delayed for 10 to 12 days. Additional delays can compromise results, but it is still worthwhile to attempt a repair up to 4 to 6 weeks after injury.

PROCEDURE

A Pure blowout fractures of the floor can be approached through an infraciliary or high eyelid (subtarsal) incision. The infraciliary incision is designed 2 to 3 mm below the cilia of the lower eyelid, just lateral to the puncta. If injuries of the malar bone must be repaired, the incision can be extended laterally into one of the "crow's foot" creases. The alternative high eyelid (subtarsal) incision is designed about 5 to 7 mm below the cilia in a crease line lateral to a line perpendicular to the pupil of the eye. Limiting the length of this incision will help minimize postoperative edema.

B–D The incision should be injected with 1% lidocaine containing 1:100,000 epinephrine to help control hemostasis. Using a sharp knife, the surgeon cuts both skin and the orbicularis oculi muscle fibers. The dissection then proceeds in a plane between the orbicularis oculi muscle and the orbital septum inferiorly, until the surgeon reaches the level of the anterior maxillary wall. Using a malleable retractor to hold and protect the septum orbitale and another retractor to pull the eyelid downward, an incision is made 5 mm below the rim through the orbicularis oculi–zygomaticus muscles and periosteal attachments. This incision should avoid injury to the infraorbital nerve and artery, which lie just medial and inferior to the area of dissection.

E,F The periosteum and attached soft tissues are released with a Joseph elevator. The subperiosteal dissection continues over the orbital rim and onto the floor of the orbit. Lighting and control of bleeding are very important, as the surgeon must be able to see each maneuver and identify the different types of tissue attached to the floor region. Using a Freer elevator, the periosteum is lifted medially and laterally to the defect. The attached or extravasated soft tissues can then be teased out with a smaller Cottle

elevator. The dissection proceeds posteriorly and, to ensure completeness of the procedure, should expose the junction of the infraorbital canal and inferior orbital fissure.

After soft tissues are elevated from the defect, the bony trap-door deformity should be reduced. This can be accomplished by dropping a small, single skin hook beneath the fragment, twisting the hook to engage the fragment, and elevating the fragment into position. Other depressed fragments are treated identically. The area of fracture is then reinforced with a piece of polyethylene (Marlex) mesh so that the mesh covers the defect and adjoining intact floor.

G,H Forced ductions are performed, and if reduction is satisfactory, the periosteum is closed with a single 3-0 chromic suture. The skin is approximated with a 5-0 subcuticular nylon suture. Prophylactic antibiotics (i.e., erythromycin or penicillin) are administered for 5 days. The patient should be evaluated at 1 week and monthly thereafter to ensure stability and uneventful healing.

PITFALLS

1. Accurate diagnosis is essential for proper management. Historical and clinical examination should be complemented by CT scans in the horizontal and coronal planes. If the patient cannot be positioned for these tests, frontal plane tomograms are indicated. An ophthalmology consultation is highly recommended.

2. Measurements of enophthalmos and hypophthalmos can be compromised by swelling of the tissues and/or a displacement of the reference point (the lateral wall of the orbit). It is therefore important that a final evaluation be delayed until the swelling has disappeared. If the wall of the orbit is displaced, projection of the globes in relationship to the cheeks and forehead can be estimated by visualizing these structures tangentially from above or below the patient.

3. Restriction of muscle activity should be suspected when there is diplopia and nonconjugate movement. Confirmation should be obtained by forced duction tests and radiographic evidence of disruption of the orbital wall near the affected muscle.

4. Contraindications to repair of the floor are hyphema, retinal tear and detachment, and globe perforation. Traumatic optic neuropathy and retinal artery inclusion are also important considerations. Surgery should also not be performed on an only-seeing eye.

5. Timing of surgery is important. Early exploration and repair coupled with an accurate diagnosis

REPAIR OF BLOWOUT FLOOR FRACTURE

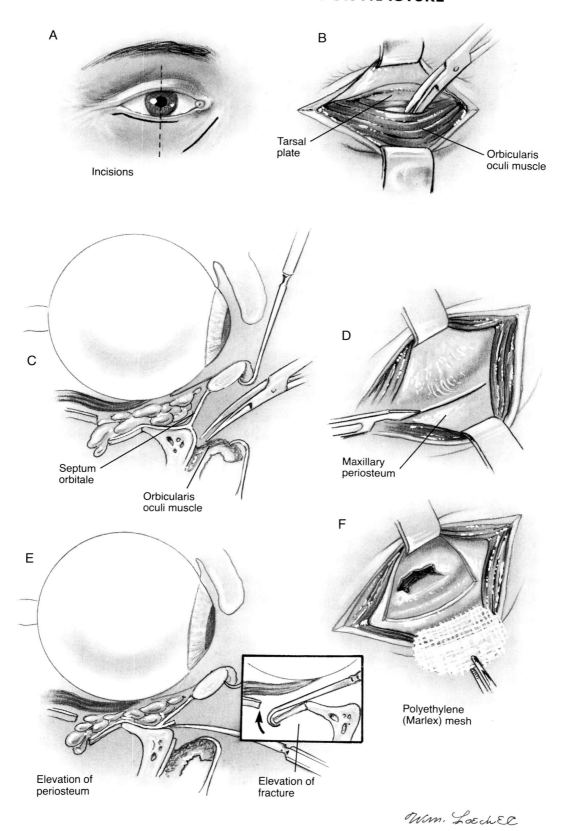

A

Incisions

B

Tarsal plate

Orbicularis oculi muscle

C

Septum orbitale

Orbicularis oculi muscle

D

Maxillary periosteum

E

Elevation of periosteum

Elevation of fracture

F

Polyethylene (Marlex) mesh

REPAIR OF BLOWOUT FLOOR FRACTURE *(Continued)*

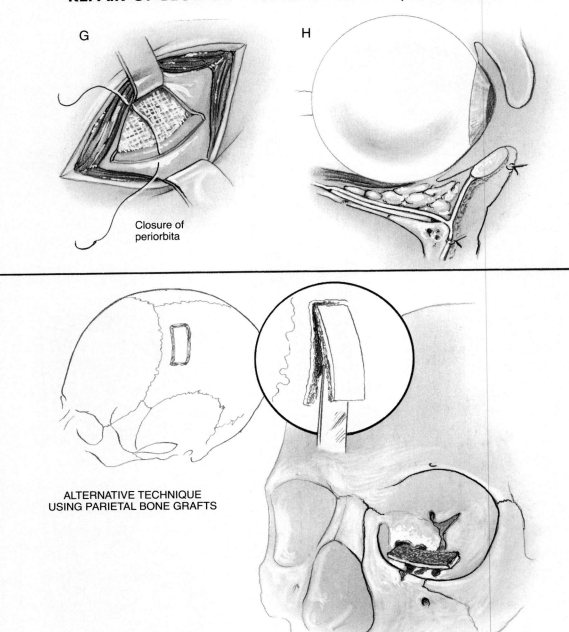

G

H

Closure of
periorbita

ALTERNATIVE TECHNIQUE
USING PARIETAL BONE GRAFTS

are necessary for successful results. An optimal time for surgery is 7 to 10 days after injury.

6. Avoid damage to the tarsal plate. The orbicularis oculi inserts onto the lower portion of the plate, and to be safe, a cuff of these tissues should be left on the plate. Scarring in and around the tarsal plate can lead to retraction of the lower eyelid.

7. Keep eyelid incisions small. Long eyelid incisions compromise lymphatic drainage and cause postoperative edema.

8. Orbital fat herniating into the sinus must be treated with atraumatic techniques. Avoid direct injury or amputation of fat, as this causes necrosis and/or resorption. Changes in intraorbital contents will ultimately affect the globe position.

9. Injury to the infraorbital artery should be avoided, but if this should occur, gentle pressure will control the bleeding. Cauterization should not be used, as this can potentially cause damage to the infraorbital nerve. As a last resort, vascular clips can be applied to the bleeding vessel.

10. Polyethylene (Marlex) mesh is the preferred implant. It has an excellent record of providing good results without the adverse sequelae reported with other types of alloplastic materials. Silastic tends to extravasate and must be anchored into position. Autogenous bone grafts, if too thin (i.e., from the anterior wall of the maxilla), tend to resorb. Autografts from the cranium tend to be too thick and are difficult to mold to appropriate wall contours.

11. When the orbital floor has undergone healing and fusion of malpositioned bone fragments, a more aggressive approach is required. These fractures may require reduction with a strong elevator. Sometimes the entrapped tissues have to be freed by cutting away areas of the depressed wall with Kerrison rongeurs. The defect can be subsequently repaired with the appropriate implant.

12. Fractures that are more posteriorly and medially oriented may require a transantral approach for adequate reduction. The anterior antrostomy should be large enough to allow the surgeon to visualize the floor region and admit a finger for palpation and reduction of the fragments. This approach ideally should be performed in combination with one of the eyelid approaches so that the floor can also be inspected from above and reinforced with polyethylene mesh. Maxillary packing is rarely indicated. If the floor fragments do not hold in a reduced position, the surgeon should consider a more substantial implant, such as a bone graft.

13. For large floor defects, polyethylene mesh will not provide sufficient support. In these cases, a bone graft must be considered. The outer parietal cortex is the preferred donor site.

COMPLICATIONS

1. Loss of vision is probably the most dreaded complication associated with a blowout fracture. This loss can occur from an injury to the lens or cornea, hyphema, retinal tear, and/or globe perforation. Optic nerve injury and/or retinal artery occlusion can develop primarily from trauma near the optic canal or secondarily from excessive retraction on the globe, retro-orbital hemorrhage, and displacement of an implant. The medical condition of the eye and results of visual tests should be recorded. Surgery should be delayed if there are factors present that would predispose to additional injury. If visual loss occurs following surgery, the condition should be recognized and treated immediately. If applicable, the surgeon should remove a displaced implant, control bleeding, remove accumulated clots, and reduce pressure on the retrobulbar area with a canthotomy and lysis of the periorbita. In addition, the surgeon can administer steroids and diuretics to relieve intraorbital and retro-orbital pressures.

2. Persistence of diplopia and/or enophthalmos may indicate an inadequate repair. In the early postoperative period, it is possible to reexplore and reduce the fracture and again reinforce the wall defect. In our experience satisfactory results can be obtained up to 6 weeks following surgery. Beyond that time, other alternatives such as orbital reconstruction with bone grafts should be considered (see Chapter 60).

3. Postoperative hypoesthesia is a common sequela following blowout fractures. The neural deficit may also be associated with paresthesia and pain over the distribution of the infraorbital nerve and its maxillary branches. Theoretically, an early and accurate reduction of the floor should prevent this complication from occurring and allow for regeneration of the nerve. If the complication persists, the surgeon can consider exploration of the nerve for a neuroma. Any compression phenomena can be treated by opening and decompressing the infraorbital canal (see Chapter 56).

4. Ectropian can usually be avoided by careful atraumatic technique. The tarsal plate should be protected and repeated cuts through the orbicularis muscle should be avoided. Reactive scarring can be minimized by closing the periosteum with only one chromic suture. If ectropian should start to develop, steroid injections (40 mg/mL) of triamcinolone should be started and the eyelid massaged daily. If the ectropian persists, the surgeon must consider lysis of the scar and/or split-thickness grafts applied to the skin.

ALTERNATIVE TECHNIQUE USING PARIETAL CORTEX GRAFTS

Occasionally the floor fracture extends along the floor to involve the medial wall and is so severely comminuted that mesh is not able to provide sufficient support. For such a condition, a bone graft is desirable. The outer cortex of the parietal bone is preferred, as the donor site is close to the affected area and the graft can be harvested with minimal morbidity. Anterior maxillary wall grafts are not as satisfactory, because they tend to resorb. Iliac crest or rib grafts can be used, but they are more difficult to obtain and are often associated with added discomfort during the postoperative period.

The parietal cortex is exposed and the bone removed as described in Chapter 60. The graft is then rotated so that the curve approximates the floor (outer surface down), and the bone is trimmed appropriately with cutting burs and rongeurs. Because the graft will be only slightly resorbed (if at all), the amount of correction must be exact. If the graft tends to raise the floor to a higher level, this will cause hyperophthalmos, and the graft should be thinned accordingly. If the graft lies at a low level, it must be reinforced with other grafts to accommodate the loss of orbital volume. The graft is usually stabilized by closing the periosteum over it with 3-0 chromic sutures. The eyelid skin is approximated with a 5-0 subcuticular nylon suture, and the patient is treated with prophylactic antibiotics for at least 7 to 10 days.

ALTERNATIVE TECHNIQUE USING THE CALDWELL-LUC APPROACH

In fractures of the floor of the orbit characterized by severe injury, comminution of fragments, and extension of the fracture to the posterior portion of the orbit (ethmoid ledge), a transantral approach may be helpful. The procedure should be carried out in conjunction with the orbital exploration from above, so that as the surgeon reduces the fragments from below, the correct position can be ensured from more than one direction.

a—d The approach is through an incision about 3 to 4 mm above the gingival margin from the first or second molar to the lateral incisor. Hemostasis is achieved with electric cautery. The periosteum is then elevated from the canine fossa superiorly onto the face of the maxilla. The dissection is continued superiorly to the level of the infraorbital canal, posteriorly to the zygomaticomaxillary buttress, and anteriorly to the nasofrontal buttress. An osteotomy is made in the anterior wall of the maxilla, and using Kerrison rongeurs, the opening is enlarged to approximately 2 × 3 cm. Blood is suctioned from the cavity, and the floor of the orbit is visualized from below.

e Assuming that the periorbita has already been elevated from the fracture site, the surgeon can then slip a finger through the antrostomy, palpate the fragments, and push the fragments into appropriate position. If the fragments do not stay in that position, the floor should be examined from above and appropriate adjustments carried out.

The surgeon may be tempted to pack the sinus from below, but this should be avoided. Packing of the maxillary sinus often leads to stasis of secretions, localized inflammation, and ultimate absorption of the floor. We prefer instead to reinforce the floor of the orbit with a cranial bone graft.

f The maxilla should be drained with a small hole (1.5 cm in diameter) made through the medial wall of the maxilla, below the inferior turbinate, and into the nose. The gingival mucosa is closed with 4-0 chromic sutures. Prophylactic antibiotics are prescribed for 7 to 10 days.

REPAIR OF BLOWOUT FLOOR FRACTURE *(Continued)*

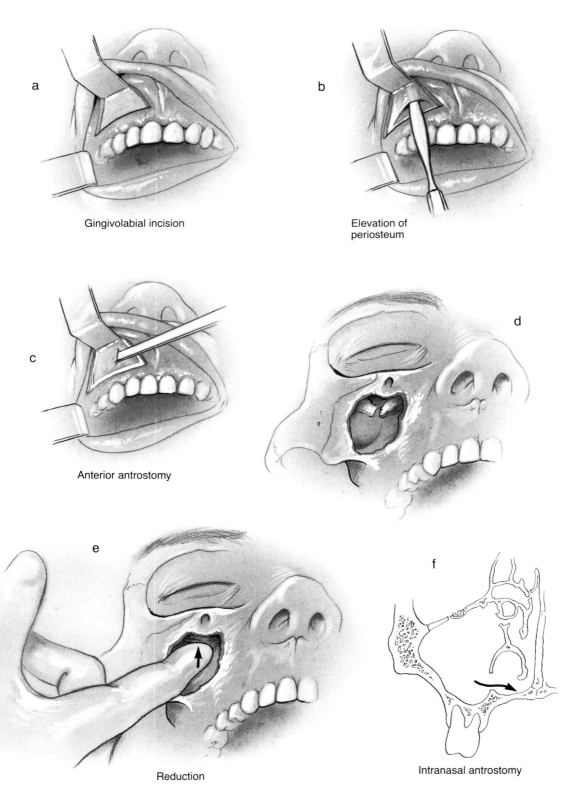

a

Gingivolabial incision

b

Elevation of
periosteum

c

Anterior antrostomy

d

e

Reduction

f

Intranasal antrostomy

Wm. Loechel

chapter 59

Repair of Medial Wall Fractures of the Orbit With Polyethylene Mesh
Alternative Technique for Repair of Junctional Injuries

INDICATIONS

The same philosophy employed in the treatment of the floor fracture is applied to the management of the medial wall (see Chapter 58). Consequently, if the surgeon has a full understanding of the pathophysiology, uses appropriate indications for surgery, and applies standard surgical techniques, medial orbital wall surgery can provide for an effective repair with minimal or no sequelae.

Pure blowout fractures of the medial wall often present with enophthalmos and/or diplopia. Defects that extend to the inferior wall (junctional type) produce significant intraorbital volume-to-content discrepancies and thus are often associated with marked retrodisplacement of the globe. Smaller defects occurring near the medial rectus muscle can cause displacement of the muscle and subsequent impairment of movement. Fractures on the deeper aspect of the medial wall can additionally affect inferior rectus functions, and if the injury extends to the optic canal, a loss of vision can occur.

Absolute indications for surgical exploration include the following:

1. Acute enophthalmos (>2 to 3 mm) and/or hypophthalmos (>2 to 3 mm).
2. Restriction of lateral (or medial) gaze associated with diplopia.

Relative indications include (1) large defects (an area of 2 to 3 cm²) associated with at least 2 to 3 mm of wall displacement; and (2) persistent diplopia on lateral gaze, presumably caused by a small defect, and mechanical changes not perceptible by forced duction tests. Such cases should have no evidence of neural injury.

Ideally the procedure should be performed when swelling has decreased and function can be accurately assessed, usually at 7 to 10 days following the injury. If there are associated fractures that require treatment (i.e., naso-orbital), the procedures should be coordinated to take place at the same time. Surgery performed too late can be compromised by malunion of small fragments of bone and scarring and contraction of soft tissues. Nevertheless, it is still worthwhile to explore and repair medial wall fractures up to 4 to 6 weeks after injury.

PROCEDURE

A The medial wall of the orbit is best approached by a curved incision approximately 2.5 cm in length placed one half the distance from the lacrimal caruncle to the dorsum of the nose. Prior injection with 1% lidocaine containing 1:100,000 epinephrine will help in hemostasis. The angular vessels should be ligated or cauterized and the periosteum incised along the frontal process of the maxilla.

B Using Joseph and, subsequently, Freer elevators, the periosteum is elevated toward the medial orbital wall. The dissection should be superior to the junction of the anterior and posterior lacrimal crests, thereby avoiding injury to the medial canthal ligament and the lacrimal sac. The trochlea is then detached from the superior orbital rim. Elevation of the periosteum along the medial wall should expose the anterior ethmoidal artery, which is often involved with the fracture. However, if the artery is intact, it should be detached and bleeding controlled with gentle pressure or vascular clips. The extent of the dissection posteriorly should be limited by the posterior ethmoidal artery.

C–F The periorbita should subsequently be teased out of the fragmented lamina papyracea. Often the periorbita is torn, and the surgeon must be careful not to injure the displaced fat. The hook technique, described in Chapter 58, can be useful for elevation of the bone fragments. Most medial orbital wall defects can be repaired by placing an appropriate

REPAIR OF MEDIAL WALL BLOWOUT FRACTURE

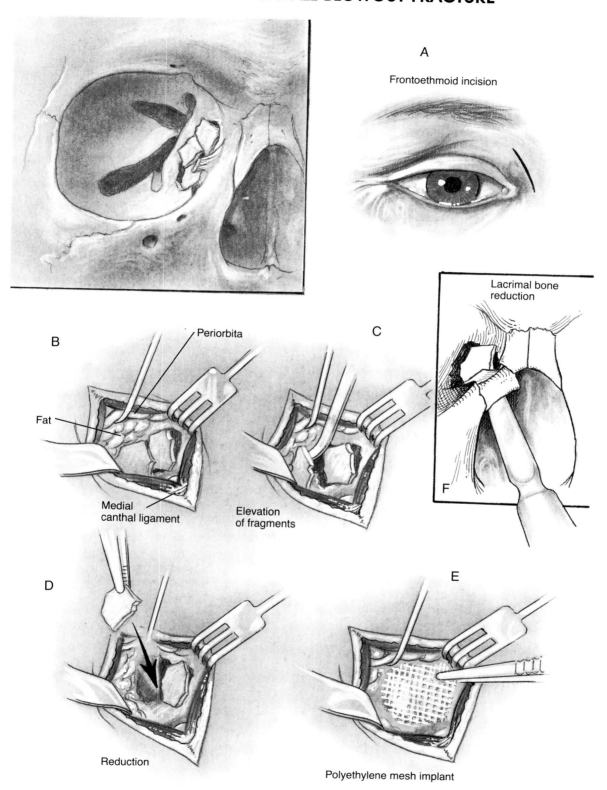

A
Frontoethmoid incision

B
Periorbita
Fat
Medial canthal ligament

C
Elevation of fragments

F
Lacrimal bone reduction

D
Reduction

E
Polyethylene mesh implant

Wm. Loechel

piece of polyethylene (Marlex) mesh of appropriate size along the defect. If the ethmoid/lacrimal complex is displaced medially, reduction can be facilitated by placing a Boies elevator along the middle turbinate and pushing the wall laterally. Adequate reduction should be confirmed with forced duction tests applied to the insertion of the medial rectus muscle.

The periosteum is closed with a 4-0 chromic suture. The subcutaneous tissues are brought together to relieve tension on the skin with a 4-0 chromic suture. The skin is closed with a 5-0 or 6-0 nylon suture. Prophylactic antibiotics (i.e., penicillin or erythromycin) are prescribed for 5 to 7 days. The patient should be evaluated at 1 week and then monthly for 6 months to ensure stability and uneventful healing.

PITFALLS

1. Patients with suspected medial wall injuries should have appropriate imaging studies performed and an accurate evaluation of globe position and eye movements. Size, site, and severity of the injury will dictate the clinical and/or surgical management. Ophthalmologic examination and consultation are highly recommended.

2. Contraindications to surgery are hyphema, retinal tear, and/or globe perforation. Traumatic optic neuropathy and retinal artery occlusion are also important considerations. Surgery should not be performed on an only-seeing eye.

3. Surgery should be timed to a period when inflammatory responses and swelling have subsided. Ideally exploration should precede bone healing and soft tissue scar contraction. If there are associated fractures that must be treated, surgery should be coordinated with those repairs.

4. Avoid injury to the medial canthal ligament and lacrimal sac. Elevation of the sac should be limited to the fundus region only, and the surgeon should preserve those ligamentous attachments that surround the body of the sac and insert onto the anterior and posterior lacrimal crests.

5. Bleeding of the anterior ethmoidal vessels can make surgery difficult and cause problems later (i.e., retro-orbital hemorrhage). Usually bleeding from the vessel can be controlled with gentle pressure. If bleeding does not stop, vascular clips can be judiciously applied.

6. The optic nerve can be damaged by the initial injury or by a too-aggressive dissection on the medial wall of the orbit. The posterior ethmoidal artery is a valuable landmark, and dissection should be anterior to this vessel. So-called "standard distances" cannot be relied on to determine the exact position of the optic nerve.

7. Large unstable defects of the medial wall probably should be treated with bone grafts. In grafting this area, the surgeon should make sure that the graft is properly contoured to the defect. A graft that is too large can cause pressure on the optic nerve and should be avoided. The nasal mucosa should be kept intact if contamination and resorption of the implant are to be prevented.

8. If the medial wall fracture extends inferiorly and is associated with a floor injury, the fracture is better repaired by an additional exposure from below. The infraciliary or high eyelid (subtarsal) incision, combined with the medial canthal incision, will provide an excellent approach.

COMPLICATIONS

1. The medial wall fracture places the optic nerve at risk at the time of injury and at the time of exploration and repair. Careful preoperative evaluation, coupled with a skillful dissection, should help minimize any injury to the nerve.

Vision disturbances occurring postoperatively must be immediately evaluated. Ophthalmic consultation should be obtained. If indicated, the surgeon can remove the implant or drain a retro-orbital hematoma. Additionally, retro-orbital pressures can be relieved by periosteal incisions and canthotomy. Steroid and diuretic administration may be helpful.

2. Persistence of diplopia should be evaluated and treated appropriately. If restriction of eye movement is not caused by neural injury, the surgeon should consider reexploration and repair.

3. Postoperative enophthalmos usually indicates an intraorbital volume-to-content discrepancy and suggests a failure in adequately reducing the orbital defect. Reexploration and repair should be considered, but if these complications persist or are noted to develop at a later time, then orbital reconstruction with strategic implantation of bone grafts (see Chapter 60) is preferred.

4. Medial canthal displacement and/or obstruction to the lacrimal system can be prevented by maintaining the anatomic integrity of this area. If telecanthus and/or epiphora develop, appropriate measures (see Chapters 62 through 69) should be taken.

ALTERNATIVE TECHNIQUE FOR REPAIR OF JUNCTIONAL INJURIES

Fractures that extend from the medial wall to the inferior wall create a unique set of problems. The defect tends to be large, there is loss of tissue into the nose and sinuses, and the potential for enophthalmos is high. The injury is not well appreciated by the medial canthal incision, and thus a combined technique becomes advantageous.

a The procedure should utilize infraciliary and medial canthal incisions. The floor dissection is carried more medially, hopefully avoiding the area anteriorly that contains the lacrimal sac and nasal lacrimal duct. From the medial canthus incision, the dissection is carried above and behind the medial canthal attachment and posterior lacrimal crest. The subperiosteal dissections should then meet at the junction of the medial and inferior walls.

b—e For the reduction of fragments, the surgeon can use the skin hook technique. If the ethmoid complex is displaced, elevation of the lateral wall of the nose with a Boies elevator, as described previously, is helpful. If the reduction cannot be stabilized with one or several pieces of polyethylene mesh, the surgeon must consider the use of bone grafts (see Chapter 60). The wounds are closed in standard fashion, and the patient is administered prophylactic antibiotics.

REPAIR OF MEDIAL WALL BLOWOUT FRACTURE *(Continued)*

ALTERNATIVE TECHNIQUES FOR REPAIR OF JUNCTIONAL INJURY

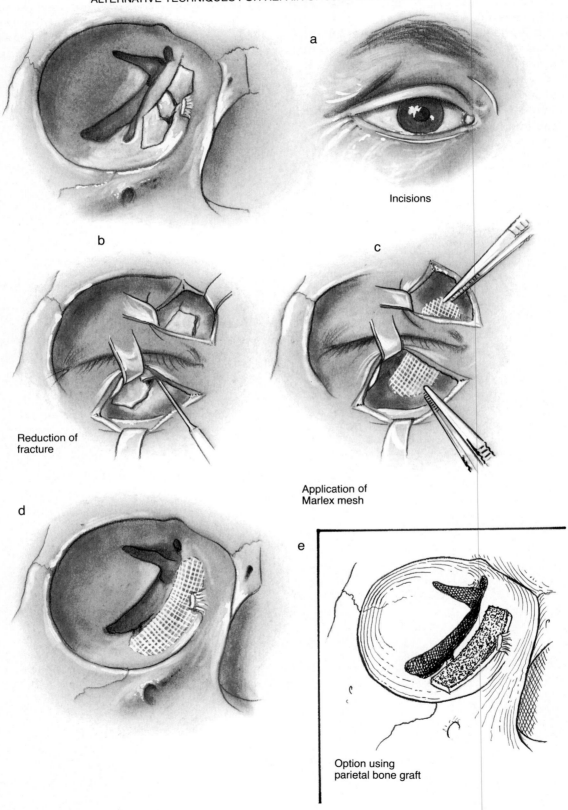

a

Incisions

b

Reduction of
fracture

c

Application of
Marlex mesh

d

e

Option using
parietal bone graft

chapter 60

Reconstruction of the Orbit Using Iliac Crest Grafts
Alternative Techniques Using Cranial Grafts and Osteotomies

INDICATIONS

Persistent or progressive enophthalmos following injury to a wall of the orbit can occur as a result of an expansion of the orbital wall, reduction in space occupied by intraorbital tissues, or a shift of fat behind the globe to a more peripheral position. Other possible, but less likely, causes are dislocation of the superior oblique muscle, cicatricial contraction of retrobulbar tissues, or rupture of the orbital ligaments or fascial bands.

Enophthalmos is frequently associated with hypophthalmos and/or diplopia. Muscle imbalance occurs as a result of muscle (or fibrous septae) entrapment, neuromuscular injury, or displacement of the axis of the globe. The inferior rectus muscle, close to the inferior wall, and the medial rectus muscle, close to the medial orbital wall, are often involved.

Early after orbital trauma, a displaced globe and restriction of muscle movement can be treated by exploration and repair (see Chapters 58 and 59). However, if these findings are observed later, there is a possibility of malposition or resorption of an orbital wall and/or atrophy and loss of soft tissues. When this occurs, the orbit must be reconstructed. The muscles and their attachments will have to be freed, and the walls will have to be rebuilt by osteotomy or onlay grafts. The soft tissues will have to be replaced or augmented by implant materials.

PROCEDURE

Our reconstructive technique is designed to reduce the size of the orbit and increase intraorbital contents by the strategic implantation of bone grafts. Soft tissue retractions are released by a 280° subperiosteal dissection, carefully sparing injury to the anulus tendineus, the superior orbital fissure, and the medial superior quadrant that contains the optic nerve and ophthalmic artery. The grafts are then placed against the orbital walls, especially along those in which there is a defect. The implants are positioned so that they displace the tissues primarily from behind the equator and along the horizontal-vertical axis of the globe.

General anesthesia and oral intubation are used, and the patient is placed in a supine position. The left hip is elevated on a pillow or sandbag. The hip and face are then prepared and draped as sterile fields. If two operating teams are available, the harvesting of the graft can be done by one team while the other prepares the orbit.

The bone graft is obtained as described in Chapter 26. The surgeon should harvest sufficient bone, and if the enophthalmos is greater than 3 to 4 mm, the surgeon should anticipate using a block of bone 1 × 3 × 6 cm. The bone should be kept in a basin containing blood until it is carved and implanted. The hip wound should be drained and closed appropriately.

The position of the eye should be remeasured, as the degree of enophthalmos can be affected by anesthesia and by the pull of gravity in the supine position. The opposite eye should be used as a reference for position, forced duction tests, and what would be palpated as "normal" tissues.

A The surgical approach is usually through three incisions: the lower eyelid, lateral eyebrow, and medial canthus. The pathologic condition often indicates which incisions are best utilized for the exploration.

B The medial wall of the orbit is explored through a medial canthal incision made one half the distance between the lacrimal caruncle and the dorsum of the nose. A local anesthetic containing epinephrine is injected for vasoconstriction effects. The angular vessels are ligated or cauterized as described in Chapter 59. The trochlea is released, while the periosteum is elevated to expose the anterior ethmoidal artery. The dissection should avoid injury to the medial canthal ligament and lacrimal sac. The anterior ethmoidal artery can be ligated or avulsed at its entry into the ethmoid bone, and hemostasis can be obtained with gentle pressure or application of vascular clips. The posterior ethmoidal vessel limits the dissection posteriorly and serves to protect the optic nerve.

C The approach to the lateral wall is through an eyebrow incision in which the area is infiltrated earlier with 1% lidocaine containing 1:100,000 epinephrine. The incision should not extend beyond the level of the hairs of the lateral eyebrow, and to avoid injury to the hairs, the incision should be beveled in a plane corresponding to the hair follicles. The orbicularis oculi is cut and the periosteum incised at the level of the zygomaticofrontal suture. Using Freer elevators, the periosteum is then elevated off the lateral wall of the orbit, relaxing the attachment of the lateral canthal ligament from the lateral orbital tubercle and elevating the lacrimal gland from its fossa. Small vessels are encountered, and bleeding can be controlled by gentle pressure.

D The lower eyelid incision is designed 2 to 3 mm below the lash line and extended into a "crow's foot" crease laterally. After injection with 1% lidocaine containing 1:100,000 epinephrine to control bleeding, the skin is incised through the orbicularis oculi to the orbital septum. The septum is then separated from the muscle, and the dissection is continued inferiorly toward the orbital rim. It is at this point, with good visualization of the rim, that the orbicularis oculi and the zygomaticus muscle insertions are released. The incision is then carried through the periosteum to the anterior wall of the maxilla.

Using Joseph elevators initially and Freer elevators later, the periosteum is elevated off the rim and floor of the orbit. By beginning in a nonfractured area, a difficult dissection is made somewhat easier. In places where there are old fractures and adhesions of the periosteum, the surgeon may have to refracture displaced fragments or even enter a plane above the periosteum. In severely injured patients, it is difficult to maintain the integrity of the infraorbital nerve and vessel, and the dissection often requires avulsion or a cutting of these tissues.

Laterally the dissection often encounters adhesions at the inferior orbital fissure. Fat can be observed coming either up through the fissure or downward from the orbital contents. In many cases, the surgeon has to dissect through the fat and adhesions, keeping as close as possible to the imaginary level of the floor.

The dissection should proceed posteriorly to the junction of the infraorbital groove of the maxilla and the inferior orbital fissure. Just medial to this junction, the orbital plate of the ethmoid forms a ledge that limits the posterior dissection and serves as a "guard" to the optic nerve. Entrapment of muscle posterior to this area is not considered surgically and safely accessible, at least from the inferior approach.

E–G The dissections should create pockets along the medial and lateral walls to the floor. The pocket along the medial wall should be posterior to the lacrimal sac and nasolacrimal duct. Superiorly and laterally, the dissection should elevate the periosteum behind the globe to a level of approximately the pupil.

H Following this extensive subperiosteal dissection, the globe should be completely mobile in all directions. The first implant is usually in the shape of a shield and placed along the floor region. As the globe is elevated, pressure will be exerted along the superior wall; this will also tend to project the globe outward. The primary effect, however, will be to elevate the globe and correct a hypophthalmos.

I–K For the most part, projection is obtained by placing a curved, crescent-shaped piece of bone through the eyebrow incision behind the equator of the globe. This graft will have the effect of pushing the eye outward, but there also will be a tendency to push it medially. The medial displacement must be corrected by placement of a pyramidal piece of bone along the medial wall. This will also add to the intraorbital contents and increase the projection of the globe. Ideally the surgeon will be aiming at an overcorrection of the hypophthalmos and enophthalmos by about 1 to 2 mm; to get these effects, the surgeon will have to either add or trim the implants. Walls with the greatest defects will obviously receive the most volume of graft.

Following placement of the grafts, there will be some tension on the globe; this should be checked by palpation. The contralateral globe is used as a reference. Because the muscles will be stretched, forced duction tests will give false impressions of binding. However, some movement is to be expected.

The periosteum is then closed with one or several interrupted 3-0 chromic sutures. A subcuticular 5-0 nylon suture is used to approximate the infraciliary incision. The other wounds are closed in layers. The eye is washed with a balanced salt solution and treated with an appropriate eye ointment. A light compression dressing of fluffs and stretch gauze is applied for 48 hours to prevent chemosis and swelling of the eyelid. Prophylactic antibiotics are pre-

RECONSTRUCTION OF THE ORBIT WITH ONLAY GRAFTS

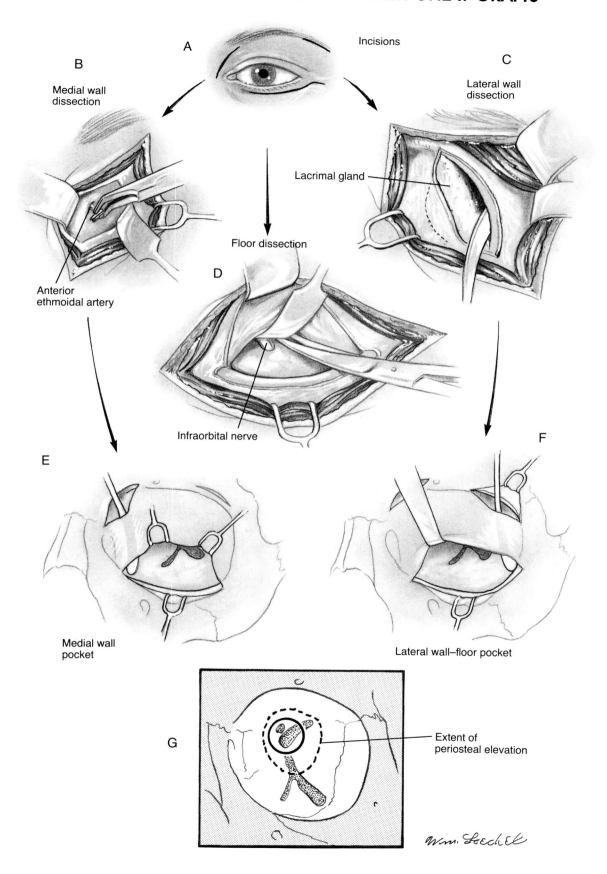

A — Incisions

B — Medial wall dissection

Anterior ethmoidal artery

C — Lateral wall dissection

Lacrimal gland

Floor dissection

D — Infraorbital nerve

E — Medial wall pocket

F — Lateral wall–floor pocket

G — Extent of periosteal elevation

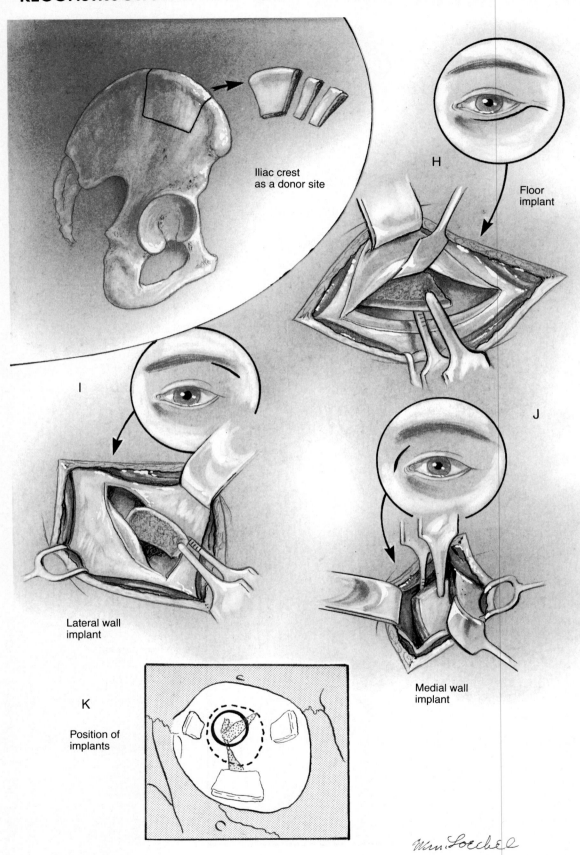

Iliac crest
as a donor site

H

Floor
implant

I

Lateral wall
implant

J

Medial wall
implant

K

Position of
implants

Wm. Loechel

scribed for 7 to 10 days. Diet and exercise are advanced as tolerated.

PITFALLS

1. Indications for the procedure, alone or in combination, are enophthalmos or hypophthalmos greater than 2 mm and/or diplopia in at least one field of gaze. These conditions can be accurately evaluated by history and physical examination and by forced duction tests used to assess globe mobility. The degree of deformity and dysfunction should be documented and quantified so that the patient and surgeon can appreciate the results of the surgical procedure.

2. An understanding of the pathophysiology is important if the surgeon is to obtain the desired correction. This information is derived from the history and physical findings, along with a complete set of imaging studies. Clues will thus be obtained on where to make the correction. The larger deficits obviously require a larger implant. Restricted muscles need to be adequately freed by the subperiosteal dissection.

3. Avoid surgery on those patients who have evidence of sinusitis. Two most dreaded complications are infection and extrusion of the grafts, and these can often be prevented by successfully treating the sinusitis before embarking on the reconstructive procedure.

4. The surgeon should not operate on an only-seeing eye. Although our experience has shown that there is little risk to vision, the risk far outweighs the benefits. All patients are informed that loss of vision is a possibility.

5. Ophthalmologic evaluation is important for diagnosis and proper treatment of the condition. The ophthalmologist is an important part of the team and should be available throughout the procedure.

6. Relative contraindications to surgery are a small contracted globe and ophthalmoplegia from retrobulbar cicatrization of soft tissues. The small globe is difficult to position. The scarring associated with ophthalmoplegia may sometimes not be completely relaxed and will limit repositioning of the globe and movement of muscles.

7. Limited degrees of dysfunction and/or deformity can often be treated with only one or two of the incisions. If a patient has only a mild to moderate hypophthalmos, a floor implant is all that is needed.

8. The hip graft is probably the best type of graft when the orbital reconstruction is associated with globe displacement greater than 3 to 4 mm. Cranial or rib grafts give only limited amounts of bone, and because they are thin grafts, the surgeon often has

to stack several pieces of bone to obtain appropriate size and contour. This can cause problems with instability and proper positioning of the graft.

9. Exposure for the procedure requires exact placement of the head and focused lighting. A surgeon-controlled table and a Lempert headlight are helpful adjuncts for the procedure.

10. The dissection must be adequate to obtain visualization of all wall deformities and relaxation of all "entrapped" tissues. Failure to achieve this degree of dissection will compromise the results.

11. The patient should be warned about the possibility of hip pain persisting for days to weeks following the procedure. Suction drains in the hip wound are best left in place until drainage is less than 20 mL per day. Early ambulation and rehabilitation are desirable.

12. Overcorrection of the enophthalmos and hypophthalmos is desirable. A sufficient amount of bone grafts will put increased tension on the globe that must be checked constantly, relating the globe pressure in the operated eye to that on the unoperated eye. Sudden increases in tension may be caused by retrobulbar hemorrhage, and the surgeon must try to distinguish these changes from those that would occur from the placement of the graft.

13. Patients who have associated injuries such as malar depressions often present with a more severe type of enophthalmos than that occurring from the blowout alone. These patients require more intraorbital grafting. In addition, the associated malar deformity must also be treated (see Chapter 61).

14. The dressing that is used to control soft tissue swelling can also mask the same conditions that cause loss of vision (i.e., retrobulbar hemorrhage, hyphema, etc.). If the surgeon is concerned that one of these complications may be developing at the time of surgery, the dressing is better left off. If the patient complains of pain in the postoperative period, the dressing should be immediately removed and the eye examined.

In applying the dressing, the eye should be well lubricated and the upper eyelid pulled down over the globe. The dressing must be tight enough to hold the upper eyelid in position. If the eyelid becomes raised, it is possible to develop a corneal abrasion. This will become suspect when the patient complains of pain and mentions that the eyelid is moving under the dressing.

COMPLICATIONS

1. Although loss of vision from this procedure is extremely rare, all patients should be told of this possibility and be prepared to accept the risk. Vision

can be compromised by increased intraorbital tension and compression of the optic nerve. This can be associated with displacement of the graft, retrobulbar hemorrhage, or retinal artery occlusion. Proper analysis and treatment should be implemented (see Chapters 58 and 59).

2. Infection of the graft is possible, and when this occurs, the patient should be treated vigorously with intravenous antibiotics. Debridement and removal of the graft may be necessary. This complication can be partially avoided by ensuring aeration of sinuses and healthy soft tissues around the graft. The dissection should also avoid exposure of contaminated areas such as the mucosa of the nose.

3. Although results are generally good with the reconstructive procedure, some degree of enophthalmos and hypophthalmos can return. This problem can occur with the resorption of bone, from infection, or from poor vascularity, but usually the malposition reflects inadequate correction with the implant. In the patient with a small contracted globe or ophthalmoplegia, the surgeon is most likely to have problems properly positioning the globe.

4. Diplopia, although often improved, can persist in some patients. If the surgeon is certain that there has been an adequate dissection and relaxation of tissues and that the globe is in an appropriate anatomic position, then it is logical to assume that there is a neuromuscular deficit or intramuscular contraction phenomenon (i.e., Volkmann's contracture). Eye muscle surgery may be helpful in correcting the problem.

5. Hip pain is to be expected. If this pain persists for more than a few weeks, consultation with an orthopedic surgeon is advisable.

6. Ectropion of the lower eyelid can occur as a result of the initial injury or as a result of surgery in those tissues that surround and support the eyelid. This complication can be somewhat avoided by careful atraumatic technique. However, if ectropion occurs, it can be treated initially with steroid injections (40 mg/mL of triamcinolone) into the contracted tissues. If this is unsatisfactory, the tissues will have to be lysed and the lower eyelid strengthened. Occasionally the tissues will need to be supported by a split-thickness graft.

ALTERNATIVE TECHNIQUE USING CRANIAL GRAFTS

For the most part, the hip graft is quite satisfactory for the reconstruction of the orbit. The donor site provides an adequate amount of bone that can be readily carved to appropriate size and shape. The grafts are stable and viable within the orbit; the main disadvantage is the hip morbidity that accompanies the procedure.

Limited dysfunction and deformity of the eye, however, can be treated satisfactorily with outer cranial cortex grafts. The procedure has minimal morbidity. The graft is well tolerated in the orbit, and its curvature fits conveniently along one of the orbital walls. However, the bone is thin, and if thicker pieces are needed, it will be necessary to stack the bone, which can cause instability. If large amounts of bone are needed, the exposure and the dissection must be expanded to include other ipsilateral and contralateral cranial bones.

a The procedure is carried out by first shaving the hair in a vertical line directly above and posterior to the auricle. This incision can be extended into a complete coronal incision if additional bone is desired from the opposite side. Infiltration of the area with 1% lidocaine containing epinephrine will help control some of the bleeding.

The incision is made through the skin, subcutaneous tissues, galea, and periosteum. Branches of the superficial temporal muscle will need to be ligated or cauterized to control bleeding. The periosteum is then elevated off the parietal bone. Self-retaining retractors are used to expose the bone and hold the tissues in position.

The surgeon should map out the location of the temporal, coronal, sagittal, and lamboidal suture lines. The dissection should stay several centimeters lateral to the sagittal suture line if the surgeon is to prevent the brisk bleeding that can occur from penetration of the sagittal sinus. The temporal bone should be avoided, as this bone is thin and extremely brittle.

b,c The harvest of bone is carried out by making parallel troughs about 1.5 cm apart through the outer cortex with cutting burs (3 mm) and saline irrigation and then joining the troughs horizontally at points lateral to the sagittal sinus and above the temporal suture line. This will provide grafts with a length of approximately 4 to 5 cm. The diploë will be more vascular and softer than the outer cortex, and the surgeon should proceed through the diploë until the more compact inner cortex is exposed. The troughs are then widened to accommodate a curved, sharp osteotome that is inserted into the diploë. With the tap of a mallet, the outer cortex is separated from the inner portion of the skull. Alternatively, the surgeon can use an offset oscillating saw. Additional grafts can be harvested as necessary from the frontal and occipital regions, and this can potentially provide grafts totaling 6 × 10 cm from one side of the head. However, it should be realized that females have thinner bone, and their cortical plates and diploë are not as well developed as those in males.

Bleeding of the diploë can be controlled by application of bone wax. The wound is closed in layers of 3-0 chromic, first approximating the periosteum and galea and then the subcuticular tissues. A 5-0 nylon suture is used to close the skin.

The bone is kept in a physiologic solution (or preferably a blood bath) until it is ready for grafting. When the surgeon has an estimate of the size and location of the defect, the bone can be carved and contoured to appropriate size and shape.

Complications from this procedure are cranial fracture, dural tear, and bleeding. If the osteotome is used as a fulcrum, it is possible to create a depressed fracture of the inner table. A small depression is probably inconsequential, but the patient should be followed postoperatively for changes of sensorium and/or other evidence of intracranial damage. Dural tears with cerebral spinal fluid leakage should be repaired. Bleeding of the dura should be brought under control. Injury to the sagittal sinus or to one of the branches of the middle meningeal artery can be quite troublesome, and if this should occur, neurosurgical consultation is immediately indicated.

ALTERNATIVE TECHNIQUE USING OSTEOTOMY

a′–c′ Reduction in size of the orbit can also be accomplished with the osteotomy technique. This method is particularly important in the relatively early period when the bones of associated craniofacial fractures (e.g., malar or naso-orbital) have just started to heal in malposition. The osteotomy ideally will recreate the fracture and usually provides an excellent opportunity for reduction and fixation with correction of the orbital wall.

It is also possible to perform an osteotomy at a later point in time, but usually the results are compromised by resorption of bone and instability of the reduction. The technique of lateral and inferior wall (malar osteotomy) is described in Chapter 54. The medial wall or medial maxillary (naso-orbital) correction is described in Chapter 39. Further improvement of the enophthalmos can often be obtained by shortening one of the orbital walls prior to repositioning the block of bone. Osteotomy can be also combined with onlay graft techniques.

ALTERNATIVE TECHNIQUES FOR RECONSTRUCTION OF THE ORBIT

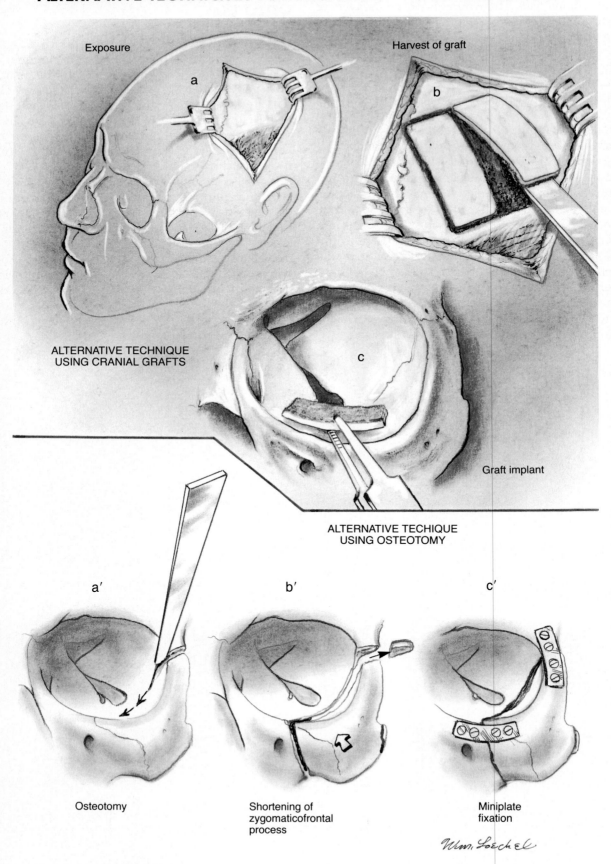

Exposure

a

Harvest of graft

b

ALTERNATIVE TECHNIQUE
USING CRANIAL GRAFTS

c

Graft implant

ALTERNATIVE TECHIQUE
USING OSTEOTOMY

a′

b′

c′

Osteotomy

Shortening of
zygomaticofrontal
process

Miniplate
fixation

chapter 61

Reconstruction of the Orbit for Combined Orbital Trauma Syndrome

INDICATIONS

If the floor fracture is associated with a malar fracture, the pathologic abnormalities can be additive, causing a more severe degree of deformity and dysfunction. In the floor fracture, the loss of the floor leads to failure in support of the globe and hypophthalmos. In the malar fracture, the suspensory ligament of Lockwood is displaced inferiorly, contributing more to the support problem. The floor fracture, when depressed, causes an increase in the volume of the orbit described by the walls, and this may be associated with some atrophy or necrosis of soft tissues; the malar fracture presents with an even greater depression and lateralization of the walls, adding to the discrepancy. It is important to recognize these effects, as the design of the procedure should be sufficient to correct them. The early repair (i.e., reduction and fixation) is described in Chapters 52, 53, and 58. The technique described here is for those patients in whom there is moderate to severe enophthalmos and hypophthalmos, with or without diplopia, associated with both a malunited blowout fracture and a malar fracture.

PROCEDURE

Essentially, the patient is prepared as for the orbital reconstruction (see Chapter 60). The graft harvested from the hip should be at least $1 \times 5 \times 8$ cm. The graft should be kept in a physiologic solution (preferably blood) until it is ready for shaping and implantation.

Eyebrow, medial canthal, and infraciliary incisions are useful approaches to the orbit. For the malar bone exposure, the surgeon can extend the infraciliary incision into one of the "crow's feet." The dissection is carried out as in Chapter 60, and the periorbita is elevated in all planes except that quadrant containing the ophthalmic artery and optic nerve. The subperiosteal dissection is also continued along the walls of the zygoma (including the frontal process of the zygoma, the anterior arch, and the zygomaticomaxillary buttress). The anterior wall of the maxilla is also exposed. If the deformity also involves the anterior wall of the maxilla, then it is necessary to extend the subperiosteal pocket to include the nasomaxillary buttress. This extended dissection frequently requires a sacrifice of the infraorbital nerve and vessel.

The bone harvested from the iliac crest must be large enough to accommodate a curved piece of bone to fit the anterior wall of the maxilla and malar eminence (A). Smaller pieces are carved to fit strategically within the orbit (B); the design of these grafts is described elsewhere (see Chapters 55 and 60). Pieces of cancellous bone should also be available and are placed between the floor and malar implants to provide a smooth contour to the rim. Additional pieces of graft may be necessary to provide a smooth transition between the malar graft and the adjoining frontal process of the zygoma.

The grafts are usually held in position by securing 2-0 or 3-0 chromic sutures to the overlying periosteum. A light compression dressing of fluffs and stretch gauze is desirable for 5 to 7 days. Prophylactic antibiotics should be given intravenously for 5 days and extended orally for an additional week.

PITFALLS

1. The same pitfalls pertain to the combined procedure as pertain to the separate reconstructions described in Chapters 55 and 60.

2. Remember that a reconstruction of the malar eminence will project the inferior wall of the orbit and create a relative enophthalmos. It is thus important that the techniques to project the eye overcompensate sufficiently to place the globe in proper relationship to the zygoma.

3. Avoid deficits that will develop between the planes of the orbital floor and the reconstruction of the malar eminence. A smooth contour should be

established with appropriate carved pieces of cancellous bone.

4. To prevent displacement of grafts in the early postoperative period, a light compression dressing should be used. The dressing can be removed in 24 hours. The malar grafts and eye functions should be examined and the dressing applied for an additional 48 hours.

COMPLICATIONS

1. Loss of vision, persistence of enophthalmos and/or diplopia, and hip pain are discussed in Chapter 60. Methods to prevent and treat displacement and/or absorption of a malar graft are described in Chapter 55.

2. Ectropion is a common complication, as the surgeon must perform an extensive dissection, and the grafts have a tendency to pull the lower eyelid downward. Measures to prevent retraction of the lower eyelid include relaxation through an extensive subperiosteal dissection and careful placement of periosteal sutures so that the tension is distributed in a natural direction. The surgeon should also provide sufficient tissues to cover the tarsal plate and should try to retain the integrity of the orbicularis oculi muscle. Excessive foreign body reaction should also be avoided by using only necessary suture material. Occasionally a Frost suture that holds the lower eyelid to the forehead superiorly is helpful. If ectropian should develop, the surgeon should first consider the use of steroid injections (triamcinolone, 40 mg/mL) and massage. Persistence of the ectropion may require oculoplastic reconstruction of the lower eyelid.

3. Hypoesthesia will develop, especially if the surgeon has to cut the infraorbital nerve. This is a "trade-off," as a pocket in this area is often necessary to hold the appropriate-sized graft.

RECONSTRUCTION FOR COMBINED ORBITAL TRAUMA

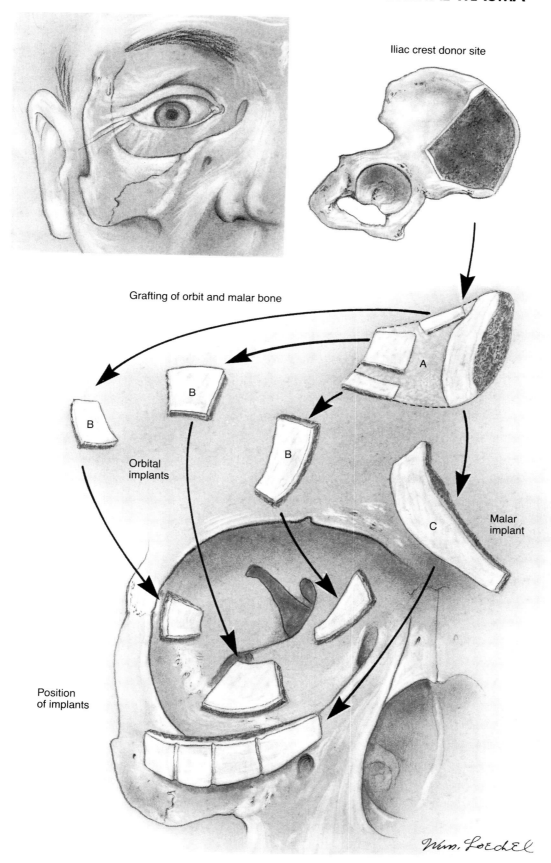

Iliac crest donor site

Grafting of orbit and malar bone

A

B

B

B

C

Orbital implants

Malar implant

Position of implants

Wm. Loechel

part seven

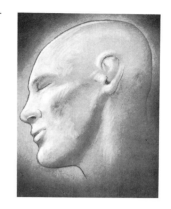

Naso-Orbital Fractures

Classification and Pathophysiology of Naso-Orbital Fractures

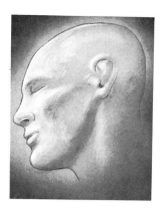

chapter 62

General Considerations

Naso-orbital fractures occur as a result of injury to the anteromedial wall of the orbit. They are commonly associated with multiple deformities and dysfunction. In many cases there is a change in appearance of the palpebral fissure, accompanied by tearing and failure of the lacrimal collecting system.

A,B The orbit is formed medially by the frontal process of the maxillary bone, the lacrimal bone, and the lamina papyracea of the ethmoid bone. The frontal and maxillary bones define the superior and inferior extent. The lacrimal fossa, in which lies the lacrimal sac, is formed by the posterior portion of the frontal process of the maxilla and the anterior portion of the lacrimal bone. Anterior and posterior crests receive insertions of the anterior and posterior slips of the medial canthal ligament and, additionally, on the posterior crest, an extension of the orbicularis oculi called *Horner's muscle.*

The anatomic relationships of the bone and soft tissues are important in understanding the pathophysiology of fractures in the region. The lacrimal collecting system, consisting of the puncta, canaliculi, sac, and duct, is intimately associated with the medial canthal ligament and orbicularis oculi muscle fibers. Tears normally enter the puncta at the medial free edge of the upper and lower eyelids and are transported through upper and lower canaliculi to a common canaliculus, which enters the sac near the junction of the body and fundus. Exit of tears is through a nasolacrimal duct that runs through the medial maxilla to the inferior meatus. The posterior portion of the orbicularis oculi, which attaches to the posterior crest, pulls the puncta against the globe. The puncta then picks up the tears from the surface of the globe. On closing the eyelids, the orbicularis oculi squeezes the tissues surrounding the lacrimal system. This causes alternating negative and positive pressures that collect and pass the tears. Failure of this pumping action as a result of trauma will result in epiphora.

The medial canthal ligament is also important in defining the palpebral opening. The medial canthal ligament is an extension of the tarsal plates. These plates also connect to the lateral canthal ligament, which attaches to the lateral wall of the orbit. The tarsal plates and ligaments receive insertions of the orbicularis oculi muscles. If the medial canthus becomes displaced or lax, the palpebral fissure becomes narrow, the medial caruncle moves laterally, and the medial aspect of the eye takes on a rounded appearance. Normally the palpebral fissure width equals the intercanthal distance and the palpebral fissure width of the other side, but with lateral displacement of the medial canthal ligament, these relationships are altered. Thus, measurements become an important part of the evaluation.

C–E Injuries to the medial wall can be classified according to the degree of deformity and dysfunction. Surgical repair can then be designed according to this classification system. Type I injury indicates that the medial canthal ligament has been displaced with a small piece of attached lacrimal bone or that the ligament has been severed completely. The patient presents with telecanthus, epiphora, blunting of the inner angle, and narrowing of the palpebral fissure. A type II injury implies that the medial wall of the orbit is comminuted and displaced. In addition to the signs and symptoms associated with the type I injury, there can be entrapment of the medial rectus muscle, cerebrospinal fluid leak, and damage to the optic nerve. In the type III injury, the medial walls of both orbits are fractured. This implies also a fracture of the nasoethmoid complex, including the nasal bones, septum, and portions of the frontal sinus. Patients with this type of injury have a flattening and widening of the nasal dorsum, nasal obstruction and epistaxis, bilateral telecanthus, blunting of the inner angle, narrowing of the palpebral openings, and epiphora. Intracranial damage and a cerebrospinal fluid leak often occur.

NASO-ORBITAL FRACTURES

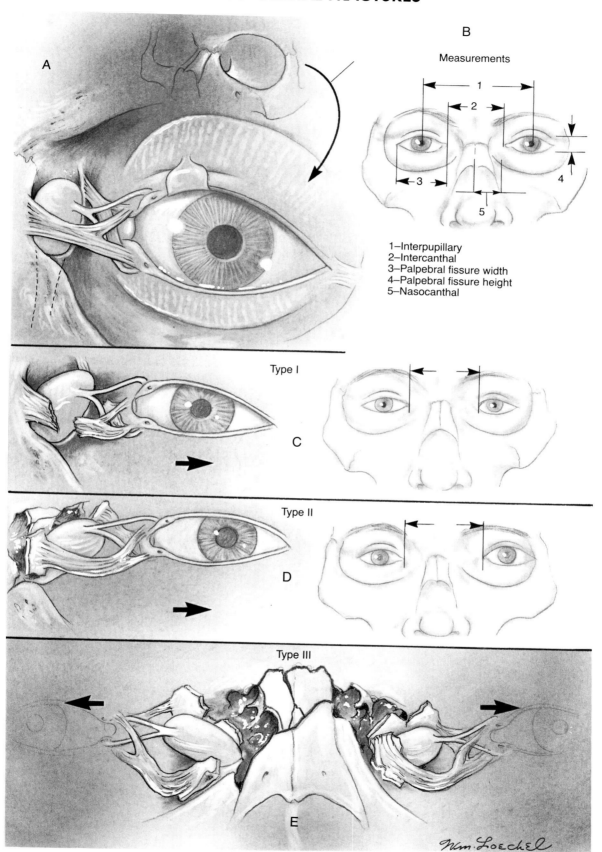

B

Measurements

1—Interpupillary
2—Intercanthal
3—Palpebral fissure width
4—Palpebral fissure height
5—Nasocanthal

Type I

C

Type II

D

Type III

E

Wm. Loechel

Management Strategies for Naso-Orbital Fractures

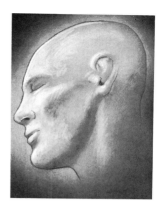

chapter 63

Open Repair of Type I Naso-Orbital Injury

INDICATIONS

Early diagnosis and repair is important in the treatment of the type I naso-orbital injury. The patient may present with a sharp penetrating wound of the medial canthus or with blunt trauma and a limited fracture of the lacrimal bone. In these patients, the palpebral fissure is narrowed, the inner angle becomes rounded, and tears collect in the lacus lacrimalis. Clinically there is telecanthus of a variable degree. The eyelids are lax, which is confirmed by pulling one of the eyelids laterally and testing for the presence or absence of tension near the attachment of the medial canthal ligament. The extent of bone involvement should be determined with appropriate imaging studies.

PROCEDURE

A Under general anesthesia, the face is prepared and draped as a sterile field. The palpebral fissure openings and nasocanthal distances are measured and recorded so that the amount of correction can be known before the start of the procedure (see Chapter 62). A curved medial canthal (frontoethmoid) incision halfway between the caruncle and dorsum of the nose is designed with marking solution. Another incision is marked in the lateral eyebrow region. Both areas are infiltrated with 1% lidocaine containing 1:100,000 epinephrine to help control hemostasis.

B,C Through the medial canthal incision, the angular vessels are either cauterized or ligated. The periosteum overlying the frontal process of the maxilla is incised, and with a Joseph elevator, the periosteum is elevated toward the margin of the medial orbital rim. The trochlea is identified, detached, and retracted laterally. The periorbita is elevated inferiorly to identify the lacrimal fossa and both crests. Additional exposure can be obtained by cutting the anterior ethmoidal vessel and retracting the soft tissues of the orbit laterally with malleable retractors. Hemostasis is achieved with gentle pressure, but if bleeding does not stop, vascular clips can be applied. The lacrimal collecting system (in particular the sac portion) should be explored and evaluated for damage.

D The repair requires relaxation of the lateral canthal ligament. This will remove the countertraction and provide an opportunity to overcorrect the position of the medial canthal ligament. For this portion of the procedure, the eyebrow incision is used, the orbicularis oculi is separated, and the periosteum of the frontal process of the zygoma is incised. The periosteum is elevated with a Freer elevator along the lateral wall and rim of the orbit. This releases the attached lateral canthal ligament. The wound is closed in layers with 4-0 chromic and 5-0 nylon sutures.

E The point of attachment for the medial canthal ligament is important. If a piece of the lacrimal bone is displaced with the ligament, the bone can be wired with 28-gauge stainless steel wires into its natural position. However, if the bone of the medial orbital wall is intact and the ligament has been severed, then the ligament should be attached with a strong ligature to the superior portion of the posterior lacrimal crest. The pull of the ligament upward and backward will facilitate improved contact of the puncta with the surface of the globe. The hole through the posterior crest can be made with a minidriver and a 0.035-inch Kirschner wire.

F–H The medial canthal ligament is next identified. The lacrimal sac and the inner caruncle are useful landmarks. The ligament can usually be found as a subcutaneous band of firm tissue that covers the lacrimal sac. To isolate the ligament, the subcutaneous tissues should be dissected over the sac for several millimeters until the surgeon meets resistance from the medial canthal ligament. These "tough" tissues can then be grasped with a forceps, and a 30-gauge stainless steel wire attached with a sharp cutting needle. This wire is then secured to the hole made on the superior part of the posterior crest. Assurance that the medial canthal ligament has been corrected can be obtained by repeating the eyelid tension test. Overcorrection is desirable. The periosteal and subcutaneous tissues are closed with 4-0 chromic sutures, and the skin is closed with a 6-0 nylon suture. Antibiotic ointment is applied to the wound.

The patient should be observed for at least 24 hours for any increase in intraorbital tension. Prophylactic antibiotics are prescribed for 5 days. The sutures are removed in 5 to 7 days.

PITFALLS

1. The best results are obtained with early diagnosis and treatment, as these will avoid the sequelae of scarring, chronic obstruction of the lacrimal system, and dacryocystitis. During the first few days, swelling will obscure the degree of injury. As the swelling disappears, the physician should continually evaluate for signs and symptoms. The eyelid tension test should be used to determine dehiscence of the medial canthal ligament.

2. Overcorrection of the medial canthal ligament is desirable and can be obtained by relaxation of the lateral canthal ligament.

3. Make sure that the traction on the ligament is upward and backward. This is best achieved by attaching the wire to the superior part of the posterior lacrimal crest.

4. Avoid the use of plates or buttons to hold the medial canthal ligament in position. These materials often cause necrosis of the skin, leave scars, and usually do not exert sufficient posterior pressure to maintain the desired position of the ligament.

COMPLICATIONS

1. Persistent or recurrent telecanthus presents a formidable problem. This complication can be avoided by early exploration and accurate attachment of the ligament. However, if this is not achieved or the wire becomes detached from the tissues, then reexploration must be performed.

2. Telecanthus that is diagnosed and treated late requires a different approach. Because of the scarring and retraction of tissues, the late surgery demands a more extensive dissection of the periorbita. Removal of bone along the medial wall of the orbit, as performed with a type II late repair (see Chapter 64), may also be required.

3. Injury to the lacrimal collecting system can result in obstruction and epiphora. Any part of the system can be compressed or twisted. Such injuries should be recognized and treated at the time of exploration. Damage to the puncta or canaliculus necessitates a repair, but if this is not successful, the surgeon can later perform a conjunctivodacryocystorhinostomy or conjunctivorhinostomy. If an outlet obstruction or infection develops, a dacryocystorhinostomy is the procedure of choice. These techniques are described in Chapters 64, 67, and 68.

TYPE I REPAIR

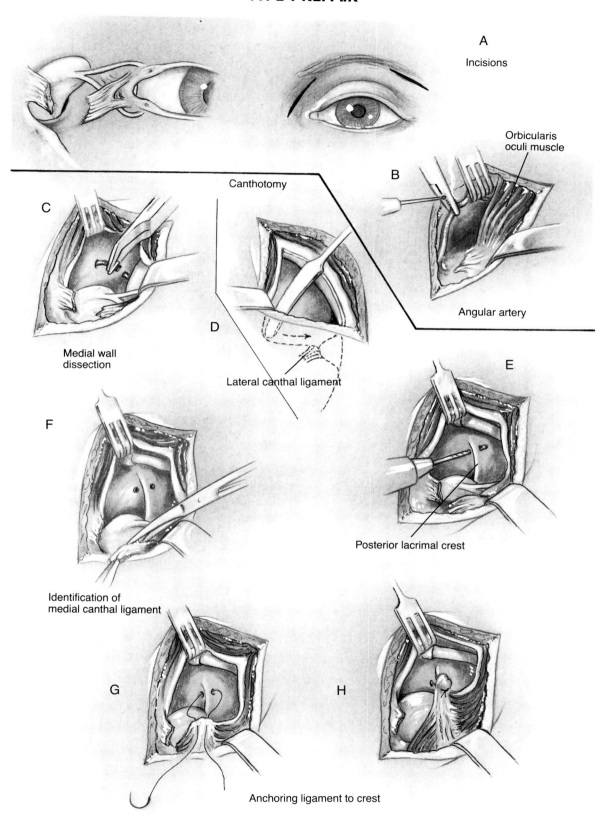

A
Incisions

Orbicularis
oculi muscle

B

Angular artery

Canthotomy

C

Medial wall
dissection

D

Lateral canthal ligament

E

Posterior lacrimal crest

F

Identification of
medial canthal ligament

G

H

Anchoring ligament to crest

Wm. Loechel.

chapter 64

Open Repair of Type II Naso-Orbital Injury With Transnasal Canthoplasty
Alternative Techniques for Late Repair

INDICATIONS

The type II injury should be identified and treated early if a successful result is to be obtained. This injury is characterized by multiple fractures involving the medial wall of the orbit. These small fragments are difficult, if not impossible, to stabilize and will not support the attachment of the medial canthal ligament. It thus becomes important to find a more suitable purchase point; this usually requires transnasal wiring to the opposite orbital wall. Patients with type II injuries present with telecanthus, blunting of the inner angle, narrowing of the palpebral fissure, and epiphora. The medial rectus and superior oblique muscles may be involved. Cerebrospinal fluid leak and compression of the optic nerve are rare but can also occur.

PROCEDURE

A,B The patient is prepared as described in Chapter 63, except that an additional medial canthal incision is marked on the opposite side. These approaches allow exploration of the medial canthal ligament and lacrimal sac on the involved side, a relaxing lateral canthotomy, and exposure of the lacrimal crests on the opposite side.

The angular vessels should be ligated and the trochlea and periosteum elevated from the medial orbital rim. The orbital soft tissues should then be retracted laterally, and with a Freer elevator, the junction of the anterior and posterior lacrimal crest should be exposed. If more relaxation is necessary, the anterior ethmoidal artery can be ligated and additional periorbita elevated off the medial wall of orbit. Displaced fragments of bone should be replaced; herniated fat and entrapped muscle should

be released and the wall, if necessary, reinforced with polyethylene mesh (see Chapter 59).

C,D The medial canthal ligament is identified as described in Chapter 63 and secured with a 30-gauge stainless steel suture. One end of the wire is then attached to a large curved needle, which is passed through the nasal septum and out through the lacrimal bone on the opposite side. The other end of the wire is passed in a similar way, but preferably through the lamina papyracea so that the wires exit on each side of the posterior lacrimal crest. The soft tissues of the orbit must be carefully protected with malleable retractors during these maneuvers.

E The 30-gauge wire is then secured to the opposite lacrimal crest in a way that ensures overcorrection of the displaced ligament. The ends of the wire are twisted flat against the wall of the orbit. The periosteum is closed using 4-0 chromic sutures; 5-0 nylon sutures are used to coapt the skin edges. The patient should be evaluated during the next several days for changes in intraorbital tension. Prophylactic antibiotics are prescribed for 5 days, and sutures are removed in 5 to 7 days.

PITFALLS

1. An accurate diagnosis is essential for successful treatment. If the surgeon tries to attach the wire to a fragmented piece of bone on the same side, the bone will slip, and telecanthus will return. If the surgeon attaches the wire to the nasal or frontal bone, it is possible that the medial canthal ligament will be pulled too far anteriorly, creating a deformity and failure of the puncta to reach the globe.

2. Some degree of "slippage" is expected and should be compensated for by a more medial placement of the medial canthal ligament. Relaxation of

TYPE II REPAIR

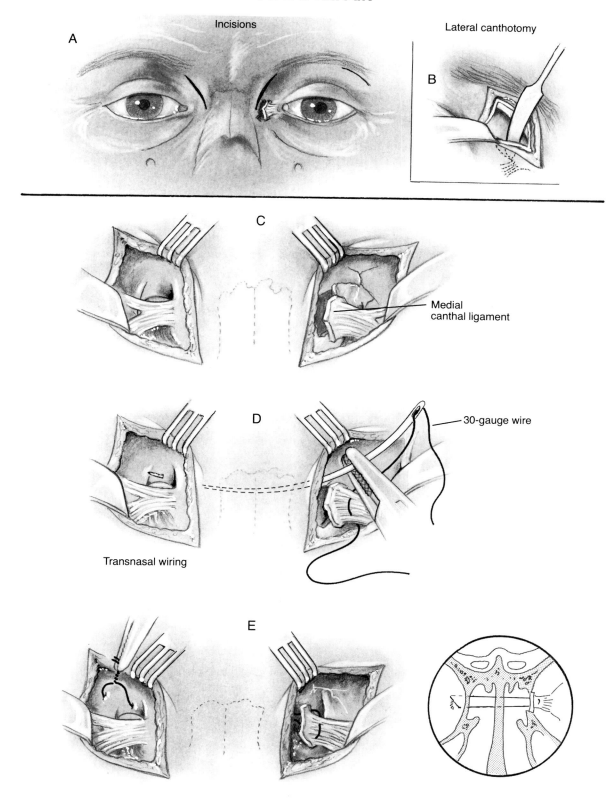

A

Incisions

B

Lateral canthotomy

C

Medial canthal ligament

D

Transnasal wiring

30-gauge wire

E

Wm. Loechel

the lateral canthal ligament will also help in the overcorrection.

3. Carefully inspect the lacrimal collecting system to make sure that there are no kinks or twists. Also, pass the fixation wire superior to the main part of the sac so that the sac is not obstructed by the wire. An ideal position is in the fundus or in the soft tissues that lie just superior to the fundus.

4. The fixation point on the opposite medial wall of the orbit must be intact and strong enough to "hold" the area. If strength is a problem, the wire should be secured to a screw or hole at the edge of the frontal process.

5. Avoid external buttons or plates, as they tend to cause necrosis of the skin and leave permanent scars. Also, it is unlikely that these materials are placed far enough posteriorly to hold the medial canthal ligaments in anatomic position.

6. For late repairs in which scarring and/or dacryocystitis develops, other techniques must be applied. These are discussed later.

COMPLICATIONS

1. Inadequate repair will result in residual telecanthus and/or epiphora. Usually this occurs when the postoperative swelling pulls the soft tissues from the wire or the wire loosens from the lacrimal bone. If this occurs, reexploration and repair are necessary. Late correction can be difficult to perform, and results are often compromised.

2. Dacryocystitis can occur from obstruction of the lacrimal collecting system. If this develops, the patient should be treated with appropriate antibiotics and the lacrimal collecting system evaluated with the Jones dye test for the degree and level of obstruction. Persistent dacryocystitis must be treated as described in Chapter 68.

3. If a cerebrospinal fluid leak persists or presents in the postoperative period, the patient should be continued on antibiotic therapy. Most leaks stop in a few days, but if a leak continues beyond 2 to 3 weeks, the site should be determined and preparations made for repair of the leak (see Chapters 84 through 87).

4. The transnasal wire technique can pull soft tissues of the involved orbit into the ethmoid sinus and potentially obstruct the nasofrontal duct. If the patient complains postoperatively of pain and swelling around the eye, appropriate radiographs should be obtained to evaluate the frontal sinus. Obstruction of the nasofrontal duct requires either reconstruction of the duct or obliteration of the frontal sinus with fat (see Chapters 72 and 76).

5. Medial canthal scars can result in web formation and deformity. This problem can be prevented by designing incisions with irregular patterns. If this complication does occur, a zigzagplasty or Z-plasty is indicated. Early injection with 40 mg/mL of triamcinolone may also be helpful.

ALTERNATIVE TECHNIQUES FOR LATE REPAIR

When treatment of the type II injury is delayed, the walls of the orbit become malunited, the periorbita is pulled into fracture lines, and the soft tissues become fixed with scar formation. Obstruction of the lacrimal collecting system causes epiphora, and long-term stasis leads to dacryocystitis. New bone often forms along the medial wall of the orbit. Under these conditions, alternative techniques must be applied.

a,b The incisions and approaches are the same as in the acute injury. Because scarring will limit the exposure, the surgeon will have to free up large areas of periorbita. This is accomplished by developing subperiosteal pockets that are extended along the floor and superior wall regions. If sufficient laxity of the tissues is not obtained, then an inferiorly placed incision and a subperiosteal dissection as described in Chapter 60 are carried out.

c—e New bone formation on the medial wall of the orbit requires removal of the bone with cutting burs and Kerrison rongeurs. The resection should accommodate the relocation of the medial canthal ligament. If the growth of scar tissue and bone tissue prevents passage of a large curved needle, the surgeon must drill holes with a 0.035-inch K wire and minidriver. The holes can be cannulated with a 14-gauge needle, and through the needle, the surgeon can then pass the transnasal wires. The process can be simplified by first passing a loop of 30-gauge wire through the needle, pulling through the end of the medial canthal–attached wire, removing the needle, and leaving the end in place. Another cannulation is then performed with an exit point just beyond the first; again, a 30-gauge wire loop technique is used to pass the other end of the medial canthal wire. The technique requires sufficient exposure of the medial walls of the orbits and retraction and protection of the globes and soft tissues with malleable retractors. Attachment of the medial canthal wire to the lacrimal crest of the opposite side, overcorrection of the medial canthal ligament, and incision closure are carried out as in the acute injury.

If the patient has a history of dacryocystitis, a dacryocystorhinostomy, described in Chapter 68,

TYPE II REPAIR *(Continued)*

ALTERNATIVE TECHNIQUES FOR LATE REPAIR

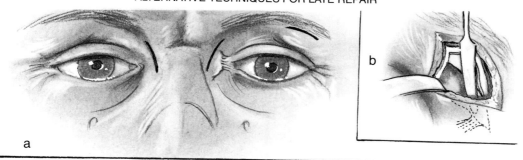

a

b

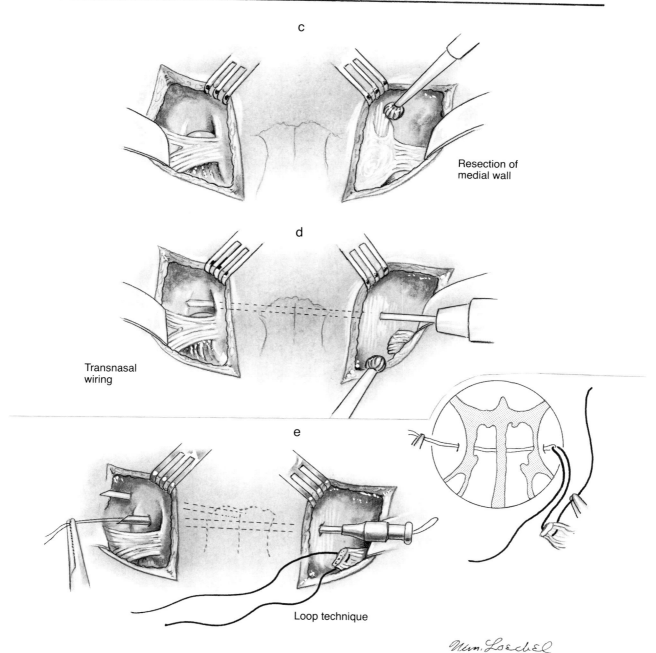

c

Resection of
medial wall

d

Transnasal
wiring

e

Loop technique

Wm. Loechel

should also be performed. Timing is important. The dacryocystorhinostomy repair should be carried out after the attachment of the wire to the medial canthal ligament, but before the wire is attached to the bone and the medial canthal ligament brought into the corrected position. If the dacryocystorhinostomy is done too early, there is a risk of pulling out the mucosal sutures with the transnasal wiring technique. If the dacryocystorhinostomy is done too late during the procedure, then the exposure will be compromised by the medially displaced orbital tissues.

chapter 65

Open Repair of Type III Naso-Orbital Injury With Transnasal Canthoplasty (Intercanthal Ligament Fixation)
Alternative Technique Using Frontal Process Fixation

INDICATIONS

The type III injury is characterized by comminution of the upper midface. The damage involves the medial walls of both orbits. Clinically there is marked bilateral telecanthus, displacement and blunting of the inner angles, narrowing of the palpebral fissures, and epiphora. The nasal bones are usually depressed. There is a history of epistaxis and unconsciousness, and often there is evidence of nasal obstruction and cerebrospinal fluid leak. Recognition of this type of injury is important, as stable bony attachments are not readily available, and the surgeon must find alternatives for attachments of the ligaments.

PROCEDURE

A The patient should be in stable medical condition for the procedure. The head and neck are prepared with antiseptic solutions and draped as a sterile field. The incision sites are injected with 1% lidocaine containing 1:100,000 epinephrine to assist in the hemostasis. The surgeon has the option of marking out bilateral lateral eyebrow incisions and standard bilateral medial canthal incisions (as described in Chapter 64) or performing the open sky approach in which the medial canthal incisions are connected with a horizontal limb to each other. The medial canthal incisions can also be extended beneath the eyebrow so that access can be gained to the anterior plate at the frontal sinus. Alternatively, the surgeon can approach the glabella angle from a coronal incision, but exposure along the medial orbital walls will be limited.

Working on one side at a time, the angular vessels are ligated or cauterized. The periosteum is incised and elevated superiorly off the glabella angle and prominence of the brow. Inferiorly the lacrimal fossa, the lacrimal collecting system, and the medial wall of the orbit are explored. Additional exposure is obtained by releasing the attachment of the trochlea and anterior ethmoidal artery. Hemostasis is carried out with gentle pressure or vascular clips. Bone fragments involving the medial wall of the orbit are reduced, and if necessary, the wall is reinforced with polyethylene mesh (see Chapter 59). The nasal and frontal bones are reduced and fixed with 28-gauge interosseous wires or bone plate techniques (see Chapters 48 and 71). Lateral canthotomies as described in Chapter 63 are performed bilaterally.

B On one side, the medial canthal ligament is secured to a 30-gauge wire with a cutting needle. Both ends of the wire are then attached to a large curved needle, which is passed through the superior portion of the septum to the opposite side. Entrance and exit on the medial walls of the orbit should be through the lacrimal bone region. The globes and soft tissues of the orbit must be protected with malleable retractors during these maneuvers. One free end of the 30-gauge wire is then attached to a fine curved needle and the needle passed through the opposite medial canthal ligament. The wire is tightened and the ends pulled together so that the ligaments pull toward each other. The twisted ends of the wire are subsequently bent back against the wall of the orbit.

Closure is in layers. The periosteum of the medial orbital and eyebrow incisions is closed with 4-0 chromic sutures. Tension-relieving 4-0 chromic sutures are applied to the subcutaneous tissues. The skin is coapted with an interrupted and/or continuous 5-0 nylon suture. Antibiotics are prescribed for at least 5 to 7 days, or for a longer time if there is any evidence of a cerebrospinal fluid leak. The sutures are removed at 5 to 7 days. The status of the frontal sinus should be evaluated with serial radiographs in the postoperative period.

PITFALLS

1. As described in the type I and II repairs, the pull on the medial canthal ligament should be upward and backward, with an overcorrection toward the midline. To achieve these relationships, the transnasal wire must be placed high along the septum. The surgeon must take precautions to avoid entering the anterior cranial fossa. A ligament placed too low will tilt the medial canthal ligaments downward and cause scleral show. Alternatively, the surgeon can place crossed transnasal wires attached to the frontal process of the maxilla (see later).

2. The transnasal wire technique requires protection of the globes during the transfer of the needle and wires from one side to the other. Large, carefully placed malleable retractors and skilled assistants are helpful during these maneuvers.

3. Avoid passing wires through the lacrimal collecting system, as this can cause obstruction. The wires should be passed high above it.

4. For the repair of injuries that have healed with deformity, drill techniques for passage of the wire are required. These methods are similar to those described for the type II repair (see Chapter 64).

5. External plates can be used for comminuted nasal fractures (see Chapter 47), but they will be of little, if any, assistance in holding the medial canthal ligaments in position. Excessive pressure from plates can cause necrosis of the skin and should be avoided.

6. Diagnosis of the degree and extent of associated frontal sinus fractures is important if the surgeon is to select and apply appropriate treatment. Anterior wall fractures of the frontal bone can frequently be managed with interosseous wires or thin plate techniques. Fractures extending to the posterior wall or floor of the frontal sinus may cause dural injury and/or obstruction to the nasofrontal duct and need to be treated differently. These conditions are discussed in Chapters 70 through 76.

COMPLICATIONS

1. Residual eyelid deformity and dysfunction of the lacrimal collecting system must be recognized and treated as soon as the complication is recognized. These sequelae can be best treated when the tissues are soft and the bones are mobile. Later, scarring, retraction, and malunion can cause significant problems in the reduction and repair. Techniques to free up the periorbita, relax orbital tissues, remove bone,

and perform a transnasal repair are described in Chapter 64.

2. Low placement of the transnasal wire can lead to a downward displacement of the medial canthal ligament and excessive scleral show. If this condition occurs, the wires should be reattached high through the septum. If there is only mild asymmetry of the medial canthal ligaments, this may be managed by VY- and Z-plasty techniques (see Chapter 69).

3. Obstruction of the lacrimal collecting system, alone or with dacryocystitis, is a common postoperative problem. Epiphora occuring early after the injury may be caused by postoperative swelling that affects the transfer of tears through the lacrimal collecting system. However, if the epiphora persists, the surgeon must seriously consider the possibility of a mechanical obstruction. Confirmation can be obtained by a fluorescein dye test. For lower system obstruction, the surgeon must consider a dacryocystorhinostomy. If the injury is confined to the cannaliculi and/or puncta, a conjunctivodacryocystorhinostomy or conjunctivorhinostomy should be performed.

4. Obstruction of a nasofrontal duct can later cause frontal sinusitis. This condition should be recognized by a failure of the frontal sinus to aerate. Occasionally the patient will complain about swelling and pain over the forehead region. If these problems develop, the surgeon has the option of reconstructing the nasofrontal duct or obliterating the frontal sinus (see Chapters 70 through 76).

5. Cerebrospinal fluid leakage can continue following surgery. If this occurs, the patient should be treated with antibiotics, and if the leak persists beyond 2 to 3 weeks, the surgeon should be prepared for evaluation of the site and closure of the area of fistula (see Chapters 84 through 87).

6. Webbing of the medial canthal incision site can initially be treated by injection of 40 mg/mL of triamcinolone. If the scars remain unsightly, Z-plasty or zigzagplasty techniques should be performed. Sometimes making an irregular medial canthal incision at the time of initial surgery will avoid this complication.

ALTERNATIVE TECHNIQUE USING FRONTAL PROCESS FIXATION

a,b The transnasal canthoplasty, attaching one medial canthal ligament to the other, is an excellent method to overcorrect placement of the medial canthal ligament. However, if the medial canthal ligament and inner angle rotates inferiorly, then the surgeon should consider attaching the wires transnasally to the opposite frontal process.

The incisions and approaches are identical to those

TYPE III REPAIR

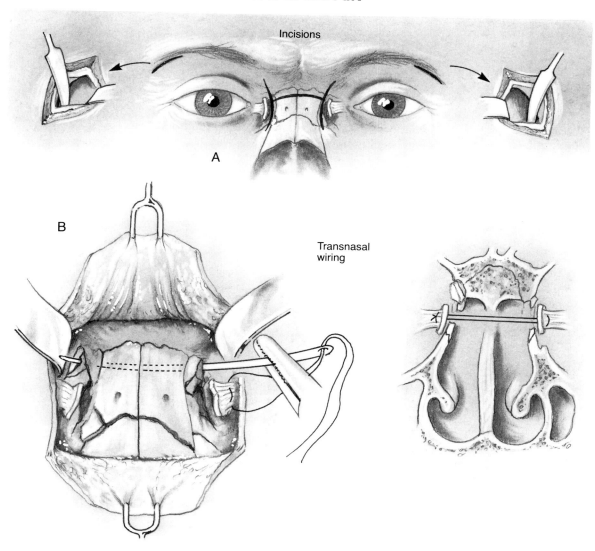

Incisions

A

B

Transnasal
wiring

ALTERNATIVE TECHNIQUE USING FRONTAL PROCESS FIXATION

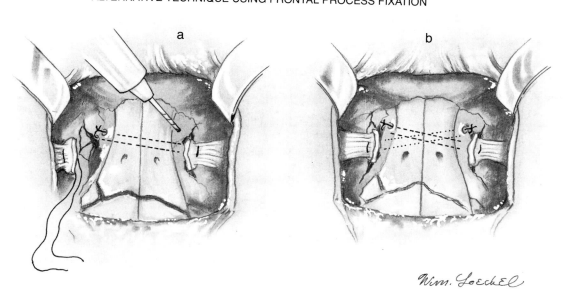

a

b

Wm. Loechel

used above. Following exposure of the medial canthal ligaments and relaxation of the ligaments by way of lateral canthotomies, a wire is passed through the medial canthal ligament transversely to the opposite wall of the orbit in the region of the upper lacrimal fossa. A drill hole is made through the anterior crest on the frontal process of the maxilla, and the wire is then passed through the hole. A similar procedure is carried out with the other end of the wire, but through a passageway several millimeters distant to the first hole. The ends of the wire are then tightened to bring the ligament into proper position. The other medial canthal ligament is secured with a similar transnasal technique. The procedure will thus effect a crossing of wires within the nasal vault. The advantage to this intercanthal wire is that one medial canthal ligament can be adjusted independently of the other. The disadvantage is that there can be asymmetry in the placement of the ligaments. Postoperative care is the same as that following the intercanthal method.

chapter 66

Open Reduction and Repair of Telescoping Naso-Orbital Injury

INDICATIONS

Instead of breaking into small pieces, the naso-orbital fracture can also be driven as a block of bone beneath the frontal bone. The medial walls of the orbit are often involved, and if the fracture extends into the lacrimal bones, the medial canthi will splay laterally. The injury causes a characteristic appearance in which the nasofrontal angle is accentuated. Frontal bone fractures are common. There is often a telecanthus and epiphora involving one or both eyes. Epistaxis, cerebrospinal fluid leakage, and intracranial damage can occur.

PROCEDURE

Under general orotracheal anesthesia, the face is prepared and draped as a sterile field. An open sky (see Chapter 65) or coronal incision (see Chapter 72) is mapped out with marking solution. The operative site should be infiltrated with 1% lidocaine containing epinephrine to help control hemostasis.

The periosteum is elevated from the nasal bones and outer cortex of the frontal bone. The medial walls of the orbits are exposed as in Chapter 63. Additional exposure can be obtained by releasing the anterior ethmoidal vessels. Bleeding can be controlled by gentle pressure or application of vascular clips.

A–C A forceful reduction is required. A small curved osteotome is inserted through the fracture line, and if the frontal bone is intact, the osteotome can be levered on the face of the frontal bone to elevate the nasoethmoid complex into correct position. If the frontal bone is also fractured or the nasoethmoid depression is severe enough to affect optimal mechanical leverage, then the nasoethmoid complex must be reduced by an anteriorly directed force. This can be accomplished by applying a towel clip to the frontal processes of the maxilla and pulling outward. Care must be taken not to be overly force-ful, or the complex will be extracted from the craniofacial skeleton.

D,E After reduction is accomplished, the medial canthal ligament is restored to anatomic position (see type I, II, and III repairs in Chapters 63 through 65). Usually the reduced frontoethmoid block of bone is stable, but if this is not the case, 28-gauge interosseous wires or plates can be applied.

The wounds are closed in layers. The periosteum and subcutaneous tissues are approximated with 4-0 chromic sutures, and the skin is closed with 5-0 or 6-0 nylon sutures. Prophylactic antibiotics are prescribed for 5 to 7 days, or longer if there is evidence of a cerebrospinal fluid leak. The sutures are removed in 5 to 7 days. Serial radiographs are obtained postoperatively to evaluate the frontal sinuses.

PITFALLS

1. Reduction is the most difficult part of the procedure. If the nasoethmoid block of bone is overcorrected, there will be a tendency for cerebrospinal fluid leakage. Extraction of the bone is also possible, especially if the surgeon does not take precautions in the amount of force exerted to effect the reduction. Overcorrection or extraction can sometimes be avoided by keeping pressure on the dorsum of the nose as the lifting is carried out. Gentle rocking can also be effective.

2. Beware of associated injuries. In addition to the telecanthus, there can be fractures extending through the cribriform plate and frontal bone. Accurate reduction of the cribriform plate will usually approximate dural tears and help seal cerebrospinal fluid leaks. However, fractures extending into the frontal bone may interfere with subsequent normal aeration and drainage of the sinus, and if there is evidence of such a fracture, it should be treated accordingly (see Chapters 70 through 77).

3. Nasal septal injury should be managed by one of the closed or open techniques (see Chapters 46

through 48). If cerebrospinal fluid leakage is also noted, packing should be avoided and the septum stabilized with polyethylene plates. Antibiotic coverage is mandatory.

4. Injuries directed to the nasofrontal angle can also transmit forces to the base of the skull and cause injury to the optic nerve. If the patient has a decrease in vision related in time to the fracture, the surgeon should consider the possibility of optic nerve compression and treat the injury as described in Chapters 80 and 81.

COMPLICATIONS

1. Failure to achieve an adequate reduction will cause a depression of the nasofrontal angle. If the bones heal in malposition, it is probably more prudent to correct the deformity by cartilage and/or onlay bone grafts to the dorsum of the nose. Osteotomies are difficult to perform and can be complicated by unstable fragments of bone, cerebrospinal fluid leaks, and damage to the nasofrontal duct.

2. Although rare, it is possible during reduction to extract the nasoethmoid complex. This complication can be avoided with gentle rocking and counter pressure by the opposite hand. If the bone is inadvertently removed, it should be replaced immediately and wired into position. Exposed and torn dura require repair. Neurosurgical consultation should be obtained.

3. Obstruction of the nasofrontal duct can be a complication of naso-orbital injury, and if it is not recognized, it can later cause a life-threatening sinusitis or mucocele. The surgeon should evaluate the extent of the fracture, and if it involves the duct, it can be treated with reconstruction of the duct or obliteration of the frontal sinus with fat (see Chapters 72 and 76). If the surgeon chooses to manage the fracture conservatively, the sinuses must be evaluated for permanent aeration.

REPAIR OF TELESCOPING NASOFRONTAL INJURY

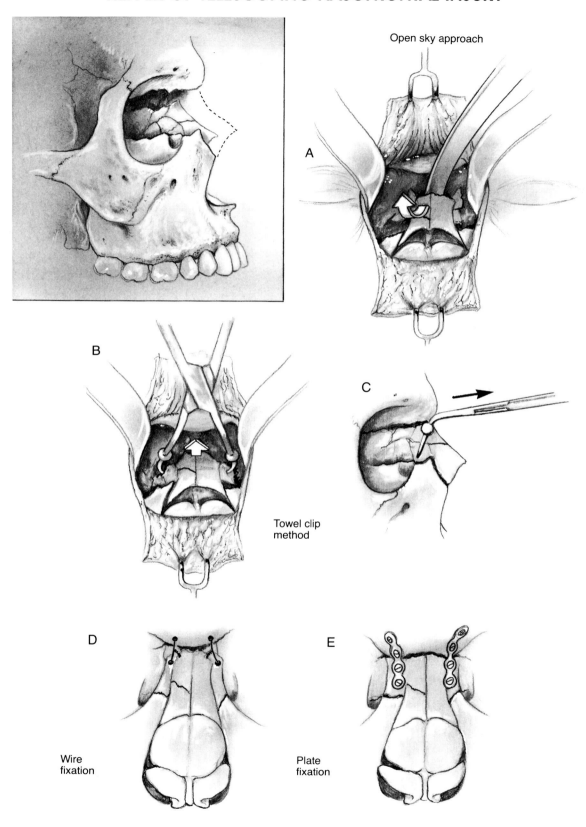

Open sky approach

A

B

Towel clip method

C

D

Wire fixation

E

Plate fixation

chapter 67

Repair of Canaliculi
Alternative Method of Conjunctivorhinostomy

INDICATIONS

Trauma to the naso-orbital region can be associated with lacerations, which, if extensive, can sever the medial canthal ligament and parts of the lacrimal collecting system. Early recognition of the injury and immediate repair are necessary if the surgeon is to restore normal anatomic relationships and physiologic functions. Damage to the lacrimal collecting system will prevent the collection of tears and, if not treated, can result in chronic epiphora. Most of the flow is through the inferior canaliculus, and it is thus important that damage be recognized and that the canaliculus be repaired early after injury. The superior canaliculus may also be repaired, but a functioning inferior canaliculus will probably suffice. Treatment of injuries to the lower (distal) portion of the lacrimal collection system is discussed in Chapter 68.

PROCEDURE

Under general anesthesia, the face is prepared and draped as a sterile field. To help with hemostasis, the medial canthal region is infiltrated with 1% lidocaine containing 1:100,000 epinephrine.

A The procedure is carried out with the operating microscope. The laceration should be irrigated with normal saline and the edges examined for the ends of the severed canaliculus. The proximal segment (near the puncta) is easy to identify, as the surgeon can dilate the puncta with lacrimal dilators and pass the probe through the canaliculus into the laceration. The probe will then point to the severed canaliculus of the opposite side. If the distal end still cannot be seen, the surgeon can then irrigate the superior canaliculus with normal saline, press on the sac, and force the fluid retrograde through the inferior canaliculus.

B–D Following identification of the ends of the canaliculus, a Silastic tube swaged on a flexible probe is passed through the superior (or inferior) canalic-

ular system into the sac and out through the nasolacrimal duct. The other swaged end is passed through the inferior (or superior) part into the sac to follow the same route as the first tube. The probes are then cut from the tubing, and the tubing is tied into a knot, which is placed on the floor of the nose. The tubing, acting as a stent, provides support while the surgeon approximates the cut ends of the canaliculus with 8-0 nonabsorbable sutures.

E–H The eyelid laceration is closed with a special suture technique. A 5-0 chromic suture is secured and buried near the edge of the tarsal border. A 6-0 silk suture is placed at the level of the meibomian gland orifices at about 1 to 2 mm from the wound margins. A second 6-0 silk suture is placed on the posterior eyelid near the junction of the skin and conjunctiva. A third 6-0 silk suture is placed in front of the first silk suture so that the needle is passed through the lashes. The sutures are then tied down and the ends brought anteriorly to be held by the most anterior suture.

Antibiotic eye ointment is applied for several days. The sutures are removed in 3 to 5 days, and stents are retained for 2 to 3 weeks. The nose should be kept clean with normal saline douches.

PITFALLS

1. The lacrimal collecting system should be carefully examined when there are lacerations through or near the medial part of the eyelid. Dehiscences of the canaliculi can be evaluated by cannulation and instillation of saline solution. The wound should also be explored, using the microscope to determine the site and degree of damage.

2. Although the lower eyelid canaliculus carries most of the tears, the surgeon should still attempt to repair the upper canaliculus. The additional function of the upper canaliculus ensures a more efficient excretion mechanism. Moreover, if the lower canaliculus fails, the upper canaliculus can take over and possibly prevent epiphora from occurring.

CANALICULI REPAIR

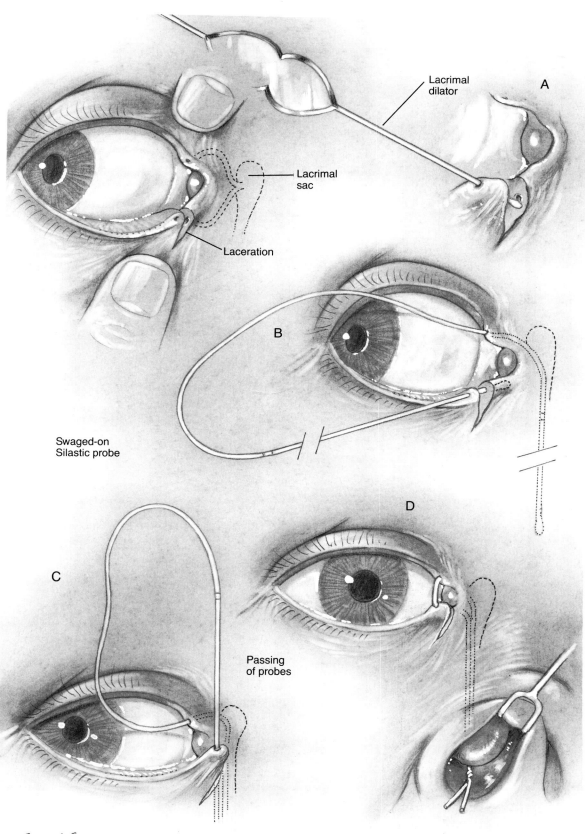

Lacrimal dilator

Lacrimal sac

Laceration

A

Swaged-on
Silastic probe

B

C

D

Passing
of probes

Wm. Loechel

CANALICULI REPAIR *(Continued)*

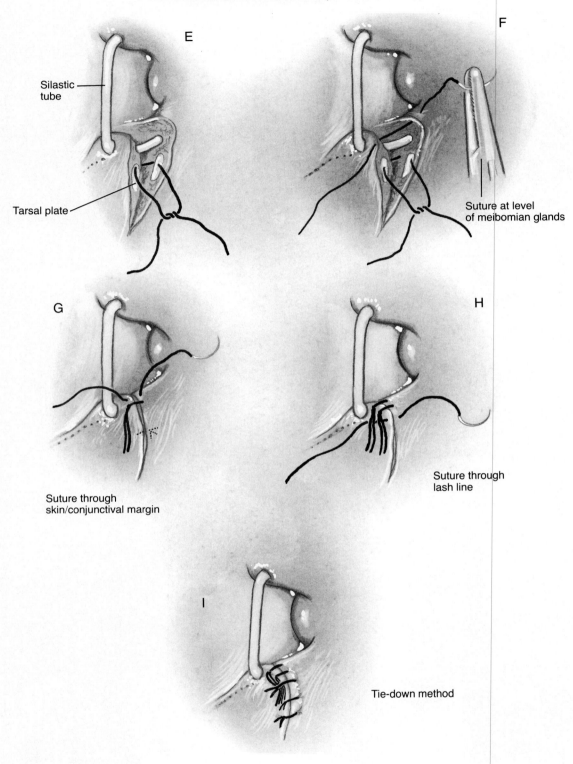

E

Silastic tube

Tarsal plate

F

Suture at level of meibomian glands

G

Suture through skin/conjunctival margin

H

Suture through lash line

I

Tie-down method

3. Canaliculus repair should be performed under the most ideal conditions. The procedure should be done within 24 to 48 hours of injury and during a time when equipment and assistants are readily available. Late repairs can be complicated by secondary infection and scarring and should be avoided.

COMPLICATIONS

1. The main complication of the canalicular repair is restenosis and failure to conduct tears. With the Silastic stent in position, function is difficult to evaluate. When the stent is finally removed several weeks later, scarring can develop, which will preclude any simple revision of the collecting system. In such cases, the surgeon should consider a conjunctivorhinostomy or conjunctivodacryocystorhinostomy. In the elderly patient, tear secretion is often reduced, and with sufficient evaporation, conservative management can be considered.

2. Displacement of the tubing can be a problem. The tubing can break and come out or, occasionally, loosen and fall into the palpebral fissure. The tubing can also erode through the canaliculus. To avoid these problems, the patient should be instructed on the correct position of the tubing. If inflammation develops, ophthalmic antibiotic drops should be administered.

3. Ectropion or entropion can be secondary problems related to the repair of the canaliculi and the eyelid laceration. These complications can be difficult to treat and are beyond the scope of this text. Ophthalmologic evaluation and consultation are desirable.

ALTERNATIVE METHOD OF CONJUNCTIVORHINOSTOMY

Failure of the upper (proximal) lacrimal collecting system following repair of the canaliculus should probably be treated with a bypass method. The diagnosis is obtained with standard fluoroscein dye (Jones) tests, described in Chapter 68. Conjunctivo-dacryocystorhinostomy, using a Jones tube, is generally effective, but the technique may be complicated by granulation tissue formation, infection from unopposed mucosal flaps, and inefficient passage of tears through scar as a result of the secondary healing. Canaliculodacryocystorhinostomy affords the advantages of physiologic reconstruction but is limited by availability of sufficient canaliculus, requires lengthy tedious dissection, and must be performed using a microscopic approach. Our method is a variant of a conjunctivorhinostomy. It provides a total lacrimal bypass and has the advantages of bipedicled mucosal flaps, optimal temporary stenting, and improvement of epiphora.

a–c Preparation consists of application of a vasoconstrictive agent to the nasal mucosa and infiltration with 1% lidocaine containing 1:100,000 epinephrine. The medial canthal incision (one half the distance between the medial canthus and the dorsum of the nose) is used for exposure. The angular vessels are ligated, and the periosteum is elevated off the nasal bones and along the medial wall of the orbit to expose the lacrimal crests and fossa. A rhinostomy is created as described in Chapter 68. The mucoperiosteum of the nose is elevated on the nasal side, and a flap is developed along the anterolateral wall of the nose. To obtain satisfactory exposure, the middle turbinate should be fractured medially. Vertical and horizontal incisions can be designed and the flap rotated through the rhinostomy defect.

d,e On the orbital side, an inferiorly based flap of approximately 1 × 2 cm is developed from the medial aspect of the bulbar conjunctiva, just lateral to the limbus. A horizontal incision is made at the inferomedial aspect of the flap in the fornix and deepened to join the original medial canthal incision. The conjunctiva is sutured (end to end) to the mucosa of the nose using 5-0 chromic sutures. As an option, the surgeon can place a Jones tube stent through the fornix into the nose. The medial canthal incision is closed with a subcuticular 4-0 chromic suture and the skin with 6-0 nylon sutures. Prophylactic antibiotics are administered for 5 to 7 days.

REPAIR OF LACRIMAL COLLECTING SYSTEM

ALTERNATIVE TECHNIQUE OF CONJUNCTIVORHINOSTOMY

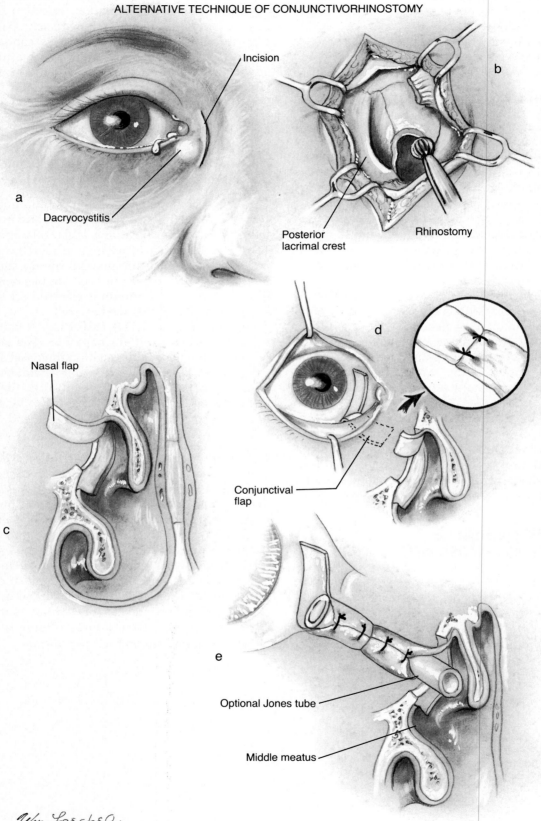

Incision

Dacryocystitis

a

b

Posterior
lacrimal crest

Rhinostomy

Nasal flap

d

Conjunctival
flap

c

e

Optional Jones tube

Middle meatus

Wm. Loechel

340

chapter 68

Dacryocystorhinostomy

INDICATIONS

Injury to the naso-orbital region has the potential to cause problems with many parts of the lacrimal collecting system. If tear collection is inadequate or obstructed, epiphora will occur. Soft tissue injuries can affect the upper collecting system (i.e., canaliculi and/or puncta); this is discussed in Chapter 67. Twisting or kinking to the lower portion of the system (i.e., nasolacrimal duct and/or sac) will cause stasis of secretions, which potentially can result in dacryocystitis. In the latter condition, there is inflammation of the medial canthus and intermittent mucopurulent discharge through the puncta. Manual pressure on the sac region will cause retrograde discharge of the mucopurulent secretions.

It is important to determine the level and degree of obstruction. In the absence of infection, a simple fluorescein dye test can be applied. The fluorescein is placed in the lower conjunctival sulcus; if the system is functioning normally, the fluorescein, on opening and closing the eyes, will be transmitted to the inferior meatus of the nose. The dye can then be examined on a pledget placed in this area. Failure of the dye to pass indicates that there is a blockage or malfunction somewhere in the system. The puncta and canaliculi should then be irrigated with saline. The appearance of the dye in the inferior meatus indicates that there was some retention of the dye in the lacrimal sac, and more force (not just natural pumping action) was necessary to pass it into the nose. These findings also suggest that the canaliculi and puncta are intact and functioning normally. For those obstructions distal to the sac, the surgeon should consider a dacryocystorhinostomy. For obstructions proximal to the sac, a conjunctivorhinostomy (or conjunctivodacryocystorhinostomy) is indicated (see Chapter 67).

PROCEDURE

A The nose should be treated preliminarily with 4% cocaine and epinephrine as described in Chapter 46. The face is prepared and draped as a sterile field.

An incision is mapped out with marking solution one half the distance between the caruncle and dorsum of the nose, but instead of the medial canthal incision described for the telecanthus repair, the incision is extended inferiorly along the inferior orbital rim. The angular vessels should be ligated or cauterized. The periosteum is incised over the frontal process of the maxilla and the periosteum released off the anterior lacrimal crest with a Freer elevator.

B–D The elevation should expose the medial or nasal side of the lacrimal sac. Working medial to the sac, the periosteum and sac are elevated from the lacrimal fossa to expose the posterior lacrimal crest. The lacrimal fossa is then fractured, and using Kerrison rongeurs, the opening is enlarged, removing the anterior and inferior portions of the anterior crest. Portions of the frontal process of the maxillary bone are also excised. The mucosa of the nose should be kept intact, and to avoid injury to the mucosa, the mucoperiosteum on the nasal side should be elevated before bone is removed. Dense, thick bone can also be excised by drilling with cutting burs. When the bone becomes thin, the remainder can be removed with Kerrison or Takahashi rongeurs.

E,F With the nasal mucosa and sac exposed, the lower canaliculus and puncta are dilated with a lacrimal probe. A No. 00 probe is then passed into the sac, and where it tents the sac, an incision is made vertically through the sac. Two 4-0 chromic sutures are passed through the posterior flap of the sac and held with a small hemostat.

G,H The nasal mucosa is tented with a clamp inserted intranasally and incised in a superior-to-inferior direction. This will also create posterior and anterior flaps. The posterior flaps of the nasal and sac membranes are subsequently attached by the chromic sutures and held loosely out of the field.

I,J At this point, Silastic tubing swaged onto flexible probes is passed through the superior and inferior canaliculi, through the opening in the sac, and into the nose (see Chapter 67). The probe wires are cut free, and the Silastic tubing is tied into a loop that

341

lies in the inferior meatus. The two sutures that had been placed through the posterior flaps are then tied securely. Two additional sutures are placed through the corresponding anterior flaps and tied down. The periosteum and subcutaneous tissues are approximated with additional 4-0 chromic sutures, and the skin is closed with a 5-0 nylon suture.

Prophylactic antibiotics are utilized for 5 days, and an ophthalmic antibiotic ointment is applied for several days. The nose is kept clean with saline douches three times a day and then daily until the tube is removed at 3 to 4 weeks.

PITFALLS

1. An incision directly over the sac, as described earlier, is helpful in exposing the lacrimal fossa and the entire sac area. The standard medial canthal incision can also be used but would make the inferior portion of the osteotomy difficult to perform. However, it is useful when combining the dacryocystorhinostomy with a telecanthus repair.

2. If the dacryocystorhinostomy is to be done in conjunction with a telecanthus repair, the surgeon must plan the timing of the procedures. If not done in the proper sequence, one procedure can adversely affect the other. We have found that the medial canthal exploration and repair and the lateral canthotomy should be done first, followed by attachment of the 30-gauge wire to the medial canthus. The wire is left loose, and preparations are made for the wire to be attached either to the upper posterior lacrimal crest or to the crest or medial canthal ligament of the opposite side. The dacryocystorhinostomy is then performed. The medial canthal ligament is subsequently pulled into position, and the wound is closed in a standard fashion.

3. Before performing a dacryocystorhinostomy, the surgeon must be certain that the puncta and canaliculi are functioning and the eyelid comes in contact with the surface of the globe. Therefore it is important that the lacrimal collecting system be first studied with a dye test and obstruction be evaluated with probe dilatations. Early injuries of the upper (proximal) collecting system can be treated with intubation and repair of the canaliculus, but if this fails, a conjunctivorhinostomy or, alternatively, a conjunctivodacryocystorhinostomy (see Chapter 67) must be considered.

4. Make sure that the nasal passageways are patent and not involved with pathologic processes. Avoid the procedure in patients with sinusitis, nasal masses, or polyps. These conditions should be controlled before performing the dacryocystorhinostomy.

COMPLICATIONS

1. Continuation or return of epiphora will occur if the lacrimal collecting system again becomes obstructed or fails to function properly. Occasionally there is still a problem with the proximal system (canaliculus and puncta), and the surgeon must be certain that these parts are patent and that the puncta is in contact with the surface of the globe. Stenosis occurring at the outlet of the lacrimal sac will cause accumulation of secretions within the sac, stasis, and infection. If this occurs, another dacryocystorhinostomy should be performed. In elderly patients in whom tearing is diminished, a dacryocystectomy can be considered. If there are associated problems with the proximal segment, a conjunctivorhinostomy (see Chapter 67) may be the procedure of choice.

2. Dacryocystitis is a serious infection that occasionally extends from the sac to involve other periorbital tissues. Orbital abscesses and orbital cellulitis can occur. If such conditions develop, the sac should be drained and the patient administered intravenous antibiotics. Cultures should be taken to evaluate microorganism susceptibility. Antibiotics should be administered until there is no longer any sign of inflammation. Subsequently (i.e., several weeks later) the patient should be considered for a repeat dacryocystorhinostomy or dacryocystectomy.

DACRYOCYSTORHINOSTOMY

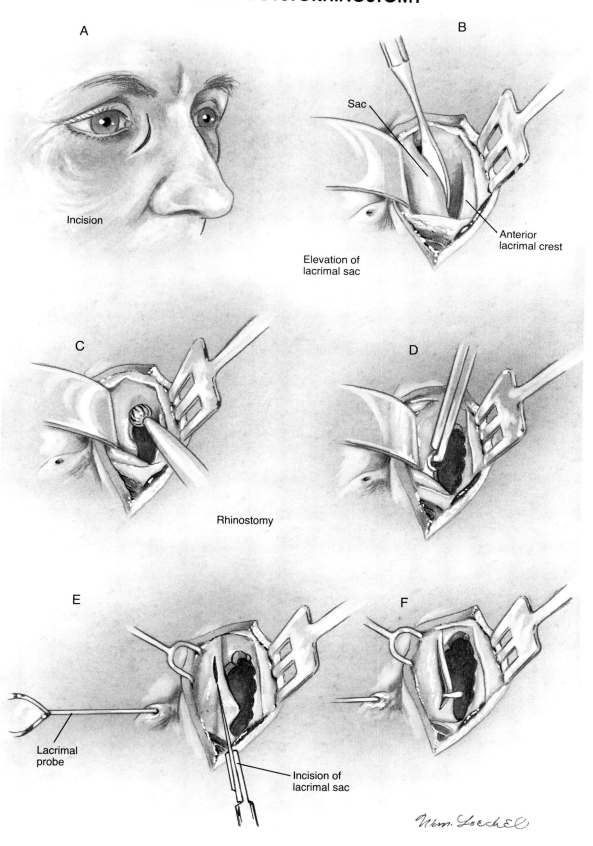

A

Incision

B

Sac

Anterior
lacrimal crest

Elevation of
lacrimal sac

C

Rhinostomy

D

E

Lacrimal
probe

Incision of
lacrimal sac

F

DACRYOCYSTORHINOSTOMY *(Continued)*

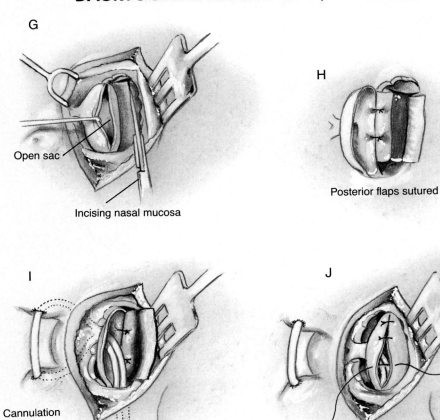

G

Open sac

Incising nasal mucosa

H

Posterior flaps sutured

I

Cannulation

Middle meatus

J

Anterior flaps
sutured

chapter 69

Repair of Widened Scars, Webs, and Displaced Angles of the Medial Canthus

INDICATIONS

Posttraumatic telecanthus can be associated with a variety of deformities that often can be corrected with limited skin surgery. A marked displacement of the inner angle and caruncle requires a formal telecanthus repair (see Chapters 63 through 65), but occasionally the displacement is minimal (i.e., 1 to 2 mm), and an advancement and/or rotation of skin flaps can provide a satisfactory result. Widened scars or web deformities can often be treated by application of zigzag- or Z-plasty techniques. If the angle of the medial canthus is displaced upward or downward, these sequelae can usually be corrected with transposition flaps (Z-plasty).

PROCEDURE

In preparation for the surgery, the palpebral fissure width and height should be measured and compared with the palpebral fissure of the opposite side. The inner angle should be symmetric, and any displacement upward or downward should be appropriately recorded. Photographic documentation should be obtained prior to the repair.

Widened Scars and Web Formation

A Usually the medial canthal incision heals well with minimal scar formation. Occasionally, however, the scar widens or contracts into an unsightly web. If these sequelae are observed early, it is possible to inject 40 mg/mL of triamcinolone to counteract the pathophysiologic processes. However, if the scar has matured, correctional surgery should be performed.

After preparation and draping of the face, the widened scar is outlined with marking solution. The area of scar is then infiltrated with 2% lidocaine. Sedation is used as necessary. If the inner angle is at the correct level, most scars can be camouflaged with a zigzagplasty. The scar is then excised with a

geometric broken line at the level of the dermis. The adjacent tissues are undermined at a subcutaneous level, advanced, and closed in layers using 5-0 colorless or white nonabsorbable suture in the subcuticular tissues and interrupted (or running) 6-0 nylon sutures in the skin.

B If the scar is contracted and appears as a web, the surgeon should consider an excision and Z-plasty technique. The excised scar should correspond to the diagonal of the Z. Arms are then created at 45° to 60° to the diagonal. The flaps are undermined and rotated into position. Closure again should utilize 5-0 nonabsorbable sutures in the subcuticular layer and 6-0 nylon sutures in the skin.

Postoperatively the wound should be kept clean with 3% hydrogen peroxide and application of antibiotic ointment. Sutures are removed at 4 to 5 days.

Displaced Angle

If the inner angle is displaced laterally, inferiorly, or superiorly, it can often be corrected by an advancement and/or transposition technique. The patient is usually prepared as for the scar revision described previously. The area is marked according to the design of the correction and infiltrated with 2% lidocaine.

C If the inner angle needs to be advanced medially, then a V-shaped incision is marked on the eyelid with the lines of the V parallel, but 1 to 2 cm below or above the eyelid margins. The point of the V is then extended as a line directed medially to form a Y. The length of this line should approximate the degree of lateral displacement and allow for 1 to 2 mm of overcorrection. The tissues are incised to the subcutaneous level and undermined approximately 0.5 to 1 cm. The flap is then advanced to the end of the Y to form a new medially displaced V, and the flap is secured with 5-0 white or colorless nonabsorbable subcuticular sutures. The skin is closed with interrupted 6-0 nylon sutures.

D If the inner angle is rotated upward or downward, then a Z-plasty should be designed to transpose the angles appropriately. One flap of the Z should contain the inner angle; the other flap should occupy space to which the inner angle will be transposed. Usually one arm of the Z will parallel the eyelid margin; the second arm will be more acutely drawn to the diagonal. The tissues are conservatively undermined and transposed. The wound is closed with 5-0 white or colorless nonabsorbable subcuticular sutures, with 6-0 nylon sutures in the skin. The incision is kept clean with 3% hydrogen peroxide and an antibiotic ointment. Sutures are removed in 4 to 6 days.

PITFALLS

1. Do not use soft tissue techniques if the lateral displacement is greater than 2 mm. For such conditions, it is probably better to perform a telecanthus procedure and reset the medial canthi into a more optimal position (see Chapters 62 through 65).

2. Avoid repeated injections of triamcinolone, as this will cause atrophy and increased vascularity within the scar. Steroid injection should be used only once or twice to alleviate web contraction or widening. If the steroid injection fails to correct the scar, revisional surgery should be carried out.

3. Local infiltration of 1:100,000 epinephrine should be avoided. Small, thin flaps will often not tolerate a reduction in blood supply caused by the vasoconstriction of the agent. For these reasons, plain 2% lidocaine should be administered and the tissues handled with great care.

COMPLICATION

The vitality of the tissues is important if the surgeon is to obtain rapid healing of the wound with minimal scar formation. The surgeon should apply atraumatic techniques and, as described earlier, avoid the use of vasoconstrictive agents. If a scar develops, steroids can be administered. Later, surgical revision should be considered.

REPAIR OF SKIN DEFORMITIES

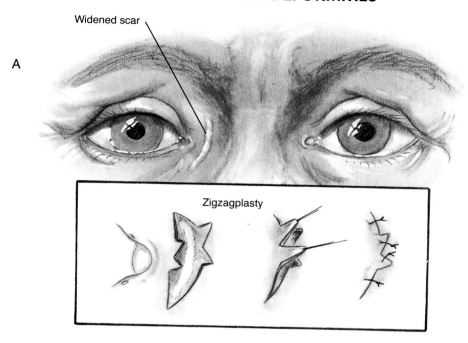

A

Widened scar

Zigzagplasty

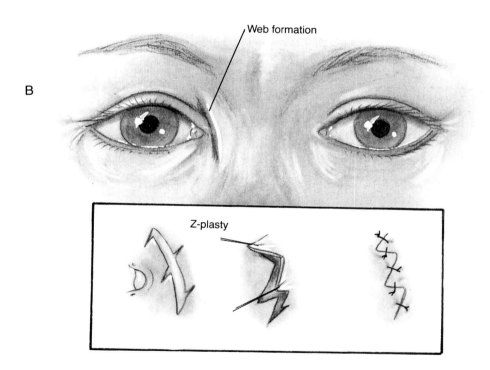

B

Web formation

Z-plasty

Wm. LoEchEl

REPAIR OF SKIN DEFORMITIES *(Continued)*

C

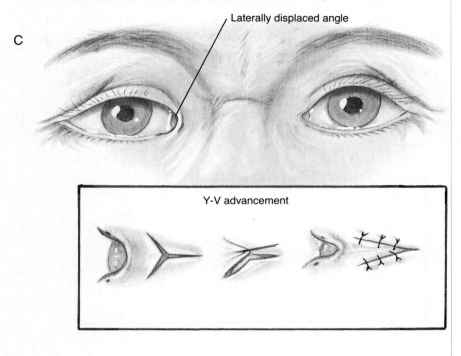

Laterally displaced angle

Y-V advancement

D

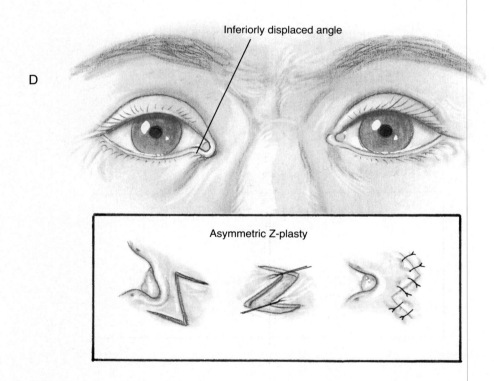

Inferiorly displaced angle

Asymmetric Z-plasty

Wm. Loechel

348

part
eight

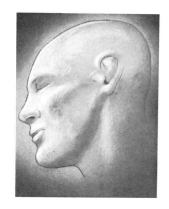

Frontal Sinus
Fractures

section I

Classification and Pathophysiology of Frontal Sinus Fractures

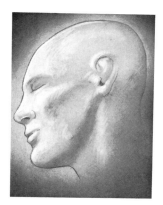

chapter 70

General Considerations

Early recognition and treatment of frontal sinus fractures is important if the surgeon is to restore normal appearance and prevent the sequelae of sinusitis and intranasal infection. Such fractures can alter the contour of the forehead and be associated with cerebrospinal fluid leakage and intracranial damage. Some injuries can cause obstruction of the nasofrontal duct, which in turn can cause stasis of secretions within the frontal sinus and sinusitis and mucocele formation. The adjacent orbital roof can be displaced, resulting in dystopia and possibly in a malfunction of the superior rectus, superior oblique, or levator muscles.

Frontal sinus fractures are classified according to anterior, posterior, or inferior wall injuries. Each takes into consideration the site and extent of the fracture, signs and symptoms, and the potential for complications.

A *Anterior wall fractures* can be linear, depressed, or comminuted. They can occur beneath intact skin, or they can be exposed through open wounds. The

fractures are usually associated with deformities involving the forehead but can also extend to the posterior wall and/or floor and present additional signs and symptoms associated with the adjacent sites of injury.

B *Posterior wall fractures* are characterized by damage to the protective shell of the cranium. These fractures may also be linear, depressed, or comminuted. Injuries to the posterior wall are usually associated with dural tears and cerebrospinal fluid leaks. Intracranial damage (i.e., epidural and intracranial hematomas) can also occur. Posterior wall fractures may be observed with the anterior and/or inferior wall injuries, and in these cases, signs and symptoms will reflect the extent and site of the fracture.

C *Inferior wall fractures* are considered primarily fractures of the anterior skull base. They have the potential to cause nasofrontal duct obstruction, stasis of secretions, and sinusitis. These injuries can also involve the cribriform and orbital plates and extend to the sphenoid bone. Dural tears, pneumocephalus, and cerebrospinal fluid leaks are common sequelae.

D One additional variation of frontal bone injury is the fracture that involves the eyebrow prominence and roof of the orbit. With such an injury, an eyebrow deformity, swelling, and ptosis of the upper eyelid can be expected. There can also be damage to levator, superior oblique, and superior rectus muscle function. Fractures extending more posteriorly can present with a blowout injury, and with such defects of the orbital plate, brain and dura can herniate into the orbit and cause a pulsating exophthalmos. If the fracture rotates upward into the anterior cranial fossa, elevation of the eye associated with an enophthalmos can occur. If the force of the fracture is transmitted farther posteriorly, the optic nerve and those vessels and nerves transmitted through the superior orbital fissure are at risk.

FRONTAL SINUS FRACTURES

A ANTERIOR WALL

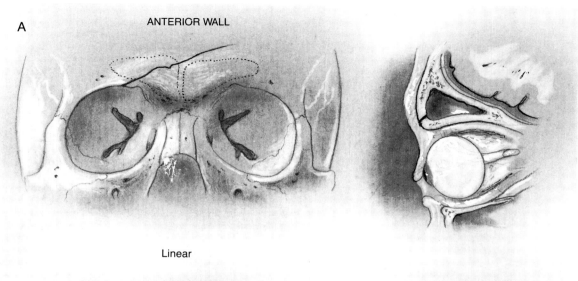

Linear

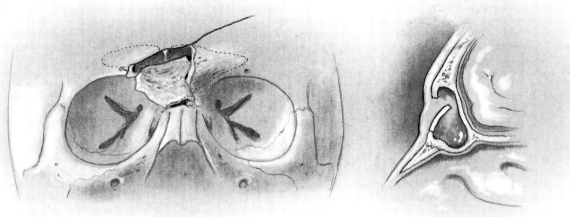

Depressed

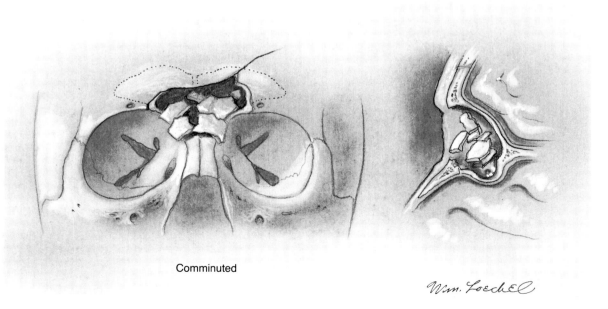

Comminuted

Wm. Loechel

FRONTAL SINUS FRACTURES *(Continued)*

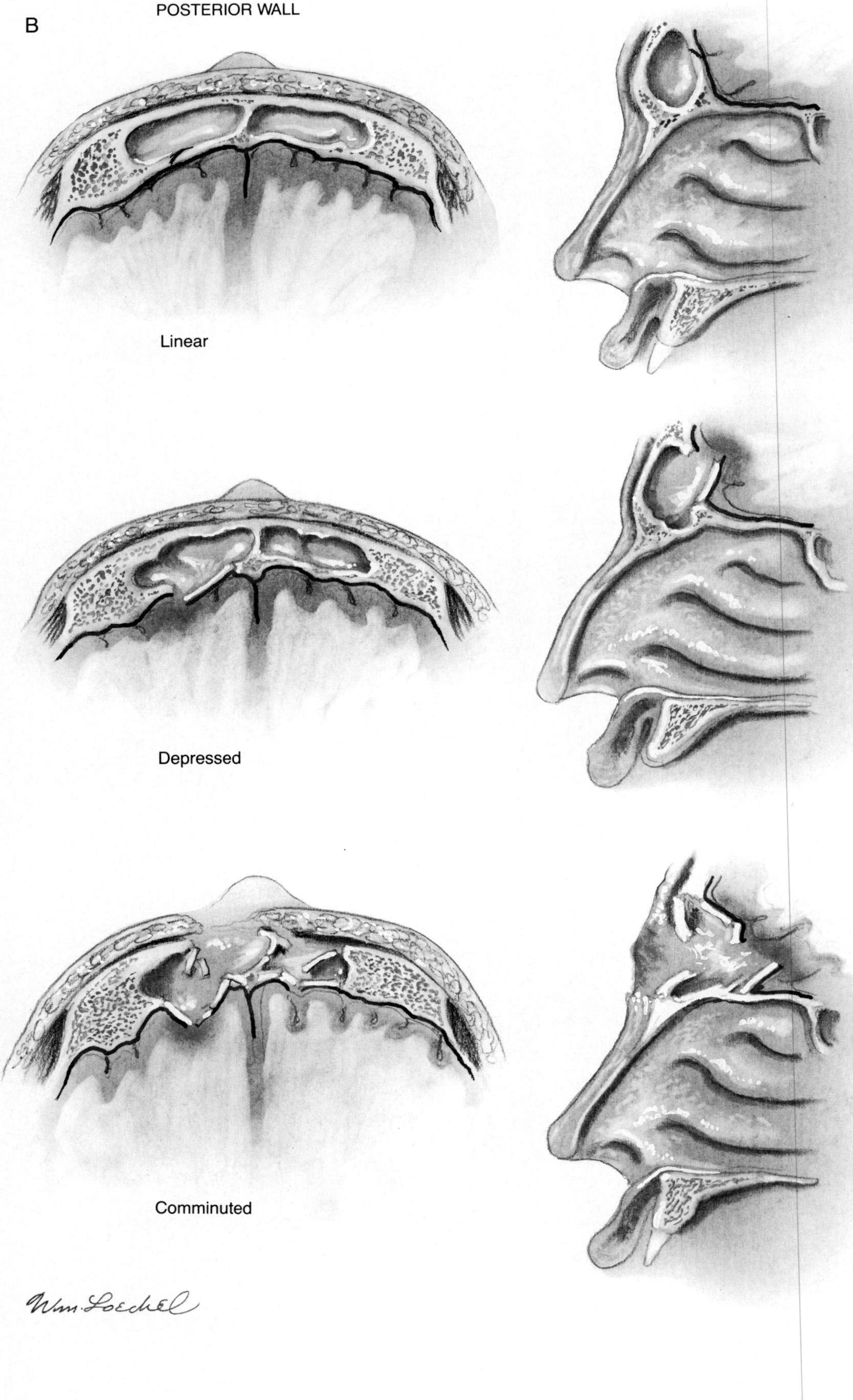
B
POSTERIOR WALL
Linear
Depressed
Comminuted
Wm. Loechel

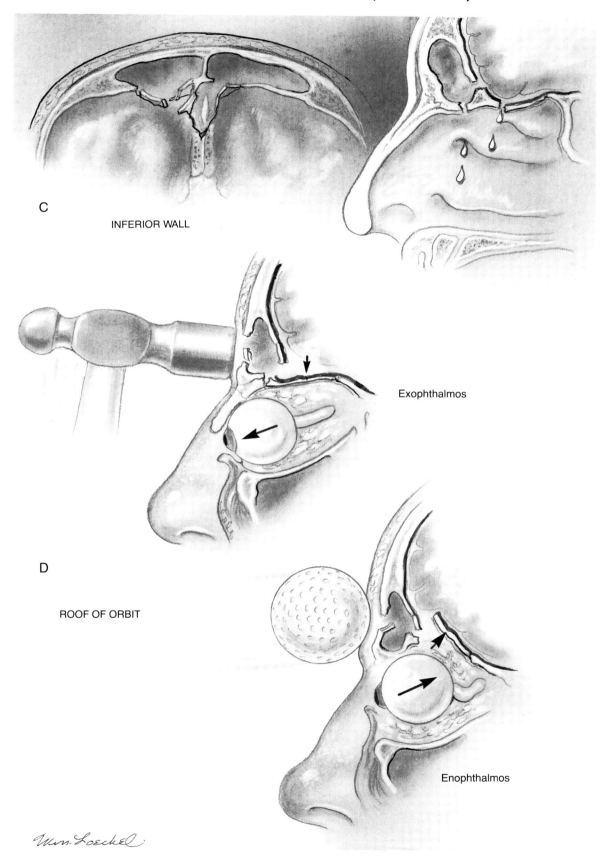

C

INFERIOR WALL

Exophthalmos

D

ROOF OF ORBIT

Enophthalmos

Anterior Wall Fractures of the Frontal Sinus

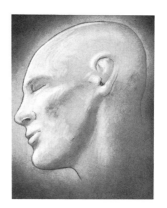

chapter 71

Repair of Anterior Wall Fracture of the Frontal Sinus With Plate Fixation
Alternative Technique Using Interosseous Wires

INDICATIONS

Fractures with minimal displacement that are confined to the anterior wall of the frontal sinus usually can be treated with conservative medical management. However, if the fracture causes a deformity, it should be reduced, and if the bones are unstable, they should be repaired with an appropriate method of fixation. There is also an opportunity during the fracture repair to explore the sinus and directly evaluate the extent of the injury.

Several methods of fixation are available. For the simple fracture in which a segment is depressed (e.g., a "trap door" type), one or several interosseous wires will be satisfactory. On the other hand, when the fracture is associated with many displaced fragments (comminuted), wire fixation tends to be unstable. The fragments tend to sway, and there is insufficient rigidity to hold their anatomic position.

Under these conditions, a thin plate fixation is the method of choice.

PROCEDURE

Lacerations of the forehead can be used for exposure, but if none are present, incisions should be planned and marked out appropriately. The surgeon has the choice of a coronal incision, as described in Chapter 72, or a more direct exposure through an "open sky" (see Chapter 65) or "butterfly" sub-brow approach. The site and length of the incision depend on the area of injury and the estimated exposure necessary for the repair.

A For most patients with anterior wall fractures, the surgeon should mark a curvilinear incision along the frontal process of the maxilla and upward to the medial part of the eyebrow. If necessary, the line of

357

incision can then be extended laterally beneath the brow or medially across the nasofrontal angle to become continuous with a similar incision of the opposite side.

B To help with hemostasis, the area of exploration is infiltrated with 1% lidocaine containing epinephrine. After 5 to 10 minutes, an incision is made through the skin and subcutaneous tissues. The angular vessels are identified and cauterized. The dissection then proceeds beneath the hair follicles, above the orbicularis oculi muscle, and across the prominence of the brow. The supraorbital and supratrochlear vessels and nerves are usually identified, and although they are kept deep and lateral to the dissection, neurovascular branches to the forehead may have to be sacrificed. The dissection then enters a plane between the galea and periosteum, and at this point, the surgeon has the option of directly exposing the fracture or continuing more superiorly until the dissection is above the area of damage. The periosteum then can be elevated retrograde to expose the fragments, but the surgeon should attempt to preserve as much as possible the vascularized periosteal attachments. The mucoperiosteal lining that lies on the deeper portion of the fracture should also be kept intact.

The defect created by the fracture is cleaned with suction irrigation, and the sinus is exposed with a focused light source. The surgeon should subsequently evaluate the possibility of the fracture extending to the posterior and/or inferior wall and resulting in cerebrospinal fluid leak. If such injury has occurred, other approaches should be considered (see Chapters 72 through 76).

C–E Fragments of frontal bone are elevated into position with skin hooks and small elevators. Thin plates are then bent to appropriate contour and adjusted so that at least two screws can be placed in solid bone adjacent to the fragment.

With the plate held against the fragments, hole positions are drawn with marking solution. Holes, confined to the outer cortex and diploë, are then made with a K wire or an appropriate-size drill. The screws should be just long enough to pass through the outer cortex and the diploë and engage the inner cortex. Because noncompression plates are usually used, the surgeon has the option of applying the screws first to the fragment and then to the adjoining bone. If there are many fragments, multiple plates will be needed to achieve a satisfactory fixation, but only the minimum number of plates necessary should be used to hold the bones in position.

For closure, the periosteum is advanced over the plates with 3-0 chromic sutures. The subcutaneous layer is closed with fine chromic sutures and the skin

with running or interrupted 5-0 nylon sutures. Incisions are covered with antibiotic ointment. A light compression dressing of fluffs and a stretch gauze is applied. Prophylactic antibiotics (i.e., ampicillin or cefazolin) are administered for 5 to 7 days. The dressings should be changed in 24 hours and the wound inspected at that time. Another dressing should be applied for at least 72 hours. Sutures are removed in 5 to 7 days.

PITFALLS

1. An accurate diagnosis, substantiated by imaging studies, is important if the direct approach to the frontal bone fracture is to be used. If the fracture extends to the posterior or inferior walls, other methods should be employed (see Chapters 72 through 76).

2. The surgeon should ensure that the wound is clean by washing the wound thoroughly with saline and mechanically removing any obvious particles or foreign material. This will help avoid postoperative infection.

3. If lacerations are present and sufficiently long, they can often be used for exposure and repair. Lacerations can also be extended in crease or furrow lines. However, if extension of the laceration would cross a crease or furrow line, then one of the sub-brow approaches should be considered.

4. Use only that part of the incision that is necessary to expose and repair the injury. If the fracture is confined to a small area, the incision should be just long enough to explore and reduce the fracture and apply the smallest plate. For displaced simple fractures, interosseous wires can be employed (see later).

5. The dissection should avoid injury to the hairs of the eyebrow, the orbicularis oculi, and the levator aponeurosis and muscle. Generally the dissection is beneath the hair follicles and above the orbicularis oculi. The periosteum of the frontal bone can be exposed above the prominence of the brow.

6. Expose only enough bone to apply a plate. The more periosteum that is attached, the more rapidly the bone will heal and the less chance there is of avascular necrosis. For these same reasons, the mucoperiosteal lining should be retained during the reduction and fixation process.

7. The surgeon should be particularly aware of cerebrospinal fluid leaks and extension of the fracture to the nasofrontal duct. Occasionally Gelfoam can be placed against the dura and an appropriate repair effected. If not, the surgeon should close the wound and use an alternate approach, such as obliteration of the sinus with abdominal fat (see Chapter 72).

PLATE FIXATION OF ANTERIOR WALL FRACTURES

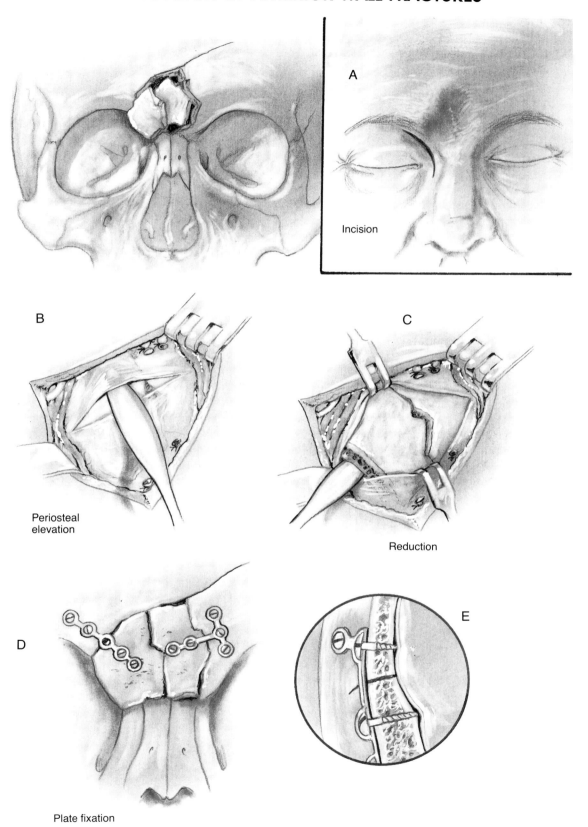

A

Incision

B

Periosteal
elevation

C

Reduction

D

Plate fixation

E

Injury to the nasofrontal duct may be treated with obliteration or reconstruction of the nasofrontal duct with a tube or one of the flap techniques (see Chapter 76).

8. Thin, malleable miniplates should be applied to the thicker areas of bone. The plate should be bent to fit closely to the forehead so that it is not palpated or seen following fixation. If this becomes a problem later, the plate may have to be removed.

9. Postoperatively there is a tendency for swelling of the forehead and brow region. These effects can be minimized by a light compression dressing of fluffs or stretch gauze. The dressing should be applied over the forehead and, to achieve proper pressure, extended over the ear region. Dressings should be removed and replaced at 24 and 72 hours, at which times the wounds are inspected for adequacy of healing.

COMPLICATIONS

1. Lacerations of the forehead are often associated with soft tissue damage and embedded foreign material. These conditions predispose to subsequent infection. To avoid this problem, wounds should be debrided and prophylactic antibiotics administered for 5 to 7 days. If an infection develops, the physician should obtain cultures and check for appropriateness of antibiotics. The area may require further debridement and drainage. Unsightly scars that develop later can be corrected with appropriate scar revision surgery.

2. Fractures extending to the posterior wall of the frontal sinus can cause dural or intracranial damage. Fractures directed inferiorly can cause obstruction to the nasofrontal duct, stasis, and sinusitis. These conditions must be recognized and treated appropri-

ately if the surgeon is to avoid and minimize the adverse sequelae (see Chapters 72 through 74).

3. The sub-brow approach unfortunately can damage branches of the supraorbital nerves and vessels that enter the forehead tissues. Loss of sensation is variable, and although return of function can be expected, the patient should be warned about the possibility of anesthesia or paresthesia of the region.

4. Depression of the frontal bone in the early postoperative period can be treated by another reduction and fixation. Later, when the bone has healed, the defect can be repaired with onlay grafts of autogenous rib or outer cortical plate from nearby parietal bone (see Chapter 78).

5. The rigid plate may be palpable or visible beneath the skin. If this occurs, the plate should be removed.

ALTERNATIVE TECHNIQUE USING INTEROSSEOUS WIRES

Interosseous wires have the advantage of being applied through a more limited incision than that used for plate fixation. The wire method is best used when there is a simple depression or when the surgeon only has to elevate a small, depressed fragment and secure it to the adjacent bone.

a–e The holes for the interosseous wires can be made with a 35-gauge K wire, a minidriver, and copious irrigation. A 28-gauge stainless steel wire is passed through the hole of the fragment; a 30-gauge wire loop is then passed through the hole of the stable bone and the loop used to pull through the 28-gauge wire. This 28-gauge wire is then twisted, cut, and rotated flat against the bone or, alternatively, into one of the bone holes. Postoperative care is the same as that used with plate fixation.

ALTERNATIVE TECHNIQUE FOR FIXATION OF ANTERIOR WALL FRACTURES USING INTEROSSEOUS WIRES

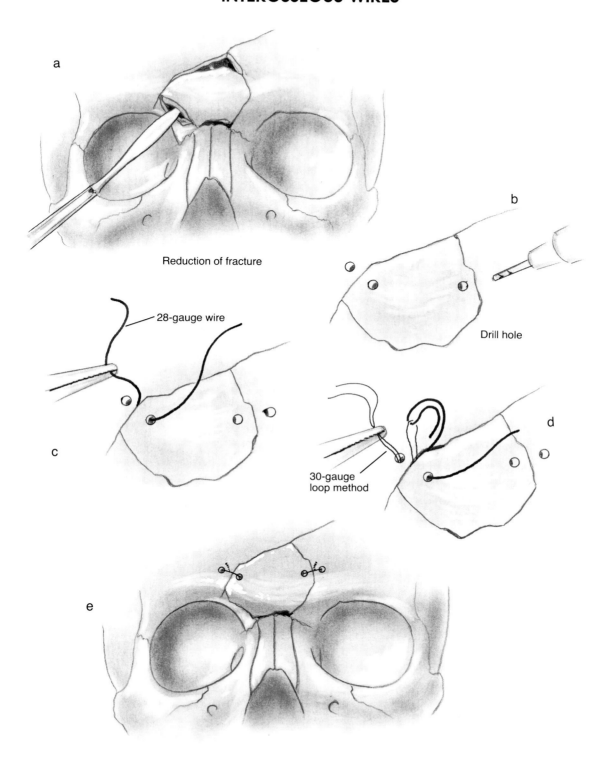

a

Reduction of fracture

b

Drill hole

28-gauge wire

c

30-gauge loop method

d

e

Wm. Loechel

section III

Posterior Wall Fractures of the Frontal Sinus

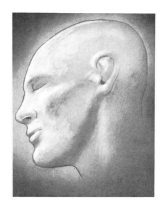

chapter 72

Repair of Posterior Wall Fracture of the Frontal Sinus With Coronal Osteoplastic Flap and Fat Obliteration

INDICATIONS

Posterior wall fractures of the frontal sinus are often associated with other fractures of the craniofacial skeleton. The diagnosis and extent of injury should be evaluated jointly with members of the neurosurgical department.

The isolated posterior wall fracture is rare, but if it is limited and nondisplaced, it can be managed conservatively. If the displacement is of a mild to moderate degree, then an external osteoplastic flap approach should be considered. For the more significant comminuted fractures that are associated with obvious dural tears, cerebrospinal fluid leaks, and pneumocephalus, a formal craniotomy may be re-

quired. When the surgeon is not certain of the degree of damage, the procedure can start with an osteoplastic flap and, if necessary, be converted (with neurosurgery) into a more formal craniotomy.

The osteoplastic frontal flap provides excellent exposure of the posterior and inferior walls of the frontal sinus. Small dural tears can be repaired, and if the surgeon is to obliterate the sinus, the mucosa can be removed and the sinus filled with fat. It is also possible through this frontal flap approach to reduce fragments on the posterior wall and repair cerebrospinal fluid leaks directly with Gelfoam or fascial plugs. The osteoplastic flap has the advantages of being vascularized and healing rapidly, with an incision that can be readily concealed behind the hairline.

PROCEDURE

The osteoplastic flap incision should parallel the coronal suture. It is marked behind the hairline in a gentle curve that is extended to a point several centimeters above the pretragal creases. The area for incision is prepared by limited shaving, antiseptic solutions, and application of drapes that keep the hair from the wound. Prior infiltration with 1% lidocaine containing 1:100,000 epinephrine will help with hemostasis.

A,B The knife blade should follow the direction of the hair follicles. The incision is made through the skin, subcutaneous tissues, and galea. Branches of the superficial temporal artery are ligated with fine silk sutures; other bleeding sites are controlled with pinpoint cauterization. The forehead flap is subsequently elevated in a plane between the galea and periosteum. Laterally the dissection is extended along the superficial temporalis fascia and inferiorly to the attachment of the fascia to the zygomatic arch. In the midline, the elevation proceeds to the eyebrows, exposing branches of the supertrochlear and supraorbital vessels that penetrate the bone flap.

C,D A template is used to make the periosteal cuts. This template is derived by cutting a replica of the frontal sinus from a "six-foot" Caldwell radiograph. The periosteum is incised at the border of the template and then elevated approximately 3 to 4 mm inferiorly. The exposed frontal bone is marked about 1 to 2 mm just beyond the edge of the periosteum. This will place the osteotomy 1 to 2 mm inside the original margin of the template. Using a medium-size oscillating saw, cuts are made obliquely so that the bevel of the cut is directed to the anterior portion of the inferior sinus. Attachments at the supraorbital ridges are released with osteotomes.

E,F A curved osteotome is then inserted beneath the bone flap at the level of the intersinus septum, and with the osteotome directed anteriorly, the anterior wall of the sinus is freed from the septum. The bone flap is then elevated, and if the procedure has been performed properly, fracture lines will develop on the superior wall of the orbit just beneath the supraorbital rim.

G,H Blood is carefully suctioned from the sinus. The mucosa is then elevated off all fragments using a Freer elevator and Takahashi rongeurs. A microscope is helpful in cleaning mucosa from the deep supraorbital crevices and cells. The posterior wall fragments are teased into position. Finally, the surface of the bone should be abraded with cutting burs and small dural tears covered with Gelfilm or fascia.

I The most popular material for obliteration of the sinus is abdominal fat. This fat is usually harvested separately in a sterile field through an oblique incision just beneath the belt line. The skin is undermined in all directions. The fat is grasped with a Babcock or Allis clamp and excised with a knife or scissors. Care is taken not to enter the underlying musculature. All bleeding should be controlled with cauterization. A small Penrose drain should be applied to the wound and secured to the edges of the incision. The incision is closed in layers, using 3-0 chromic for the subcutaneous tissues and 5-0 nylon for the skin.

J,K Before inserting the fat into the sinus, the sinus is again inspected for cerebrospinal fluid leaks and mucosal remnants. The mucosa at the nasofrontal duct is turned down into the duct system. The fat is then placed into the sinus, filling all crevices and openings. The flap is replaced, and any fat that protrudes through the osteotomy is excised.

Using 3-0 chromic sutures, the periosteum of the bone flap is then tightly secured to the periosteum of the frontal bone. The forehead flap is repositioned and closed by application of 3-0 chromic sutures to the galea and 3-0 or 4-0 chromic sutures to the subcutaneous tissues. The skin is closed with a running 5-0 nylon suture. Drains are used if there is a question of blood accumulation. A light compression dressing of fluffs and stretch gauze is applied across the forehead and temples and around the ears. The dressing is inspected at 24 hours, replaced, and left on for another 72 hours. Such a dressing usually reduces postoperative swelling. Antibiotics (i.e., cefazolin or ampicillin) are prescribed for 5 to 7 days, or longer in the case of a repair complicated by cerebrospinal fluid leakage.

PITFALLS

1. Many patients with posterior frontal wall fractures have intracranial damage. The surgeon should ensure that their medical status is stable and that there is reasonable certainty the procedure will not cause additional problems. Neurosurgical consultation is helpful.

2. Fracture of the anterior wall of the frontal sinus may compromise the development of the osteoplastic flap. In such cases, the surgeon can sometimes use the fracture line to create a smaller flap. After obliteration of the sinus, the anterior wall fracture can be repaired with a wire or plating technique (see Chapter 71).

3. The initial frontal osteotomy should not enter the dura. An accurate template is mandatory, and the physician should make sure the Caldwell radiograph is taken at six feet. The size of the sinus can

CORONAL OSTEOPLASTIC FLAP FOR POSTERIOR WALL FRACTURES

A

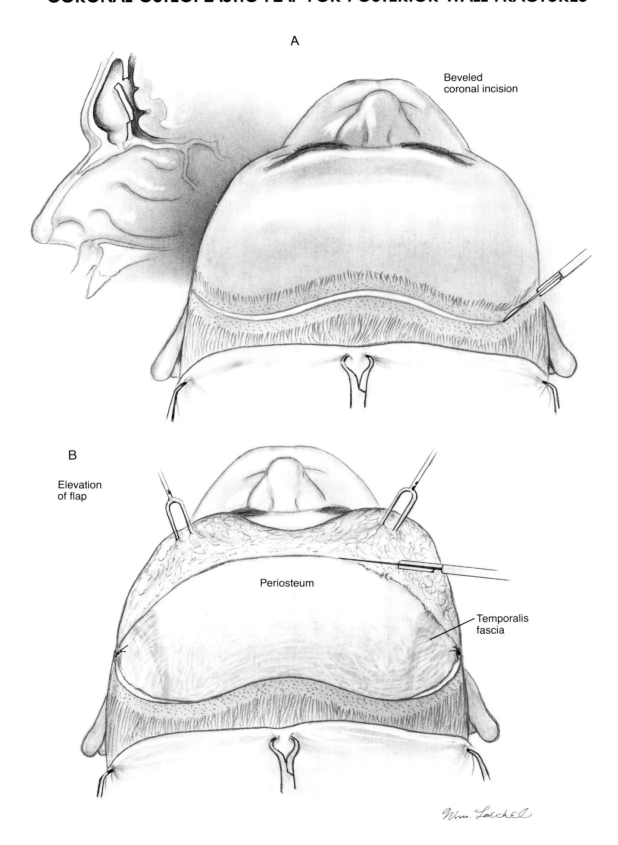

Beveled
coronal incision

B

Elevation
of flap

Periosteum

Temporalis
fascia

C

Measuring frontal sinus

X-ray template

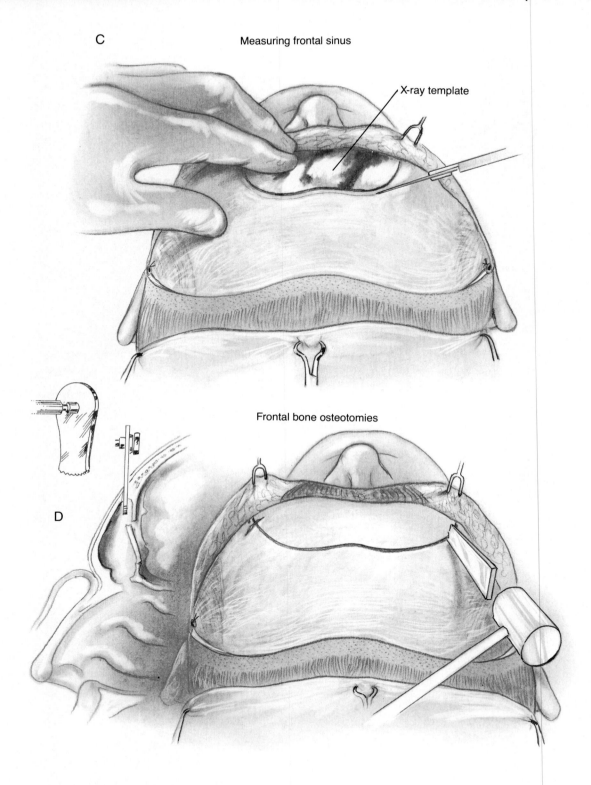

Frontal bone osteotomies

D

Wm Loechel

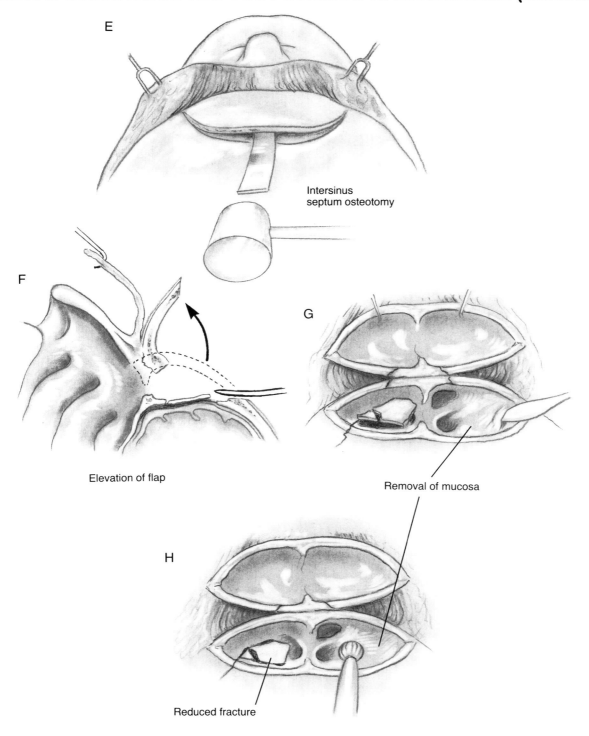

E

Intersinus
septum osteotomy

F

Elevation of flap

G

Removal of mucosa

H

Reduced fracture

CORONAL OSTEOPLASTIC FLAP FOR POSTERIOR WALL FRACTURES *(Continued)*

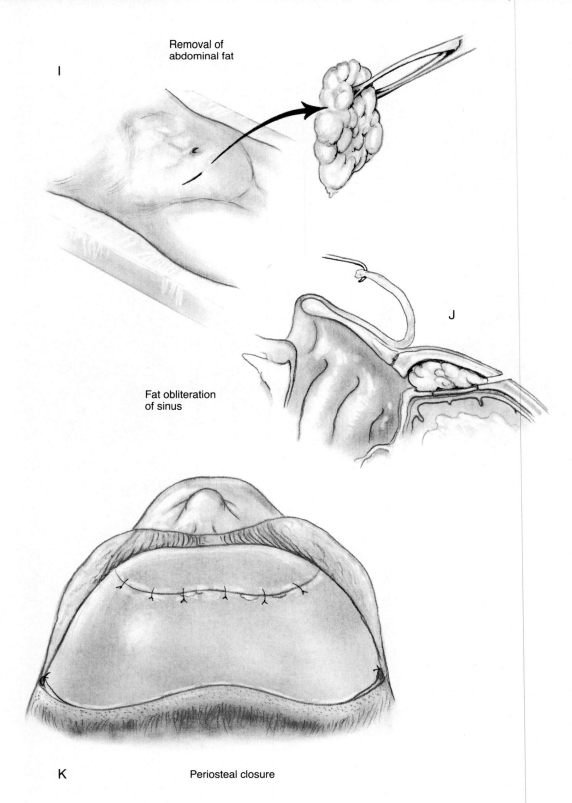

Removal of
abdominal fat

I

Fat obliteration
of sinus

J

K   Periosteal closure

also be evaluated by companion imaging studies. Starting the osteotomy 2 mm beneath the outline of the template and beveling the osteotomy while entering the sinus is helpful. Use of the oscillating saw also provides a margin of safety.

4. Make sure all mucosa is removed from the sinus. Failure to do so can later lead to mucoceles or mucopyoceles. Use of the microscope and removal of a layer of bone with the cutting burs ensures that the bone has been completely cleaned of mucous membrane. If multiple comminuted fragments make it impossible to remove all mucous membrane, the surgeon should consider a frontoethmoidectomy and reconstruction of the nasofrontal duct (see Chapter 76). The surgeon still has the option, if the frontal sinus does not clear, to later perform an osteoplastic flap and fat obliteration procedure.

5. Before obliterating the sinus with fat, the surgeon should ensure that the bones are in correct position and that dural tears have been repaired. If a significant cerebrospinal fluid leak is still present, it is more prudent to lift up the bone and suture the dura closed or have a neurosurgeon assist through a standard neurosurgical approach.

6. After replacing the bone flap, make sure that all fat is removed from the osteotomy site. Fat left between bone fragments will prevent fusion of the bone and cause instability and possibly a forehead deformity at a later time.

7. Periosteal coverage of the osteotomy will help in the healing process. This can be facilitated by making the osteotomy several millimeters from the edge of periosteum, and at the end of the procedure, the periosteum can be advanced over the bone defect.

8. Light compression dressings applied to the forehead region can be used to prevent edema. If dressings are not used, the patient can develop a supraorbital swelling that can persist for 4 to 6 months following surgery.

9. Make sure that the abdominal wound is dry and well drained. Infections are common but can be prevented by taking measures to avoid accumulation of blood and serous fluid.

10. Radiographs should be obtained at prescribed intervals following surgery to ensure completeness and persistence in obliteration. The fat can be measured by computed tomographic (CT) absorption criteria. If the fat disappears and the patient is asymptomatic, no treatment is necessary. However, the patient must be watched cautiously for signs and symptoms of sinusitis and cerebrospinal fluid rhinorrhea. Follow-up appointments should be scheduled quarterly. If the fat persists in the sinus, periodic evaluations can be carried out on an annual or biannual basis.

COMPLICATIONS

1. Sinusitis is possible, especially if there has been tissue damage and contamination. Under such conditions, the surgeon should consider debridement of the wound and alternative methods of repair (see Chapter 76). If obliteration is performed, the surgeon must carefully apply atraumatic techniques, completely close all dead space, and administer intravenous antibiotics. If sinusitis develops, the infection should be cultured and treated with appropriate antibiotics. Chronic infection should be managed by reexploration, removal of diseased tissue, and reobliteration or reconstruction of the nasofrontal duct.

2. Loss of fat grafts can potentially lead to mucocele formation. Mucosa can grow from the nasofrontal duct into the sinus, and without adequate drainage, mucoceles or mucopyoceles will develop. This complication can be avoided by making sure that the fat is in contact with a well-vascularized bed and the grafts are handled in a relatively atraumatic fashion. If the fat should be absorbed, the sinus must be studied carefully by serial radiographs for the development of sinusitis and mucocele formation.

3. Deformity of the forehead can develop, especially if there is an associated fracture of the anterior table. This can be avoided by noting such fractures on radiographs prior to the initiation of the procedure and by using appropriate reduction and treatment methods. Forehead deformities, however, are also possible as a result of the osteotomy. Therefore the osteotomy should be made as thin as possible and beveled so that the bone flap will not slip. If the bone flap becomes depressed beneath the level of the frontal bone, interosseous wires should be applied directly to the outer cortical plates. Correction of a late deformity is discussed elsewhere (see Chapter 78).

4. Cerebrospinal fluid leaks are usually controlled by direct closure of the dura and/or fat obliteration. If the patient continues to have a cerebrospinal fluid leak or evidence of pneumocephalus, it is possible that other fractures are present or the obliteration is not satisfactory. Imaging studies should be obtained to determine the cause of the problem. If the condition does not improve with conservative management, additional repair procedures should be considered.

5. Anesthesia and hypoesthesia of the forehead are common following the osteoplastic flap. Some patients experience a return of function; others do not. Loss of forehead movement also can occur from damage to the frontal branch of the facial nerve. Such injury can be avoided by gentle retraction of tissues and keeping the planes of dissection close to the temporalis fascia.

chapter 73

Cranialization Technique for Posterior Wall Fractures of the Frontal Sinus

INDICATIONS

Posterior wall injuries can occasionally be isolated to the posterior wall and skull base, but they more often appear as through-and-through fractures with contamination and comminution of bone. In this latter type of injury, the viability of the soft tissues and bone may be questionable, and following debridement, there can be a significant defect. Under such conditions, a reasonable option is to fill the sinus with a vascularized obliteration.

Several techniques are available. The surgeon can remove the anterior and posterior walls of the frontal sinus and collapse the forehead tissues onto the anterior fossa. He or she can also reconstruct the anterior wall of the frontal sinus and fill the sinus with a transposed temporalis muscle galea flap (see Chapter 74) or, as an alternative, remove the posterior wall of the frontal sinus and obliterate or cranialize the sinus with the anterior displacement of brain. The collapse of the forehead (often called a *Reidel procedure*) causes a severe deformity that is difficult to correct at a later time. Filling of the defect with a temporalis muscle galea flap provides a limited amount of tissue and causes a depression of the temple region. It can also predispose to alopecia over the donor site. The cranialization procedure eliminates the sinus and allows for expansion of the injured brain. Meanwhile, it provides for protection of the frontal lobes and a normal appearance of the forehead. The disadvantage of the cranialization technique is that the anterior fossa will be located above the nasofrontal duct, and this relationship can predispose to contamination of the cranial cavity from the respiratory tract below.

PROCEDURE

Using general orotracheal anesthesia, the approach is identical to that carried out for the coronal incision and osteoplastic flap (see Chapter 72). Intravenous antibiotics are administered during and after the operative procedure.

A–C After exposure of the sinus, all depressed bone fragments from the posterior wall are removed. Necrotic brain tissues are debrided, and the dura is repaired with fine nonabsorbable sutures and/or fascial grafts. The remaining mucosa of the sinus is elevated and excised from the floor and anterior wall. The frontal intersinus septum is removed with burs and rongeurs. A layer of bone is excised from the walls of the sinus with cutting burs.

D If the anterior wall is fractured, fragments are wired or plated, as described in Chapter 71. The nasofrontal duct mucosa is pushed into the duct, and the duct is then plugged with temporalis muscle or fascia. The frontal osteoplastic flap is returned to its normal position. The periosteum is closed with 3-0 chromic sutures. The superficial layers of soft tissue are approximated and treated with topical antibiotic dressings. Postoperatively the patient should receive intravenous antibiotics for 3 to 5 days and oral antibiotics for at least an additional 10 days. A light pressure dressing is maintained for 5 to 7 days to control edema, but it should be checked and replaced during the first 24 hrs and 2 to 3 days thereafter. Sutures are removed at 7 days. Radiographs are obtained at several weeks and every few months until the physician is assured of a stable reconstruction.

PITFALLS

1. The anterior wall of the frontal sinus must be reconstructed to restore normal forehead contour and to protect the brain. Most fragments should be kept attached to the periosteum, especially because the overlying mucosa will be removed. Small, loose, contaminated fragments of bone can be treated with a povidone-iodine solution, followed by a wash in physiologic saline. They can be stabilized using appropriate methods of fixation. Plate fixation often

CRANIALIZATION TECHNIQUE FOR POSTERIOR WALL FRACTURES

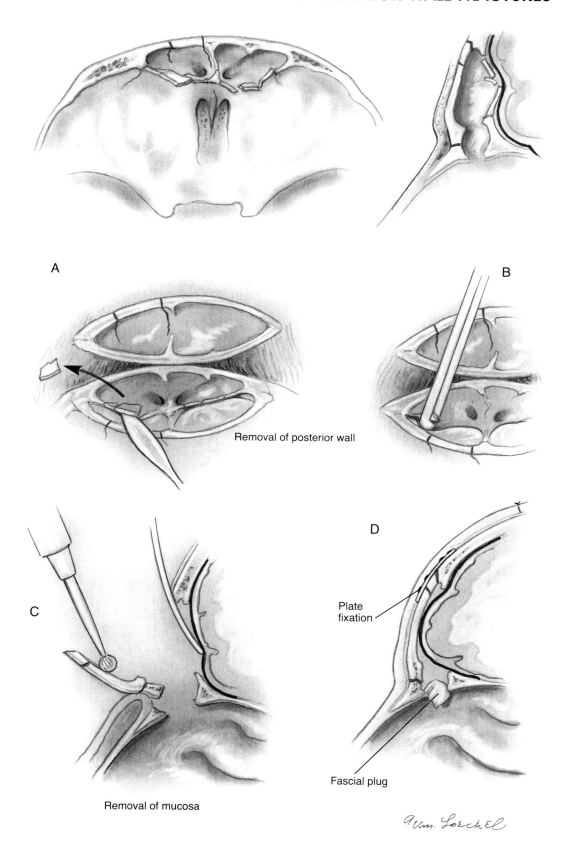

A

Removal of posterior wall

B

C

Removal of mucosa

D

Plate
fixation

Fascial plug

provides the best stability, but the surgeon must avoid extension of the screws beyond the inner table and injury to the underlying dura.

2. Complete obliteration of the sinus and nasofrontal duct is very important if the surgeon is to avoid infection. Bony ledges that restrict anterior displacement of the frontal lobes should be excised, and all mucosa should be removed from the walls of the sinus. The opening of the nasofrontal duct should then be packed with fascia to ensure complete closure.

3. The patient must be treated with prophylactic antibiotics and watched carefully for intracranial complications. Intravenous antibiotics should be started early during the procedure and continued postoperatively. Because the patient has essentially had a craniotomy, he or she should be watched closely for 24 to 48 hours for any changes in sensorium that would indicate bleeding, infection, or other damage to the brain.

COMPLICATIONS

1. As with other frontal sinus procedures, the patient may later develop sinusitis and/or mucoceles. These complications can be avoided by removal of all mucosa, obliteration of the nasofrontal duct with fascia, and complete obliteration of the sinus with brain tissue. If the sinus is large and the brain displacement only sufficient to obliterate a portion of the sinus, vascularized periosteal or temporalis muscle galea flaps should be used to fill the defect (see Chapter 74).

Postoperative radiographs should be obtained to evaluate the completeness and permanence of the procedure. If infection or a mucocele develops, then reexploration, exenteration, and obliteration with fat and/or muscle should be contemplated. Acute infection should be treated with appropriate antibiotics.

2. Deformity of the forehead can be a problem, especially if the anterior wall of the frontal sinus has been comminuted. This complication can be minimized by keeping the fragments well vascularized with periosteum and achieving an accurate (and stable) fixation. Plate fixation is usually helpful in obtaining rigidity and protection of the anterior fossa.

3. Intracranial infections can occur, especially if the forehead tissues are severely damaged, the dura is torn and accompanied by a cerebrospinal fluid leak, and the wound is open or contaminated by foreign material. To prevent meningitis and/or brain abscess, foreign material must be removed and devitalized tissue debrided. The dura must be directly closed or patched with fascia. A complete obliteration and adequate antibiotic coverage will also help avoid these adverse sequelae.

Repair of Posterior Wall Fractures of the Frontal Sinus With a Temporalis Muscle Galea Flap

INDICATIONS

Severe damage to the posterior wall of the frontal sinus associated with anterior wall injury, dural tears, and brain damage requires special techniques. As described in Chapter 73, the main objective is to separate the cranial cavity from the aerodigestive tract. Dural replacement and obliteration of dead space must be provided. The forehead tissues can be collapsed, the posterior wall of the sinus removed, and the brain allowed to expand forward (see Chapter 73), or the sinus can be filled with flap tissue. Free grafts (i.e., fat or muscle) probably should be avoided, as these grafts require a well-vascularized bed, and if this is not available, the tissues will not survive. A flap with its own blood supply is thus preferred.

Flap coverage can be obtained from several sources. Adjacent musculocutaneous flaps can be used, but these rotations cause deformity and additional scars. Pericranial flaps developed from forehead periosteum are available, but these flaps are limited in length and require a passageway anteriorly through the frontal bone. The temporalis muscle galea flap appears to be an effective, easy, accessible alternative for soft tissue coverage over skull base defects in which a reliable separation of cranial and facial compartments is desirable.

The temporalis muscle galea flap has several unique advantages over other methods. This flap is well vascularized, receiving contributions from the superficial temporal artery, the middle temporal branch of the superficial artery, and the anterior and posterior deep temporal arteries. Its length can be increased by extending the flap to include the parietal (and occipital) pericranium and galea. It can be used to repair cranial defects either alone or in combination with skin, cartilage, or bone grafts. Disadvantages are that the flap dissection is tedious and there can be loss of hair, skin, and/or sensation in the parietal region overlying the area of surgery. Although one flap can usually cover more than one half of the floor of the anterior cranial fossa, additional areas to be repaired require another flap from the opposite side.

PROCEDURE

A,B Surgery is performed under general anesthesia. The parietotemporal area is shaved, and the skin is prepared with a standard antiseptic solution and draped as a sterile field. The surgeon then marks out the incision lines for development of the temporalis galea flap. If a coronal incision is chosen as an approach to the frontal sinus injury, then a limb is extended posteriorly, at a right angle to the coronal incision, about 5 to 6 cm above the pinna. If a butterfly (sub-brow) approach is chosen, then a hemicoronal incision and a posterior limb should be employed. The design of the flap should protect the superficial temporal artery.

C,D The osteoplastic frontal flap should be planned so that the periosteum can be attached to the bone fragments and the bone later repaired with miniplates (see Chapter 71). The sinus should be cleaned of blood and examined and the extent of damage noted. Fragments should be elevated from the posterior wall, and necrotic brain should be debrided. Dural tears should be repaired when possible with fine nonabsorbable sutures or fascial patch closure.

All mucosa should be removed from the sinus and an extra margin of ensurance obtained by excising a layer of bone with cutting burs. The intersinus septum should be removed. At the frontonasal duct, the mucosa should be stripped and inverted down into the duct.

E—G The temporalis muscle galea flap is prepared by cutting through the scalp markings into a subcutaneous plane. Skin flaps are then developed superiorly and inferiorly at a level that preserves the hair follicles but does not damage the underlying temporalis muscle, galea, or superficial temporal vessels. With the skin flaps retracted superiorly, inferiorly, and posteriorly, the galea is incised. Up to 10 × 20 cm of tissue, based on the temporalis muscle, can be prepared.

The flap incision should be carried through the galea to the surface of the pericranium. The flap is then elevated anteriorly in a plane between the galea and pericranium, and at the superior temporal line, the periosteum is elevated, allowing the temporalis muscle to be elevated from the temporal fossa. The temporalis fascia, temporalis muscle, and periosteum of the temporal fossa are then rotated toward the forehead. Additional relaxation is obtained by severing the temporalis muscle just lateral to the frontal process of the zygoma. The deep temporal artery and branches of the superficial temporal artery should be preserved.

The galea and temporalis muscle are subsequently rotated to obliterate the sinus and cover any dural defect. If necessary, the galea is sutured directly to the dura with nonabsorbable sutures. A nonconstricting passageway into the anterior fossa is obtained by removing portions of the frontal, greater swing of the sphenoid and the squamous portion of the temporal bone with bone cutting rongeurs. The opening should be large enough to accommodate the flap pedicle and provide for some swelling in the postoperative period.

H The fractures of the anterior wall are repaired with plates and/or interosseous wires. The frontal osteoplastic flap is replaced with interrupted heavy chromic sutures through the periosteum. The subcutaneous tissues are approximated with 4-0 chromic sutures and the skin with 5-0 nylon sutures. If there is any oozing of blood, a Penrose drain should be placed for 24 to 48 hours at the inferiormost portion of the coronal incision. The surgeon should avoid dressings that compress the flap pedicle, but a light dressing should be applied. Prophylactic intravenous antibiotics are used both during the procedure and afterward for 5 days. The patient is then continued on oral antibiotics for 7 to 10 days. Sutures are removed at 7 days.

PITFALLS

1. The dissection of the temporalis muscle galea flap can potentially injure the hair of the parietal region. To prevent alopecia, the dissection should be carried just beneath the roots of the hair follicles.

2. Avoid injury to the superficial temporal artery. In making the incision, proceed cautiously through the skin. The superficial temporal artery usually lies in a subcutaneous plane very close to the skin.

3. Retain vascular attachments between the galea/pericranium and the temporalis fascia. The layers decussate near the edge of the temporal fossa at the superior temporal line, but if the surgeon performs a subperiosteal dissection into the fossa, damage can be minimized. The dissection should be limited to an area above the zygomatic arch, as a deeper dissection may injure the deep temporal artery.

4. Transfer of the flap into the anterior fossa requires a passageway through the frontal, sphenoid, and temporal bones. In designing this defect, the surgeon should allow for swelling of the muscle and fascial tissues.

5. Remove all mucosa of the frontal sinus and invert the mucosa near the area of the nasofrontal duct into the duct. The bone should be debrided completely with a cutting bur. The flap, combined with anterior displacement of the dura and brain, should completely obliterate the sinus.

COMPLICATIONS

1. Alopecia will develop if the hair follicles are damaged. This complication can usually be avoided by carefully dissecting between the hair follicles and the deeper subcutaneous tissues. Gentle handling of the skin flaps will preserve the blood supply to the area. A temporary alopecia is often seen near the incision lines. If alopecia persists, the surgeon can undermine and advance the tissues or, if the area of hair loss is large, employ a skin expander and sequentially advance the hair-bearing areas over the area of deficit.

2. A mass representing the muscle that is rotated into the anterior cranial fossa will appear in the temporal fossa. This projection of soft tissue will become less noticeable with time. If the deformity is bothersome and persists beyond 6 months, the base of the temporalis muscle flap can be incised and rotated back into its normal position. The distal portion of the flap should retain viability from its new attachment to the frontal sinus and anterior cranial fossa structures.

3. The flap reconstruction of the sinus is susceptible to all of the problems associated with obliteration of the sinus by other techniques. These complications are discussed in Chapters 72 and 73.

OBLITERATION WITH TEMPORALIS MUSCLE GALEA FLAP

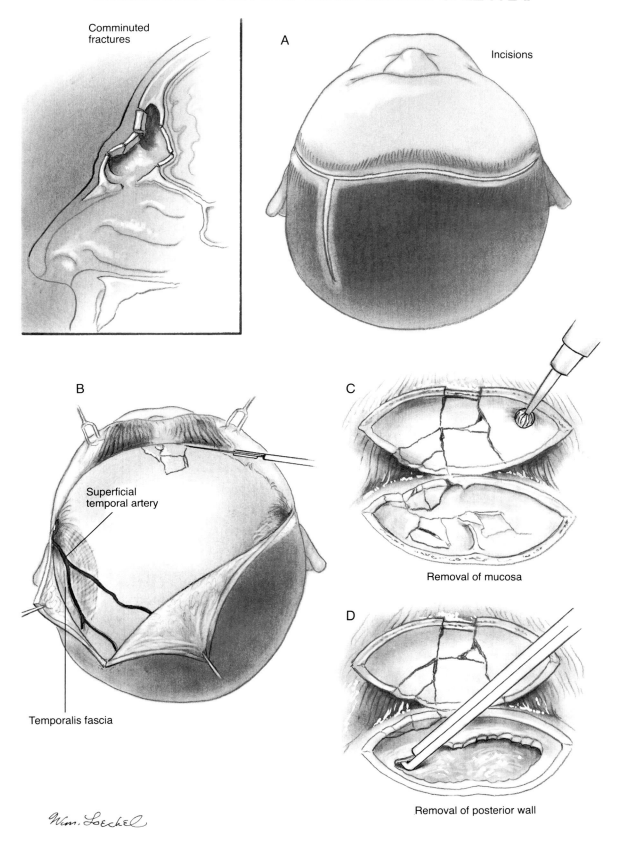

Comminuted fractures

A
Incisions

B
Superficial temporal artery

Temporalis fascia

C
Removal of mucosa

D
Removal of posterior wall

Wm. Loechel

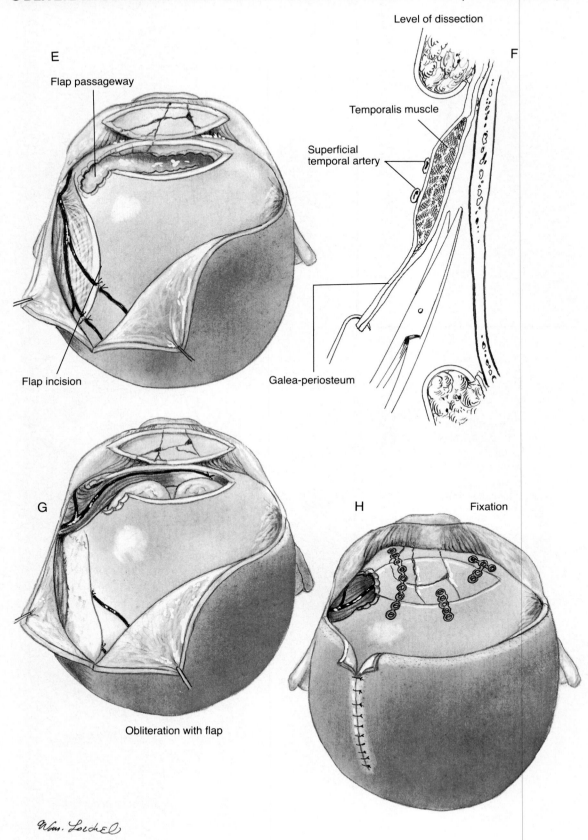

E

Flap passageway

Flap incision

Level of dissection

Temporalis muscle

Superficial temporal artery

Galea-periosteum

F

G

Obliteration with flap

H   Fixation

Wm. Loechel

section IV

Inferior Wall Fractures
of the Frontal Sinus

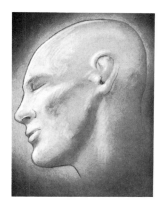

chapter 75

Fat Obliteration of Inferior Wall Fracture of the Frontal Sinus Using a Coronal Osteoplastic Flap

INDICATIONS

Inferior wall fractures can potentially interfere with the function of the nasofrontal duct. Obstruction of the duct can subsequently cause failure to aerate the sinus, stasis of secretions, and sinusitis. The infection can spread by way of Breschet's veins to the cranial cavity and through fracture lines to the orbit and adjoining structures. Thus with inferior wall fractures, obliteration of the sinus and reconstruction of the nasofrontal duct are important considerations.

The procedure of choice is dictated by the conditions associated with the injury. In nondisplaced, limited fractures, the surgeon can easily explore the sinus from below, enlarge the duct orifice, and either stent the duct with a chest tube or reconstruct it with a flap derived from the lining of adjacent nasal mucous membranes (see Chapter 76). When there is also damage to the anterior and/or posterior wall,

the coronal osteoplastic flap is better suited for evaluating and correcting the pathologic abnormality; the mucosa can then be removed and the sinus obliterated with fat.

PROCEDURE

A–D The techniques of coronal incision and osteoplastic flap are described elsewhere (see Chapter 72). As in other frontal fractures, it is important to ensure that the fragments are exposed and there is complete removal of the sinus mucosa. This often requires a microscopic dissection and removal of a layer of bone with cutting burs. The mucosa of the nasofrontal duct should be inverted and the duct plugged with fat or additional fascia. The sinus is then obliterated with fat and the flap returned to a normal position. Postoperative care is similar to that used in other obliteration procedures.

377

CORONAL OSTEOPLASTIC FLAP FOR INFERIOR WALL FRACTURES

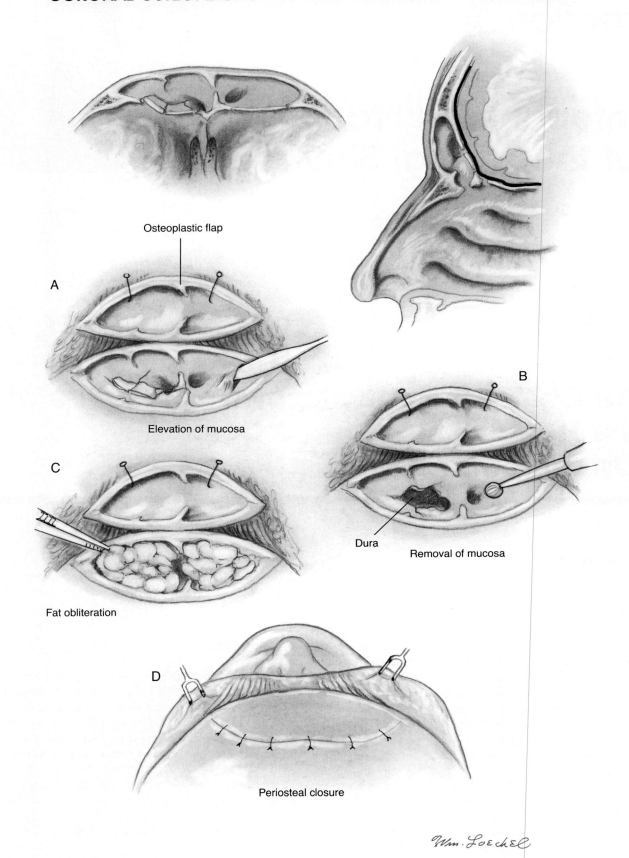

Osteoplastic flap

A

Elevation of mucosa

B

Dura

Removal of mucosa

C

Fat obliteration

D

Periosteal closure

Wm. Loechel

378

PITFALLS

1. Fractures of the inferior wall rarely occur alone. For this reason, the surgeon must be prepared to repair concurrent injuries of the anterior and/or posterior wall and also fractures that extend to the cribriform and orbital plates.

2. Care must thus be taken in manipulation or removal of bone fragments. Bone along the floor of the frontal sinus is thin and firmly attached to the dura. Thus when removing the bone, the surgeon must be careful not to tear or penetrate the underlying dura. If the dura is torn, it should be repaired with Gelfoam and/or fascial plugs.

3. If the surgeon chooses to obliterate the sinus, all mucosa should be removed. The bone should be cleaned of mucosa with a microscope, and additional layers of bone should be removed with a cutting bur. If it is not possible to do this, then a reconstruction of the nasofrontal duct should be considered (see Chapter 76).

4. Some anatomic variations preclude removal of all mucosa. Occasionally the mucosa lies deep within supraorbital crevices that extend beyond the orbit. The boundaries of the mucosa are not easily determined, and in such cases, obliteration should then cover only the anterior cells. The deep extensions of the sinus usually drain through a posterior group of cells that should subsequently function in a normal fashion.

COMPLICATIONS

1. Acute sinusitis is an important complication, as infection can spread into the meninges and orbit.

The surgeon should avoid obliteration of a contaminated open wound. Antibiotic prophylaxis is mandatory. The patient should be followed during the postoperative period for infection and treated accordingly.

2. Chronic sinusitis, characterized by mucoceles and mucopyoceles, can develop at any time following the procedure. For these reasons, patients with inferior wall injuries should be followed with radiographs for infection and/or persistence of fat and cyst formation. If the patient develops these complications, medical therapy should be initiated. Failure to control the disease process should prompt appropriate surgical procedures.

3. Cerebrospinal fluid leaks can continue or develop in the postoperative period. Most leaks will stop within 2 weeks, but if the leak persists, its exact anatomic location should be determined. Most leaks can be repaired from the osteoplastic frontal flap or frontoethmoid approach (see Chapter 86).

4. Loss of smell is commonly associated with the inferior wall injury. It is suspected that there is a disruption of the neural elements as they pass through the cribriform plate. The prognosis for recovery of smell is poor, and no known medical or surgical measures are available to treat this complication.

5. Deformity of the forehead can occur as a result of associated injury to the anterior plate of the frontal sinus and/or displacement of the osteoplastic flap. These complications are discussed in Chapter 78.

chapter 76

Treatment of Inferior Wall Fracture of the Frontal Sinus by Reconstruction of the Nasofrontal Duct

Alternative Technique Using Nasal Mucosal Flaps

INDICATIONS

Fractures of the frontal sinus that extend to the inferior wall threaten the integrity and function of the nasofrontal duct. This opening and passageway is essential for removal of secretions and aeration of the sinus. Failure of the duct system can cause stasis of secretions and sinusitis. There is also the possibility of developing a mucocele or mucopyocele. Infection can potentially spread through the transosseous veins to the cranial cavity and orbit.

If the inferior wall fracture appears to compromise the nasofrontal duct, the surgeon can obliterate the sinus with fat, brain, and/or muscle flaps, as described in Chapters 72 through 75, or proceed with reconstruction of the nasofrontal duct. When the frontal sinus injury is associated with contamination and infection threatens the free graft obliteration, duct repair should be considered. Also, if it is impossible to remove all of the mucosa, which can happen in severely comminuted injuries, then it is more prudent to avoid obliteration and fabricate a new duct. However, it should be recognized that duct patency following reconstruction may fail many years later, and for this reason, the surgeon should evaluate the sinus for clearing and aeration regularly during the postoperative period.

PROCEDURE

Reconstruction of the nasofrontal duct can be approached through the coronal osteoplastic frontal flap (see Chapter 72) or through a Lynch frontoethmoid incision. Exposure using the frontoethmoid approach is relatively faster; it also provides an opportunity to create an adjacent mucosal flap.

A Using general anesthesia, a curvilinear incision

is mapped out one half the distance from the medial caruncle to the dorsum of the nose. The area is then infiltrated with 1% lidocaine containing 1:100,000 epinephrine. Pledgets of 4% cocaine containing epinephrine (see Chapter 46) are applied to the nose to help in the control of bleeding.

B,C The incision is carried through the skin and subcutaneous tissues. The angular vessels are either cauterized or ligated. The periosteum overlying the nasal bones and the frontal process of the maxilla is incised and elevated with Joseph elevators to expose the nasal bones, nasofrontal suture line, and a portion of the anterior frontal bone. The trochlea is then detached, and the periosteum is elevated off the medial wall of the orbit. Bleeding from the anterior ethmoidal artery is controlled with gentle pressure or a vascular clip. The posterior ethmoidal artery, a landmark for the location of the optic nerve, is kept intact.

The floor of the frontal bone is then opened by elevating the fragments or cutting through them with burs. The opening is enlarged to expose the floor region to at least the nasofrontal duct. Exenteration of the posterior ethmoidal cells ensures that the duct has been opened and enlarged appropriately. A complete external ethmoidectomy can be accomplished with curettage and Kerrison and Takahashi rongeurs.

D,E The nasal cavity is entered inferiorly. The anterior portion of the middle turbinate and portions of the frontal process of the maxilla and nasal bone should be removed to provide a passageway that will accommodate a No. 26 chest tube. At the same time the surgeon should avoid injury to the anterior and posterior lacrimal crest and lacrimal sac.

Oozing of blood should be treated with a 4% cocaine packing containing epinephrine or with bi-

NASOFRONTAL DUCT RECONSTRUCTION

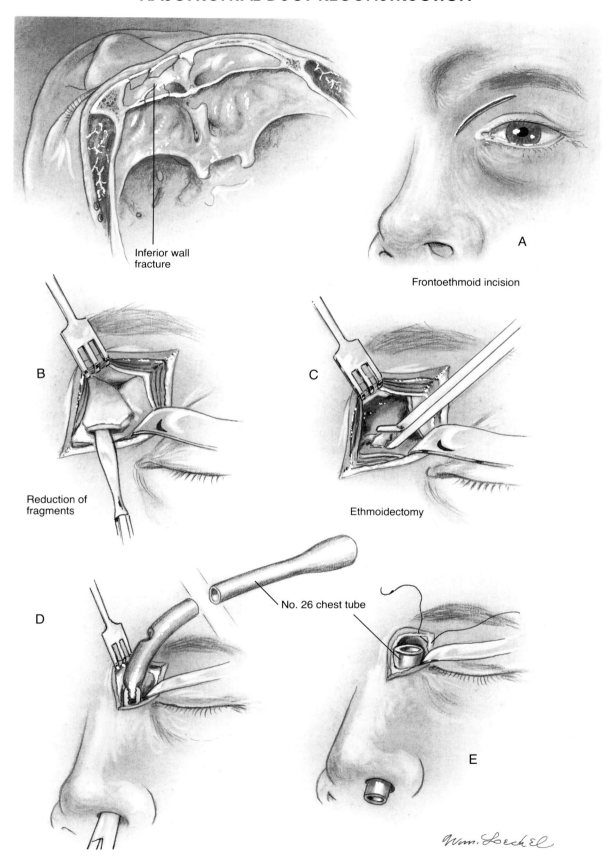

Inferior wall fracture

A

Frontoethmoid incision

B

Reduction of fragments

C

Ethmoidectomy

D

No. 26 chest tube

E

polar cauterization. Once the passageway is adequate, a No. 26 chest tube can be inserted from the sinus opening into the nose. The tube is grasped with a clamp and pulled inferiorly so that the flange rests on the floor of the frontal sinus. A high flange should be avoided and excess flange removed with scissors. The other end of the tubing should be cut so that it projects just beyond the nares. The chest tube is then secured to the intermembranous septum with a 2-0 silk suture.

The periosteum over the osteotomy is closed with a 3-0 chromic suture. The subcutaneous tissues are approximated with 4-0 chromic sutures, and the skin is coapted with 6-0 nylon sutures. The nose should be kept clean with cotton-tipped applicators and 3% hydrogen peroxide. If blood clots form in the tubing, they should be removed with 3% hydrogen peroxide and suctioning. Antibiotics (i.e., ampicillin or cefazolin) are prescribed for 10 to 14 days. Sutures are removed at 7 days and the tube at 4 to 6 weeks.

PITFALLS

1. Avoid placing the tube next to an area of dural injury. The tube should be contoured and positioned so that it stents and drains but does not come in contact with the exposed dura.

2. The opening from the sinus into the nose must be large and either stented or reconstructed with flaps if it is to provide a permanent airway. A No. 26 chest tube generally will keep the passageway open, and within 4 to 6 weeks, a reepithelialized fistula will have occurred. The surgeon has the option of developing nasal flaps, which can be rotated and immediately used to layer the edges of the opening with mucosa (see later).

3. Blood clots will form and must be removed from the tube. Failure to do so will cause swelling and periorbital pain. Blood clots can often be avoided by placing the flange of the tube at a low level within the sinus. Also, the surgeon should avoid through-and-through sutures that will cause debris to collect in the tube. Small clots can usually be removed with forceps and suction tips.

4. Keep the nares clean postoperatively with 3% hydrogen peroxide and cotton-tipped applicators. Crusts tend to develop around the suture, and if they are not removed, infection can occur.

5. The tube should be kept in position for at least 4 to 6 weeks. Usually the tube will be "caught" at the osteotomy site, but it should still be held firmly to the intermembranous septum or columella with a 2-0 silk suture.

6. Close the periosteum over the frontal process of the maxilla with a heavy chromic suture. This will return the trochlea to its normal position and reduce the incidence of postoperative diplopia.

COMPLICATIONS

1. Indwelling tubes can be associated with an infection, such as sinusitis, meningitis, and periorbital cellulitis. This complication can be avoided by strategic placement of the tube for drainage and by keeping the tube open and free from clots during the postoperative period. The surgeon should also avoid irrigations that tend to force bacteria into the adjoining tissues. Prophylactic antibiotics will help prevent infection, but if infection does develop, adequate drainage must be instituted and new cultures obtained to determine the appropriate specific treatment of the bacteria.

2. Cerebrospinal fluid leaks may be seen in the postoperative period, but most will stop within several days. Prophylactic antibiotics should be used. If the leakage persists for more than 2 weeks, exploration and repair should be considered (see Chapter 86).

3. Diplopia following frontoethmoidectomy should be transient, and vision should return to normal as the trochlea reattaches to the wall of the orbit. If diplopia persists, an ophthalmologic consultation is advised.

4. Although long-term results with tube reconstruction of the nasofrontal duct are excellent, there is also a possibility of developing obstruction of the duct, sinusitis, and sequelae such as mucocele and meningitis. These complications can be avoided by establishing an opening of more than adequate size and by providing epithelialization around the tube with a local mucosal flap. Failures can be attributed to extensive local damage or inflammatory conditions of the nose, such as rhinitis and polyps. If the sinuses fail to show signs of aeration, then the surgeon must consider obliteration with fat and/or local or regional flaps.

5. Hypertrophic scars, although rare, can develop in the frontoethmoid incision line. This problem can sometimes be prevented by making an irregular line of incision. If an unsightly scar develops, it can be treated with local injections of triamcinolone (40 mg/mL). If the scar is still unsatisfactory, then zigzagplasty or Z-plasty revision should be performed (see Chapter 69).

ALTERNATIVE TECHNIQUE USING NASAL MUCOSAL FLAPS

Although there are advantages to using a tube in the reconstruction of the nasofrontal duct, some disadvantages must also be considered. Placement of the tube may be difficult, and if the tube comes in contact with damaged dura and with cerebrospinal fluid leakage, there can be a problem with bacterial contamination and meningitis. Injury of the dura is also possible, and in such a situation, it is more prudent to reconstruct the duct with local flaps.

a—c The exposure is identical to that obtained for the tube reconstruction procedure. However, the surgeon must avoid injury to the nasal mucosa that lies beneath the nasal bones and anterior and inferior to the middle turbinate. Working through the nose, parallel incisions about 2 cm apart are made along the upper nasal vault. These incisions are extended inferiorly to the level of the lower lateral cartilages. The tissues are then cut horizontally, and a flap based superiorly is elevated and rotated on itself into the frontal sinus. Closure of the periosteum and wound and postoperative care are identical to those used for the chest tube placement technique.

NASOFRONTAL DUCT RECONSTRUCTION *(Continued)*

ALTERNATIVE TECHNIQUE
USING NASAL MUCOSAL FLAP

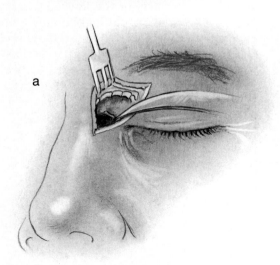

a

Frontoethmoid approach

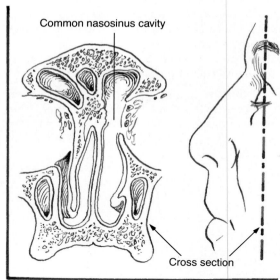

Common nasosinus cavity

Cross section

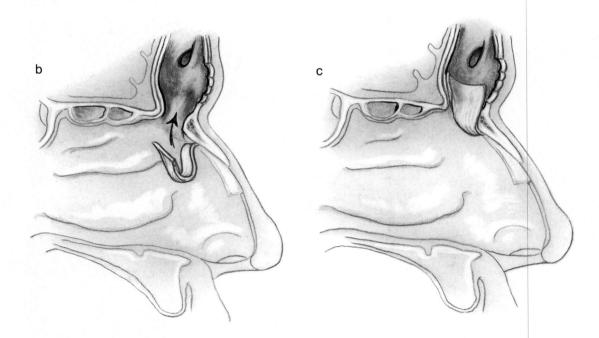

b   c

Development and rotation of flap

section V

Superior Orbital Wall Fractures

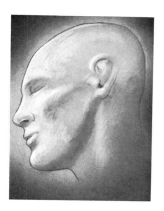

chapter 77

Repair of Superior Orbital Wall Fractures Using a Transorbital Approach
Alternative Technique Using Frontotemporal (Frontopterional) Craniotomy

In Consultation With L. Murray Thomas, MD

INDICATIONS

Fractures of the orbital plate of the frontal bone can be isolated injuries or associated with fractures of the frontal sinus or zygoma that extend into the orbit. If the frontal sinus is small, the fracture will usually involve the orbital roof and floor of the anterior cranial fossa. If the frontal sinus is large, the fracture can cause damage to the inferior wall of the sinus and adversely affect the function of the naso-frontal duct.

Fracture of the superior orbital wall will often effect changes in orbital volume and displacement of the globe, clinically apparent as enophthalmos or exoph-

thalmos. In fractures extending to the anterior fossa, there is usually a history of unconsciousness, and the patient may appear with pulsations of soft tissues within the orbit. Proptosis as a result of brain herniation can also be a problem. Fractures occurring more medially can present with cerebrospinal fluid leaks. Levator and superior rectus injuries are also possible.

Superior orbital wall fractures that are confined to the rim and frontal sinus can often be explored and repaired by a direct transorbital sub-brow approach or a frontal osteoplastic flap approach (see Chapter 75). For more extensive areas of injury, the surgeon should consider a frontotemporal (frontopterional) craniotomy. This provides an excellent exposure with which to repair other areas of the anterior fossa and, if necessary, to carry out decompression of the superior orbital fissure and/or optic nerve (see Chapters 81 and 82).

PROCEDURE

Under orotracheal anesthesia, the face is prepared and draped as a sterile field. The eyes should be exposed so that the surgeon can evaluate the relative position and mobility of the globes. Incisions can be designed either through the lateral eyebrow or as in a sub-brow approach in which an incision is made about 3 cm in length beneath the medial part of the eyebrow. The incisions should then be infiltrated with 1% lidocaine containing 1:100,000 epinephrine for assistance in hemostasis.

A To avoid injury to the hair follicles, the skin should be incised either below or parallel to the orientation of the hair follicles. The incision is then carried through the orbicularis oculi. Angular vessels should either be ligated or cauterized. The periosteum is incised and elevated off the rim toward the orbit. Laterally the surgeon should elevate the lacrimal gland off the lacrimal fossa. Medially the trochlea is released from its attachment. Additional exposure is obtained by elevating the periosteum off the frontal bone. If possible, the branches of the supraorbital and supratrochlea nerves and arteries should be preserved.

B–D If the fracture does not involve the nasofrontal duct and displacement of the fracture is minimal without any evidence of cerebrospinal fluid leak, then the rim of the orbit should be reduced, reinforced if necessary with a piece of polyethylene mesh, and wired (or alternatively plated) into position. Drill holes are placed with a 0.035 K wire and minidriver through the anterior plate. A 28-gauge wire is then passed through the hole of the loose fragment. A 30-gauge loop is subsequently passed through the hole of the adjacent stable fragment, and with this wire loop, the 28-gauge wire is attached and passed. Other fractures are managed in a similar way. All wires are then twisted so that the fragment is secured to the craniofacial skeleton.

The periosteum and subcutaneous tissues are closed with 4-0 chromic sutures. The skin is coapted with a 6-0 nylon suture. A light pressure dressing consisting of eye ointment, eye pads, stretch gauze, and fluffs is helpful in controlling postoperative edema. The wound should be evaluated at 24 and 72 hours. Prophylactic antibiotics (i.e., ampicillin or cefazolin) are recommended for 5 days. Skin sutures are removed at 5 to 7 days.

PITFALLS

1. An accurate diagnosis is essential for application of proper treatment. If the fracture involves the nasofrontal duct, a coronal incision, osteoplastic flap, and obliteration of sinus with fat or reconstruction of the duct are preferred (see Chapters 75 and 76). If the fracture involves the anterior fossa, the surgeon must consider combining the exploration and reduction of the frontal fracture with a craniotomy (see later).

2. Forces applied to the orbital rim can be transmitted posteriorly, resulting in compression of the optic nerve. For these reasons, vision must be evaluated preoperatively. During the reduction, the surgeon should be careful to elevate the orbital rim forward and avoid any posterior displacement of the fractures.

3. If the orbital rim is severely comminuted, the surgeon should consider holding the reduced fragments with a tight periosteal closure or, alternatively, with miniplates applied across the region of injury. In using the miniplate, the surgeon should place holes just through the outer cortex and not into the frontal sinus or anterior fossa. Small fragments can be "basketed" by stabilizing adjoining fragments.

4. In patients with enophthalmos and/or exophthalmos, the surgeon has to consider a defect involving the anterior cranial fossa. The orbital plate can be displaced either upward or downward. In such situations, an osteoplastic flap or craniotomy (as described later) should be utilized for the repair.

5. Dystopia of the globe can be caused by downward or upward displacement of the superior orbital wall, alone or in combination with a floor injury. In planning reconstruction of the superior orbital wall, the surgeon should release those pressures that cause a downward displacement of the globe. Malar and inferior orbital rim fractures should be concurrently reduced and repaired to help in the support of the orbital tissues.

COMPLICATIONS

1. The initial fracture or the repair of the supraorbital rim can result in hypoesthesia or anesthesia of the forehead. When performing surgery, the surgeon should attempt to identify and avoid injury to the supraorbital nerve. In many patients function will return, whereas in others, there will be paresthesias and even permanent loss of sensation. Additional medical or surgical intervention has not proven to be effective.

2. If the orbital rim is not accurately reduced and stabilized, a brow deformity can occur. In the early

TRANSORBITAL REPAIR OF SUPERIOR WALL FRACTURES

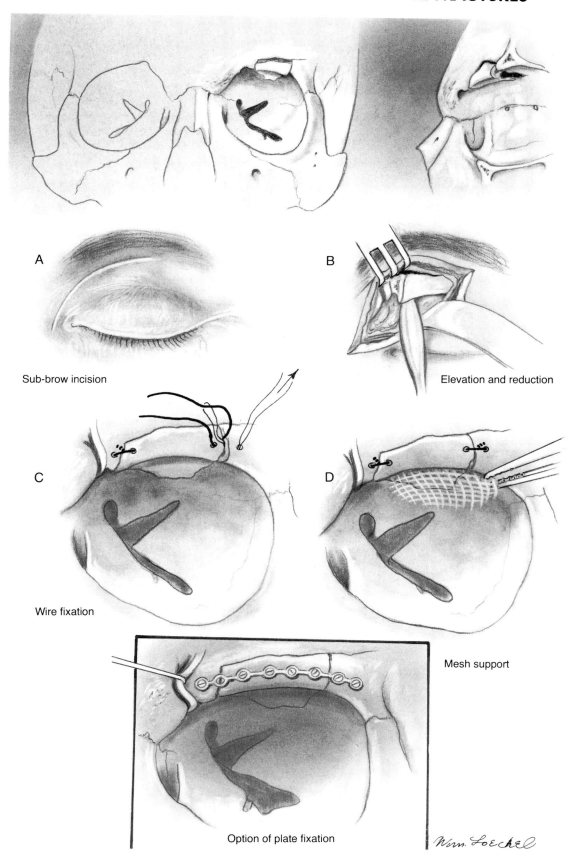

A

Sub-brow incision

B

Elevation and reduction

C

Wire fixation

D

Mesh support

Option of plate fixation

Wm. Loechel

postoperative period, open reduction, refracture, and repair are indicated. If healing of the bone has been completed, the surgeon must then consider removing projections with a cutting bur and filling in the defects with cranial bone grafts (see Chapter 78).

3. Most swelling of the eyelid and weakness of levator function will improve with time. A subperiosteal dissection along the orbital rim should avoid injury to the neuromuscular units. If ptosis continues to be a problem, ophthalmologic consultation is advised.

4. Fractures extending to the nasofrontal duct and the anterior fossa can later be associated with sinusitis and/or cerebrospinal fluid leaks. These complications are described in Chapter 72.

ALTERNATIVE TECHNIQUE USING FRONTOTEMPORAL (FRONTOPTERIONAL) CRANIOTOMY

a,b The frontotemporal craniotomy and repair of the superior orbital wall (roof) is indicated when there is a suspicion of a large dural tear (i.e., cerebrospinal fluid leak and/or pneumocephalus) and displacement of the roof affecting position of the globe (i.e., hypopthalmos). For this procedure, a coronal skin flap is designed 2 cm behind the hairline. A small area of hair is shaved, and the head is prepared and draped as a sterile field. The incision is beveled in the direction of the hair follicles, and a plane is developed below the galea. The flap is elevated and rotated inferiorly and held in position with fish hooks or self-retaining retractors. The temporalis fascia and muscle are cut and reflected inferiorly.

Bur holes are then placed to develop a bone flap. One bur hole is made just behind the frontal process of the zygoma, another about 2 cm laterally and posteriorly in the temporal bone, and a third just above the frontal sinus and 3 to 4 cm lateral to the midline. The dura is then elevated around and between the bur holes with a special malleable dissector. Injury to the middle meningeal artery may occur and will require electrocoagulation. A craniotome or Gigli saw is used to divide the bone. The bone flap is removed providing exposure to the anterior and middle fossa. Bone wax should be used as necessary to control small bleeders within the bone.

c,d The dura is carefully elevated from the orbital roof and the dissection extended to the cribriform plate area. Fragments of bone on the roof may be removed or elevated and replaced in anatomic position. No fixation is necessary. The dura should be meticulously closed with 4-0 nonabsorbable sutures. If a defect is present, a piece of temporalis fascia or fascia lata may be used to close and reinforce the area.

e In most cases, the bone flap is replaced and secured to adjacent bone with strategically placed angulated drill holes and 2-0 nonabsorbable sutures. The temporalis muscle and forehead flap are closed in layers, and a head dressing is applied. Prophylactic antibiotics (i.e., nafcillin and gentamicin or cefazolin) should be administered for at least 5 days following surgery. The skin sutures can be removed on the seventh to tenth postoperative day.

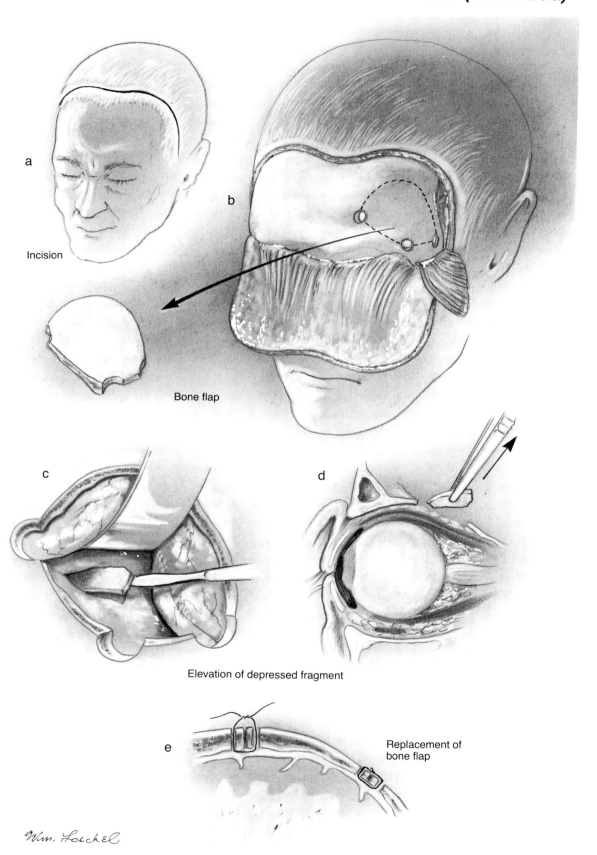

a

Incision

b

Bone flap

c

d

Elevation of depressed fragment

e

Replacement of bone flap

Wm. Loechel

section VI

Forehead Deformity

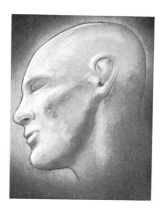

chapter 78

Repair of Forehead Deformity With Bone Grafts
Alternative Technique Using Methylmethacrylate

In Consultation With L. Murray Thomas, MD

INDICATIONS

A posttraumatic deformity involving the fronto-orbital region can develop as a result of inadequate reduction and fixation and/or from absorption of bone. The defect is usually not noticeable early after the repair, but the affected patient will return months or years later complaining of a projection or depression of the frontal or brow region. For a small defect, we prefer recontouring of the forehead with cutting burs and application of onlay split cranial grafts. For the larger defects, an alloplastic graft (e.g., methylmethacrylate) is employed.

PROCEDURE

For most patients, a coronal incision and elevation of the forehead flap will provide optimal exposure. Nevertheless, for those patients with scars already present over the forehead region or for those who are balding, direct approaches should be considered (see Chapter 71).

A The coronal incision and method to expose the anterior plate of the frontal bone are described in Chapter 72. If the deformity involves the orbital rim, additional exposure can be obtained by extending the dissection along the zygomaticofrontal process and the frontal process of the maxillary bone. To provide for the harvest of the graft, the dissection should also be extended posteriorly over the parietal bone and upper portion of the temporal bone. The periosteum along the frontal bone should be incised just above the area of deformity, as this will later provide for a periosteal closure over the area of reconstruction.

B The deformity should be measured by cutting a 4 × 4 gauze sponge to the size of the defect and

391

transposing this sponge to the donor site. The area to be harvested is then outlined with a marking solution.

The donor bone is obtained by forming an island of bone with cutting burs. A "trough" is developed by removing additional bone from around the donor site. The block of outer cortical bone is then removed with curved osteotomes or an oscillating saw. Bleeding is controlled by application of bone wax to the inner table of parietal cortex.

C,D The graft is subsequently placed over the defect to be repaired and contoured with burs so that it fits the defect. The recipient site can also be carved to help with the fit. The periosteum is then closed with heavy chromic (2-0 or 3-0) sutures; usually this closure will hold the graft in desirable position. Postoperative care is the same as that described in Chapter 77.

PITFALLS

1. In preparing for the reconstruction, the surgeon should ensure that the sinus is completely obliterated or functioning normally. The patient should be free of cerebrospinal fluid leaks or other defects of the anterior fossa. Care should also be taken during the preparation of the recipient site to avoid injury to the sinus and/or underlying dura.

2. Always harvest a larger graft than anticipated. Donor bone should then be carved in phases until the bone fills and fits the defect. If too much bone is removed in the shaping of the graft, additional small pieces can be harvested and inserted into the forehead gaps.

COMPLICATIONS

1. Deformity can develop when the graft is too small or too large or when the bone undergoes resorption. If a defect is noticed, additional bone grafting can be considered. If there is excess of bone, the surgeon can remove the projected areas with cutting burs. Revisional surgery, however, should be delayed until the grafted site area has stabilized, which may take from 6 months to 2 years after the repair.

2. A graft affected by infection is unusual, but if this complication occurs, the graft will have to be removed and the area treated with appropriate drainage. Intravenous antibiotics should be administered. Prophylactic antibiotics and aseptic techniques should help prevent this complication from occurring.

3. Dural injury, intracranial bleeding, and other complications associated with harvest of the cranial graft are described in Chapters 55 and 60.

ALTERNATIVE TECHNIQUE USING A METHYLMETHACRYLATE PLATE

The methylmethacrylate technique is best used when a craniectomy results in a large frontal bone deficit, with or without involvement of the orbital rim. The procedure should be performed under ideal conditions, and this means that the area of surgery must be clean. If there is an open wound, the wound should be closed and the procedure delayed for several months.

a Exposure of the fronto-orbital defect is usually obtained through a coronal forehead flap. The incision is about 2 cm behind the hairline, with a potential extension to the supraauricular areas. The incision line should be shaved and the patient's head prepared and draped as a sterile field.

The incision is carried into a subperiosteal plane. Hemostasis is achieved with electric cautery and with the optional use of hemostatic clips. Laterally the dissection is superficial to the temporalis fascia. The flap (with frontal bone periosteum) is then elevated forward and rotated over the face and is held in position with fish hooks or self-retaining retractors.

b–d The defect to be corrected is cleaned of soft tissues. Any projections beyond the desired contour are removed with a cutting bur. Methylmethacrylate powder and liquid are mixed according to directions. When the polymer has a pasty consistency, it is rolled out like pie dough between sheets of plastic and then molded into the defect. It will get hot as it cures, and the temperature can be controlled with saline irrigation. After the plate has hardened, drill holes can be made in the plate and adjacent bone; the plate is then held in place with four or five 3-0 nonabsorbable sutures. Any irregularities of the plate can be corrected with a cutting bur.

For more extensive and complex defects, a copper mold, which is fabricated preoperatively to fashion the acrylic implant, can be used. To make the mold, the surgeon must obtain the external dimensions of the defect or estimate them from a six-foot Caldwell radiograph. A copper sheet is then hammered to the proper contour and fitted over the defect and the adjacent cranio-orbital structures. The copper should extend at least 0.5 to 1 cm beyond the defect. Intraoperatively methylmethacrylate, in paste form, is rolled out and placed into the mold. The mold and polymer are then pressed over the defect and against the adjoining bone. The mold is held into position

GRAFTING FOR A FOREHEAD DEFORMITY

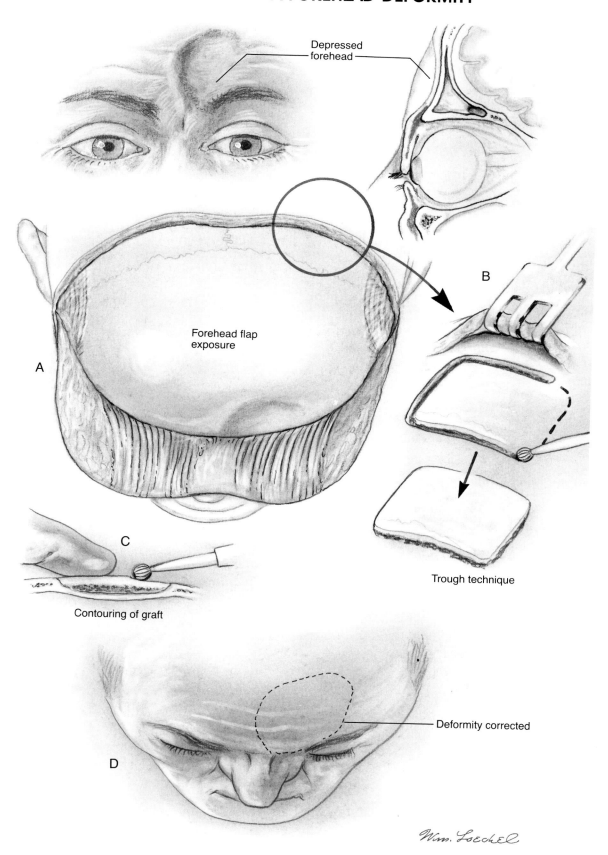

Depressed forehead

Forehead flap exposure

A

B

Trough technique

C

Contouring of graft

D

Deformity corrected

Wm. Loechel

until the acrylic hardens. Cooling can be facilitated by saline irrigations.

The wound is closed in layers. A bulky head dressing is applied, and the patient is treated with prophylactic antibiotics (i.e., nafcillin and gentamicin or cefazolin) for 5 to 7 days. Subgaleal fluid collections are usually prevented by careful hemostasis and a bulky compression dressing, but if fluids accumulate, they can be removed with needle aspiration using a sterile technique. Small fluid collections usually resorb without treatment.

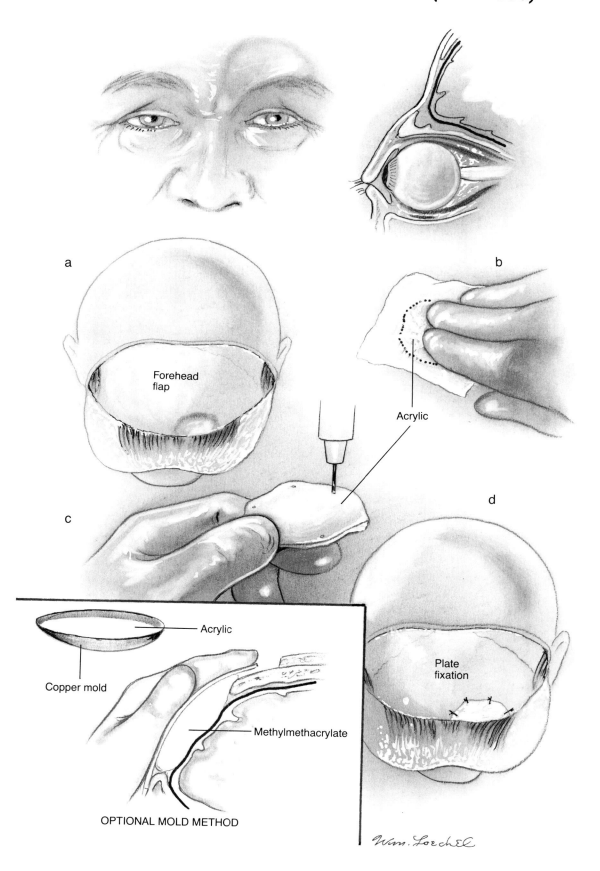

a

b

Forehead
flap

Acrylic

c

d

Acrylic

Copper mold

Plate
fixation

Methylmethacrylate

OPTIONAL MOLD METHOD

Wm. Loechel

part nine

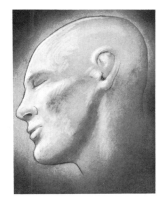

Sphenoid Fractures

section I

Classification and Pathophysiology of Sphenoid Fractures

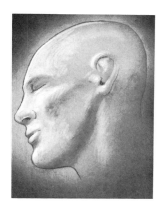

chapter 79

General Considerations

The sphenoid bone appears to be protected by its central position within the craniofacial skeleton, but its multiple attachments to the cranium and face make it particularly vulnerable to fracture. Sphenoid injuries are commonly associated with maxillary, zygomatic, ethmoid, frontal, and temporal bone fractures, and thus the sphenoid injury often presents with a variety of additional deformities and neural and vascular deficits. Successful management depends on early diagnosis and appropriate medical and surgical regimens.

Sphenoid fractures often present with specific syndromes. Injury to the body of the sphenoid can cause a cerebrospinal fluid leak from the nose and/or damage to the optic nerve. Fractures involving the greater wing of the sphenoid and superior orbital fissure can result in injury to the recurrent branch of the lacrimal artery; the superior and inferior ophthalmic veins; the oculomotor (III), trochlea (IV), and abducens (VI) nerves; and the lacrimal, frontal, and nasociliary

branches and sympathetic fibers of the ophthalmic nerve (V_1). The multiple neuropathies generally affect pupillary and extraocular functions. Also, a greater wing fracture can extend to the foramen ovale and foramen spinosum and cause problems with the maxillary and mandibular nerves, the middle and accessory meningeal arteries, and the lesser petrosal nerve, resulting in problems with jaw strength and facial sensation. Pterygoid plate displacement can affect mastication, and if the hamulus is involved, the tensor veli palatini will fail to open and close the eustachian tube. This can lead to fluid and/or blood accumulation within the middle ear.

The location and extent of the sphenoid bone fracture are best evaluated by a combination of plain radiographs, tomograms, and computed tomography (CT) scans. Clinical management depends specifically on the problem created by the injury. In most cases expectant waiting with appropriate prophylactic antibiotic therapy is indicated. In others, there is a need for immediate, aggressive medical and/or surgical decompression of one or several nerves. Persistent cerebrospinal fluid leakage may require exploration and repair of a dural tear. Diplopia may require reduction of one of the orbital walls, prisms, and/or exercises with eye muscle surgery. Masticatory dysfunction may require a reduction of the pterygoid plates, but if a neural deficit is the cause, it is probably best treated with prosthetic and rehabilitative techniques.

SPHENOID FRACTURES

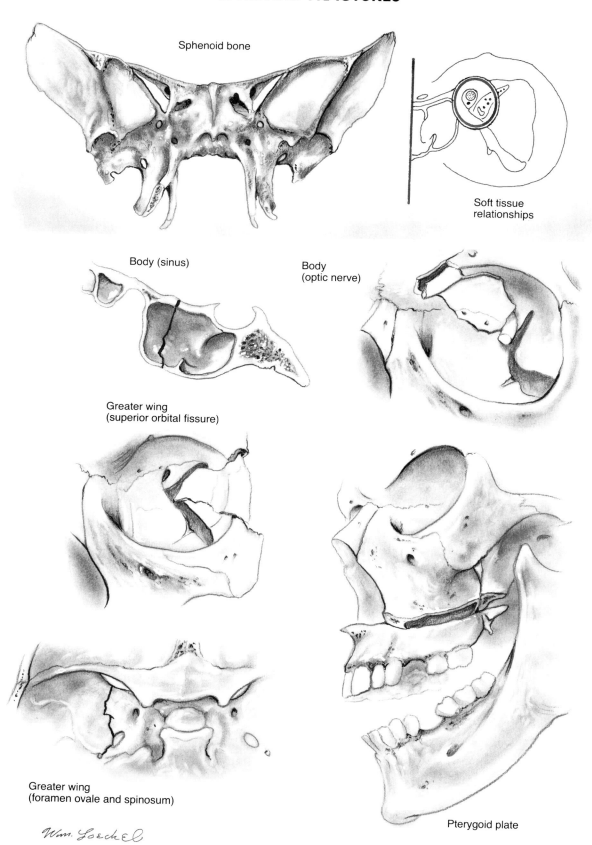

Sphenoid bone

Soft tissue
relationships

Body (sinus)

Body
(optic nerve)

Greater wing
(superior orbital fissure)

Greater wing
(foramen ovale and spinosum)

Wm. Loechel

Pterygoid plate

Optic Nerve Injury

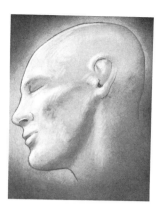

chapter 80

Decompression of the Optic Nerve Using a Transethmoidal Approach

INDICATIONS

Sudden or progressive loss of vision in the absence of globe injury often indicates optic nerve damage. The patient may demonstrate a Marcus Gunn pupil (afferent pupillary defect), but the physician should not expect optic nerve pallor or atrophy for several weeks. Evoked visual potentials are often markedly diminished or absent. The clinical picture may be complicated by other ocular injuries, and the impact these injuries have on vision must be determined.

A variety of mechanisms have been used to describe optic nerve damage. The optic nerve may be mechanically impacted by displacement of adjacent bone fragments, or it may be contused or compressed by blood clots or swelling within the optic canal. There is also a possibility that the nerve has been lacerated and severed from its attachments.

From a treatment standpoint it is important to evaluate whether the nerve is severed or compressed, but this is often impossible to determine by clinical and/or radiographic methods. An immediate loss of vision suggests a laceration or cutting, whereas a gradual loss is more consistent with a compression phenomenon. Major displacements of sphenoid bone fragments may imply an impaction or tearing of the nerve. All of this information is helpful, but because the surgeon cannot be certain of the pathologic condition, medical and/or surgical trials of therapy are indicated.

Our usual approach is to evaluate the history, physical examination, and radiographic information (sinus radiographs, coronal tomography, and horizontal and coronal computed tomographic [CT] scans). Ophthalmologic consultation is obtained. Most patients are started on megadose steroids (i.e., 100 mg dexamethasone followed by 50 mg every 6 hours for three doses). If the patient responds, the steroids are tapered. If the patient does not respond or there is a relapse after a gradual improvement, then the steroids are stopped (or tapered), and a surgical decompression is considered.

The transethmoidal approach is preferred when the injury to the sphenoid also involves the medial and inferior walls of the orbit. The exposure is indicated when there is a need to repair other facial fractures. The intracranial approach is best employed when there are associated cranial bone injuries and, in particular, dural tears, frontal bone fractures, and injury to the orbital plate (see Chapter 81).

PROCEDURE

The patient is placed in a supine position, and anesthesia is provided by way of an orotracheal tube. The nasal mucous membranes are treated with 4% cocaine containing epinephrine (see Chapter 46), and the medial canthal area is injected with 1% lidocaine containing 1:100,000 epinephrine. The head is extended, and the patient is placed in Trendelenburg's position. The head and neck are then prepared with antiseptic solutions and draped as a sterile field.

A With the surgeon sitting at the head of the table, a curvilinear incision is made one half the distance between the inner caruncle of the eye and the dorsum of the nose. The incision is carried through the subcutaneous tissues; the angular vessels are ligated, and bleeding is stopped with cautery. The incision can also be extended to the shadow area beneath the brow.

B,C The periosteum is elevated off the nasal bones and the frontal process of the maxilla. The lamina papyracea and lacrimal bones are exposed, and the lacrimal sac is retracted laterally. The trochlea is released from its attachment. The periosteum is elevated off the medial wall of the orbit with a Freer elevator. The anterior ethmoidal artery is clipped or avulsed, and bleeding is controlled by gentle pressure. Posteriorly the dissection should expose, but not injure, the posterior ethmoidal artery.

D,E A frontoethmoidectomy is then performed by removing portions of the floor of the frontal sinus, the nasal bone, and the frontal process of the maxilla. The frontal sinus is opened by a small drill hole and enlarged with Kerrison rongeurs. The inferiorly located ethmoid cells are then removed with Takahashi rongeurs. The curved posterior wall of the frontal bone should be visualized and followed inferiorly and posteriorly along the base of the skull. The undersurface of the cribriform plate is exposed.

F–H The operating microscope with a 300-mm lens is used for the remainder of the procedure. Self-retaining retractors are helpful in holding the soft tissues of the orbit from the sinus cavity. We prefer to open the sphenoid sinus with Hajek rongeurs, which in turn exposes the intersinus septum and those landmarks that identify the optic nerve and carotid artery. The transverse bulge superiorly shows the course of the optic nerve; a wider bulge laterally and posteriorly represents the carotid artery canal.

With the optic nerve bulge identified within the sphenoid sinus and the posterior ethmoidal artery visualized within the orbit, the posterior ethmoidal artery is clipped or treated with a bipolar cautery. The bone along the posteromedial wall of the orbit is then removed, exposing more of the sphenoid sinus. The periorbita is elevated 1 or 2 mm at a time, and immediately posterior to the posterior ethmoidal artery, the surgeon will see the optic nerve sheath entering the optic canal. The entrance to the canal (ring) is quite thick, and diamond burs on a long drill handle should be used to open this area. The more posteriorly and medially directed portion of the canal is thinned with burs and extracted with small elevators. Approximately one half to three fourths of the canal is opened. Any displaced bone spicules are removed.

Bleeding should be minimal, and nasal packing should not be needed. The periosteum is closed with 3-0 chromic sutures, and the trochlea should be returned to its anatomic position. The subcutaneous tissues and skin are closed in layers.

The patient should be treated with prophylactic antibiotics (i.e., cefazolin or ampicillin) and the eye checked periodically for visual function and for changes in pressure on the globe. The patient can be discharged in 24 to 48 hours.

PITFALLS

1. The optic nerve decompression procedure requires exquisite attention to detail. The patient must be in an appropriate position; therefore a motorized table and mechanical chair should be available for rapid, frequent, and exact changes in position of the patient and/or surgeon during the procedure. Overhead lighting should be supplemented by a bright, adjustable headlight. Self-retaining retractors; long, thin suctions; and microinstruments, such as those used in pituitary and/or ear surgery, are helpful. A long-handled, smooth-cutting drill is also important. As soon as the surgeon penetrates the sphenoid sinus and/or posterior ethmoidal cells, lighting and magnification through a microscope will help in the visualization and dissection.

2. There are two important methods of defining the location and extent of the optic nerve. Although distances measured from the orbital rim can be variable, the posterior ethmoidal artery and its relationship to the nerve are fairly constant, and in almost all cases, the nerve lies 3 to 10 mm directly posterior to the artery. The bulge on the superior wall of the sphenoid sinus is also a reliable landmark. Thus if the surgeon works below the posterior ethmoidal artery and toward this bulge, the optic nerve and ring should be readily discernable.

TRANSETHMOIDAL DECOMPRESSION OF THE OPTIC NERVE

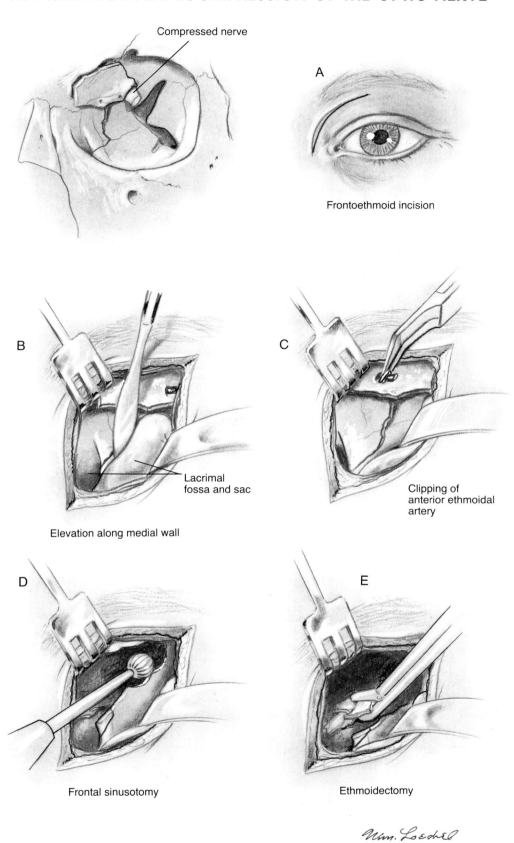

Compressed nerve

A

Frontoethmoid incision

B

Lacrimal
fossa and sac

Elevation along medial wall

C

Clipping of
anterior ethmoidal
artery

D

Frontal sinusotomy

E

Ethmoidectomy

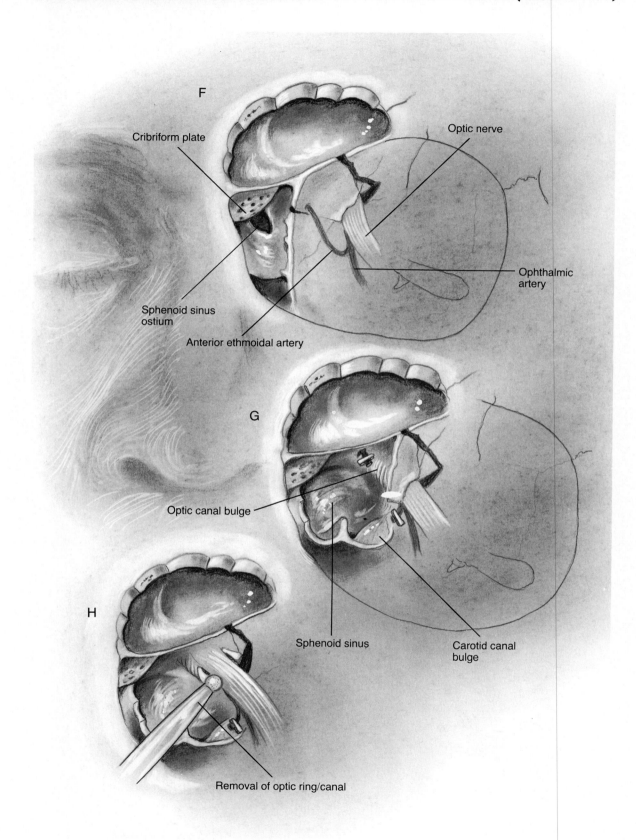

F

Cribriform plate

Optic nerve

Ophthalmic artery

Sphenoid sinus ostium

Anterior ethmoidal artery

G

Optic canal bulge

Sphenoid sinus

Carotid canal bulge

H

Removal of optic ring/canal

3. Avoid injury to the carotid artery. The carotid canal lies on the lateral wall of the sphenoid, below and posterior to the optic canal. Once this bulge is identified, the surgeon should keep the drill a distance from this area.

4. Although the optic nerve can be visualized by a pure transethmoidal/transsphenoidal approach, the additional orientation obtained by removing all or part of the medial wall of the orbit is desirable. The posterior ethmoidal vessel is easily identified and can act as a "pointer" directly to the nerve. The procedure rarely requires removal of the lateral wall of the nose or entrance through the anterior wall of the maxilla; these additional exposures may cause more bleeding and morbidity.

5. Removal of the medial wall of the orbit will cause an enlargement of the orbit to some degree, and this will predispose the patient to a postoperative enophthalmos. The amount of wall removed often determines the degree of enophthalmos. Generally the resection should be as conservative as possible, yet still expose the important landmarks. If necessary, the surgeon can remove a portion of the wall and then replace it into the area of deficit following the procedure. It should also be noted that with practice, sections of the medial wall can be retained, and eventually only that section between the posterior ethmoidal vessel and optic nerve will have to be resected.

6. The question of whether to open the optic nerve sheath is controversial. Removal of one half to three fourths of the optic canal makes the nerve fairly mobile. This suggests that with an adequate decompression, an opening of the sheath is probably not necessary. Moreover, a cut through the sheath often causes a cerebrospinal fluid leak, and there is always the possibility that this leak may persist or cause complications in the postoperative period.

7. Bleeding can be avoided by ligature of the vessels with vascular clips or by letting the vessels clot off with gentle pressure. If cautery is to be used, we prefer the bipolar cautery applied directly to the ends of the vessels. This avoids additional injury to the optic and other cranial nerves.

COMPLICATIONS

1. If the medial wall of the orbit is removed, enophthalmos will most likely occur. This complication can be avoided by limiting the resection of the wall, replacing the wall, or (in experienced hands) removing only a small portion of the wall in front of and behind the posterior ethmoidal artery. If enophthalmos develops and is a problem to the patient, the surgeon can later reconstruct the orbit with bone grafts (see Chapter 60).

2. Postoperative bleeding can cause accumulation of blood in the retro-orbital space. Significant amounts of bleeding can compromise and obstruct the ophthalmic vessels and thereby further threaten visual acuity. The problem is suspected when increasing proptosis is observed, and if this occurs, the incision should be opened and the blood removed. Hemostasis should be obtained with a bipolar cautery.

3. Epistaxis can often be controlled by judicious use of nasal packing. Nasal tampons or ¼-inch gauze treated with bacitracin ointment, placed appropriately within the nose, are standard methods of control (see Chapter 46).

chapter 81

Decompression of the Optic Nerve Using a Transfrontal Craniotomy

In Consultation With L. Murray Thomas, MD

INDICATIONS

Sphenoid fractures associated with optic nerve injury can be treated by a transethmoidal approach (see Chapter 86) or by a transfrontal craniotomy. The rationale and indications for the surgical decompression are discussed in Chapter 79. The craniotomy technique is useful when injury of the optic canal is associated with fractures of the greater and lesser wings of the sphenoid. The approach is also indicated when there is damage to the dura, frontal sinus, and orbital roof. It has an advantage over the frontoethmoid approach when important craniofacial landmarks along the base of the skull are lost or distorted by the injury.

PROCEDURE

A,B The surgery is carried out under general anesthesia. Coronal skin flaps are marked behind the hairline, and about 2 to 3 cm of hair is shaved along the incision line. The incision is carried to a subperiosteal plane. Hemostasis is achieved with electric cautery and/or hemostatic clips. The scalp flap is then rotated forward and held in place with fish hooks or self-retaining retractors.

The craniotomy is best performed through a frontotemporal (frontopterional) approach (see Chapter 77). One bur hole is made just behind the frontal process of the zygoma, another about 2 to 3 cm laterally and posteriorly in the temporal bone, and a third just above the frontal sinus, 3 or 4 cm lateral to the midline. The dura is then elevated around the bur holes and from the deep surface of the bone with special malleable dissectors. Injury to the middle meningeal artery may occur, particularly at the transition from the bony portion to the epidural part. Electrocautery and bone wax are used for control. A craniotome or Gigli saw is used to divide the bone and remove the flap.

C,D The dura is elevated from the floor of the frontal fossa. Medially the surgeon should avoid injury to the dura over the area of the cribriform plate, as the olfactory fibers cannot be adequately elevated without tearing the fibers and entering the dura. Often it is not even necessary to dissect this area.

On exposure of the roof of the orbit, the dural elevation should be carried medially and posteriorly to the edge of the lesser wing of the sphenoid. The orbital roof is then opened with a small osteotome or high-speed drill, and a portion of the roof is removed. The dissection is directed toward the optic canal. All bone fragments and splinters should be carefully removed, and the dura of the optic canal should probably be opened. When the anatomy is obscure, it may be safer to open the anterior fossa dura and visualize the optic nerve before a decompression is carried out.

Bleeding should be controlled with electric cautery and bone wax. Dural openings and tears should be carefully repaired and openings into the sinuses closed with muscle, fat, or periosteum.

The bone flap is held in place with four or five 3-0 nonabsorbable sutures, and the scalp flap is closed with interrupted and inverting galeal 3-0 chromic sutures. Staples or nonabsorbable sutures can be used for the skin. Antibiotics (i.e., nafcillin and gentamicin or cefazolin) are administered for 5 to 7 days. The head dressing can be removed at 48 hours, and sutures/staples can be removed at 7 to 10 days.

PITFALLS

1. If the craniotomy is more than 1 cm from the midline, the sagittal sinus should not present a problem. If more exposure is necessary to repair the frontal fossa and a bilateral bone flap is needed, then the sagittal sinus will be at risk. In such cases, we

TRANSFRONTAL OPTIC NERVE DECOMPRESSION

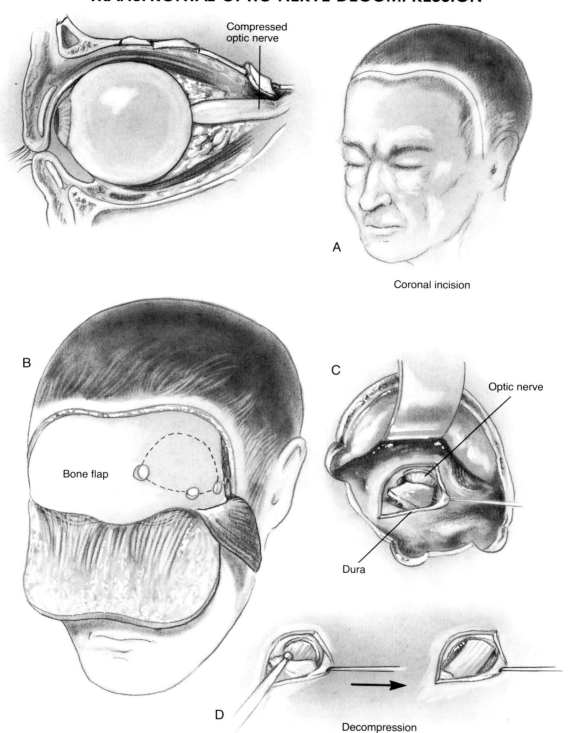

Compressed optic nerve

A

Coronal incision

B

Bone flap

C

Optic nerve

Dura

D

Decompression

prefer to place a bur hole on each side of the sinus, 1.5 cm lateral to the midline and posterior to the planned bone flap. The cut between these bur holes should be made last. If the sinus bleeds, a large piece of Gelfoam placed over the sinus and covered with a cottonoid pledget will usually provide sufficient hemostasis.

2. If the bony dissection is confined to the orbital roof and the roof of the optic canal, the carotid artery should not present a problem. If a greater dissection is needed, this portion should be done transdurally with direct visualization of the structures.

3. Cerebrospinal fluid leaks can be prevented by meticulous closure of the dura in all areas. Dural leaks into the orbit are ordinarily not a problem, but if the leak does extend over a sinus, cerebrospinal fluid rhinorrhea can occur. Thus an opening into the air-bearing sinuses should be carefully closed with muscle, fat, or periosteum.

4. Protection of olfaction is provided by doing a unilateral craniotomy and by staying away from the cribriform plate and the olfactory fibers.

COMPLICATIONS

1. Dural tears may occur when the dura is dissected from the bone flap, when the craniotomy flap is cut, and when the dura is elevated from the floor of the frontal fossa. Careful dissection will decrease the possibility of a dural tear, but if one does occur, prudent management is to provide a watertight closure with fine nonabsorbable sutures.

2. Postoperative epidural or subdural hematomas result from inadequate control of bleeding. Careful use of the electrocautery and bone wax is mandatory. A hematoma presents clinically as a decrease in conscious state or a progressive neurologic deficit. The diagnosis should be confirmed by a nonenhanced CT scan. Immediate evacuation of the hematoma is the treatment of choice.

3. Cerebrospinal fluid leaks may be prevented by meticulous closure of dural tears and careful closure of openings into the sinuses. If a leak occurs, treatment consists of bed rest with the head elevated 30°. Occasionally lumbar puncture drainage may be helpful. If the leak does not stop, a craniotomy is necessary for repair of the dura. The use of prophylactic antibiotics to prevent meningitis is controversial.

section III

Superior Orbital Fissure Injury

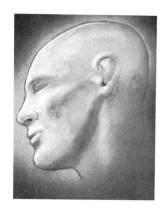

chapter 82

Decompression of the Superior Orbital Fissure Using a Frontotemporal Approach

In Consultation With L. Murray Thomas, MD

INDICATIONS

Sphenoid fractures associated with frontozygomatic injuries can often involve the lateral superior orbital wall, causing injury to the superior orbital fissure. Such a fracture can affect nerves III, IV, and/ or VI and result in various degrees of ophthalmoplegia. Sometimes there is an associated optic nerve injury, ocular injury, or dural tear.

In those patients in whom the orbital injury is localized to the superior orbital fissure (and optic nerve) and in whom the eye is otherwise salvageable, a decompression procedure can be contemplated. Generally we prefer a trial of an 18- to 24-hour course of high-dose steroids (100 mg dexamethasone followed by 50 mg every 6 hours for three doses); if there is no response, surgical decompression is performed. The frontotemporal approach is direct and also offers the opportunity to decompress the optic

nerve and/or repair other associated cranial base fractures.

PROCEDURE

A–C The surgery is performed under general anesthesia. An incision is marked from the preauricular crease upward to curve forward and end in the hairline lateral to the midline. The head or a small area of hair is shaved; the face and scalp are draped as sterile fields.

The incision line is first injected with 1% lidocaine containing 1:100,000 epinephrine to help control hemostasis. An anterior flap is elevated in a subperiosteal plane just deep to the temporalis fascia. If necessary, the superficial temporal vessels are ligated with fine silk sutures. The dissection should be anterior enough to expose the lateral wall of the orbit. The zygomatic arch is stripped of periosteum and divided from its attachment to the body of the zygoma and temporal bone. The arch is then retracted downward with its masseter muscle. The temporalis muscle is split and reflected posteriorly off the coronoid process.

D–F An opening is made into the greater wing of the sphenoid and parietal bone with cutting burs. Mannitol is infused intravenously. The dura is elevated off the lateral wall of the orbit and the floor of the middle fossa. Loose fragments from the lateral orbital wall are reduced, and the area around the superior orbital fissure is opened with Kerrison rongeurs.

G The operative defect is obliterated with the bulk of the temporalis muscle. The frontal process of the zygoma and the frontal bone are reduced and stabilized with interosseous 28-gauge wires and/or miniplates. The zygomatic arch is returned and wired into place.

The facial flap is positioned, and the wound is closed in layers. Light compression dressings of fluffs and stretch gauze are applied to the eye, cheek, and lateral face areas for 2 to 3 days. Prophylactic antibiotics (i.e., nafcillin and gentamicin or cefazolin) are used for 5 to 7 days. The sutures are removed at 7 days. Jaw exercise is initiated within several days after surgery and continued as necessary.

PITFALLS

1. Because the procedure has the risk of a craniotomy, it should be performed only when the patient is stable and eye functions can be expected to return to normal. The procedure should not be carried out if there is changing vision or any vision-threatening damage to the globe. A short trial of high-dose steroids should be used prior to the surgery.

2. The osteotomies of the zygoma provide good exposure to the inferior portion of the middle fossa. If more exposure is needed superiorly, the lateral orbital rim can be osteotomized and repaired after decompression. This direct approach also provides an opportunity to explore both sides of the orbital wall.

3. Although the facial nerve is well protected in the soft tissues and is located anterior to the incision, the surgeon should still be careful with excessive pressure from the retractors.

4. Avoid extensive dissection of the temporalis muscle. The superficial blood supply will be interrupted with the facial flap, and the deep blood supply beneath the muscle flap should be protected.

COMPLICATIONS

1. Dural tears may occur when the craniotomy is cut and the dura is elevated from the floor of the middle fossa. Careful dissection will decrease the possibility of a dural tear. If a tear occurs, the tear can be closed with sutures or covered with a temporalis muscle flap. The patient should subsequently be confined to bed with the head elevated 30°. If a leak develops, lumbar puncture drainage may be helpful. If the leak does not stop, a craniotomy may be necessary for repair of the dura. Prophylactic antibiotics to prevent meningitis may be administered.

2. Postoperative epidural or subdural hematomas result from inadequate control of bleeding. Careful use of the electrocautery and bone wax is mandatory. A hematoma usually presents as a decrease in consciousness or a progressive neurologic deficit. The diagnosis can be confirmed with a nonenhanced computed tomographic (CT) scan. Immediate evacuation of the blood is the treatment of choice.

DECOMPRESSION OF SUPERIOR ORBITAL FISSURE

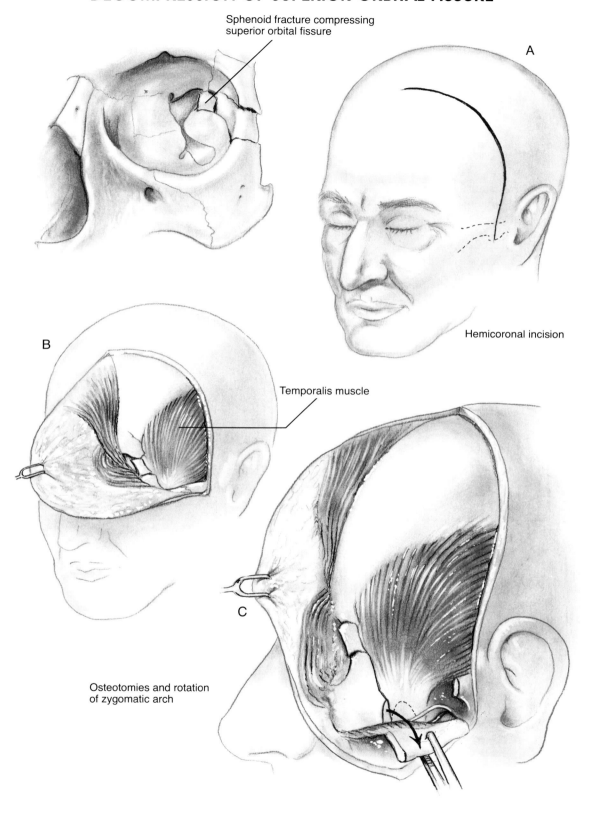

Sphenoid fracture compressing superior orbital fissure

A

Hemicoronal incision

B

Temporalis muscle

C

Osteotomies and rotation of zygomatic arch

DECOMPRESSION OF SUPERIOR ORBITAL FISSURE *(Continued)*

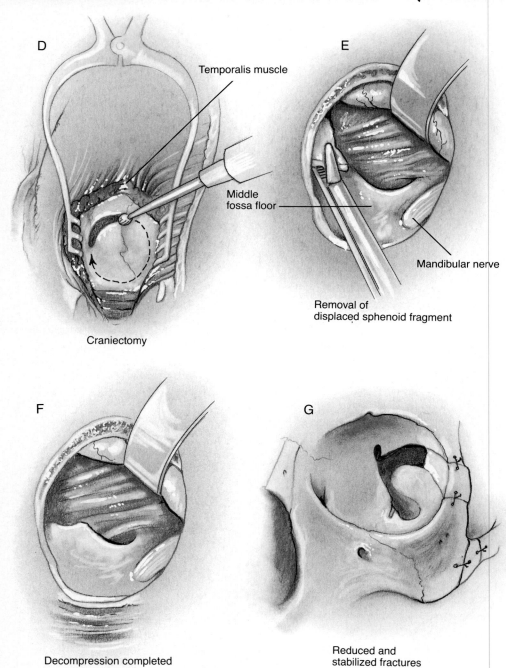

D

Temporalis muscle

Middle
fossa floor

Craniectomy

E

Mandibular nerve

Removal of
displaced sphenoid fragment

F

Decompression completed

G

Reduced and
stabilized fractures

section IV

Cerebrospinal Fluid Leaks

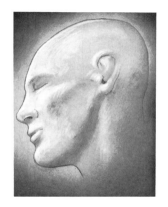

chapter 83

Transseptal Repair of a Sphenoid Bone Cerebrospinal Fluid Leak

INDICATIONS

Fractures through the body of the sphenoid can be associated with dural tears, pneumocephalus, and cerebrospinal fluid leakage. Early recognition of this problem is important if the sequela of meningitis is to be avoided. The injury should be delineated by imaging studies, and special intrathecal tests should be used to demonstrate the site and degree of the leak. The pathophysiologic and diagnostic considerations are discussed in Chapters 84 and 85.

In general, the patient is treated first with reduction and fixation of the facial fractures; antibiotics are administered to prevent meningitis. Most cerebrospinal fluid leaks cease within 1 to 2 weeks, but if the leakage persists, a surgical repair must be considered.

Three popular approaches for repair of a sphenoid bone cerebrospinal fluid leak are (1) transseptal, (2) frontoethmoid (see Chapter 86), and (3) frontal craniotomy (see Chapter 87). The transantral-ethmoidal approach is also possible but provides little, if any,

advantage over the others and can lead to greater instability when there are facial fractures. The transseptal dissection is time-proven, easy to perform, and associated with minimal morbidity. It does not have the potential problems of diplopia and enophthalmos found with the frontoethmoid procedure or the morbidity associated with craniotomy and exploration of the anterior fossa. Results are generally good, and if there should be a recurrence or persistence of the leak, the surgeon can consider an alternative method.

PROCEDURE

For the sphenoidotomy, the nose is prepared as for a septorhinoplasty (see Chapter 49). A motorized table is preferred; the head is later extended and the patient placed in Trendelenburg's position. A microscope and microinstrumentation should be available.

A–C The procedure is initiated by a sublabial degloving incision from the molar-to-molar region. The periosteum is elevated off the premaxilla to expose the anterior nasal spine and piriform apertures. A septal/columella incision with extension along the nostril sills provides for additional elevation of tissues and wider entry into the vestibule of the nose.

D,E The septal cartilage and bone are exposed by a subperichondrial and subperiosteal dissection. First, the mucoperichondrium is elevated off the quadrilateral plate; the mucoperiosteum is subsequently lifted off the perpendicular plate of the ethmoid and vomer. The dissection is continued along the maxillary crest, and after cutting the decussating fibers, the mucosal flaps are elevated off the floor region. Cottle elevators and speculae may be helpful. An identical procedure is carried out on the opposite side of the nose.

F With the septum completely exposed, the quadrilateral plate is separated from the maxillary crest and ethmoid and swung to the side as a "swinging-door" flap. The perpendicular plate of ethmoid and vomer are removed by to-and-fro rotation and fracture with Takahashi ronguers. Additional exposure is obtained by excising portions of the maxillary crest, anterior nasal spine, and piriform aperture with sharp osteotomes.

G–I At this stage, a large self-retaining speculum is inserted and the patient placed into Trendelenburg's position. With the surgeon sitting at the patient's head, the microscope is positioned, and the sphenoid sinus is inspected. The rostrum and ostia of the sphenoid are identified, and after the mucosa is elevated laterally along the basisphenoid, the anterior wall is removed with Hajek and Takahashi rongeurs. The remainder of the midline septum of the sphenoid is removed, and the mucosa is stripped from the walls of the sphenoid sinus with elevators and a Takahashi rongeur.

J The cerebrospinal fluid leak should then be identified. The surgeon can, if necessary, inject fluorescein into the spinal fluid (see Chapter 85) to distinguish the spinal fluid from other tissue fluids. Fascia lata and muscle from the leg (approximately 3 × 3 cm) are harvested. A small piece of fascia is then cut and pushed into the hole to plug the intracranial side of the defect. Additional muscle and fascia are then placed on the sinus side against the defect. The sphenoid sinus is filled with additional tissue (muscle and fascia). The speculum is removed, and the mucosal flaps are placed back into original position.

The septal/columella incision is closed with interrupted 4-0 chromic sutures. The mucosa of the sublabial incision is approximated with additional chromic sutures. The nose is then packed bilaterally with nasal tampons or ½-inch gauze treated with bacitracin ointment.

Postoperatively the patient is placed in the head-up position and told to avoid any straining, sneezing, coughing, or blowing of the nose. The patient is given a stool softener and placed on antibiotics (i.e., cefazolin or ampicillin) for approximately 2 weeks. The nasal packing is removed at about 5 days, and the nose is treated with saline mists at least three times daily.

PITFALLS

1. Exposure of the sphenoid sinus requires accurate placement of the patient, surgeon, and microscope. Microinstruments for sphenoid and ear surgery should be available.

2. The sphenoid sinus lies in the midline, on a line drawn 30° from the floor of the nose. The rostrum is an important landmark. The position of the midline septum of the sphenoid, however, is quite variable, and the anatomy of the septum should be evaluated on computed tomographic (CT) scans. Once in the sphenoid sinus, the surgeon should recognize the optic nerve ridge and projection of the carotid artery. These landmarks are described in detail in Chapter 80.

3. Although placement of the fascia on the intracranial side of the dura is helpful, there is an excellent opportunity to treat sphenoid sinus leaks by completely obliterating the sinus. Remember that for obliteration, all mucosa must be removed. If this is not possible, the area of defect should be treated with a small piece of fascia and the sphenoid sinus packed with Gelfoam, rather than tissue grafts.

COMPLICATIONS

1. Failure to stop the leakage can result in meningitis and/or pneumocephalus. All patients should be followed closely after the procedure, and if meningitis is suspected, a CT scan should be used to reevaluate the defect and intracranial tear. A lumbar puncture should be performed to analyze the spinal fluid and obtain cultures for appropriate antibiotic therapy.

2. Recurrent or persistent cerebrospinal fluid leakage requires reevaluation and repair. However, the surgeon should make sure that the leak is from the same place as before and there are no other leaks compounding the clinical picture. Imaging studies and intrathecal tests should be considered. A repair from below is still desirable, as the intracranial exposure carries more risk for morbidity and complication. The sphenoidotomy can be repeated, or

TRANSSPHENOIDAL REPAIR OF CEREBROSPINAL FLUID LEAK

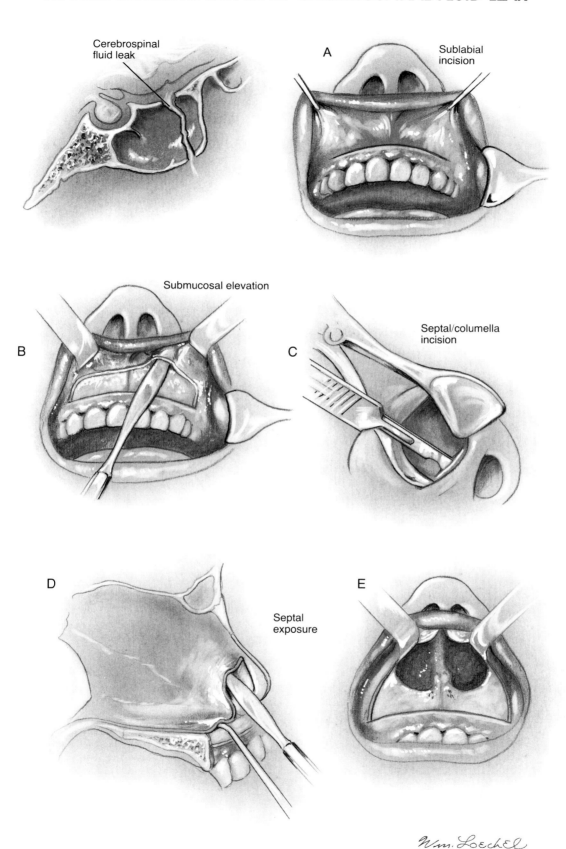

Cerebrospinal fluid leak

A

Sublabial incision

Submucosal elevation

B

C

Septal/columella incision

D

Septal exposure

E

Wm. Loechel

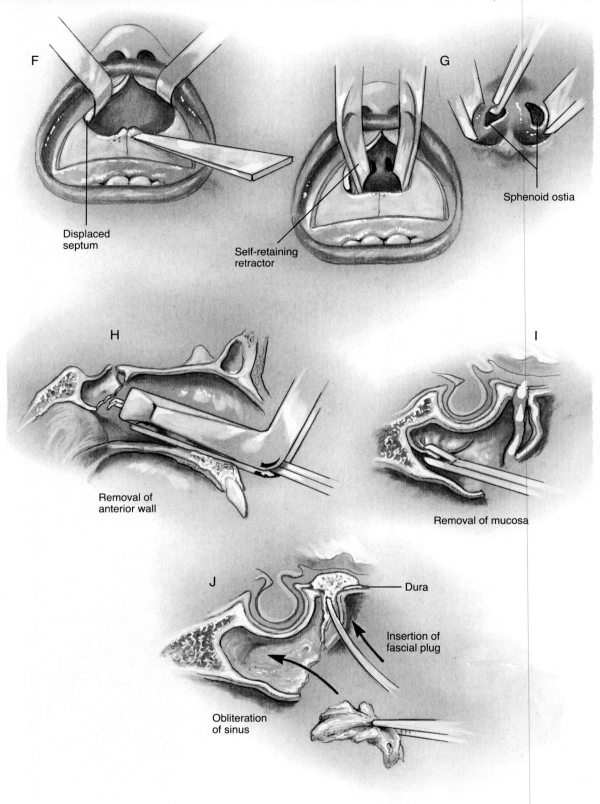

F

Displaced
septum

Self-retaining
retractor

G

Sphenoid ostia

H

Removal of
anterior wall

I

Removal of mucosa

J

Dura

Insertion of
fascial plug

Obliteration
of sinus

alternatively, the surgeon can consider the fronto-ethmoidectomy or transantral ethmoidectomy approaches.

3. Injury to the optic nerve and/or carotid artery can be avoided by an appreciation of the anatomic relationships. Exposure provided by magnification and lighting from the microscope is important, and such an approach should delineate the anatomy of the walls (see Chapter 80). The mucosa should always be stripped under direct visualization, as this will help avoid injury to any of the adjacent structures.

part
ten

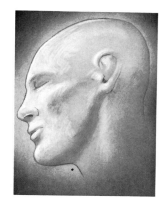

Ethmoid
Fractures

Classification and Pathophysiology of Ethmoid Fractures

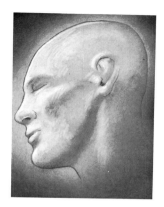

chapter 84

General Considerations

The tentlike ethmoid bone can be fractured at its central support (the nasal septum), its lateral support (the lamina papyracea), or its roof (the cribriform plate). Damage involving the cribriform plate is often associated with anosmia, cerebrospinal fluid leak, pneumocephalus, and loss of consciousness. The cerebrospinal fluid leak can also result in untoward sequelae such as meningitis or brain abscess, requiring immediate treatment. The care of septal and lamina papyracea injuries is discussed in Chapters 45 through 49, 57, 59, and 60.

As for the cerebrospinal fluid leak, several pathophysiologic processes can take place. If the dura is torn, pressure differences will force the fluid into the upper respiratory–digestive tract. If the dura is partially torn, constant intracranial arterial and respiratory pressures can slowly separate the dural fibers and cause a delayed presentation of the leak. A hematoma may form over the area of injury, and as it dissolves, the fluid becomes noted.

Many dural tears heal spontaneously without sequelae. The main problem with a cerebrospinal fluid leak is that there is no way to predict which leak will stop and which will be associated with intracranial infection. Thus for most patients, it is important to localize the site and nature of the injury and, if the leak does not stop, to prepare for surgical exploration and repair. The leak of the cribriform plate must be distinguished from other leaks in the frontal sinus, the sphenoid sinus, the roof of the orbit, and temporal bone.

A–D The history and physical examination are helpful. Gushing clear fluid from the nose associated with a change in head position suggests a fluid collection in one or several of the paranasal sinuses. Anosmia is often associated with leaks through the cribriform plate. Visual problems suggest injury to the tuberculum sella, sphenoid sinus, or posterior ethmoidal sinus. Loss of cochlear, vestibular, or facial nerve function indicates a temporal bone injury. Paresthesia or anesthesia of the face and forehead suggests damage to one or several branches of the trigeminal nerve.

On physical examination of the nose, the surgeon should shrink the mucous membranes with ¼% oxymetazoline hydrochloride (Neo-Synephrine) and observe for a clear fluid discharge. Leakage superiorly from the vault area and/or from the superior meatus is indicative of a cribriform plate, ethmoid, or sphenoid injury. Leakage from the middle meatus is often associated with a flow of fluid from the frontal sinus by way of the nasofrontal duct. Fluid coming from behind the inferior turbinate may indicate a eustachian tube transit from a dural tear of the temporal bone. In most patients, the cerebrospinal fluid flow can be increased by placing the patient in the head-down position; a stream or drops of fluid may be observed at the tip of the nose. In some patients, fluid may be seen behind the tympanic membrane.

With small leaks, cerebrospinal fluid may be difficult to collect and analyze. However, if the fluid can be collected, it should be evaluated in the laboratory and compared chemically and physically to the known properties of spinal fluid. Glucose-sensitive sticks are not usually diagnostic, as glucose can vary in cerebrospinal fluid and in lacrimal and nasal secretions. A handkerchief test in which the surgeon observes different rings can be suggestive; mucus generally will cause rings, and in contrast to a cloth soaked with spinal fluid, the handkerchief will stiffen with drying.

The site and size of the defect must be obtained by special imaging and/or dye studies. Plain radiographs of the facial bones, polytomography, and coronal and horizontal computed tomographic (CT) scans are useful in demonstrating fracture sites. The studies may also show the accumulation of fluid in adjoining sinuses. Metrizamide in combination with a CT scan is very helpful in defining the larger leaks. Sodium iodide I-123, ytterbium Yb-169 pentetate, In-111, and technetium Tc-99m tests are sensitive, but because of high background counts, interpretation can be difficult. Fluorescein dye is also a useful method, but the surgeon must be aware of a potential reaction to the intrathecally placed substance.

Patients with cerebrospinal fluid leaks should have an early reduction of any associated facial fractures, and most of the time the leak will stop in 2 to 3 weeks. Although there is controversy regarding the use of prophylactic antibiotics, we prescribe them at least during the early observation period. If the cerebrospinal fluid leak persists beyond several weeks, we assume that it will not stop, and for these leaks, site localization and surgical repair must be considered.

SITES AND SIGNS OF CEREBROSPINAL FLUID LEAK

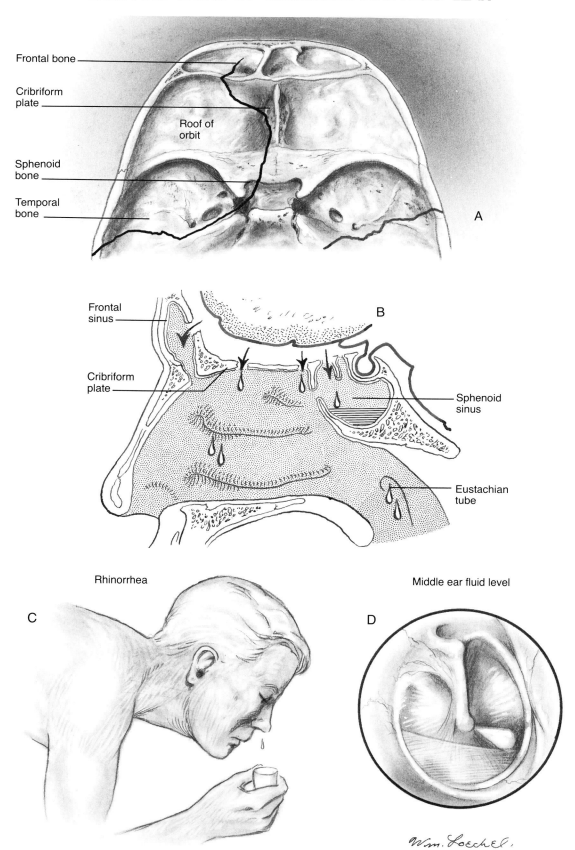

Frontal bone

Cribriform plate

Roof of orbit

Sphenoid bone

Temporal bone

A

Frontal sinus

B

Cribriform plate

Sphenoid sinus

Eustachian tube

Rhinorrhea

C

Middle ear fluid level

D

Wm. Loechel.

section II

Cerebrospinal Fluid Leaks

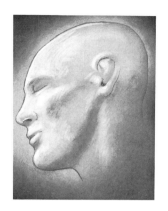

chapter 85

Examination of Cerebrospinal Fluid Leak Using Intrathecal Fluorescein Dye

INDICATIONS

A small cerebrospinal fluid leak may be difficult to diagnose. In many patients, the surgeon cannot be certain that there is a leak, and the site of dural tear may not be evident. Some clues can be obtained from the history and physical examination of the patient. Imaging studies are particularly important for evaluating fractures and accumulation of fluid within the paranasal sinuses. The identification of a leak, however, requires special intrathecal tests that rely on contrast (radioactive materials or colored dyes).

Many methods are available. A contrast material such as metrizamide is excellent for showing large leaks; the material will also accumulate within the adjacent sinuses or upper aerodigestive tract. Radioactive materials with a small molecular structure (e.g., sodium iodide I-123, ytterbium Yb-169 pentetate, and indium In-111) are useful in identifying very small leaks, but interpretation of data is often confounded by high background counts of contami-

nated blood and/or secretions. Iodinated I-131 serum albumin (RISA) is quite accurate in showing leaks but can be reactive and is not recommended (or approved by the Food and Drug Administration) for routine use. Some of the dyes that are visually detectable provide sensitive methods of evaluation, but these substances carry a risk of central nervous system reactions. Thus each test substance has its own risk-benefit relationship, and although this may vary among individual patients, the information should be shared with them. Our preference is to first use metrizamide; if a leak is not demonstrated but is still suspected, we usually proceed to an intrathecal fluorescein dye test.

PROCEDURE

Sedation should be light, as patient cooperation is important in performing the test. Special equipment such as a mechanical table or chair, headlight, nasal preparation tray, and lumbar puncture tray should be available.

For the patient in the sitting or recumbent position, the nose is sprayed with 4% lidocaine and ¼% oxymetazoline hydrochloride (Neo-Synephrine). The nasal mucous membranes are then treated with 4% cocaine containing epinephrine, and the nose is blocked with 1% lidocaine containing 1:100,000 epinephrine. This nasal preparation is identical to that used in the preparation for rhinoplasty (see Chapter 49).

A The pledgets are removed from the nose after approximately 10 minutes and replaced with cottonoids (approximately ½-inch × ½-inch square pads) moistened in saline. Cottonoids are placed on both sides of the nose. The first set is placed superiorly in the vault near the superior meatus. They should lie very close to the cribriform plate and anterior wall of the sphenoid sinus. Another set is placed in the middle meatus and a third set along the floor posteriorly near the eustachian tube. The strings are left hanging loosely from the nose.

The patient is then placed in a sitting or a lateral knees-up position for the lumbar puncture. The lumbar area is prepared with antiseptic solution, and the skin over the area of L4-5 is infiltrated with 2% lidocaine. A neurosurgeon or neurologist usually performs the puncture. With the index finger of the hand on the iliac crest, the thumb palpates the fourth lumbar interspace. A 22-gauge needle is then inserted between L4 and L5 and directed slightly upward. Proper penetration is assured by a free flow of spinal fluid. A 10-mL syringe is then filled with ½ mL of 5% fluorescein and attached to the spinal needle. The fluorescein is gradually diluted with the withdrawal of 9.5 mL of spinal fluid (barbotage technique). One or two milliliters of the diluted solution are then injected and the syringe is again filled with aspirated spinal fluid. This is repeated several times until the dilution does not change color within the syringe. The remainder of the fluid is then injected and the area covered with an adhesive dressing.

B The positioning of the patient will depend on the site and degree of leakage that is suspected. If a major leak is suspected, the cottonoids are left in place for approximately 7 to 10 minutes and then inspected visually with an ultraviolet (Wood's) light. If no fluorescein is observed, the cottonoids are replaced and the patient placed into the prone position. In about 10 to 15 minutes, the pledgets are again inspected. If there is still no evidence of a leak, new cottonoids are placed and the head of the table tilted approximately 20°. If the cottonoids remain clear after this positioning, another clean set is placed and the patient tilted even further to about a 45°

angle. Failure to see the dye at about 45 to 60 minutes signifies a negative test. If a small leak is suspected, the surgeon can proceed more rapidly to the later phases of the test but must still wait 30 to 45 minutes for the dye to mix and appear in the leaking spinal fluid.

Cottonoids placed in the nasal vault that are positive for fluorescein suggest a defect in the cribriform plate and/or sphenoid sinus. Cottonoids within the middle meatus that are colored with dye are consistent with a frontal sinus or ethmoid leakage. Pledgets that are positive along the floor are suggestive of a basisphenoid, eustachian tube, or temporal bone leakage.

PITFALLS

1. Fluorescein can cause reactions such as paresthesias, weakness, and seizures. The lumbar puncture can be associated with moderate to severe headaches for several days to several weeks. The patient should be informed of these potential sequelae but should also be told that the effects are usually temporary and there should be no permanent damage.

2. Patient cooperation is important for a valid test. The patient will be asked to move into specific positions and to hold still during the spinal puncture and during the insertion and removal of the pledgets.

3. The fluorescein should be diluted and injected very slowly, and no more than 0.5 to 1.0 mL should be used. The dilution should have a concentration of no more than 0.5 mL of fluorescein to 10 mL of spinal fluid, and even at that concentration, only a few milliliters should be injected. The solution within the syringe is again diluted and the process repeated until the color of the fluid is not changed by the aspirated spinal fluid.

4. The intrathecal mixing of fluorescein takes approximately 30 minutes. If a significant leak is suspected from the history, the surgeon should gradually approach the head-down position. If there is a moderate to severe leakage of spinal fluid, the pledgets will tend to contaminate each other, which will cause confusion in interpretation of the results. If the leakage is small, the surgeon should proceed more quickly to the head-down position. Pledgets should be changed every 10 to 15 minutes for at least 45 minutes.

5. The patient should be observed after the test for adverse sequelae from the intrathecal substance. If the patient has a history of seizures, antiseizure medications should be utilized preoperatively and adequate levels of medication maintained during and after the test. If the patient develops signs or symptoms of inflammation, administration of steroids may be indicated.

INTRATHECAL DYE TEST

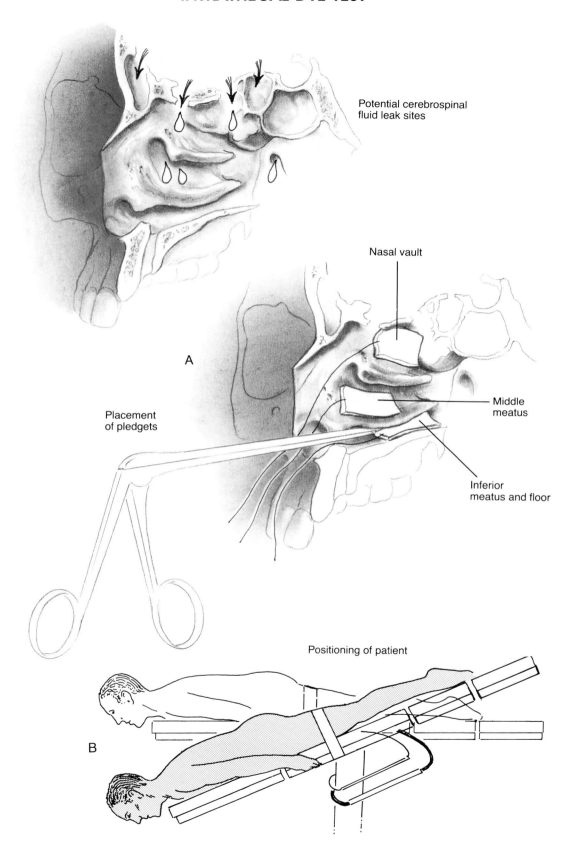

Potential cerebrospinal fluid leak sites

Nasal vault

A

Placement of pledgets

Middle meatus

Inferior meatus and floor

Positioning of patient

B

COMPLICATIONS

1. Although the threat of impending meningitis necessitates early identification and control of the fistula, the test itself may cause meningitis. The mechanism is not well understood. Meningitis can occur from just the lumbar puncture, from a reversal of the flow through the fistula, and/or from contaminated fluorescein solutions. If evidence of meningitis develops, cultures should be obtained and the patient immediately treated with appropriate antibiotics.

2. The lumbar puncture can be associated with headache. The complication is not predictable, and although the amount of aspirated spinal fluid is sometimes related to the degree and length of time that the headache persists, this will vary among subjects. The headache can be reduced by having the patient lie flat in the postoperative period. Analgesics should be administered and the patient kept well hydrated.

3. Intrathecal fluorescein has been reported to cause reactions within the central nervous system (e.g., paresthesias, weakness of the extremities, and seizures). It appears that the complications probably can be minimized or avoided by using small amounts of dye, diluting the dye, and injecting it slowly. Patients who have a history of seizures should be maintained on antiseizure medications before and after the procedure. Adequate levels of the antiseizure drug should be maintained throughout the day. Steroids may be injected, if necessary, to control some of the inflammatory phases of the reaction.

chapter 86

Repair of a Cribriform Plate Cerebrospinal Fluid Leak Using a Frontoethmoidal Approach

INDICATIONS

Cerebrospinal fluid leakage following trauma can occur in many sites along the skull base but is commonly found associated with dural tears along the cribriform plate. Early management requires reduction of facial fractures and antibiotic coverage. If the leakage persists for more than several weeks, the site of leakage should be determined and the repair carried out by either an intracranial or extracranial approach. Brain herniation evident on a computed tomographic (CT) scan and associated with a leak is also an indication for exploration and repair.

For uncomplicated cerebrospinal fluid leaks, we prefer an extracranial frontoethmoid approach. The surgery is often easier to perform and is associated with less morbidity and a high success rate. The extracranial approach is also useful when there are other midfacial injuries that require further reduction and fixation (see Chapter 87). A craniotomy is reserved for those patients with herniation of brain tissues and displaced fragments of the skull base in which an open reduction is required. Also, the intracranial approach must be considered when the extracranial procedure fails to repair the leak.

PROCEDURE

With the patient under general anesthesia and in the supine position, a curvilinear incision is marked one half the distance between the caruncle and the dorsum of the nose. The nose is prepared with both topical and local anesthetic (i.e., treatment of the mucous membranes with 4% cocaine containing epinephrine, along with a block consisting of 1% lidocaine containing 1:100,000 epinephrine) (see Chapter 46). The medial canthal incision is also infiltrated with the anesthetic solution. The face is washed with antiseptic solution and isolated with towels as in a sterile field.

A–C A microscope using a 300-mm lens is then brought into position. The surgeon can sit at the head of the table or stand to the side. The standard external frontoethmoidectomy is performed as described in Chapters 76 and 80. The opening into the ethmoid and frontal region is enlarged with rongeurs and cutting burs so that there is adequate exposure of the posterior wall of the frontal sinus. The curvature of the frontal sinus plate is then followed inferiorly toward the cribriform plate. Additional ethmoid cells are removed, as well as portions of the lamina papyracea. The superior and middle turbinate are examined and, if necessary, removed to provide sufficient exposure. Tissues adjacent to the cribriform plate should be salvaged and used later for flap closure. Bleeding is controlled by packing with ½-inch gauze soaked in the 4% cocaine solution. Larger vessels such as the anterior ethmoidal artery are cauterized with a bipolar cautery.

D,E Using magnification, the cribriform plate is cleaned free of mucosal attachments. As the plate is exposed, the surgeon should inspect carefully for evidence of cerebrospinal fluid leakage. If the presence of leakage or the site of leakage is uncertain, it is possible to dye the spinal fluid with fluorescein, as described in Chapter 85.

The cribriform plate should be completely exposed by removing all adjacent cells and mucosa with Takahashi rongeurs and cleaning the area with a diamond bur. The hole over the leakage should be devoid of mucosa and opened slightly to expose the dural tear. We prefer to then harvest several small pieces of temporalis fascia and force one of the pieces through the hole with either a duckbill elevator or an alligator forceps so the fluid and pressure from within the cranium keep the fascia in position and close the defect. Another piece of fascia is then placed, using similar ear instruments, on the undersurface of the cribriform plate. Additional coverage is obtained by rotation (and/or advancement) of a flap of adjacent mucosa or turbinate. If these tissues are not available, then Gelfoam is packed over the deficit. Layers of ½-inch gauze treated with bacitracin ointment are used to hold the tissues in position.

The periosteum over the frontoethmoidectomy is closed with 3-0 chromic sutures. The subcutaneous tissues are closed with 4-0 chromic and the skin with 5-0 nylon sutures. The patient is kept with his or her head elevated for 5 days. When the packing is removed, the nose is treated with saline mists. The patient is maintained on antibiotics (i.e., cefazolin or ampicillin) for approximately 2 weeks and during this time is told to refrain from lifting, sneezing, straining, or blowing the nose. A stool softener is provided. Follow-up examination should be performed weekly during the first month and then monthly for at least 6 months.

PITFALLS

1. Exposure is an integral part of the extracranial approach. The incision must be large enough to allow evaluation of the anteroinferior portion of the skull base. A motorized table and mechanical chair provide opportunity to position the patient's head and surgeon in optimal positions. A microscope is important for visualization and lighting and for identification and repair of the leak. Ear and sphenoid instruments should be helpful in placing the fascial graft and rotating mucosal flaps.

2. If the surgeon finds that the leakage is coming from the sphenoid sinus, the anterior wall of the sphenoid sinus should be removed to show the defect. Once the leakage is identified, treatment is very similar to that following the sphenoidal approach (see Chapter 83).

3. Although the surgeon may know preoperatively that the leak is at the cribriform plate, it may be difficult to find the leak at the time of surgery. Fluorescein dye injected into the spinal fluid, as described in Chapter 85, should be helpful in distinguishing the cerebrospinal fluid leakage from other fluids.

4. The three-layer closure of the deficit is important. The intracranial placement of fascia acts as a plug, and the external fascia and flap provide protection and coverage to the defect.

5. Do not allow the patient to participate in any activities that will increase the cerebrospinal fluid pressure. During the postoperative period, the patient's head should be elevated, and the patient should be given instructions to avoid sneezing, blowing the nose, and straining.

COMPLICATIONS

1. Failure to close the leakage may result in meningitis and/or pneumocephalus. For this reason, the patient must be maintained on antibiotics and vital signs followed closely for several days. Any change in clinical status should be evaluated by CT scan, and if meningitis is suspected, a lumbar puncture should be performed. Additional spinal fluid should be obtained for cell counts and for cultures to determine appropriate antibiotic treatment.

2. Recurrence or persistence of the cerebrospinal fluid leak requires additional attempts at closure. In general, a failed extracranial procedure indicates a need for a subsequent intracranial approach. However, the surgeon should make sure that the leak is still in the same place as originally suspected and that there are no additional sites. More testing with intrathecal substances may be necessary.

3. The complications noted from frontoethmoidectomy also pertain to the cribriform plate repair (see Chapter 76). Diplopia from malalignment of the trochlea is rare. A limited resection of the lamina papyracea should prevent enophthalmos, and hypertrophic scarring can be avoided by atraumatic techniques and tensionless closure.

FRONTOETHMOIDAL REPAIR OF CEREBROSPINAL FLUID LEAK

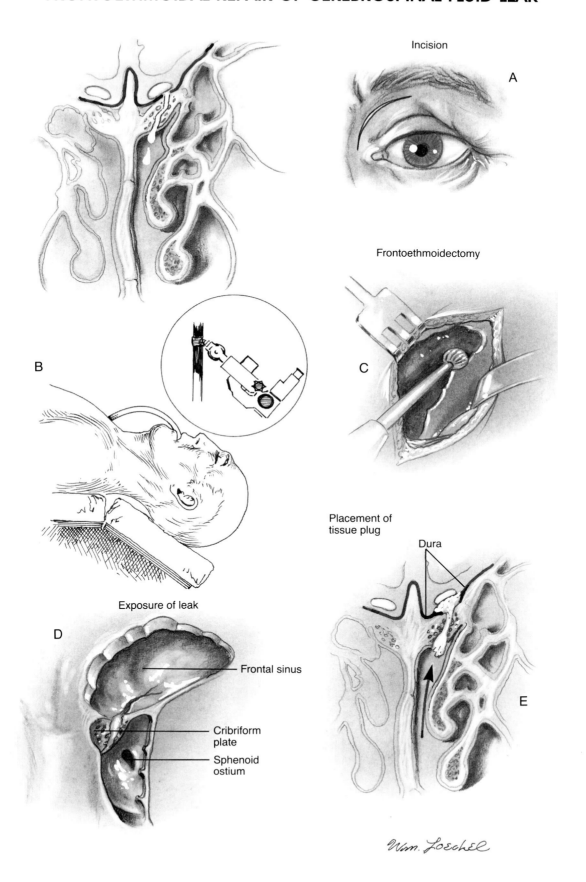

Incision

A

B

Frontoethmoidectomy

C

Placement of tissue plug

Dura

E

Exposure of leak

D

Frontal sinus

Cribriform plate

Sphenoid ostium

Wm. Loechel

Repair of a Cribriform Plate Cerebrospinal Fluid Leak Using a Frontotemporal Approach

In Consultation With L. Murray Thomas, MD

INDICATIONS

Cerebrospinal fluid leaks require repair if they persist following craniofacial trauma. Indications for the frontoethmoid approach are discussed in Chapter 86. The cranial approach becomes important when the frontoethmoid repair fails or when there is a significant injury to the skull base resulting in dural tears, displaced fragments, and compression of cranial nerves. The frontotemporal (or frontopterional) bone flap is an excellent method to expose and repair the damage to the floor of the anterior fossa.

PROCEDURE

A,B The operative approach is identical to that used for the repair of the roof of the orbit (see Chapter 77). The coronal (bifrontal) flap, if needed, is discussed in Chapter 81.

The dura is carefully elevated off the frontal bone, orbital roof, and cribriform plate with duckbill elevators and cottonoid sponges. If the elevation causes more tearing of the dura, the surgeon should consider an incision through the dura with exposure of the dura from the intradural side. Ideally the dura should have a watertight closure with fine (5-0) nonabsorbable sutures. If this is not possible, muscle is placed between the dura and bone, and fascia is laid over the intracranial side of the dura. Intracranial fluid pressure will usually press the grafts against the dura and bone and allow healing to occur.

Significant bony defects should also be repaired with fat, muscle, and/or suitable tissue plugs. Large defects may require the use of split cranial bone, which can be obtained from the bone flap.

Closure is accomplished by suturing the bone flap into place with 3-0 nonabsorbable sutures. The skin flap should be closed in layers, using galeal investing sutures and 5-0 nylon sutures or staples on the skin. The use of prophylactic antibiotics (i.e., nafcillin and gentamicin or cefazolin) for 5 days is desirable. A bulky dressing is left on the head for 48 hours, and sutures are removed at 7 to 10 days.

PITFALLS

1. As with the frontoethmoid approach, the site of leakage should be determined preoperatively. The leak may be difficult to identify at the time of surgery, and preoperative studies that provide the exact location of the leak are extremely helpful.

2. Tears over the cribriform plate pose special problems. Sometimes these tears are small and difficult to see but may be the cause of the leak. On the other hand, the cribriform area may be normal and may only appear pathologically abnormal as the surgeon elevates and separates the olfactory filaments. Any obvious tears must be repaired with suture or grafts.

3. Tears or fractures that extend to the posterior ethmoid, sphenoid, and sella area are difficult to repair. Tissue patches should be applied, but if the leak persists postoperatively, the surgeon must consider a frontoethmoidal or transphenoidal exposure and a packing from the undersurface of the cranium (see Chapters 83 and 86).

COMPLICATIONS

1. Occasionally the surgeon fails to eradicate the cerebrospinal fluid leak, or the leak recurs following surgery. The surgeon may repair the area suspected to be the source of the leak, but the leak may actually be coming from a different area. This is why an

FRONTOTEMPORAL REPAIR OF CEREBROSPINAL FLUID LEAK

A

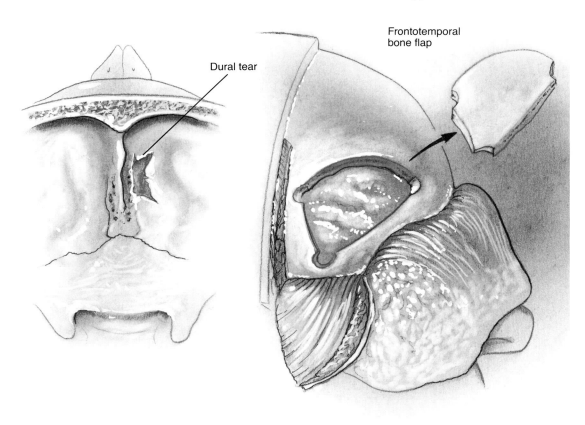

Dural tear

Frontotemporal
bone flap

B

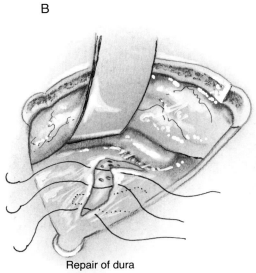

Repair of dura

OPTIONAL METHOD
USING TISSUE PLUG

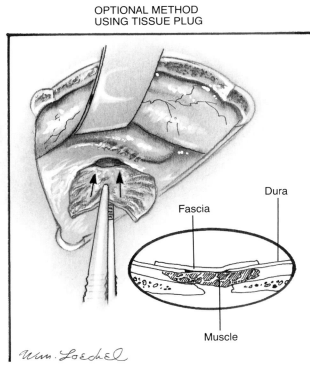

Fascia

Dura

Muscle

accurate preoperative evaluation is necessary for a successful repair.

Sometimes the closure is not sufficiently watertight, or the patch does not hold. In such cases, a short period of bed rest, elevation of the head, and lumbar drainage may be indicated. The patient should avoid nose-blowing. Antibiotic coverage is optional. If the leak continues after these conservative measures, the surgeon should repeat localization studies. The location of the leak often requires a new operative approach.

2. Infection can present clinically as meningitis in the postoperative period. This often signifies a continuation of the leak, and identification and localization studies should be carried out. If a leak is present, it should be treated with standard medical or surgical methods. The bacteria associated with meningitis should be cultured by obtaining cerebrospinal fluid from a lumbar puncture and the patient subsequently treated with antibiotics appropriate for the organism.

part
eleven

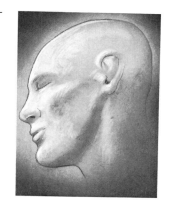

Temporal Bone
Fractures

section I

Classification and Pathophysiology of Temporal Bone Fractures

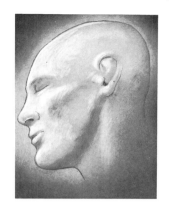

chapter 88

General Considerations

A Temporal bone fractures can cause damage to the brain, ear, and facial nerve. There can also be injury to the ossicular chain and tympanic membrane. Although a "pure" fracture is rare, about 20% of temporal bone fractures are transversely oriented to the base of the skull; the rest are longitudinal.

The transverse temporal bone fracture often occurs from a blow to the occiput. This fracture begins in the foramen magnum and crosses the petrous pyramid, ending in or lateral to the region of the foramen spinosum or lacerum. The labyrinth is involved, resulting in anacusis, vestibular damage, and possibly a facial nerve paralysis. The fracture may traverse the jugular foramen, hypoglossal canal, and/or internal auditory canal. Blood and cerebrospinal fluid can sometimes be seen in the external auditory canal and in the tympanum.

The longitudinal fracture usually results from a blow to the side of the head. The fracture begins in the squamous part of the temporal bone and runs through the external auditory canal, annulus, and tegmen tympani. It then passes along the carotid canal near the foramen spinosum or lacerum. The fracture usually crosses anterior to the labyrinth, and therefore it often spares the facial nerve and sensorineural auditory and vestibular functions of the ear. The patient with a longitudinal fracture usually has blood and cerebrospinal fluid in the external auditory canal, hematotympanum, and conductive hearing loss.

B,C The most common type of middle ear injury is fracture-dislocation of the incus and/or stapes. Rarely is the malleus involved. The fracture can also extend across the middle ear space to involve the facial nerve. The incus can be displaced into the hypotympanum or mastoid region, and the tympanic

439

membrane may be folded onto itself or torn, with lacerations extending toward the anulus.

To make the diagnosis, the surgeon should question the patient about loss of consciousness and onset of auditory and/or facial nerve dysfunction. Tuning fork tests are helpful in evaluating the presence or absence of conductive and/or sensorineural hearing loss. A formal audiogram should be obtained if the tuning fork tests are inconclusive or surgery is planned. Labyrinthine injury, as evidenced by a horizontal jerk nystagmus, should be confirmed by caloric tests, but such tests should be avoided if there is a cerebrospinal fluid leak or tympanic membrane perforation. The time of onset and degree of facial paralysis should be documented. Special electrostimulatory and acoustic reflex tests should be initiated and can be followed (if desirable) to document the changing status of the facial nerve. Computed tomographic (CT) scans are invaluable for determining the location of the fracture, but even CT scans can fail to document a fracture in the temporal bone. If cerebrospinal fluid leakage is suspected, the fluid should be tested for its physical and biochemical characteristics (see Chapter 84).

Little can be done for sensorineural auditory and vestibular deficits. Sedatives should be employed to control vertigo. Permanent losses can potentially be habilitated with hearing aids and/or vestibular exercises. Surgical repair for conductive hearing losses should be performed on an elective basis.

There is much controversy regarding facial nerve injury. If there is evidence of the nerve being transected, immediate exploration and repair are indicated. If the nerve is compressed by edema and there is a slow, gradual loss of function, medical decompression with steroids, control of infection, and avoidance of hypoxia and hypotension are appropriate. If there is radiologic evidence of displaced bone spicules and/or electrodiagnostic evidence of degeneration and the area is surgically accessible, the surgeon should consider exploration and reduction of the fracture and/or decompression of the nerve.

TEMPORAL BONE FRACTURES

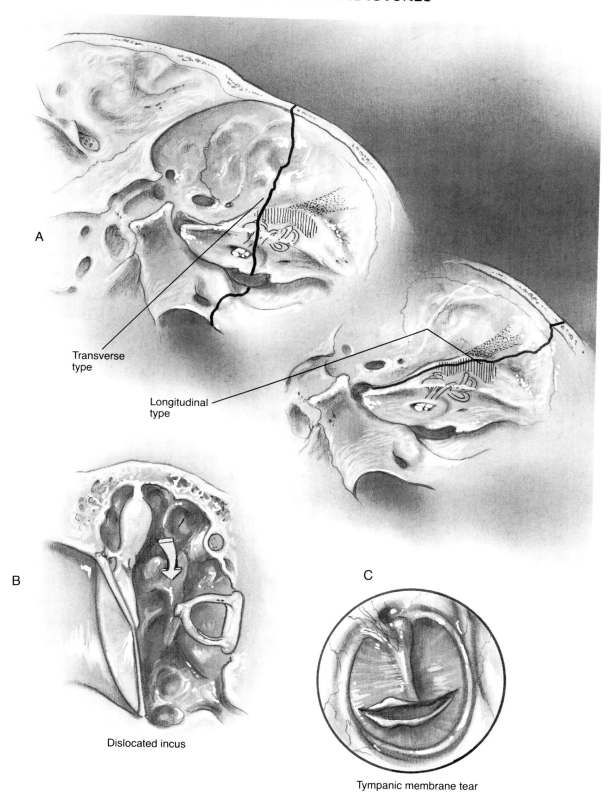

A

Transverse
type

Longitudinal
type

B

Dislocated incus

C

Tympanic membrane tear

Wm. Loechel

section II

Management Strategies for Temporal Bone Fractures

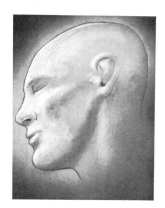

chapter 89

Decompression of the Facial Nerve Using a Transmastoid Approach
Alternative Technique of Middle Fossa Decompression

In Consultation With Brian W. Blakley, MD, PhD

INDICATIONS

The facial nerve may be transected or compressed by bone fragments in any part of its intratemporal course. Patients with an immediate loss of function should undergo decompression and/or repair of the nerve. When the onset of paralysis is delayed and there are electrodiagnostic signs of degeneration (see Chapter 107), a decompression may help alleviate the postinjury fibrosis that may occur under these conditions.

For the most part, facial nerve injuries that are definitely confined to the vertical (mastoid) or horizontal (tympanic) portions should be explored using a mastoidectomy and facial recess approach. When the injury lies medial to the middle ear, a middle fossa decompression should be performed. If there is uncertainty about the site of damage to the nerve, then a middle fossa decompression should be combined with the transmastoid decompression. However, the surgeon can choose not to explore the middle fossa if the acoustic reflexes are normal or nearly normal, or if the patient or guardian does not agree to the middle fossa portion of the procedure.

PROCEDURE

A The patient is positioned in the supine position, the neck is extended 15°, and the head is rotated so that the operative ear is addressed by the surgeon. Prophylactic antibiotics are administered preoperatively and during the procedure. The postauricular area and external auditory canal are infiltrated with 1% lidocaine containing 1:100,000 epinephrine to help control with hemostasis.

A simple mastoidectomy is carried out through a postauricular incision placed 3 to 4 mm posterior to the postauricular crease. The skin, subcutaneous tissues, and mastoid periosteum are incised, and bleeding is controlled with an electric cautery. The periosteum is elevated anteriorly and posteriorly, exposing the mastoid process to the lateral aspect of the external auditory canal. Self-retaining retractors are applied in such a way that the external auditory canal is not entered.

B,C Using burs, a microscope, and irrigation, the external cortex of the mastoid is removed. The mastoid air cells are exposed. The antrum, sigmoid sinus plate, and tegmen plate should be identified. The dissection is deepened to define the sinodural angle, the solid angle, and the lateral semicircular canal. The head is rotated to expose the incus, the fossa incudis, and the dome of the lateral semicircular canal.

D Next the facial recess approach is performed. Using the short process of the incus as a landmark, drilling is started 3 mm inferior to the attachment of the short process of the incus. Using the small cutting bur, more bone is removed, making the opening larger as progress is made anteriorly. Medially the facial nerve should be carefully sought, as the opening into the middle ear is made just lateral but parallel to the tympanic part of the nerve. Laterally the surgeon should look for and avoid injury to the tympanic membrane and chorda tympani nerve.

E,F Looking through the opening into the facial recess, the facial nerve can be followed to the geniculate ganglion. The incus is not removed. Bone is excised from the lateral aspect of the tympanic part of the nerve and the posterior aspect of the mastoid part of the nerve. When the nerve is just visible, the final layer of bone is removed with a hook or curet. The perineurium is not incised.

The pathologic condition should dictate the handling of the nerve. If the nerve has been bruised or crushed by the fracture, the overlying bone is removed from the canal. If the nerve is transected, the edges of the nerve are freshened with a sharp knife and approximated with at least two 10-0 nylon su-

tures. If there is a deficit between the edges, a small graft harvested from the great auricular nerve (see Chapter 107) can be interposed between the segments. Usually fibrin from the blood clot will act as a sufficient supporting scaffold. We usually leave the perineurium intact.

After copious irrigation, the wound is closed with 4-0 absorbable sutures through the periosteum and subcutaneous layers and 5-0 nylon sutures in the skin. A mastoid dressing is applied and then removed the following morning.

PITFALLS

1. Mastoidectomy requires special expertise and a knowledge of temporal bone anatomy. The surgeon must first recognize the landmarks of the temporal bone (i.e., the sigmoid sinus plate, tegmen, sinodural angle, antrum, and semicircular canals). The facial nerve can then be identified either at the bend inferior to the lateral semicircular canal or at the stylomastoid foramen, where the foramen meets the digastric ridge. Either approach is satisfactory in exposing and exploring the remainder of the nerve.

2. Remember that the facial nerve derives its blood supply from the fallopian canal, and therefore the surgeon should retain as much of the canal as possible. We prefer to keep at least 50% of the deep portion of the canal intact.

3. We do not cut back or incise the perineurium, although this is controversial. The perineurium provides the blood supply to the nerve; we prefer to keep it in contact with the fallopian canal.

4. If the incus and stapes are not intact, the middle ear should be explored at the same operation (see Chapter 90).

5. A facial nerve that has been traumatically transected between the brain stem and the internal auditory canal can rarely be identified and isolated proximal or distal to the injury. Repair of the nerve in such cases is not feasible.

COMPLICATIONS

1. Permanent and complete loss of facial nerve function can still occur, but in many patients, there is recovery with some degree of weakness and synkinesis. The nerve will repair itself at a rate of about 1 mm per day, and the more intact the axon cylinders are, the better the prognosis. As to the decompression, the surgeon should remove all areas of obstruction while ensuring a sufficient blood supply for the reparative processes. Special techniques must be used for those cases characterized by disruptive or avulsive neural injury.

TRANSMASTOID DECOMPRESSION OF FACIAL NERVE

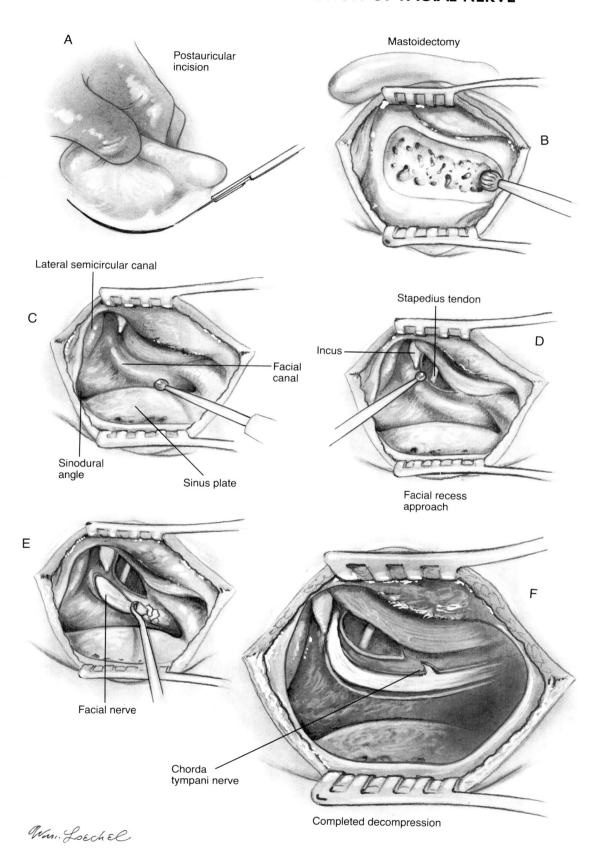

A Postauricular incision

Mastoidectomy B

C Lateral semicircular canal

Facial canal

Sinodural angle

Sinus plate

Stapedius tendon

Incus

D Facial recess approach

E

Facial nerve

F

Chorda tympani nerve

Completed decompression

Wm. Loechel

2. Ossicular chain damage is a possibility as a result of the original injury. Disruptions and/or tympanic membrane tears should be recognized and treated at the time of the facial nerve repair. If the incus is detached, it can be replaced in its original position (see Chapter 90).

3. Infection is a rare complication. Otitis media, meningitis, and brain abscesses are prevented in part by irrigating the wound with saline and by treating the patient prior to, during, and after surgery with prophylactic antibiotics. If there is any evidence of wound infection postoperatively, the incision should be opened and the wound cultured and drained. External packing with antibacterial gauze is indicated.

ALTERNATIVE TECHNIQUE OF MIDDLE FOSSA DECOMPRESSION

For injuries that involve the geniculate ganglion and portions of the facial nerve in the internal auditory canal, the middle fossa approach is the treatment of choice. The middle fossa approach can also be combined with the transmastoid decompression, especially if there are multiple sites of injury.

The middle fossa decompression is performed with the patient in the supine position. A shoulder roll is placed and the head rotated so that the squamous portion of the temporal bone lies in a horizontal plane. Mayfield percutaneous pins are used to hold the head in position and to hold the retractors. The scalp is shaved, prepared, and draped appropriately. The surgeon sits at the head of the table.

a,b The operative site is infiltrated with 1% lidocaine containing 1:100,000 epinephrine. An incision is made through the skin and subcutaneous tissues, 1 cm in front of the helical root and upward for about 6 cm over the temporal fossa. The temporal muscle is incised, elevated anteriorly and posteriorly, and held with a self-retaining retractor. A 3 × 3–cm rectangular craniotomy is then performed with a drill so that about two thirds of the removal is anterior and one third posterior to the external auditory canal. Useful landmarks are the squamous parietal suture superiorly and the zygoma inferiorly. The dura is then elevated and held with self-retaining retractors.

c–e Under microscopic visualization, the region of the middle meningeal artery is identified; the greater superficial petrosal nerve is found 1 cm medially and traced posterolaterally to the geniculate ganglion. By using a diamond bur and constant irrigation, a small opening is made into the middle ear space. This helps with orientation and with the removal of bone from the nerve. With the arcuate eminence in view, the bone is removed laterally and posteriorly to the geniculate ganglion and into the internal auditory canal.

Once the decompression is completed, the surgeon should ensure meticulous hemostasis with bipolar cautery. Self-retaining retractors are removed, and the temporal lobe is allowed to reexpand. The craniotomy flap is usually replaced, and the temporalis muscle and subcutaneous tissues are closed in layers. The skin is approximated with either a nylon suture or staples.

TRANSMASTOID DECOMPRESSION OF FACIAL NERVE *(Continued)*

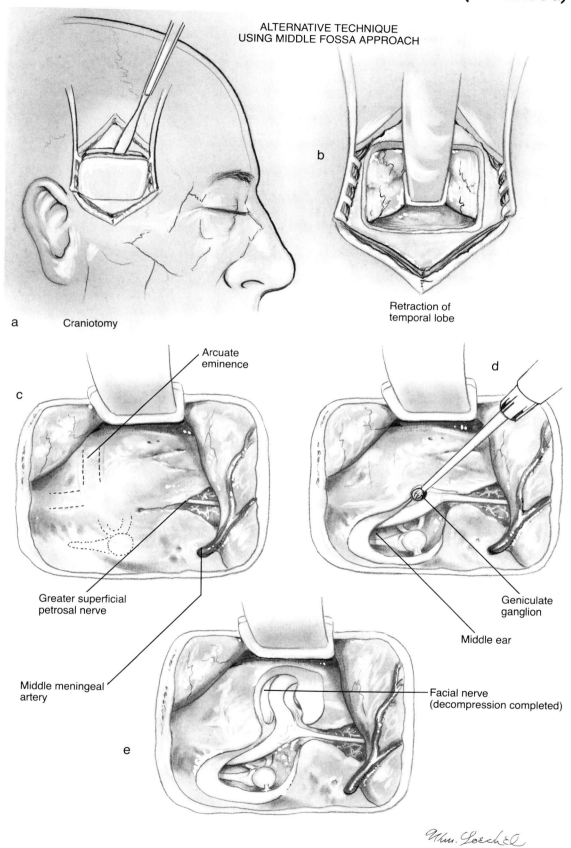

ALTERNATIVE TECHNIQUE
USING MIDDLE FOSSA APPROACH

a   Craniotomy

b

Retraction of
temporal lobe

c

Arcuate
eminence

d

Greater superficial
petrosal nerve

Middle meningeal
artery

Geniculate
ganglion

Middle ear

e

Facial nerve
(decompression completed)

chapter 90

Repair of the Ossicular Chain

INDICATIONS

Craniomaxillofacial injuries can damage the ossicular chain and cause conductive hearing loss. The ossicles can be fractured and/or dislocated. Scar tissue can cause impairment of the conductive mechanism.

The most common injury is a separation of the incudostapedial joint. The incus is often dislocated and can be displaced into the hypotympanum or mastoid antrum. Fracture of the stapedial arch can also occur. Rarely is the malleus involved with the injury.

The diagnosis is not easy to establish. Early following injury, the middle ear is filled with blood, fluid, and debris. The tympanic membrane may also be injured. The suggestion of an ossicular chain abnormality will only become obvious as the fluid clears, the membrane appears intact, and conductive loss exceeds that expected in the postoperative period (i.e., greater than 30 dB). Tympanometry may be helpful. Some patients require a trial of tympanostomy tubes to secure the diagnosis.

Exploration and repair of the ossicular chain should usually be performed on an elective basis. The patient can always use a hearing aid or, presumably, the other useful ear. The reparative procedures are generally successful, but there can be postoperative sequelae of sensorineural hearing loss, tinnitus, and/or dizziness. Although these complications are very rare, they must be explained to the patient.

PROCEDURE

A Local and/or general anesthesia (preferably without muscle relaxants) is used, and the patient is placed in the supine position. The external auditory canal is injected with 1% lidocaine containing 1:100,000 epinephrine to minimize bleeding. The neck is extended 15° and the head rotated to expose the operative ear. The ear is prepared and draped as a sterile field.

A tympanomeatal flap is then elevated from approximately the 6 o'clock to the 12 o'clock position, making first the vertical incisions and then the horizontal incision just beneath the vibrissae. The flap is elevated with a duckbill elevator. Adhesions are cut with microscissors, and the flap is rotated to the level of the annulus. Cotton pledgets containing 1:10,000 epinephrine are used to control hemostasis.

B The membranous annulus is elevated from the bony annulus posteriorly and inferiorly along the circumference of the canal. The drum head is then rotated anteriorly. The middle ear space is suctioned clear of fluid and blood, and the ossicular chain is inspected.

The evaluation should be carried out in an orderly fashion. The stapes is first inspected. The incus is palpated, and normal stapes motion is determined. A round window reflex will ensure the adequacy of the movement. The malleus is then palpated, and transmission of movement is noted across the incus. Again, the round window reflex is elicited. If the surgeon has difficulty in making these determinations, additional exposure can be obtained by taking down a portion of the attic with small curets.

C Depending on the pathologic condition, various procedures can be carried out. If the incus has been dislocated, it is loosened with sharp picks and replaced in its natural position. However, there are many options. If the lenticular process of the incus or the head of the stapes has been damaged, a small hole is drilled into the head of the incus, and using a transposition technique, the head is placed onto the stapes. The short process of the incus will fit under the malleus handle. If the stapes is fractured, the short process of the incus can be repositioned so that it fits in between the crura of the stapes; the head of the incus should then project upward beyond the facial nerve ridge. If the incus cannot be found, the surgeon must consider a cortical bone graft or a partial ossicular replacement prosthesis.

D Usually the middle ear is packed lightly with Gelfoam containing steroid-antibiotic otic drops. The tympanic membrane is placed back in its normal position, and the external auditory canal is packed loosely with a few strips of Gelfoam. Prophylactic antibiotics are prescribed for 2 days. The patient is

REPAIR OF OSSICULAR CHAIN

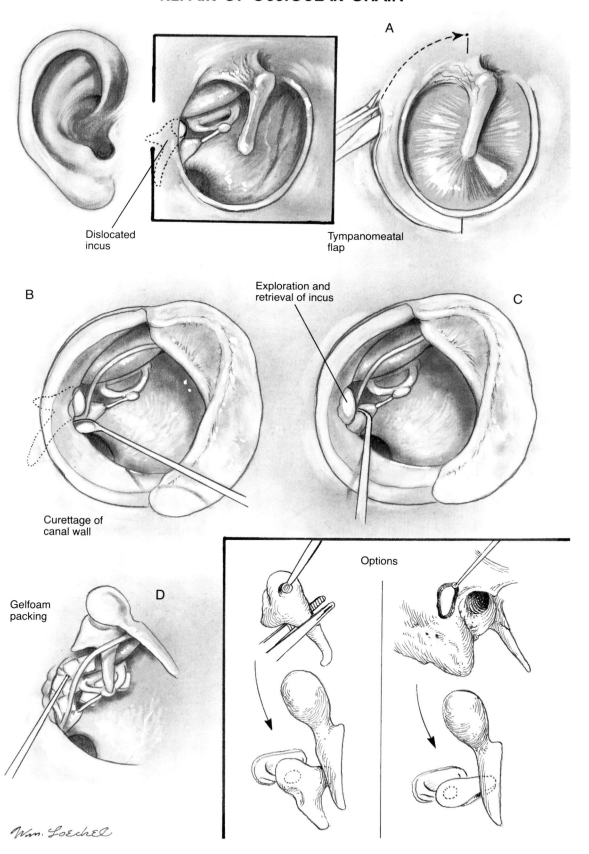

Dislocated incus

Tympanomeatal flap

A

B Curettage of canal wall

Exploration and retrieval of incus

C

Gelfoam packing **D**

Options

Wm. Loechel

cautioned about the possibility of dizziness, and he or she is asked to avoid straining or nose-blowing for 10 days.

PITFALLS

1. Making the diagnosis is very important. Many variations of ossicular chain displacement and many pathologic conditions can impair movement. The surgeon should be aware of the possibility of malleus fixation, and if this occurs, the attic attachments must be released and a piece of Silastic inserted between the malleus head and scutum. Stapes fixation should also be evaluated, and if this is apparent, the stapes will have to be mobilized or removed and replaced with a prosthesis.

2. Make sure that the incus is in good position. The bone is easily displaced and can later be dislocated with newly formed scar tissues. The incus transposition technique provides a time-proven, stable union.

3. Occasionally the surgeon finds a cerebrospinal fluid leak. In such situations, the defect should be filled with soft tissue (i.e., fat). If there is a leak in the oval window, the mucosa should be removed from the edges of the defect and the oval window layered with autogenous fat.

COMPLICATIONS

1. Probably the most common complication following reconstructive ear surgery is conductive hearing loss. The surgeon can expect a success rate of about 70%, but if the procedure fails, it is probably because of a displaced ossicle or infiltration with scar tissues. Early after surgery some loss can be expected from the Gelfoam and/or fluid. After 6 to 8 weeks, if the loss persists, the procedure should be deemed a failure, and reoperation or a hearing aid must be considered.

2. Sensorineural hearing loss and vertigo following middle ear surgery is very rare. These symptoms usually follow an infection that spreads to the inner ear. If this develops, the patient should be placed on a broad-spectrum antibiotic (i.e., ampicillin). Bed rest and intravenous fluids are important adjunctive measures.

3. In those patients with persistent unsteadiness and vertigo, the surgeon must be aware of the possibility of perilymph fistula. In such patients, symptoms will be aggravated by changes in position and especially by pressure changes within the middle ear. Hearing loss may be progressive. Treatment may require exploration, identification of the leak, and plugging of the leak with autogenous tissues.

Repair of the Tympanic Membrane Using an Overlay Technique

In Consultation With Brian W. Blakley, MD, PhD

INDICATIONS

Although most tympanic membrane perforations heal spontaneously, a small number persist and cause problems with middle ear hygiene and loss of hearing. It thus becomes important to evaluate and determine which perforations will not heal; once this is known, these can be repaired on an elective basis.

All tympanic membrane perforations should be examined with microscopic visualization. Perforations that are small (less than 25%), clean, and central in position will probably heal without sequelae. On the other hand, larger perforations characterized by irregular tears and involvement of the annulus may not heal. They are often associated with other kinds of middle ear injury and cholesteatoma. In general, if the perforation does not heal within 3 months, repair must be considered. If there is a significant conductive hearing loss, the middle ear will also require exploration.

PROCEDURE

Repair of a perforation is usually performed under local and/or general anesthesia. The ear area is infiltrated with 1% lidocaine containing 1:100,000 epinephrine. The local anesthetic will help control hemostasis and reduce the need for analgesia. The neck is extended 15°, and the head is rotated so that the operative ear faces upward. The ear is prepared and draped as a sterile field.

A For the larger perforations without conductive hearing loss, the overlay technique is desirable. An incision is made 3 to 4 mm behind the postauricular crease. A piece of temporalis fascia is exposed, cut, cleaned, and pressed for later use in grafting. The postauricular incision is closed in layers with 4-0 chromic and 5-0 nylon sutures.

B,C The perforation is freshened by removing the margins with a straight pick. The epithelium of the external surface of the drumhead is separated from the fibrous layer. This can be accomplished by careful dissection, beginning at either the margin of the perforation or in the posteroinferior aspect of the tympanic membrane, where the epithelial layer is usually less adherent. If there is some limitation provided by the anterior canal wall overhang, this is removed with cutting burs. Visualization can be improved by elevating the anterior canal wall skin from medial to lateral. The drumhead is inspected, and any epithelial remnants are carefully removed from its surface.

D,E The middle ear is filled with pieces of Gelfoam soaked in a steroid-antibiotic otic solution. The piece of fascia is then fitted over the perforation and just onto the canal walls. The epithelial remnant that was removed can be placed over the fascia, but it may not survive. Care is taken to be certain that the fascia is in the correct position anteriorly.

The external auditory canal is packed either with steroid-antibiotic–soaked Gelfoam or a "rosebud" dressing containing fine mesh silk/rayon and cotton balls soaked in steroid-antibiotic otic solution. The external meatus is packed with ½-inch gauze treated with bacitracin ointment. The pinna is returned, and the wound is closed in layers. A mastoid dressing of fluffs and stretch gauze is applied. Prophylactic antibiotics are prescribed for 2 days, and sutures are removed at 7 days. The packing is removed from the external auditory canal and ear in about 10 days.

PITFALLS

1. Most perforations with large conductive hearing losses are better treated with middle ear exploration combined with an overlay technique. Other, usually smaller, perforations can be managed by packing the middle ear with Gelfoam and placing a small piece

of fascia underneath the perforation. In this procedure, the drumhead is then advanced anteriorly to close over the defect.

2. The drumhead should be cleaned of all epithelial remnants. Failure to do so can cause small areas of skin growth, which can eventually lead to a cholesteatoma. Initially these will be small, pearl-like lesions; ultimately the cholesteatoma can lead to an erosive destructive lesion of the external auditory canal.

3. Make sure that the fascia fits around the defect and onto the drumhead. The fascia is easier to manipulate if it is thinned and dried, and properly prepared fascia will provide for a thinner drumhead and improved acoustic properties.

4. The skin graft and fascia should be in contact with the vascular supply from the external auditory canal. The blood supply around the perforation may be limited; a better vascular supply may be found on the walls of the canal.

5. Make sure that the fascia is tightly "sandwiched" to the anterior portion of the annulus. Failure to do so may lead to retraction and foreshortening of the drumhead. Tight packing will help prevent this from occurring.

6. The external packing should be left in place for 10 to 14 days. The packing acts as a scaffold, and under such conditions, the epithelium will grow around and across the area of perforation.

COMPLICATIONS

1. Infection is a dreaded complication, as it can cause the dissolution of the graft and potentially a toxic/sensorineural hearing loss and meningitis. For the most part, infection can be prevented by sterile atraumatic techniques. The middle and external ear should be packed with antibiotic-soaked dressings, and prophylactic antibiotics should be used for 2 days. If the patient develops signs of infection, the packing should be removed, cultures obtained, and the ear treated with appropriate antibiotic drops.

2. As with any ear surgery, hearing may be worse following this procedure. Tinnitus and dizziness may occur. The diagnosis and prevention of these complications are addressed in Chapter 90.

3. A new perforation is always a possibility. If the eustachian tube fails to function properly, the middle ear will develop fluid and cause undue pressure on the new tympanic membrane. This can cause a graft failure. If the surgeon suspects that this has occurred, the patient must be checked out for rhinosinusitis, obstruction in and around the eustachian tube (i.e., adenoids), and obstruction caused by deflection of the septum. These conditions must be treated prior to embarking on another repair procedure. The patient can also be given the option of living with the perforation and/or using a hearing aid.

4. Although rare, graft surgery can cause a cholesteatoma. This complication develops from a failure to remove all of the epithelial remnants from the drumhead and/or middle ear space. If a cholesteatoma develops, the area should be cleaned of epithelial remnants and a new tympanic graft placed.

REPAIR OF TYMPANIC MEMBRANE PERFORATION

A

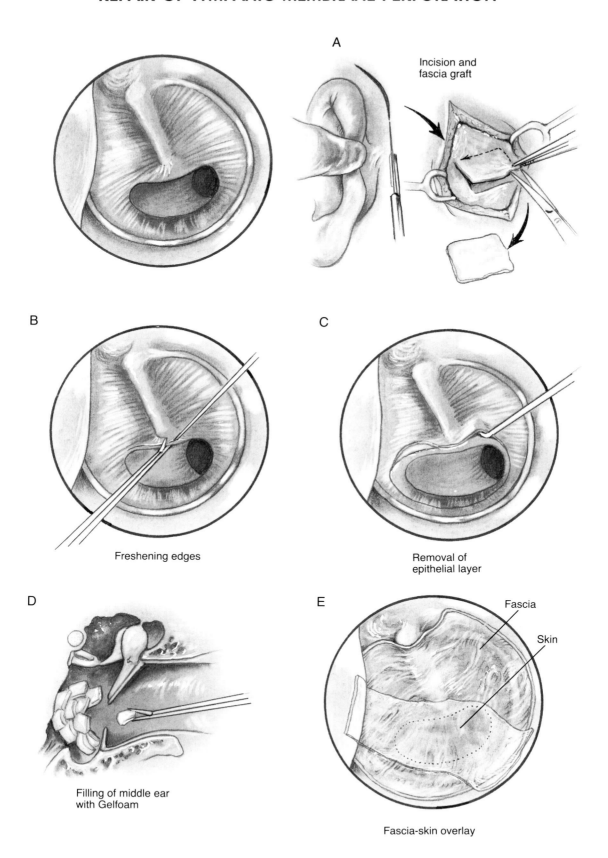

Incision and fascia graft

B

Freshening edges

C

Removal of epithelial layer

D

Filling of middle ear with Gelfoam

E

Fascia

Skin

Fascia-skin overlay

453

part
twelve

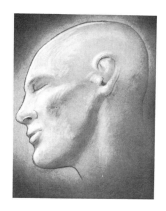

Laryngeal
Injuries

section I

Classification and Pathophysiology of Laryngeal Injuries

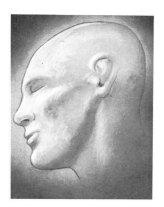

chapter 92

General Considerations

A The larynx, by virtue of its anterior position in the neck, is susceptible to both blunt and penetrating trauma. The risk is even greater when the neck is hyperextended, as the mandible and sternum no longer provide a natural protection in this position. Moreover, the larynx can be easily crushed against the rigid cervical spine.

From an anatomic standpoint, the larynx can better tolerate a lateral blow. The vertically oriented muscular and ligamentous slings provide some freedom of mobility and, consequently, protection from laterally directed forces. Laryngeal calcification and rigidity, which are related to age, can also be factors. Additional pathophysiologic considerations include (1) the soft tissue contents and shape of the neck that define a protective cushion and (2) the lamina angle that describes the projection of the larynx and point of potential impact.

Although laryngeal injury can occur alone, it is often associated with other types of trauma. The cervical spine can be damaged and must be evaluated early when a laryngeal fracture is suspected. Displacement of the larynx can also be associated with a laryngotracheal separation, pharyngoesophageal tears, and damage to the recurrent laryngeal nerve. Penetrating injuries of the neck can tear the laryngeal skeleton and, additionally, cause damage to a variety of nerves and vessels that pass through the cervical region.

Laryngeal injuries are usually classified according to site of soft tissue and skeletal damage. Supraglottic, glottic, subglottic, and laryngotracheal patterns are described, but more commonly, a variety of combinations can occur. The diagnosis is usually made on the basis of a careful examination and imaging studies. Laryngoscopy is used to confirm pathologic findings. The classification that follows is useful in defining and understanding the injury and planning for specific treatment protocols.

B SOFT TISSUE. Soft tissue injury commonly develops from blunt trauma and manifests as edema and/or hematoma involving the aryepiglottic folds, arytenoids, and false and true vocal cords. In addition, superficial lacerations of the laryngeal mucosa can occur.

C SUPRAGLOTTIC. Supraglottic injuries are fractures of the hyoid bone and thyroid cartilage that are usually oriented in a caudal-cephalic direction. The injury is generally associated with a depression or widening of the thyroid notch and loss of the thyroid prominence. If there is a disruption of the thyrohyoid membrane and/or thyroepiglottic ligament, the epiglottis and soft tissues of the anterior larynx can be displaced posteriorly. Tears of the false cords, aryepiglottic folds, pharyngeal walls, and ventricles are common. The injury pattern is often complicated by avulsion-dislocation of the arytenoid cartilages.

D TRANSGLOTTIC. Transglottic injuries are injuries of the vocal cord region and are usually divided into anterior and posterior types. The anterior glottic damage is characterized by midline vertical fractures of the thyroid cartilage with lacerations that extend into the true cords, false cords, and aryepiglottic folds. The larynx is foreshortened in the anteroposterior diameter, and vocal cord mobility is affected. If the lateral walls of the larynx are involved, there can be posterior displacement of the thyroid ala into the piriform sinus, with ipsilateral avulsion-dislocation of the arytenoid.

Fractures isolated to the posterior larynx present with disruptions of the interarytenoid and thyroarytenoid muscles. They are often associated with dislocation and exposure of the arytenoid cartilages. Compression-induced cricoarytenoid damage to the recurrent laryngeal nerves can occur.

E SUBGLOTTIC. Isolated injuries to the subglottic larynx are unusual and are often seen in combination with thyroid cartilage injuries or the laryngotracheal separation pattern. Typically, anterior cricoid arch fractures occur in the midline or paramedian position and result in loss of the cricoid prominence. Displacement of cartilage fragments and submucosal edema often compromises the subglottic lumen. Both cricothyroid and cricotracheal membrane tears may be seen. One or both cricoarytenoid joints can be affected.

F LARYNGOTRACHEAL. Laryngotracheal injuries develop from excessive shearing forces with the neck in a hyperextended position (i.e., a "clothesline" injury). The cricotracheal separation often involves damage to the strap muscles, the recurrent laryngeal nerves, and even the anterior esophageal wall. Characteristically the trachea retracts substernally, whereas the larynx migrates upward for a distance of approximately 6 to 10 cm.

Most laryngeal injuries are managed conservatively, but if there are significant mucosal lacerations and tears and/or displacement of cartilage, open reduction and fixation must be considered. The objectives of surgery are to restore respiration and/or phonatory function. The degree of injury and prognosis should direct the individual evaluation and treatment protocol.

LARYNGEAL INJURIES

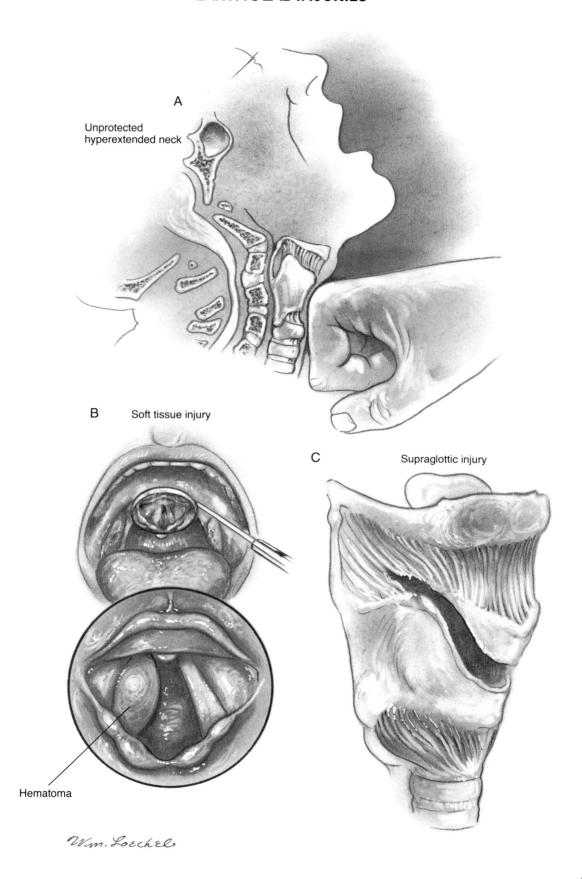

A

Unprotected
hyperextended neck

B Soft tissue injury

Hematoma

C Supraglottic injury

Wm. Loechel

459

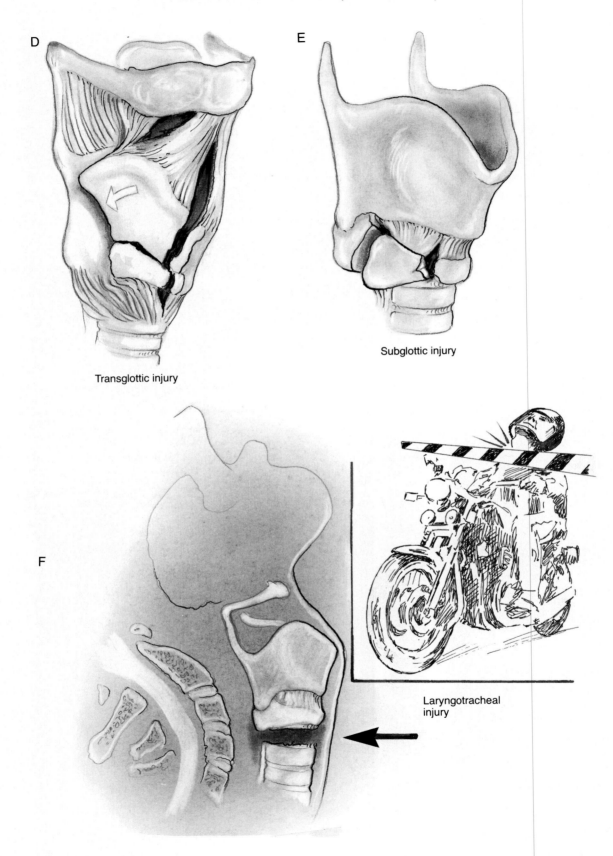

D

Transglottic injury

E

Subglottic injury

F

Laryngotracheal
injury

General Techniques for Laryngeal Injury

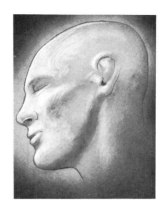

chapter 93

Open Reduction and Repair of Endolaryngeal Injury by Thyrotomy

In Consultation With Richard Arden, MD

INDICATIONS

Adequate evaluation and proper treatment of endolaryngeal injury are essential if the surgeon is to preserve both phonatory and sphincteric functions and prevent the sequela of laryngeal stenosis. A secure airway is the first priority and is usually achieved by tracheostomy under local anesthesia (see Chapter 4). Endoscopic evaluation (direct laryngoscopy/esophagoscopy) soon follows to assess the extent of injury.

The main goals of surgery are to restore normal laryngeal skeletal relationships while providing for an epithelium-lined internal covering. Open reduction and repair are often indicated when there is (1) airway obstruction necessitating tracheotomy, (2) progressive subcutaneous emphysema, (3) fracture-dislocation of cartilaginous structures, and/or (4) endolaryngeal laceration or mucosal disruption that is

seen or suspected. The traditional approach is through a midline thyrotomy, which is easy to perform and provides excellent exposure of the internal larynx. Most injuries can be evaluated directly and subsequently repaired with a variety of reconstructive techniques.

PROCEDURE

A,B Control of the airway is often obtained with a tracheostomy or anode tube. After preparation and draping of a sterile field, a 5- to 7-cm transverse skin incision is marked in a natural neck crease halfway between the hyoid bone and inferior border of the cricoid cartilage. Subcutaneous infiltration with 1% lidocaine containing 1:100,000 epinephrine will optimize hemostatic control. The skin incision is made and deepened to the level of the superficial cervical fascia, just deep to the platysmal layer. Superior and inferior subplatysmal planes are developed to the level of the hyoid superiorly and to the level of the first tracheal ring inferiorly. The placement of two opposing self-retaining retractors will assist in this exposure.

C–E The cervical fascia is incised in the midline to expose the perichondrium of the thyroid and cricoid cartilages. By using a combination of sharp and blunt dissection techniques, the strap muscles are dissected from the larynx, and self-retaining retractors are reset to hold the skin flaps and strap muscles laterally. Marking solution is used to outline the thyrotomy incision in the midline. If fracture of the thyroid cartilage already exists in the median or paramedian plane, it can be used for the endolaryngeal exposure. The thyrotomy is performed with an oscillating saw, taking care not to prematurely enter the larynx. Depending on the patient's needs, vertical midline incisions can be extended through the thyrohyoid and cricothyroid membranes. Using wide double skin hooks for lateral retraction of the thyroid ala, the surgeon then incises the inner perichondrial layer. Usually the incision begins at the cricothyroid membrane "window" and cuts the anterior commissure in the midline. Above the anterior commissure, the incision follows the inferolateral border of the epiglottis (depending on the side of injury) and proceeds superiorly along the aryepiglottic fold. This procedure maximizes exposure and preserves epiglottic mucosa.

F At this point, the surgeon should assess the extent of endolaryngeal injury and plan the repair. As a matter of principle, the mucosa should be handled delicately with noncrushing forceps. Whenever possible, the tissues should be approximated primarily with 4-0 chromic sutures on a small, sharp needle.

A careful inspection of the arytenoids is next carried out. If the arytenoid is simply subluxated, an attempt should be made to reposition it onto the cricoid facet. With severe disruptive injuries, submucosal resection of the arytenoid is advised, followed by a careful mucosal closure. Presuming that the contralateral vocal cord is mobile, the affected cord (minus the arytenoid) is fixed to the midline by suturing the vocal process of the arytenoid to the middle of the posterior cricoid cartilage.

Advancement flaps can be designed and adjusted to fill small areas of endolaryngeal defect. For larger areas of damage, the surgeon can use a variety of epiglottic flaps (see Chapter 101). If the mucosal injury is large and cannot be covered with a flap, the surgeon should consider mucosal or split thickness grafts applied to an internal soft stent (see Chapter 94). Debridement should always be conservative, and rarely should a cartilaginous fragment be removed.

Fractures of the hyoid bone, thyroid, and cricoid can be fixed with heavy chromic, polyglactin, or wire sutures and replaced in their anatomic positions. The surgeon can then apply internal stents, T tubes, or keels (see Chapters 94 through 96).

G The thyrotomy is closed by approximating the outer perichondrium with interrupted 3-0 chromic sutures or by bringing the ala together with 30-gauge stainless steel wire. A figure-of-eight technique will help prevent overriding and slippage of the laminae. The strap muscles are next approximated loosely with 3-0 chromic suture and a two-layered skin closure is accomplished with 4-0 chromic and 5-0 nylon sutures. A ¼-inch Penrose drain is placed in the deeper layers. Prophylactic antibiotics are given for 7 to 10 days.

PITFALLS

1. Surgery should ideally be performed within 48 to 72 hours of injury. The tissues of the larynx have a poor blood supply and are prone to infection and necrosis, and the sooner the repair, the less chance there is of contamination and further injury.

2. Failure to precisely divide the junction of the vocal cords in the midline can lead to transection of a portion of the anterior membranous vocal cord and a foreshortening and alteration in vibratory characteristics. Excessive mucosal disruption can predispose to anterior glottic webbing.

3. Overtightening or undertightening the sutures applied to the thyroid ala can lead to overriding of the cartilaginous anterior segments and can also cause vocal cord asymmetries. Using a figure-of-eight technique with the wires crossed between cartilage fragments can prevent the sliding effect and any overriding of the segments.

4. Failure to approximate the mucosal edges, improper mucosal handling, or inadequate assessment of the need for mucosal free grafting can lead to cartilage exposure with subsequent chondritis and laryngeal stenosis. Use of a stent with a mucosal graft is discussed in Chapter 94.

5. Recognition of comminuted cartilaginous fragments and collapse of the airway is important. If such a condition develops, the surgeon must consider an internal keel or stent fixation technique (see Chapters 94 through 96).

6. Injuries to the cricoid require extension of the incision to include the cricoid area. These techniques are described in Chapter 98.

COMPLICATIONS

1. Stenosis of the airway is possible after laryngeal injury and must be avoided by careful application of

REPAIR OF LARYNGEAL INJURY USING THYROTOMY APPROACH

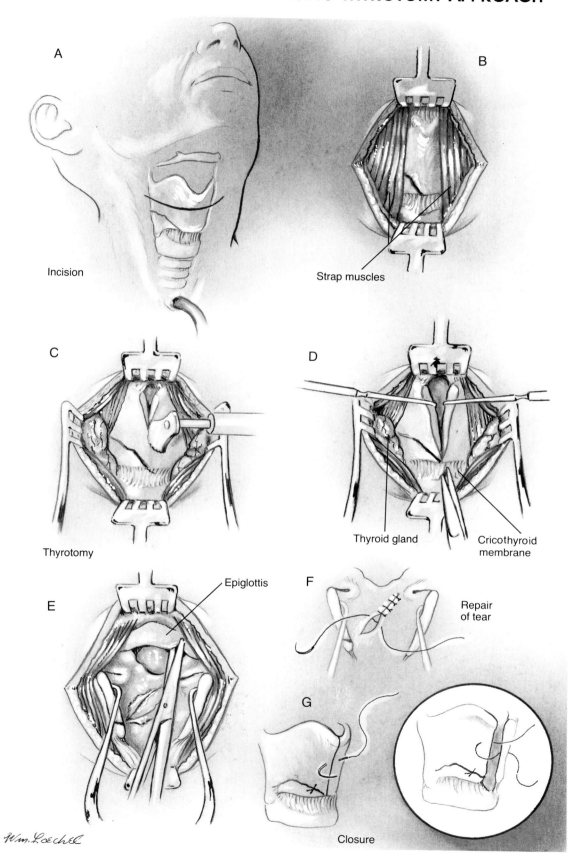

A

Incision

B

Strap muscles

C

Thyrotomy

D

Thyroid gland

Cricothyroid membrane

E

Epiglottis

F

Repair of tear

G

Closure

Wm. Loechel

reduction and fixation techniques. If this complication develops, the surgeon should dilate the area of constriction. If this is not successful, a thyrotomy and formal reconstruction can be carried out (see Chapters 101 through 105). Occasionally arytenoidectomy with or without a vocal cord resection is indicated.

2. Granulation tissues can form following the thyrotomy and repair. This complication can be prevented by carefully advancing mucosa and/or mucosal or skin grafts to cover all raw areas and by adjusting or removing stents so that they do not rub or cause pressure on adjoining tissues. If the granulations become excessive, they should be removed by way of an endoscope with a cupped forceps or laser technique. Broad-spectrum antibiotics should be used as an adjunctive measure.

3. Vocal cord paralysis and fixation are potential complications that affect both voice and respiration. The physician must distinguish between the two by careful examination of laryngeal–vocal cord movements and by palpation of the arytenoid (and/or vocal cord) under anesthesia. Electrodiagnosis may also be helpful. In the case of a unilateral vocal cord paralysis, the surgeon should wait at least 6 to 9 months for a return of function. If vocal cord function does not return, then a Teflon or cartilaginous interposition can be considered (see Chapter 99). For bilateral vocal cord paralysis, a unilateral arytenoidectomy or pedicled omohyoid flap is preferred (see Chapter 100). If fixation of the cord occurs, the surgeon should consider surgical relaxation of the stenotic area, arytenoidectomy alone, or arytenoidectomy in combination with partial cordectomy (see Chapters 100 and 101).

chapter 94

Internal Fixation of a Laryngeal Injury With a Soft Stent
Alternative Technique Using the Montgomery Silicone Stent

In Consultation With Richard Arden, MD

INDICATIONS

The internal laryngeal soft stent usually provides skeletal support when there is extensive comminution of laryngeal fractures or when, following open reduction and internal stabilization, the fracture segments remain unstable. The stent can also be used to stabilize skin or mucosal free grafts to denuded areas of the larynx and to prevent mucosal web formation across two opposing raw surfaces. Ideally the stent should be rigid enough to provide internal support but resilient enough to permit restoration of epithelial bridging without compromising "graft take." The stent should move with the larynx during respiration and deglutition but should also be well tolerated by the host. It should be easy to place and easy to remove once healing has been completed.

Although a wide variety of conforming alloplastic laryngeal stents have been described, each type is for a different purpose. A soft stent is useful in supporting free mucosal or skin grafts or more relatively stable fractures in the glottic-subglottic region. The prefabricated Montgomery silicone stent (see later) is indicated when there is a need to support unstable fractures. The Montgomery T tube works well for injuries of the trachea and cricoid. In patients with an uncomplicated midline glottic injury, avulsion of the true or false cords (or both), and the potential for anterior web formation, we often choose a Teflon keel (see Chapter 96).

PREPARATION AND TECHNIQUE OF SOFT STENT FABRICATION

A The soft stent is made from a finger cot or a size 8 or 6 surgical glove finger, depending on the size of the larynx. The "container" is internally supported and stretched with opposing Trousseau dilators or an open nasal speculum while a surgical prep sponge is cut to appropriate size, rolled, and inserted into it with bayonet forceps. The stent should be checked to ensure that it is soft and conforming. A 2-0 silk suture is then secured around the open end of the stent to retain the sponge and is cut long to allow for uncomplicated endoscopic retrieval at a later date. Depending on need, a split-thickness skin (0.0014-inch), dermal, or mucosal graft can be wrapped around the stent, trimmed, and secured with 4-0 chromic suture.

B–D The stent is transfixed within the larynx by passing an 18-gauge spinal needle through the skin, platysma, thyrohyoid muscle, and thyroid lamina at a level superior to the glottis and anterior to the arytenoids. The needle is then passed through the upper aspect of the stent and out through the contralateral thyroid lamina, strap muscles, and soft tissues of the opposite side. Two No. 0 polypropylene sutures are subsequently passed through the cannula (needle), the cannula is withdrawn, and the ends of the suture are secured with Silastic buttons. A similar maneuver is performed at a level below the site of injury through the lower aspect of the stent. The second set of sutures is also held into position with button fixation. The surgeon can also secure the buttons to the laryngeal skeleton, but although this will fix the stent to the mobile cartilages, it will also require additional surgery for removal. The wounds are then closed in layers.

The stent is usually retained for approximately 10 to 14 days but can be left in for longer periods of time when severe comminution is a problem. A broad-spectrum antibiotic or penicillin is provided intravenously for 2 days, and then the antibiotics are given orally while the stent is in place. To remove the stent, the patient is anesthetized through the tracheostomy tube. The suture underlying a skin button is snipped, and the opposite button is pulled to extract the suture. The stent can then be removed endoscopically.

PITFALLS

1. Avoid overpacking the stent. A "soft" stent can thus be converted to a "hard" stent, with the resulting potential for pressure necrosis of the surrounding mucoperichondrium and free graft. Under such conditions, infection can occur, causing loss of soft tissues and chondritis of the laryngeal skeleton.

2. Stents that are underpacked or improperly contoured can also cause problems. Mucosal or skin grafts may not be in contact with denuded surface, leading to uncovered cartilage with its inherent sequelae. Poorly fitted stents with inadequate internal support can predispose to displacement of the cartilaginous fragments within the laryngeal lumen; this can cause cross-bridging of mucosal edges and laryngeal stenosis.

3. Using a stent to carry mucosal or skin grafts will help produce epithelial coverage. The skin will "take" on raw areas and disappear on those areas that are covered by healthy mucosa. This will provide for an early coverage of exposed tissues.

4. Overtightening of sutures on the skin can lead to ischemic changes and permanent skin markings. On the other hand, if the wires holding the stent become loose or break, the stent can migrate and cause respiratory obstruction. To avoid these problems, the wires should be checked weekly and the position of the stent ensured by indirect laryngoscopy. If a wire breaks, a new one should be affixed immediately.

5. The procedure to remove the stent should not be taken lightly. The stent can break up or even become displaced inferiorly. Under endoscopic control, the stent should be grasped with a large forceps. The hold of the forceps should be retained until the fixation suture is loose and the stent is removed from the larynx.

COMPLICATIONS

1. Granulation tissues often occur adjacent to the stent. This reaction is partially the result of stasis of secretions and contact of tissue with a foreign body. Antibiotic coverage is helpful. The stent should also be removed as soon as it has fulfilled its purpose. Residual granulations can be managed by endoscopic surgery or laser removal. Recurrence of granulations and/or collapse of the endolarynx may require reinsertion of another stent or keel.

2. Stenosis can also follow laryngeal injury and stent fixation. If it is recognized early, dilatation and/or reinsertion of the stent for a longer period may be successful. However, if the stenosis persists and affects respiration and/or phonatory functions, surgical removal of the stenosis and reconstruction with or without stents or keels may be indicated.

3. Skin ulceration and scars can develop from the buttons and wires used for stabilization. Such areas on the skin should be kept clean with application of 3% hydrogen peroxide followed by antibiotic ointment. Unsightly scars can later be revised by excision and reorientation of the scars in crease lines.

ALTERNATIVE TECHNIQUE USING THE MONTGOMERY SILICONE STENT

a Although a "hard" stent can be used with skin or mucosal grafts sutured to the deficit, we prefer soft stents, with the graft secured to the stent and placed in apposition to the raw area. The hard silicone Montgomery stent is reserved for those patients who require primarily stabilization of a reduced laryngeal skeleton. Such stents are available in a variety of sizes to fit almost any larynx in a patient of any age, male or female.

b Essentially the procedure for inserting the hard stent is the same as that described for the soft stent. However, we reinforce the stent with a No. 26 wire, as experience has shown that the silk frays in the larynx and often comes apart when it is time to remove the stent. This can be dangerous, especially when the Silastic is wet and slippery and tends to migrate inferiorly.

c The Montgomery stent is positioned so that the contour fits the vocal cords and isthmus of the larynx. The stent is fixed to the skin with the button suture technique. The patient is placed on prophylactic antibiotics while the stent is in place. We prefer to remove the stent in 2 to 3 weeks to prevent necrosis and granulation tissues. Longer periods of fixation may be necessary, however, when the injuries are characterized by loss of tissue and/or comminution of the laryngeal skeleton.

REPAIR OF LARYNGEAL INJURY WITH STENTS

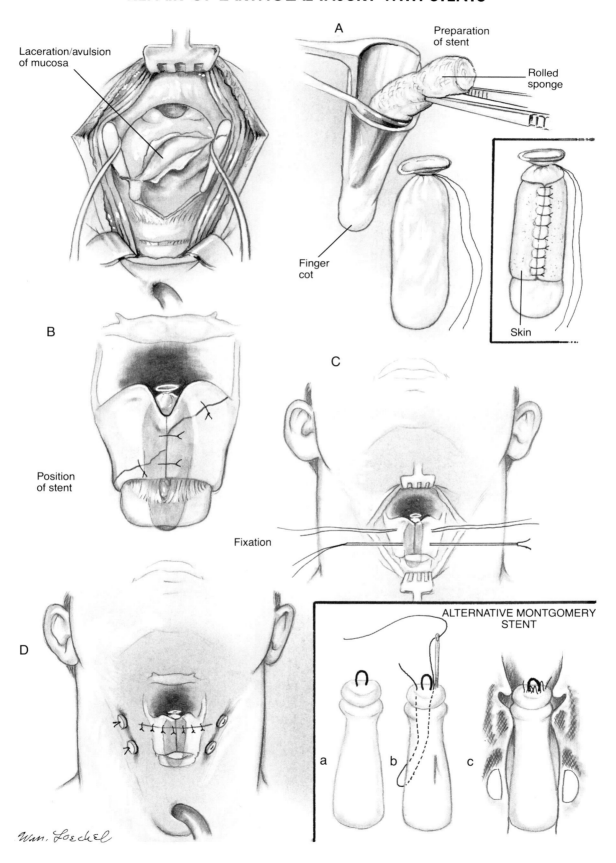

A

Laceration/avulsion of mucosa

Preparation of stent

Rolled sponge

Finger cot

Skin

B

Position of stent

C

Fixation

D

ALTERNATIVE MONTGOMERY STENT

a   b   c

Wm. Loechel

chapter 95

Internal Fixation of a Laryngeal Injury With a Montgomery T Tube

In Consultation With Richard Arden, MD

INDICATIONS

The silicone Montgomery tracheal T tube is best applied to the management of complex tracheal and subglottic injuries. Its primary role has been to serve as a lumen keeper, but it is also useful in stenting segmental subglottic resections and comminuted cricoid fractures. The T tube is also employed for tracheomalacia, with the expectation that long-term stenting will encourage the development of fibrocartilage, strengthening of tissues, and resolution of a collapsing cartilaginous framework.

PROCEDURE

A The T tube is a flexible, hollow silicone tube in the shape of a T that comes in a variety of lengths and diameters (8 to 16 mm). Its superior and inferior vertical sections are of unequal length. The horizontal limb is of a smaller diameter. The tube can be further adjusted by trimming one or several of the parts.

In sizing the T tube, the largest outer diameter stent that is readily accommodated by the airway should be selected. The superior and inferior limbs of the tube should be cut so that their ends overlie a normal laryngotracheal mucosa. When this technique is selected for subglottic stenting, the stent should be extended just slightly below the glottis. This allows the supraglottic and glottic valves to function and prevents aspiration.

B—E Insertion of the T tube requires a tracheostomy and endolaryngeal exposure. The tracheostomy is usually created below the site of injury. If a tracheostomy tract already exists, it may require dilatation intraoperatively, or it can be prepared preoperatively by sequential insertion of progressively larger tracheostomy tubes.

Topical anesthesia with sedation is preferred. Intravenous lidocaine and application of 4% cocaine to the laryngeal mucosa will help control bronchospasm and laryngospasm. A No. 8 ventilating bronchoscope is passed, and the airway is secured. The anode or tracheostomy tube is removed. The T tube is grasped with a hemostat near the junction of the upper vertical and horizontal limb so that the curve of the hemostat is in a position to direct the lower vertical limb inferiorly through the tracheostoma. With continued advancement of the hemostat, the superior limb of the stent will become intraluminal; this can be confirmed bronchoscopically. While holding the tube in position, a second, much smaller hemostat is applied to the horizontal limb. This will prevent dislodgement of the tube into the tracheobronchial tree. The first hemostat can then be released. Usually the tube will position itself in the airway, but if adjustments are necessary, an alligator forceps can be passed through the bronchoscope and the upper limb directed into the appropriate position.

Postoperatively the patient is placed on penicillin (or erythromycin) for 5 to 7 days. To reduce the likelihood of crusting and obstruction, the horizontal limb of the T tube is corked as soon as possible. If crusts form, application of mucolytic agents may be helpful. In general, the T tube should remain in place for 6 to 12 months, with interval changes for cleaning made every 3 months until removal. This can be done under local anesthesia and sedation or under general anesthesia by simply tugging steadily on the horizontal limb and pulling anteriorly. At the time of decannulation, it is recommended that the T tube be replaced with a small tracheostomy tube (No. 4 cuffless) for at least 4 weeks to allow adequate time to reassess the airway for possible restenosis. Decannulation is then carried out by occluding the tracheostomy tube, and if this is tolerated, the tube can be

INTERNAL FIXATION WITH MONTGOMERY T TUBE

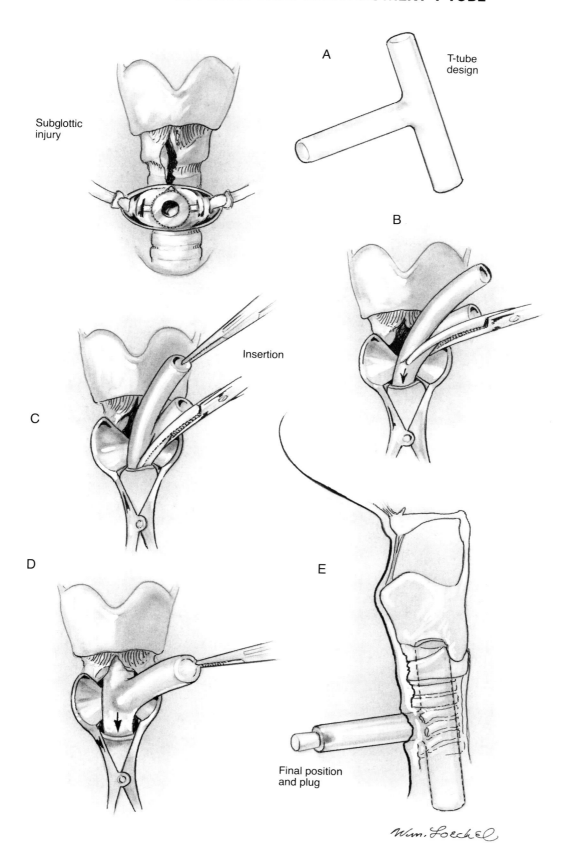

Subglottic
injury

A

T-tube
design

B

C

Insertion

D

E

Final position
and plug

Wm. Loechel

removed from the stoma. These decannulation procedures are also addressed in Chapter 4.

PITFALLS

1. Working through a small stoma makes T tube insertion and manipulation difficult, if not impossible. Employ proper dilatation techniques before attempting insertion.

2. A tube that is too small in diameter will not provide adequate internal stenting; a tube that is too large will be difficult to manipulate into position and is likely to result in significant mucosal trauma and possible displacement of skeletal segments.

3. A long upper limb can interfere with epiglottic closure, resulting in aspiration. If the cut end sits too close to the vocal cords, it may result in mucosal irritation and ulceration, with the potential for granulation tissues and laryngeal stenosis.

4. Do not use the T tube technique with free mucosal or skin grafts. The manipulations required for insertion predispose the graft to shearing and displacement. An open procedure using a conforming silicone stent or a soft sponge stent is recommended for subglottic injuries of this type (see Chapter 94).

5. A close cooperative and communicative effort between the surgeon and the anesthesiologist is essential during the procedure to ensure safe and controlled airway management.

6. The horizontal limbs of the T tube should extend 3 to 4 cm beyond the surface of the skin. Short limbs can predispose to retrodisplacement of the tube during vigorous coughing. Newer tubes with external ring cuffs help overcome this problem.

COMPLICATIONS

1. Displacement of mucosal and cartilaginous segments may occur during insertion. For this reason, direct visualization by bronchoscopy and careful guidance of the upper limb with laryngeal instrumentation will aid in a smooth and precise manipulation.

2. Aspiration can occur. Under such conditions, the patient should be fed a clear liquid diet. An efficient cough can be facilitated by occluding the horizontal limb of the tube. Usually the patient learns to compensate, and as aspiration is diminished or disappears, the patient can progress to a regular diet.

3. Restenosis may occur following T tube removal and can be managed early with dilatation. Failure to keep the airway open may necessitate a more formal reconstructive procedure (see Chapter 105).

4. The T tube can become displaced with coughing and choking. If the tube enters a bronchus and/or kinks, the patient can develop respiratory difficulty. If this occurs, the surgeon can open the tracheostomy with a nasal speculum, grasp the edge of the tube, and extract the tube. For tubes that are displaced even farther down the trachea, the surgeon will have to completely excise the tracheostomy site and gain control of the airway just beneath the area of tracheostomy.

5. Secretions can thicken, harden, and become obstructive. Management includes interval changes, administration of mucolytic agents, and appropriate suction techniques. For firmly adherent crusts, bronchoscopic removal may be necessary.

chapter 96

Internal Fixation of a Laryngeal Injury With a Teflon Keel

In Consultation With Richard Arden, MD

INDICATIONS

The alloplastic keel is best applied in those cases of blunt laryngeal trauma in which uncomplicated vertical fractures of the thyroid cartilage result in lacerations or mucosal disruptions of the anterior commissure and/or both vocal cords. Because of opposing raw mucosal surfaces, these cases have the potential for anterior web formation. By interposing a thin conforming keel that possesses low tissue reactivity, spontaneous epithelialization may ensue without significant fibrous cross-bridging between the vocal cords. A properly fitted keel should permit intelligible speech when the tracheostomy is plugged and should not interfere with swallowing functions.

PROCEDURE

The application of a keel is often preceded by a prophylactic tracheostomy (see Chapter 4) and placement of an anode tube. The keel is then aligned according to the size of the endolarynx. The length of the keel should correspond to measurements from the superior aspect of the thyroid to the top of the cricoid cartilage. The depth of the keel should be about the distance from the anterior commissure to the vocal process of the arytenoid. Ready-made keels are available, but the keel can also be made from standard septal splints that are trimmed according to the previously taken length and width measurements.

A–D In patients treated with open techniques, the keel is inserted just prior to closure of the thyrotomy. The true and false vocal cords should be secured to the edge of the thyroid cartilage. The keel is then brought into position and held with a No. 0 polypropylene suture. The placement of the suture is such that the external flanged surface of the keel lies on the thyroid cartilage, and the superior leading edge lies between the vocal cords. The suture is subsequently passed through one flange of the keel, the thyroid cartilage, and the opposite flange of the keel. The needle is returned in a similar fashion to create a figure-of-eight configuration. The needle is then cut off from the suture, and the ends are tied over the thyroid prominence. A similar procedure is performed over the lower part of the thyroid laminae. The thyroid cartilages are then approximated with heavy chromic sutures, and the platysma and skin are closed in layers. Placement of a subplatysmal Penrose drain (½-inch) for 1 to 2 days is desirable. Prophylactic antibiotics are given during keel retention, which is usually 2 to 3 weeks. The keel is easily removed transendoscopically after exposing and cutting the laryngeal sutures.

PITFALLS

1. The keel should be used only when injury involves the anterior commissure. For patients who also have damage to the arytenoids or vocal cords, the surgeon should consider a soft stent with or without a graft (see Chapter 94).

2. After securing the retention sutures, it is imperative to check for proper seating of the upper and lower ends of the keel. The leading keel angle should fit into the anterior commissure, and excessive tension should be avoided as the sutures are tied down.

3. Make sure that the vocal cords are secured to the thyroid cartilage at the same level. Vocal cord apposition following removal of the keel is the primary determinant of voice quality.

COMPLICATIONS

1. Granulation tissue formation may occur at the upper and lower ends of the keel and may develop, in part, from movement of the keel against opposing

mucosa. If not corrected, this inflammatory process can also lead to web formation. Fixing the keel to the laryngeal skeleton and then removing the sutures later using an open technique will reduce the possibility of such sequelae.

2. The keel, if improperly placed, can cause exposure of thyroid cartilage and subsequent chondritis. This complication can be avoided by making sure the keel fits the opening (i.e., not too large or too small). Tight fixation should also prevent movement and further irritation of the tissues.

3. Aspiration may be a problem in some patients who are treated with a keel that is too large. One or several factors can contribute to the complication. The device itself can interfere with epiglottic closure and approximation of the true and false cords. An open tracheostomy will reduce subglottic pressures and afford little, if any, protection against entry of food or drink into the upper airway. Temporarily plugging the tracheostomy tube during eating or drinking may be helpful. If aspiration continues, the surgeon should consider either a redesign of the keel or an alternative technique.

INTERNAL FIXATION WITH TEFLON KEEL

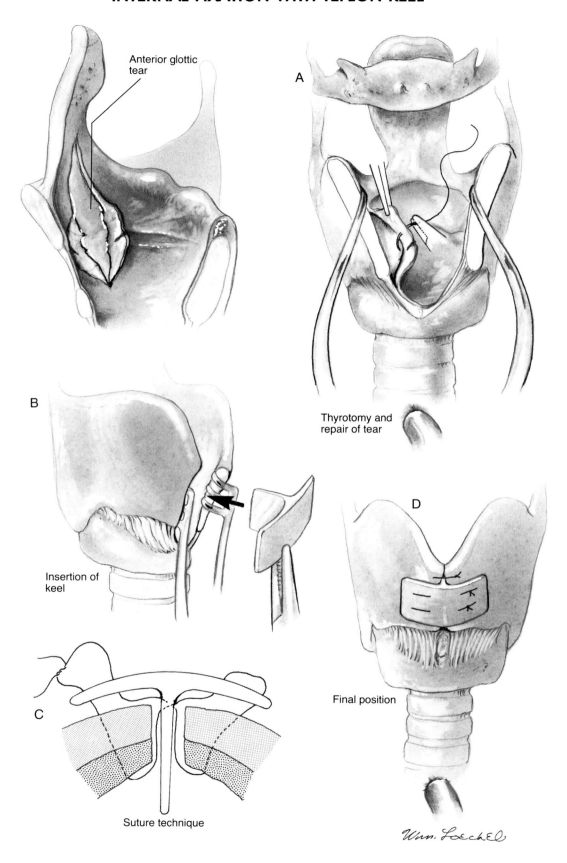

Anterior glottic tear

A

Thyrotomy and repair of tear

B

Insertion of keel

C

Suture technique

D

Final position

Wm. Loechel

section III

Supraglottic Injury

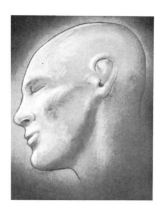

chapter 97

Treatment of Supraglottic Injury With Supraglottic Laryngectomy
Alternative Techniques of Anterior Pharyngotomy With Partial Supraglottic Resection and Epiglottic Base Resection

In Consultation With Richard Arden, MD

INDICATIONS

The surgical approach and method of repair used for a supraglottic injury characterized by avulsion and/or laceration require an understanding of the extent of injury and the degree of vocal cord mobility. The epiglottis is important for the supraglottic valve mechanism that protects the larynx from aspiration. In its absence, the valve must be compensated with a more posterior excursion of the tongue, a more anterior displacement of the larynx, and complete closure effected by the true and false vocal cords. Attempts should thus be made to preserve the epiglottis, but when this is not possible, complete or partial resection must be considered.

If there is an extensive comminution of the thyroid ala in which repair of the cartilage is not feasible, a conventional supraglottic laryngectomy is indicated. If the thyroid cartilage fracture is limited to its superior half and vocal cord mobility (and glottic competence) can be established, the supraglottic injury can be managed by an interfragmentary repair and a partial supraglottic resection. If true vocal cord mobility is impaired and the epiglottis is dislocated only, it is probably advisable to resect the inferior portion (petiole) and reattach the epiglottic base to the superior margin of the thyroid cartilage.

TECHNIQUE

Anesthesia is provided by an endotracheal tube, with conversion at the end of the procedure to a tracheostomy (see Chapter 4). Alternatively, the sur-

475

geon can control the airway with an initial tracheostomy followed by placement of an anode tube. A nasogastric tube is also inserted.

A–C A transverse skin incision is made in a skin crease at the midthyroid cartilage level. Subplatysmal flaps are elevated both superiorly and inferiorly to expose the hyoid bone and cricoid cartilage. Assuming a pure supraglottic injury, the strap muscles are carefully mobilized from the thyroid ala and underlying cricoid. Sharp division of these muscles at a level just above the thyroid cartilage is carried out, followed by incision of the thyroid cartilage perichondrium at its superior border. A subperichondrial flap is developed inferiorly with a Freer elevator, and the thyroid cartilage is exposed to visualize all fracture lines. Depending on the level of these fracture lines, transverse cartilage cuts are outlined between the superior thyroid notch and the attachment of the vocal cords, which occurs just below the midthyroid level. Vertical cuts are then made at least 1 cm medial to the superior horns to intersect with the transverse cuts on the thyroid cartilage. This should protect the internal laryngeal nerves and superior laryngeal arteries that penetrate the thyrohyoid membrane.

D–H The suprahyoid muscle attachments are next released with a dissection close to the hyoid. The superior and inferior horns are cut from the body. The hyoid is grasped with an Allis clamp and excised. The hypopharynx is then entered by sharp dissection through the base of the vallecula (or piriform sinus), and the tip of the epiglottis is secured with an Allis clamp. An incision is carried out across the vallecula. The thyrohyoid membrane cuts are then completed, and with appropriate counter rotation, endolaryngeal cuts are made through the aryepiglottic folds, just above the arytenoids and the false vocal cords toward the thyroid angle. By sectioning intervening tissues, the supraglottic larynx is mobilized and extracted.

Mucosal tears within the larynx should be carefully approximated with 4-0 chromic sutures. If primary repair cannot be implemented because of devitalized or avulsed segments of mucosa, the surgeon can use grafts with stents or, preferably, local flaps from the interarytenoid or piriform sinus region (see Chapter 101). Fractures of the remaining thyroid laminae should be identified and, if noted to be unstable, reduced and fixed with 28- or 30-gauge stainless steel wires. If the region is still unstable, the surgeon must consider an internal fixation technique (see Chapter 94).

I Two additional procedures can be used to minimize aspiration: laryngeal suspension and cricopharyngeal myotomy. Laryngeal suspension can be carried out by drop sutures from the mandibular symphysis adjusted to elevate the larynx 2 cm and thereby distribute the tension load. The net effect is anterosuperior rotation of the larynx, with protection from aspiration afforded by the overlying base of the tongue. Cricopharyngeal myotomy is carried out sharply with the No. 15 scalpel blade against a finger inserted on the mucosal surface of the cricopharyngeus muscle.

J,K Closure of the larynx is completed by approximating the thyroid cartilage perichondrium with the base of the tongue superiorly and the remnants of the thyrohyoid membrane laterally with interrupted 2-0 chromic sutures. A second layer of closure is accomplished by approximating the strap muscles loosely in the midline and to the tongue with interrupted 3-0 chromic sutures. A ½-inch Penrose drain is inserted, and the platysma and skin are closed with interrupted 3-0 chromic and 5-0 nylon sutures. Prophylactic antibiotics are given for 10 days.

PITFALLS

1. As in resection for neoplastic disease, supraglottic laryngectomy may be contraindicated in those elderly or debilitated persons or those with chronic lung disease who would otherwise not tolerate aspiration.

2. Care must be taken during the lateral part of the resection to preserve the superior laryngeal nerves. Sensory denervation can lead to aspiration problems.

3. Instability of the remaining cartilaginous laryngeal framework (after wiring), the presence of opposing raw mucosal surfaces (especially anteriorly), or separation of the inner perichondrial layer or intrinsic laryngeal musculature from the thyroid cartilage should be recognized and supported with an internal soft stent (see Chapter 94).

4. Avoid tension on mucosal closures. If such a condition develops, it is more prudent to use flaps or free mucosal grafting with internal soft stents (see Chapter 94).

COMPLICATIONS

1. Supraglottic laryngectomy effectively removes the supraglottic valve mechanism during swallowing and predisposes to aspiration. This complication is more prone to occur in patients who have inadequate vocal cord mobility and poor lung function; in such patients, the procedure should be avoided. Aspiration can also be minimized by suspension techniques and cricopharyngeal myotomy. If it should occur in spite of these precautions, the surgeon must consider

LARYNGEAL INJURY TREATED WITH SUPRAGLOTTIC LARYNGECTOMY

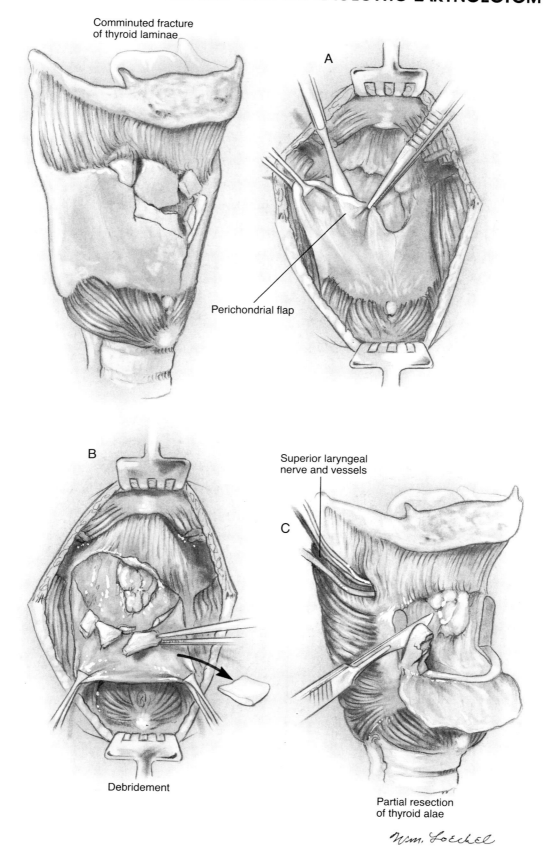

Comminuted fracture of thyroid laminae

Perichondrial flap

A

B

Debridement

Superior laryngeal nerve and vessels

C

Partial resection of thyroid alae

Wm. Loechel

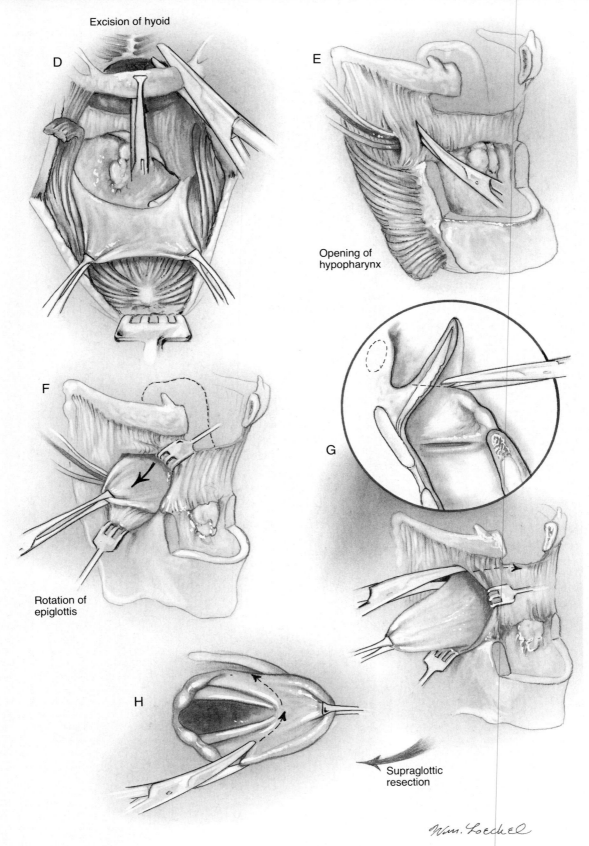

Excision of hyoid

D

E

Opening of
hypopharynx

F

G

Rotation of
epiglottis

H

Supraglottic
resection

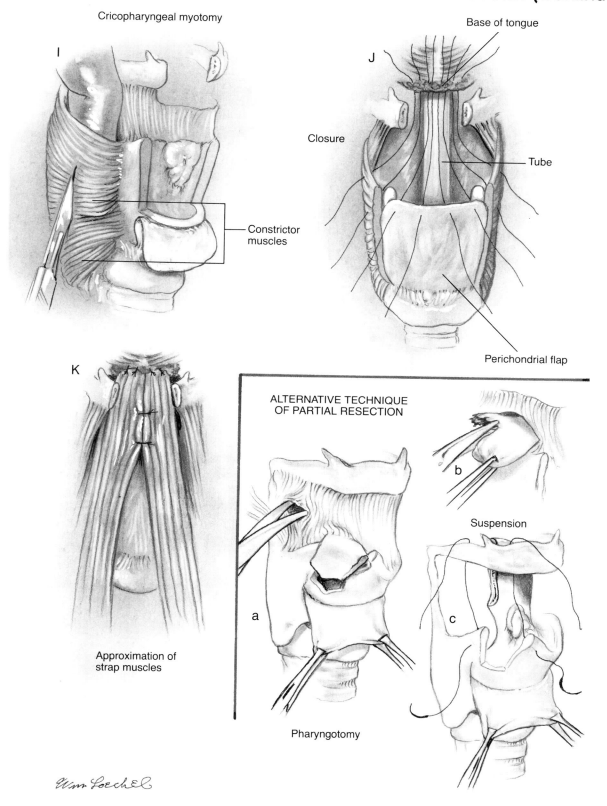

Cricopharyngeal myotomy

I

Constrictor muscles

Base of tongue

J

Closure

Tube

Perichondrial flap

K

Approximation of strap muscles

ALTERNATIVE TECHNIQUE OF PARTIAL RESECTION

a

b

Suspension

c

Pharyngotomy

Wm Loechel

training the patient in supraglottic swallowing and appropriate modifications in diet.

2. Some degree of respiratory obstruction may be noted following supraglottic resection. Usually this is the result of swelling of the arytenoids and false cords, and in such cases, improvement will occur with time. Excessive folds or granulations can be removed microsurgically or with a laser technique.

ALTERNATIVE TECHNIQUE OF ANTERIOR PHARYNGOTOMY WITH PARTIAL SUPRAGLOTTIC RESECTION

A modified supraglottic resection for limited injuries to the supraglottic larynx can be carried out using suprahyoid, transhyoid, or infrahyoid approaches. The goal of this surgery is the conservative removal of devitalized segments while preserving epiglottic and vocal cord functions.

a,b The skin incision is placed in a transverse skin crease line near the upper border of the thyroid cartilage. Superior and inferior subplatysmal flaps are developed, and the strap muscles are separated away from the laryngeal complex. The insertions of the sternohyoid and a portion of the thyrohyoid muscles are sharply divided at the inferior border of the hyoid bone and reflected inferolaterally. An inferiorly based flap of thyrohyoid membrane incorporating perichondrium covering the thyroid laminae is developed to a level sufficient to expose the fracture lines of the superior part of the thyroid. Comminuted or unstable segments are resected; fractured but stable segments can be reinforced by interchondral sutures or wires.

An anterior pharyngotomy is then made by transversely incising the thyrohyoid membrane near its midportion, being careful to visualize and protect the neurovascular pedicle entering laterally. The surgeon then resects the area of irreversible injury (i.e., epiglottis, aryepiglottic folds, or false cords).

C In preparation for closure and laryngeal suspension, 28-gauge stainless steel wires are passed around the hyoid in front of the thyrohyoid membrane flap and through the anterior edge of the remaining thyroid ala. If the hyoid is fractured and unstable, the segments are removed, and suspension is em-

ployed from the mandibular symphysis. Closure of the pharynx is then carried out by approximating the base of the tongue to the inferior thyrohyoid membrane flap. If possible, the superior flap should be imbricated and closed with 2-0 chromic sutures over the lower flap. The tension on the suspension wires is adjusted and the wires are tied to provide for laryngeal elevation and a decrease in tension on the suture line. The strap muscles are reattached and approximated in the midline with 3-0 chromic sutures. A two-layered closure with drainage completes the procedure.

ALTERNATIVE TECHNIQUE OF EPIGLOTTIC BASE RESECTION

The approach to the epiglottic base is initiated in a manner similar to that described for thyrotomy (see Chapter 93). Essentially the surgeon resects the base and closes the defect with advancement of the remaining epiglottis. This technique is useful in repairing a defect or stenosis of the anterior glottic area (see Chapter 10).

a–d A midline laryngofissure or a paramedian fracture line can provide appropriate access. Following careful separation of the thyroid ala and after appropriate endolaryngeal assessment and mucosal repair, a conservative resection of the preepiglottic space fat adjacent to the epiglottic base is carried out. A transverse mucosal incision is then made at the level of intended cartilage resection, and a submucoperichondrial plane is developed superiorly about 5 mm onto the anterior surface of the epiglottis. Epiglottic mucosal flaps are developed on the anterior cartilaginous surface and then on the posterior surface just above the level of the original mucosal incision. The epiglottic base is resected while protecting the mucosal flaps with malleable retractors. A 2-0 chromic suture is next passed between the thyroid ala and the remaining epiglottic base from anterior to posterior and then back again to the contralateral ala in a horizontal mattress fashion. The epiglottis is tacked with additional sutures to the thyroid cartilage. The remainder of the closure and postoperative care are as described for thyrotomy (see Chapter 93).

ALTERNATIVE TECHNIQUE OF EPIGLOTTIC BASE RESECTION

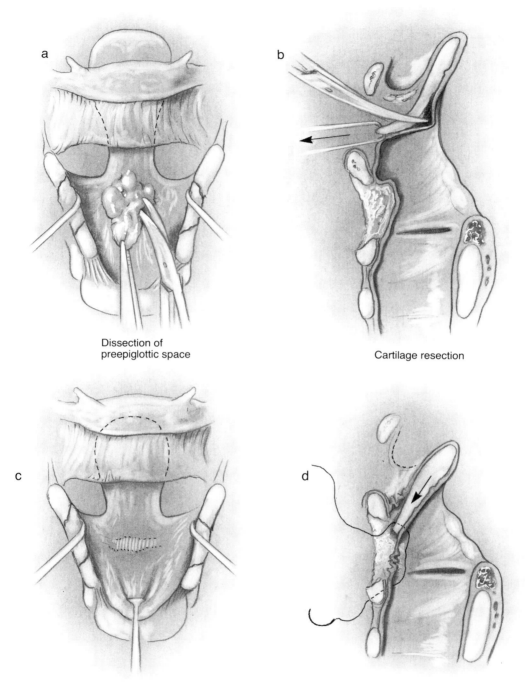

a

Dissection of
preepiglottic space

b

Cartilage resection

c

d

Advancement of epiglottic base

section IV

Subglottic Injury

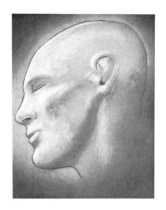

chapter 98

Open Repair of Subglottic Injury
Alternative Technique of Hyoid Interposition Graft

In Consultation With Richard Arden, MD

INDICATIONS

Acute subglottic injury is often an emergency characterized by early obstruction and respiratory distress. In such situations, control of the airway takes priority. Any cervical spine injury and the degree and extent of subglottic damage are subsequently evaluated by endoscopy and appropriate imaging techniques.

A spectrum of injuries are recognized, including isolated cricoid fracture, comminution of the cricoid arch, and laryngotracheal disruption. In general, limited cricoid arch fractures are managed by open reduction with optional soft stenting. Cricoid comminution requires a composite hyoid arch transposition or a resection with a thyrotracheal anastomosis. Laryngotracheal disruption is often managed with a direct cricotracheal repair.

PROCEDURE

A Following a tracheostomy at the third or fourth tracheal ring (see Chapter 4), a transverse collar neck incision is outlined over the lower half of the thyroid cartilage. Superior and inferior subplatysmal flaps are developed to allow exposure of the thyroid and cricoid cartilages, as well as the first and second tracheal rings. An effort should be made to maintain soft tissue between the newly created tracheostomy site and the area of cricoid repair.

B–D The investing and pretracheal fascia are incised in the midline; the thyroid isthmus is divided, and the thyroid lobes are retracted laterally to expose the cartilaginous laryngeal structures. Because endoscopy has already been performed, a determination will have been made regarding the necessity of opening into the larynx (e.g., for denuded mucosa requiring free grafting or grossly displaced fracture segments). If mucosal continuity has been essentially maintained with minor displacements of the fracture segments, then reduction using the tip of the rigid bronchoscope or application of a tissue-holding clamp can facilitate appropriate repositioning. If the larynx must be entered, the surgeon should extend the incision from the fracture line into the cricotra-

483

REPAIR OF CRICOID INJURY

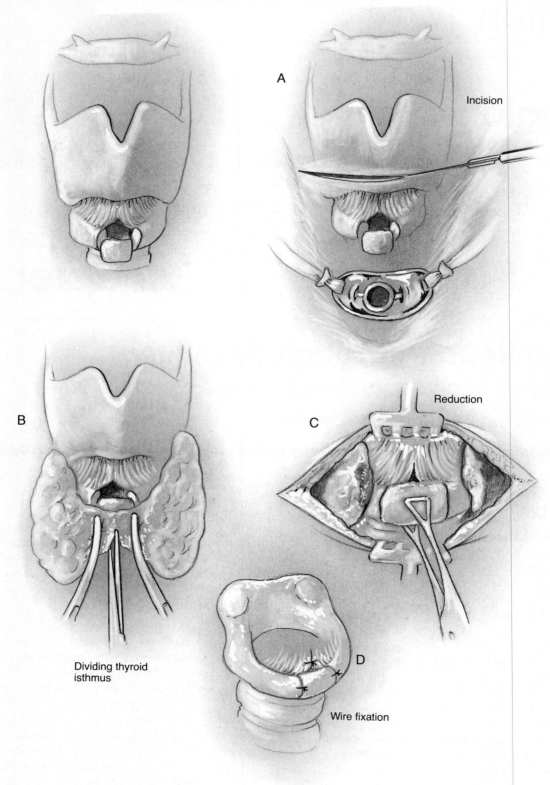

A

Incision

B

Dividing thyroid
isthmus

C

Reduction

D

Wire fixation

Wm. LoechEl

cheal/cricothyroid membranes. Additional cuts through the thyroid cartilage in the midline will provide the necessary exposure for free grafting, mucosal repair (4-0 chromic suture), reduction of cartilage segments, and soft stent placement (see Chapter 94). Fractures are usually stabilized extralumenally with 30- to 32-gauge stainless steel wire. Comminution of fractures and instability of the cricoid area should be treated with either rotation or free flaps from the hyoid with appropriate fixation (see later) and/or long-term placement of a T tube (see Chapter 95). Cricopharyngeal separation should be repaired by suturing the first ring of the trachea to the cricoid with strategic placements of 3-0 chromic sutures.

The cricothyroid membrane is repaired with 3-0 or 4-0 chromic sutures. A small drain is placed and the overlying soft tissues are approximated with additional 4-0 chromic sutures. The skin is closed with a 5-0 nylon suture, and prophylactic antibiotics are employed for 7 to 10 days.

PITFALLS

1. Failure to recognize associated injuries such as arytenoid dislocation, esophageal rupture, or cervical spine trauma can lead to complications of glottic incompetence, fistula, or neurologic injury. For this reason, the patient must be carefully evaluated with a detailed history, physical examination (including indirect laryngoscopy), sequential endoscopy, and computed tomographic (CT) scans in the horizontal plane.

2. The integrity of the cricoid arch is essential for respiration. For these reasons, debridement should be minimized and reconstruction limited to simple techniques that will not disrupt the blood supply of the tissues. The larynx should not be entered for exploration unless there is a strong indication of failure in reduction and/or repair of intralaryngeal injury.

3. Make sure that the dissection of tissues is limited to the central portion of the cricoid, as the recurrent nerve can be injured laterally. This should be avoided.

4. An internal stent should be employed any time stability of the framework is in question. The T tube (see Chapter 95) is a very popular technique and is often indicated. Failure to stent can lead to a retro-displacement of fracture segments and stenosis.

COMPLICATIONS

1. Subglottic stenosis is probably the most common significant complication following cricoid injury.

Appropriate reduction of the fragments and fixation should help avoid this occurrence. Early stenosis can be treated with dilatation and steroid injections. Persistent stenosis may require resection of the involved segment and either an interposition graft or a fresh cricotracheal anastomosis.

2. Vocal cord paralysis and/or fixation is possible with cricoid injury. An accurate diagnosis should distinguish between the various conditions. If paralysis is present and vocal cord function does not return, then a cartilage interposition or Teflon implant is indicated (see Chapter 99). For bilateral paralysis, an arytenoidectomy or neuromuscular pedicle procedure is preferred (see Chapter 100). Fixation and stenosis require dilatation and injection of steroids; if this does not work, resection of the involved area (i.e., arytenoidectomy and/or cordectomy) may have to be considered.

ALTERNATIVE TECHNIQUE OF HYOID INTERPOSITION GRAFT

Owing to its regional proximity and strength, the hyoid bone is well suited for interpositional grafting. The gentle curve and thickness of its body is helpful in reinforcing an anterior cricoid arch deficiency. In using the hyoid autograft, we prefer to raise it based on a vascularized muscle pedicle composed of sternohyoid muscle with or without attached omohyoid (depending on the length of graft needed). In contrast to a free graft technique, the vascularized graft should provide optimal conditions for healing, thus lessening the chances of resorption and fibrous tissue replacement.

a–d In preparation for the graft, all devitalized cartilage fragments should be removed, preserving as much inner perichondrium as possible. Endolaryngeal mucosal tears are meticulously repaired with 4-0 chromic sutures, and the larger, more viable, cartilaginous segments are retained and stabilized with 30- or 32-gauge stainless steel wires. Next the length of the cricoid defect is measured with a ruler, keeping the defect's anterior convexity in mind. This length is then mapped out over the body of the hyoid, but if necessary, it can extend beyond the lesser cornus laterally. The suprahyoid muscular attachments overlying the donor segment to be used are released. Working from below, posterolaterally to anteromedially, the layers of fascia that invest the sternohyoid (and omohyoid) muscle are preserved and followed to the level of the hyoid. Care must be exercised to avoid injury to the superior laryngeal neurovascular bundle. Using sharp bone cutters, hyoid osteotomies are created at the previously marked points. The underlying thyrohyoid muscle is

REPAIR OF CRICOID INJURY *(Continued)*

ALTERNATIVE TECHNIQUE OF HYOID GRAFT

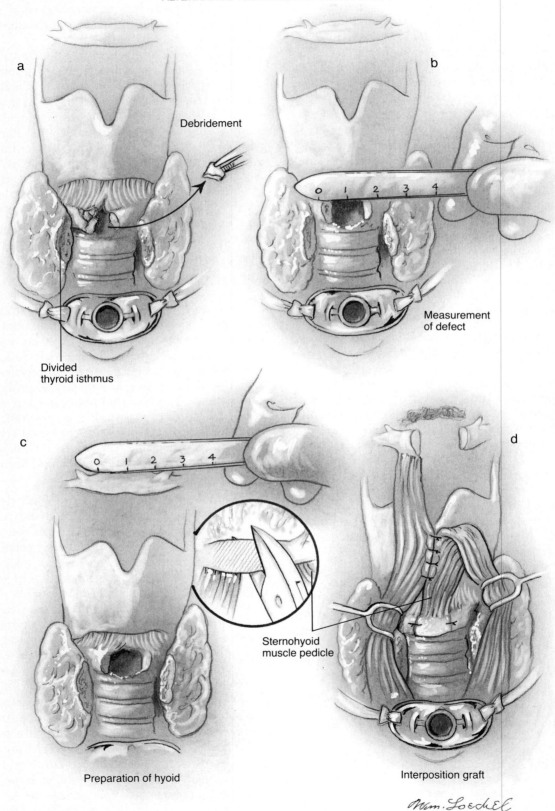

a

Debridement

Divided
thyroid isthmus

b

Measurement
of defect

c

Preparation of hyoid

Sternohyoid
muscle pedicle

d

Interposition graft

Wm. Loechel

next divided sharply, and its attachments to the overlying strap muscles are released. The compound hyoid bone–muscle pedicle graft is then rotated into the cricoid defect.

If the graft is oriented vertically, 30- or 32-gauge stainless steel wire, placed extralumenally, can be used to secure it to the thyroid cartilage above and the first tracheal ring below. If the graft is to be oriented horizontally, it is secured to the ends of the remaining cricoid cartilage. Additional graft stability can be provided by approximating the medial borders of the sternohyoid muscles to each other with absorbable sutures. A standard two-layer closure with drainage is employed, and prophylactic antibiotics are given for 7 to 10 days.

section V

Vocal Cord Paralysis

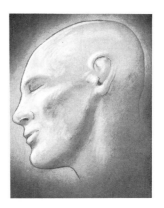

chapter 99

Treatment of Unilateral Vocal Cord Paralysis With Teflon Injection
Alternative Technique of Cartilaginous Interposition

INDICATIONS

Recurrent laryngeal nerve injury is often a consequence of laryngeal trauma, especially when there has been a laryngotracheal separation or cricoarytenoid compression. Paralysis limited to one side causes a weak voice and, in some patients, aspiration of food or drink. In bilateral paralysis, the voice remains strong, but the adducted vocal cords may compromise the airway and often cause obstruction.

Unilateral vocal cord paralysis is sometimes difficult to evaluate and distinguish from posterior glottic scarring. Moreover, the diagnosis of vocal cord paralysis can be confounded by associated injuries to the superior laryngeal nerve and swelling, laceration, and hematoma in and around the glottic chink.

The patient with cervical trauma should be evaluated for adequacy of the airway, and if there is obstruction (present or impending), he or she should be treated with cricothyrotomy or tracheostomy (see

Chapters 3 and 4). The cervical spine should also be checked for injury. The vocal cords can then be inspected by mirror examination, carefully recording their appearance and function. At a later time, the surgeon will want to palpate the mobility of the arytenoid joint by way of endoscopy and assay the thyroarytenoid muscle electrically with electromyography. Videotaping and voice recordings are desirable. Computed tomographic (CT) scans should be used to elucidate the anatomic integrity of the glottic area.

Isolated unilateral vocal cord paralysis should not cause any urgent problems, but the patient may complain of a weak voice, hoarseness, and occasionally, aspiration of fluids. Speech therapy may help, but vocal cord function that does not return within 6 to 9 months suggests a poor prognosis, and the surgeon should consider a surgical method of rehabilitation. Teflon injection is an easy-to-perform and popular technique. Alternatively, interposition of a cartilage graft can be considered.

PROCEDURE

Ideally the Teflon injection procedure is performed on a sedated patient. The oral cavity, pharynx, and larynx are treated with 4 mL of a 4% cocaine solution; if the cocaine is applied with cotton pledgets, it will be diluted by saliva, and up to 8 mL of the solution can be used. We prefer the following stepwise approach:

1. One or two sprays of the cocaine to the oral cavity and pharynx.
2. Cocaine painting (with cotton pledgets) of the lips, tongue, oral and buccal mucosa, tonsillar fossae, palate, and oropharynx until the gag reflex is depressed.
3. Forceps application of cocaine-soaked pledgets into the piriform sinuses and valleculae.
4. Instillation of the remainder of the cocaine solution with a laryngeal syringe and mirror on the vocal cords and through the glottic chink.

The patient is then placed in the supine position, and a laryngoscope is introduced into the larynx. The larynx is reevaluated and the laryngoscope fixed to a holder. A microscope with a 400-mm objective lens is then focused onto the vocal cord area.

A–C The patient is asked to phonate, and cord mobility is evaluated. The aim of the vocal cord injection is to move the paralyzed vocal cord to the midline, but not beyond that point. The injection should thus be placed lateral to the thyroarytenoid muscle and anterior to the vocal process of the arytenoid. A pistol-grip syringe with a long laryngeal needle is loaded with Teflon paste. A spatula is used to lateralize the false vocal cord, exposing the ventricle. The needle of the syringe is then inserted and directed just lateral to the true vocal cord. The needle depth should be approximately 2 to 3 mm beneath the mucosa. A small amount of Teflon is introduced, and the surgeon then waits 1 to 2 minutes for it to leave the syringe. If the medial displacement of the vocal cord is less than desirable, additional amounts of Teflon are injected, again injecting very small amounts each time. The degree of infiltration is observed, and the ability of the cords to phonate is checked after each of the injections by having the patient say "e." Ideally the vocal cords should just meet along the anterior two thirds of their free surface. The injected cord should not pass the midline or be displaced in a caudal-cephalic direction.

Postoperatively the patient is checked for respiratory difficulty. If the patient has any problem with breathing, steroids should be administered and the patient placed under close observation. If there are no complications, voice use can be restored as soon as the effects of anesthesia have disappeared.

PITFALLS

1. The diagnosis of vocal cord paralysis is important. The physician must be certain that the problem is a true recurrent laryngeal nerve paralysis, free of arthritis or stenosis. A normally functioning superior laryngeal nerve is preferred. Any question of fixation or stenosis should be resolved with electromyographic studies.

With regard to timing, the surgeon must wait at least 6 to 9 months for return of vocal cord function. If the patient is severely incapacitated by voice weakness and/or aspiration, it is possible to inject Gelfoam, which will provide short-term, temporary effects. If, after 9 months, there is no return of function, the Teflon injection can be considered.

2. Neurorrhaphy of the recurrent laryngeal nerve is controversial. If there is evidence of transection of the recurrent nerve, it is probably prudent to explore the recurrent laryngeal nerve and effect a microscopic repair. However, it should be noted that results are variable, and the Teflon injection still may be needed at a later time.

3. Injection of Teflon is ideal for the small to moderate deficiency. However, if the defect is large (e.g., following atrophy or removal of the vocal cord), the Teflon injection often is not sufficient. Under such conditions, the surgeon should consider the cartilaginous interposition technique (see later).

4. Avoid overinjection of the Teflon. The syringe has a tendency to extrude material even after pressure has been released. A few practice squirts into the drapes prior to injection will give the surgeon a better appreciation of the pressure and the amount of Teflon that will be injected.

5. Avoid injection that is too deep or through the vocal cord. The Teflon can fall into the bronchi, and to avoid this complication, the surgeon should move the vocal cord to the side and inspect the subglottic area. Any excess Teflon can be removed with laryngeal suction. Injection of the material into the conus elasticus should be avoided, as this can cause narrowing of the subglottic region, which can potentially cause respiration obstruction.

COMPLICATIONS

1. Teflon injections must be accurate. Experience with the syringe will help control the amount and placement of the injection. Underinjection can easily be corrected by repeat injections at later times. An overinjection, however, can result in excessive me-

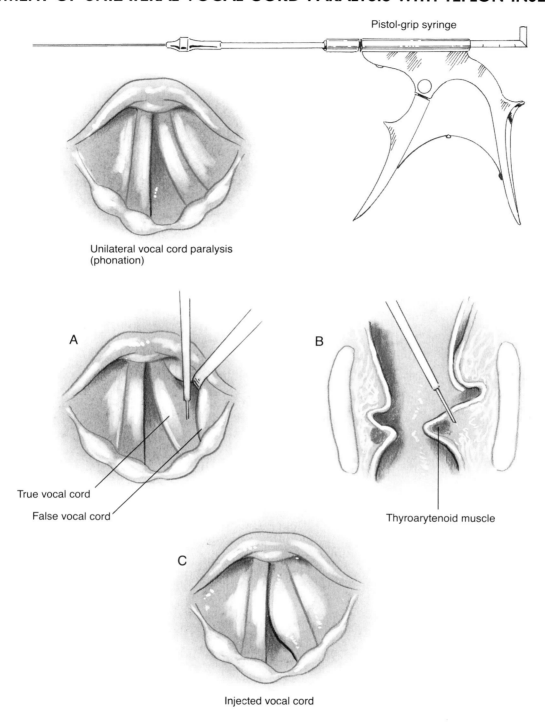

Pistol-grip syringe

Unilateral vocal cord paralysis
(phonation)

A

True vocal cord

False vocal cord

B

Thyroarytenoid muscle

C

Injected vocal cord

dialization or bulging of the vocal cord, causing phonatory and respiratory problems. If such a situation develops, the surgeon must be prepared to remove the Teflon, either by surgical or laser techniques. Injection below the cord must be recognized and the material removed, or the Teflon will enter the bronchi. Injection into the conus elasticus can be avoided by inspecting the subglottic area following each injection of the Teflon and by keeping the needle 2 to 3 mm below the upper surface of the mucosa.

It is also important that the Teflon not be introduced lateral to the vocal process. If this should occur, there can be more medialization posteriorly than anteriorly, causing a defect between the anterior two thirds of the cords. Occasionally this can be corrected by injecting additional amounts of Teflon just lateral to the thyroarytenoid muscle or by removal of the Teflon that has been overinjected lateral to the vocal process.

2. Teflon, although generally considered inert, can occasionally cause reactions. If the vocal cord swells following injection and the swelling is associated with pain and redness, the patient should be treated with a short course of steroids. Respiratory difficulty may require hospitalization, and if there is dyspnea, a tracheostomy may have to be considered.

ALTERNATIVE TECHNIQUE OF CARTILAGE GRAFT

Adduction paralysis, complicated by loss of vocal cord tissues or an opening that is too large and not corrected by Teflon, should prompt the consideration of a cartilage graft. Its main advantage is that autologous material, which is less apt to undergo reaction or displacement, is used. However, the effects are not constant, and if resorption occurs, the vocal cord defect will return.

A tracheostomy is desirable for anesthesia, as it provides excellent access and evaluation of the glottic chink. Moreover, if the glottis swells and causes obstruction, postoperative control of the airway will be possible.

The thyrotomy is performed through a horizontal curvilinear incision that is marked at the midportion of the thyroid cartilage. The tissues are infiltrated

with 1% lidocaine containing 1:100,000 epinephrine. The incision is carried through the superficial layers and into a subplatysmal plane that is developed superiorly and inferiorly. The thyrohyoid muscles are retracted laterally to expose the prominence of the thyroid cartilage.

a The perichondrium of the thyroid cartilage is incised in the midline and then horizontally across the lamina of the affected side. Using an oscillating saw, the thyroid is split in the midline (thyroidotomy), and from a tunnel just beneath the lower portion of the thyroid, scissors are used to cut the mucosa and the anterior commissure. A subperichondrial pocket is created just beneath the true vocal cord.

b—e The periosteum is then elevated external to the thyroid lamina, and the thyrohyoid muscle is retracted superiorly. Care is taken not to injure the superior laryngeal nerve, which lies just above the upper border of the lamina. The internal periosteum is subsequently freed from its attachment to the upper half of the thyroid cartilage, and with an oscillating saw or knife, a portion of cartilage is isolated and removed. The lower portion and midportion of the thyroid cartilage are then retracted laterally, and with visualization of the affected vocal cord, the cartilage graft is inserted beneath the perichondrium and directly lateral to the vocal cord. The perichondrium is closed with 3-0 chromic sutures, and the thyroid lamina is approximated with 2-0 chromic sutures.

At this point, the opening within the larynx is checked with a laryngoscope. If the medialization of the vocal cord is satisfactory, the investing layers of fascia, subcutaneous tissues, and skin are closed in layers. A small Penrose drain is usually retained for 24 hours. If the displacement of the vocal cord is less than optimal, the cartilage should be removed, its size adjusted, and closure and evaluation repeated.

The patient should be given prophylactic antibiotics for about 5 days. The tracheostomy is retained until the surgeon is assured that the postoperative swelling has subsided and the airway is adequate for respiration. If the implant becomes displaced or causes problems with phonation or respiration, removal may be required. Insufficient closure of the glottic chink can sometimes be corrected with Teflon injection.

TREATMENT OF UNILATERAL VOCAL CORD PARALYSIS *(Continued)*

ALTERNATIVE TECHNIQUE OF CARTILAGE GRAFT

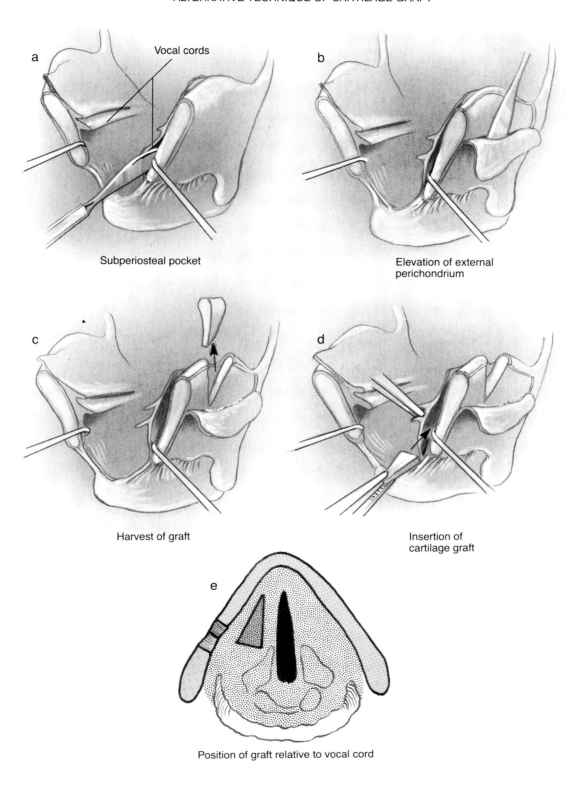

a
Vocal cords
Subperiosteal pocket

b
Elevation of external perichondrium

c
Harvest of graft

d
Insertion of cartilage graft

e
Position of graft relative to vocal cord

Wm. Loechel

Treatment of Bilateral Vocal Cord Paralysis With Arytenoidectomy by Way of Thyrotomy
Alternative Techniques of Endoscopic Arytenoidectomy and Neuromuscular Pedicle Reinnervation

INDICATIONS

The presumed mechanism of bilateral vocal cord paralysis following trauma is a crush injury or an associated laryngotracheal separation. In most patients, there is a mild dyspnea with a strong voice; in others, there can be a moderate to severe respiratory obstruction. In this latter group, intubation and/or tracheostomy must be employed.

Although it is not predictable, many patients recover vocal cord function. The patient's prognosis can usually be established at about 6 to 9 months following injury, and it is at this time that plans can be made for static or dynamic lateralization of the vocal cord. The condition must be distinguished from fixation, and for this evaluation, the surgeon should perform endoscopic mobility studies. Electromyography, videotaping, and voice recordings are desirable.

Bilateral vocal cord paralysis is treated with an arytenoidectomy or a neuromuscular reinnervation procedure. Arytenoidectomy can be performed either through a thyrotomy or through a laryngoscope using microscopic or laser techniques. The thyrotomy provides excellent exposure but can be complicated by postoperative hematoma and/or infection. The endoscopic method is easier to carry out but can be compromised by incomplete removal of the arytenoid and subsequently, an incomplete lateralization of the vocal cord.

The neuromuscular pedicle reinnervation method is more controversial than the arytenoidectomy. It has the advantage of being a dynamic method of rehabilitation, but the results are variable and less reliable. Nevertheless, if the procedure fails, there is still an opportunity to perform an arytenoidectomy. The neuromuscular pedicle reinnervation procedure will not work if there is any arytenoid ankylosis or interarytenoid fibrosis, and in patients with these conditions, the surgeon has a better chance of success with an arytenoidectomy.

PROCEDURE

The thyrotomy is usually performed under general anesthesia by way of a tracheostomy. The neck is prepared and draped as a sterile field. A transverse incision is marked across the thyroid and then infiltrated with 1% lidocaine containing 1:100,000 epinephrine for control of hemostasis.

A The incision should be extended through the platysma and a plane developed superiorly and inferiorly to expose the strap muscles. The sternohyoid and sternothyroid muscles are identified and retracted laterally. The thyroid cartilage perichondrium is incised in the midline, and a small opening is made in the cricothyroid membrane. The thyroid cartilage is then split with an oscillating saw, and from the subglottic space, the mucosa is incised in a cephalic direction between the vocal cords. Above the vocal cords, the incision can be directed to the side of the petiole. The thyroid laminae are retracted laterally with self-retaining retractors to expose the posterior wall of the larynx.

B,C The affected arytenoid is identified, and a vertical-to-oblique incision (1.5 cm) is made over the cartilage. The vocal process is exposed and freed from the thyroarytenoid muscle with small scissors. The vocal process is then grasped and pulled forward. The perichondrial tissues and the extrinsic arytenoid musculature are separated from the cartilage. Finally, the joint is cleaved and the arytenoid extracted from the wound. The mucosa is closed with two 4-0 chromic sutures.

D,E Lateralization of the vocal cord can be im-

ARYTENOIDECTOMY FOR BILATERAL VOCAL CORD PARALYSIS

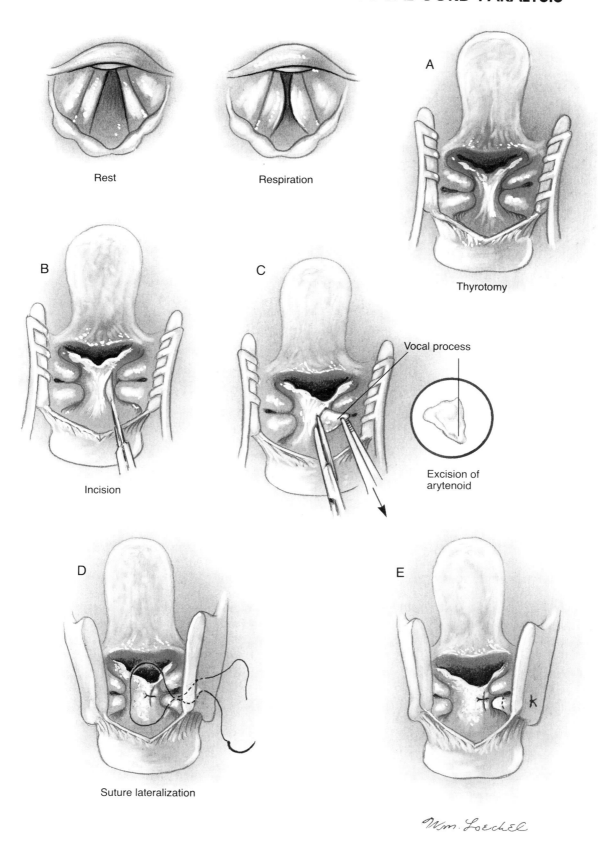

Rest

Respiration

A

Thyrotomy

B

Incision

C

Vocal process

Excision of arytenoid

D

Suture lateralization

E

Wm. Loechel

proved by suturing the vocal cord laterally to the thyroid lamina. For this procedure, the sternohyoid and sternothyroid muscles are retracted laterally from the thyroid laminae, and with a large curved needle, a 3-0 nonabsorbable suture is passed through the lamina and through the upper mucosal surface of the vocal cord. The needle should be directed several millimeters anterior to the arytenoid wound. The needle is then withdrawn and returned through the same mucosal hole to run submucosally around the vocal cord and then back out through the thyroid lamina. The suture is tied laterally to the thyroid lamina, and the position of the vocal cord is checked with a laryngoscope and adjusted accordingly.

The thyroid cartilage and perichondrium are approximated with 2-0 chromic sutures. The wound is then closed in layers, using 4-0 chromic and 5-0 nylon sutures, respectively, through the platysma and skin. A small Penrose drain should be used for 1 to 2 days. Prophylactic antibiotics are prescribed for 5 days. The tracheostomy can be removed when postoperative swelling is no longer a problem and the patient tolerates the plugging of the tube for at least 24 to 48 hours.

PITFALLS

1. Bilateral vocal cord paralysis must not be confused with fixation. The patient must be evaluated for arytenoid mobility and the absence of interarytenoid or subglottic stenosis. Electromyographic recordings may be a valuable adjunct in confirming the diagnosis.

2. Make sure that the arytenoid is completely removed and the vocal cord is adequately lateralized. Sometimes the arytenoid can be removed, and the vocal cord still remains near or across the midline. The degree of lateralization should be confirmed endoscopically before termination of the procedure.

3. A drain is important, as the wound is often contaminated, and there is a possibility of saliva leaking through the mucosa into the subcutaneous tissues. The drain can usually be removed in 24 to 48 hours.

4. The tracheostomy is helpful in establishing an airway and reducing subglottic pressures. The tube should be retained until healing is complete and the surgeon is assured that coughing or sudden increases in intrathoracic pressures will not disrupt the soft tissue closure. The timing of extubation is governed by plugging and exercise tolerance.

COMPLICATIONS

1. Infection and/or fistula formation are rare but can occur. To prevent these sequelae, prophylactic antibiotics should be prescribed and a drain employed for 1 to 2 days. The tracheostomy should be retained until healing is complete. If an infection develops in the postoperative period, the soft tissues of the neck should be opened and packed with antibiotic-treated gauze. Cultures should be obtained to determine the appropriate antibiotic treatment of specific pathogens.

2. Incomplete lateralization is probably one of the most common complications and can usually be avoided by complete removal of the arytenoid and the suture lateralization technique. However, if the vocal cord slips back into its original position, the surgeon can remove a portion of the cord with a partial cordectomy through microscopic or laser surgery.

3. Although rare, too much lateralization of the vocal cord can cause aspiration. For most patients, this will improve with time. If it continues, the physician should consider the Teflon injection technique (see Chapter 99).

ALTERNATIVE TECHNIQUE USING ENDOSCOPIC ARYTENOIDECTOMY

The arytenoid can also be removed endoscopically by way of laser or surgical resection. The procedure requires expertise and special instrumentation. Exposure can be limited by a small mouth and elements of trismus, and bleeding can be difficult to control. Because of these problems, the arytenoid may be only partially removed, and it may be difficult to achieve accurate positioning of the affected cord.

a,b Usually a tracheostomy is performed preliminarily to control anesthesia and prevent respiratory obstruction in the postoperative period. An operating laryngoscope is introduced to expose the glottic chink. An incision is made over the arytenoid, and the arytenoid is grasped with a laryngeal forceps. The cartilage is dissected free from the surrounding tissues. Bleeding can be controlled with an electric cautery, which will also cause more than usual tissue damage and will help develop more scarring and retraction of the vocal cord in the postoperative period. The mucosa is allowed to fall back into its normal position. Transcutaneous wire sutures can be used to lateralize the vocal cords, but because the amount of lateralization from the cauterization cannot be predicted, the lateralization procedure should be used sparingly. The laser method of removal requires special precautions and instrumentation. For this technique, a suitable laser surgery text should be consulted.

ALTERNATIVE TECHNIQUE USING NEUROMUSCULAR PEDICLE REINNERVATION

The lateralization procedure using a neuromuscular pedicle reinnervation requires a careful evaluation of vocal cord mobility. The procedure is contraindicated when there is arytenoid fixation. Results are variable, and the mechanism is still unclear. Although reinnervation may appear to be present, there is some evidence that the airway is actually tethered by the extralaryngeal muscle, and it is this contraction that opens the airway.

a' Tracheostomy is the preferred anesthesia route. The neck is prepared and draped as a sterile field. An incision is made at the midthyroid cartilage level and extended horizontally into a crease on the left side to later expose the left omohyoid muscle.

b' After infiltration with 1% lidocaine containing 1:100,000 epinephrine, the skin is incised through the platysma musculature. The omohyoid is identified at the anterior border of the sternocleidomastoid muscle. Using a blunt dissection, the sternocleidomastoid muscle is retracted posteriorly, exposing the jugular vein and fascia surrounding the vessel. Within this fascia, strands of ansa cervicalis will be found, and a nerve stimulator should be employed to help with this identification. The nerve and some fascia are then freed on a pedicle and kept attached to the omohyoid muscle. Using a microscope with a 250-mm objective lens, a 5 × 5–mm piece of omohyoid innervated by the nerve is excised and allowed to retract into the wound with the nerve pedicle.

c',d' The larynx is then rotated to the opposite side, and using the posterior edge of the lamina as a guide, the thyropharyngeal muscles are incised. A Senn retractor is used to rotate the lamina further, exposing the cricoarytenoid musculature. The arytenoid is palpated beneath the soft tissues. An incision is then made perpendicular to the long axis of the posterior cricoarytenoid muscle. Using the microscope, the omohyoid muscle pedicle is inserted into the defect and held with several 6-0 silk sutures. Tension should be avoided. The thyropharyngeal muscle is reattached to the lamina with chromic sutures (3-0) and the wound treated with a small Penrose drain. The platysma is closed with 4-0 chromic sutures and the skin with 5-0 nylon sutures.

Postoperatively a light dressing is applied. The dressing is removed in 24 to 48 hours. The patient is maintained on prophylactic antibiotics for 5 days. At about 1 or 2 weeks, attempts should be made to plug the tracheostomy tube. Extubation and exercise tolerance dictate the success of the procedure.

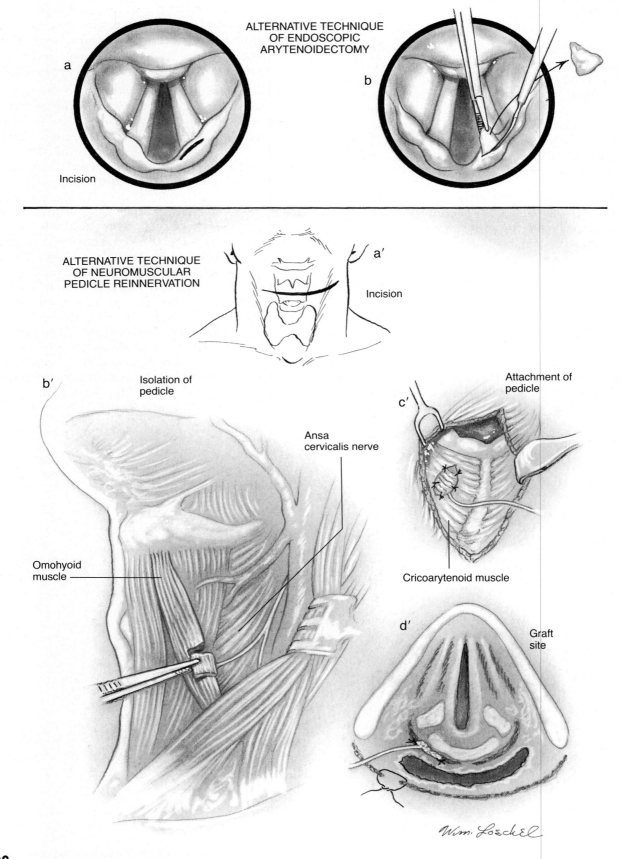

ALTERNATIVE TECHNIQUE OF ENDOSCOPIC ARYTENOIDECTOMY

a

Incision

b

ALTERNATIVE TECHNIQUE OF NEUROMUSCULAR PEDICLE REINNERVATION

a′

Incision

b′

Isolation of pedicle

Ansa cervicalis nerve

Omohyoid muscle

Attachment of pedicle

c′

Cricoarytenoid muscle

d′

Graft site

Wm. Loechel

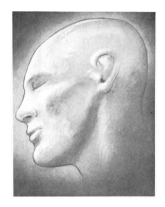

Treatment of Anterior Glottic Stenosis With Advancement of Mucosa, Skin Grafts, and Epiglottic and Interposition Grafts

INDICATIONS

Depending on the site and degree of injury to the larynx, there can be a variety of soft tissue contractions and stenoses. Supraglottic stenosis is usually caused by a retrodisplacement of the epiglottis and is often associated with injury to the hyoid and upper portions of the thyroid cartilage. An anterior midthyroid cartilage injury will cause shortening of the larynx as thyroid cartilage and soft tissues fill the anterior commissure. Injury to the arytenoid can cause scarring and limitation of vocal cord motion. Below the vocal cords, cricoid or tracheal injury will present with narrowing and/or web formation.

In general, patients with stenosis at any level of the larynx complain of a weak voice, hoarseness, and reduced exercise tolerance. Severely injured patients have respiratory distress and have been previously treated with intubation and/or tracheostomy.

Management of stenosis in the anterior and supraglottic region requires thoughtful design and implementation. A variety of procedures are available, but most focus on resection of the scar and prevention of new scar formation. The majority of the defects can be closed by advancement or rotation of mucosal flaps. More severe injuries in which the airway has been compromised will need interpositional grafts. Posterior glottic and subglottic stenosis, which can complicate the glottic injury, are discussed elsewhere (see Chapters 102 through 105).

PROCEDURE

Most approaches to laryngeal scarring will be through a standard thyrotomy (see Chapter 93). A tracheostomy is employed to provide general anesthesia and to control the airway during the postoperative period. A headlight or, even better, a microscope with its own lighting is valuable in performing the procedure.

A,B For the patient with limited supraglottic and anterior glottic stenosis, the thyroid laminae should be separated with self-retaining retractors. The larynx is entered, and small areas of scar tissue are removed. The surgeon has the option of applying a keel, as described in Chapter 96, or undermining and advancing the mucosal tissues with a primary closure using 4-0 or 5-0 chromic sutures. If the area of defect is larger than can be covered with such flaps, a full-thickness skin graft is harvested from the supraclavicular fossa and carefully sutured with 5-0 or 6-0 chromic sutures to the edge of the normal mucosa. The surgeon can consider a soft or firm stent for holding the graft (see Chapter 94).

C In patients with more extensive damage, the epiglottis can be used to provide the mucosal covering. Through the same thyrotomy exposure, incisions are carried laterally along the superior edge of the thyroid laminae, separating the thyrohyoid membrane from the laminae. The preepiglottic space is entered and a dissection carried out through the vallecula and laterally along the hyoepiglottic fold. The petiole of the epiglottis is then pulled inferiorly, and the soft tissues are used to close the defect created by resection of the scar tissues. If the anterior portion of the thyroid lamina is deficient, the flap is sutured directly to the edge of the thyroid lamina with 3-0 absorbable sutures. If the defect mostly involves the mucosal and soft tissues, portions of the petiole can be resected and the flap advanced into the anterior glottic space. Several sutures can be placed through the soft tissues to secure the flap into position. The more superior edges of the flap are attached also to the thyroid lamina (see Chapter 97). In either case, the result should be a lining of the larynx with the laryngeal surface of the epiglottis.

D If the thyroid laminae are severely damaged, hyoid interposition graft must be considered. The thyrotomy again provides a reasonable approach. The area of scarred tissue (and damaged cartilage) is resected. The hyoid bone is palpated and skeletonized in the midline. The suprahyoid muscles are released with a sharp scissors by cutting very close to the surface of the cartilage. The posterior and medial borders of the sternohyoid and omohyoid muscles are freed up, carefully avoiding injury to the deeper superior laryngeal nerve. The hyoid is cut medially and laterally with a bone-cutting instrument. The deeper thyrohyoid muscle is separated from the hyoid bone. The hyoid and muscle pedicle are then rotated and tested in the laryngeal defect. If there is a denuded surface internally, it should be treated with splints and covered with mucosa or skin grafts. The cartilage graft can then be stabilized with permanent sutures (30-gauge stainless steel wires); the muscle pedicle is attached with 3-0 chromic sutures to the strap muscles of the opposite side. A Penrose drain is used; the platysma and skin are closed in layers.

Patients having anterior glottic reconstructive procedures should be treated with prophylactic antibiotics for 5 to 7 days. If stents are used to stabilize the laryngeal skeleton, they should be removed in 3 to 4 weeks. If they are used only to hold a skin and mucosa graft, they should be removed in 7 to 10 days. Such an approach will minimize the development of granulation tissues. Healing should be evaluated by direct and indirect laryngoscopy. The tracheostomy should be plugged on a trial basis, and when the airway is adequate and there is no aspiration, it can be removed.

PITFALLS

1. If possible, the surgeon should retain viable healthy tissues and try not to use stents or keels. Unfortunately the mucosa may be difficult to undermine and advance over the defect, and when the defect is greater than 0.5 to 1 cm, a graft/stent technique will have to be applied.

2. The epiglottic mucosa provides a reasonably healthy flap that can be manipulated into a variety of defects of the anterior larynx. On the other hand, the anterior displacement of the epiglottis will affect the valve closure, and some aspiration can be expected to occur. This complication is usually transient and should disappear with time as the "supraglottic swallow" is learned. Intermittent plugging of the tracheostomy tube may be helpful.

3. The interposition hyoid graft should be secured to the thyroid laminae in such a way that it does not project or have the potential to become dislodged posteriorly into the larynx. Intralaryngeal stents will offer some security, but the grafts should still be stabilized with nylon or fine wire sutures to the thyroid laminae.

4. Avoid transposing too much tissue into the anterior larynx with the epiglottic and transposition techniques. If this should occur, the vocal cords may remain separated, the voice may be weak, and aspiration may occur. Therefore it is prudent to place just enough tissue to compensate for the soft tissue defect.

COMPLICATIONS

1. Infection can destroy the local tissues, flaps, and/or grafts and cause recurrent scarring. To protect against this occurrence, the wound should be drained for 24 to 48 hours. Prophylactic antibiotics should be used for 5 to 7 days. External stents and keels should be used sparingly and removed as soon as possible.

2. Stenosis associated with voice change and respiratory problems can occur. Early recognition of the

GLOTTIC REPAIR USING FLAPS AND GRAFTS

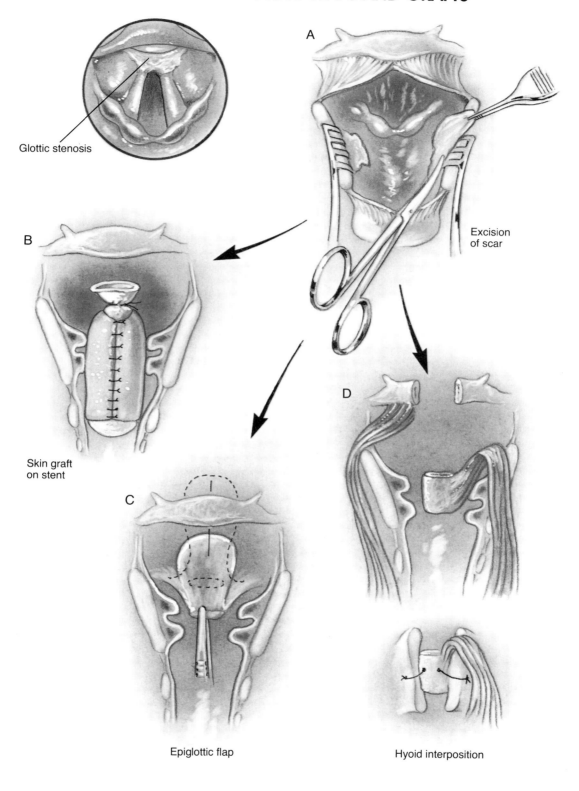

Glottic stenosis

A

Excision of scar

B

Skin graft on stent

C

Epiglottic flap

D

Hyoid interposition

developing scar tissues should prompt the use of intralesional steroids and dilatation. Endolaryngeal surgery (with or without use of a laser) may be helpful. If a reoperation is necessary, the surgeon will have to consider a wider resection and use of skin/mucosal graft techniques.

3. Aspiration will sometimes occur when the glottic chink has been made too wide. This occurs primarily with epiglottic flaps and interpositional hyoid grafts. The complication can be avoided by placing just enough tissue to fill the defect. If the cords are only slightly lateralized, it might be possible to endoscopically remove some of the intervening tissues or even inject the cord to a more medial position with Teflon (see Chapter 99).

chapter 102

Treatment of Posterior Glottic Stenosis With Interarytenoidopexy and Excision of Subglottic Webs

INDICATIONS

Vocal cord paralysis and fixation must be distinguished from each other if the surgeon is to select and apply the appropriate form of treatment. On indirect examination of the vocal cords, the paralyzed vocal cord will be associated with a "still arytenoid," and if seen sometime later, there will be atrophy and thinning of the vocal cord. If the patient with arytenoid fixation phonates, the corniculate process and the aryepiglottic fold will tend to move. The vocal cords will retain their anatomic appearance. Scarring may be observed in the interarytenoid space or in the posterior subglottic region. On direct laryngoscopy, the paralyzed vocal cords will separate on gentle pressure, and the arytenoid can be easily moved to a lateral position with a spatula. When the patient has a fixed cord, the vocal cord will be stiff and the arytenoid difficult to move in any direction. On electromyography, the fixed cord will be characterized by normal action potentials, whereas with paralysis, there will be fibrillation and polyphasic potentials.

The treatments of the two conditions are quite different. Bilateral vocal cord paralysis is often treated with a lateralizing procedure (see Chapter 100), whereas bilateral fixation requires removal of scar tissues between and below the arytenoid and either a flap or skin or mucosal graft coverage. Additionally, the patient may need a cordectomy with or without arytenoidectomy. Unilateral paralysis is generally treated with a Teflon or autogenous implant (see Chapter 99), whereas the unilateral fixed cord requires removal of scar tissue and resurfacing of the mucosa. If this latter procedure fails, the surgeon will also have to consider an implant technique.

PROCEDURE

A tracheostomy is performed to assist in anesthesia and provide a safe airway in the postoperative pe-

riod. The neck is prepared and draped as a sterile field. A microscope is sometimes helpful in carrying out this reconstruction.

A After infiltration with 1% lidocaine containing 1:100,000 epinephrine, a horizontal incision is made at the level of the inferior aspect of the thyroid cartilage through the platysma to expose the thyroid cartilage, the cricothyroid membrane, and the cricoid. As described in Chapter 93, a vertical anterior splitting incision is made through the cricothyroid membrane and thyroid laminae. The mucosa is then cut in the midline. The thyroid laminae are separated with a self-retaining retractor, the pathologic condition is evaluated, and a procedure is designed to deal with the condition.

For the patient with interarytenoid scarring, the scar is outlined with marking solution. The scar is subsequently excised, and if the underlying interarytenoid muscle is involved, it is conservatively removed with the scar. Bleeding is controlled with an electric cautery.

B–D If the defect is large and involves the surface of the arytenoids, a free graft of skin or mucous membrane should be considered. The graft can be retained by temporary placement of an intralaryngeal soft stent (see Chapter 94). For a more limited injury, the defect can be closed by designing a sliding flap based on the postcricoid mucosa and/or by advancement of local tissues. The mucosa is approximated with 5-0 chromic sutures.

In patients in whom the stenosis is caused by a subglottic web, the scar should be completely resected. The mucous membranes should be undermined, mobilized off the posterior tracheal wall, and advanced superiorly to close over the defect. The mucosa should be approximated with 5-0 or 6-0 chromic sutures. Larger subglottic areas of scarring are discussed in Chapter 105.

Following repair of the larynx and/or subglottic

INTERARYTENOIDOPEXY FOR GLOTTIC STENOSIS

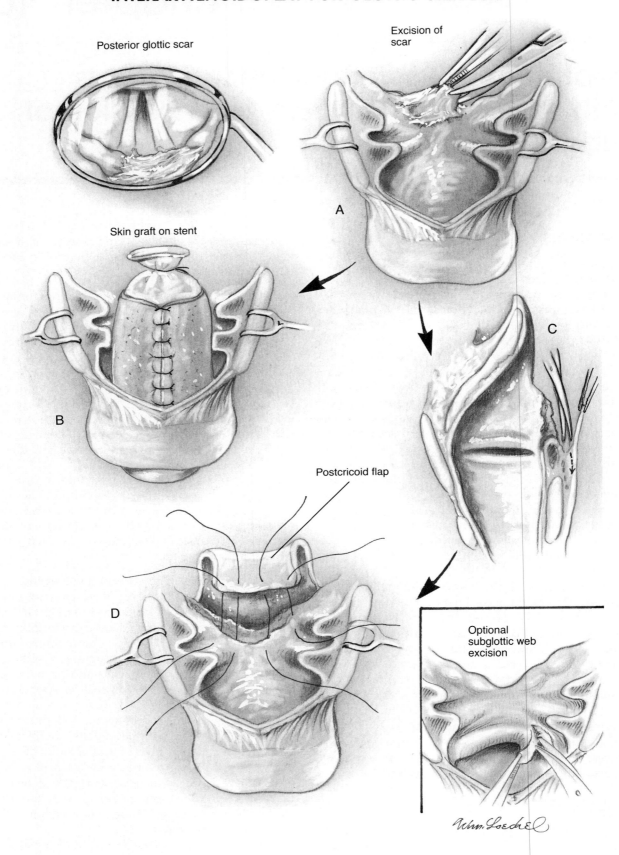

Posterior glottic scar

Excision of scar

Skin graft on stent

A

B

C

Postcricoid flap

D

Optional subglottic web excision

area, the thyroid laminae are approximated with 2-0 chromic sutures. The perichondrium and platysma are closed with 3-0 chromic sutures and the skin with 5-0 nylon sutures. A subplatysmal ¼-inch Penrose drain is usually retained for 24 to 48 hours.

Postoperatively the patient is treated with prophylactic antibiotics. A light dressing is applied. The laryngeal stent should be evaluated and removed at approximately 7 to 10 days.

PITFALLS

1. An accurate diagnosis and understanding of the pathologic condition are essential for planning of the reconstructive procedure. When stenosis is present, but there is normal recurrent nerve function, the surgeon should use methods that resect the scar or muscle and apply a mucosal reconstruction. Arytenoidectomy should be avoided, because if the arytenoid is resected with intact recurrent nerve function, the adductors may be unopposed and the glottic chink will tend to remain closed. This condition may later require a cordectomy to maintain an open airway. If the patient has a vocal cord paralysis associated with stenosis and there is an airway problem postoperatively, the surgeon will have to consider an arytenoidectomy and then decide whether to resect the vocal cord.

2. Mucosal flaps have a limited blood supply and must be handled with the utmost caution. The flaps should be designed with a broad base. Simple advancement flaps work best, and pedicle rotation flaps have less chance of survival. Closure should be meticulously performed with fine chromic sutures.

3. Avoid stents or splints. Small grafts can often be successful with just suture fixation. Splints tend to rub and cause pressure necrosis; they should only be used when the defects and grafts are large and there is a need to stabilize the larynx (i.e., with fractures of the larynx).

COMPLICATIONS

1. Failure of the technique will result in restenosis, a weak voice, and possibly respiratory difficulty. If such a complication appears to develop, it is probably prudent to perform laryngoscopy, dilate the area of stenosis, and inject the area with triamcinolone. If these attempts to prevent scarring are not successful, the surgeon will have to consider endoscopic and possibly open surgical approaches to effect a satisfactory result.

2. Infection can be avoided by prophylactic antibiotics and drainage of the subplatysmal space. If the patient develops an infection, the neck should be debrided and the wound packed with antibiotic-treated gauze. Cultures should be obtained and appropriate antibiotics administered.

chapter 103

Treatment of Subglottic Stenosis With Endoscopic Removal and Dilatation

INDICATIONS

Stenosis of the subglottic region can result from external blunt trauma, intubation, and/or tracheotomy. Children, because of their narrow subglottic area, are prone to this type of injury; congenital stenosis itself may be an etiologic factor. Tube irritation, pressure necrosis, and infection are also important pathophysiologic considerations.

Early subglottic stenosis can usually be treated with endoscopic forceps or laser resection or by dilatation and intralesional injections of steroids. Failure of treatment may prompt the use of a stent, usually a T tube. If the T tube is not effective in relieving obstruction, the surgeon may have to proceed with external approaches, interpositional grafts, and/or other reconstructive techniques (see Chapters 104 and 105).

PROCEDURE

A low tracheostomy is performed preliminarily to gain control of the airway and provide for anesthesia during the treatment of the stenosis (see Chapter 4). Ideally the tracheostomy should be several centimeters below the area of stenosis so that secretions do not accumulate and predispose to infection. The low tracheostomy also protects the operative site from repeated trauma caused by suctioning and/or manipulation of the tube.

An operating laryngoscope, suitable for the patient's age and mouth opening, is inserted orally and into the larynx. The tip of the scope is then used to spread the vocal cords, and the subglottic area is evaluated. Bronchoscopy may also be applied to help determine the site and extent of injury. Microscopic control and stabilization with a laryngoscope holder are desirable.

A,B Using fine suction tips and a laryngeal forceps, scar and/or granulation tissues are excised. Bleeding is controlled with pledgets of 4% cocaine solution.

Electrocauterization can be used, but only if bleeding cannot be controlled with cocaine and pressure. Following removal of the tissue, bronchoscopes are passed, and the size of the largest bronchoscope that effectively dilates the area is recorded. The subglottic region is then injected through the cricothyroid membrane with a 21-gauge needle containing 40 mg/mL of triamcinolone. The adequacy of the injection is checked with the laryngoscope or bronchoscope.

After the endoscopy, the patient should be maintained on a tracheal cleansing regimen. The tracheostomy should not be plugged until the surgeon is assured of an adequate airway. Prophylactic antibiotics are desirable. Reevaluation of the stenosis should be performed in about 2 weeks. The procedure can then be repeated, but if the subglottic region becomes progressively stenotic, the surgeon should consider a long-term lumen keeper (see Chapter 95).

PITFALLS

1. Treatment of subglottic stenosis should be based on the site and degree of injury and the maturity of scar formation. Soft scar and granulation tissues can usually be removed with endoscopic laser or surgery. Mature scarred areas may require a more aggressive approach (see Chapter 104).

2. The surgeon must ensure that the procedures are progressively enlarging the airway. This can be quantitated by bronchoscopic measurements and, if the surgeon chooses, by noting the size of the dilatator and/or bronchoscope that is used to pass through the area.

3. Failure to obtain progressive enlargement should prompt other techniques. The use of a T tube and/or resection must be considered (see Chapters 95, 104, and 105).

COMPLICATIONS

1. Restenosis is the most common complication. This can be avoided by making sure the tracheostomy

ENDOSCOPIC EXCISION OF SUBGLOTTIC STENOSIS

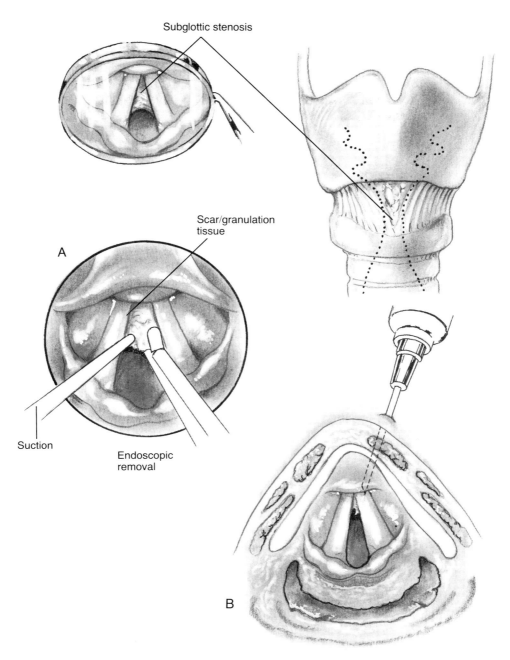

Subglottic stenosis

Scar/granulation tissue

A

Suction

Endoscopic removal

B

Injection of corticosteroids

is several centimeters below the area of endoscopic surgery, and the patient is covered prophylactically with broad-spectrum antibiotics. Reevaluation of the stenosis should take place at about 10 to 14 days, with the option of then excising more tissue and/or injecting the scar with steroid solution. Failure of these techniques should prompt laser methods or application of T-tube and/or resection procedures.

2. Bleeding can develop during and after the procedure. Intraoperative bleeding can be controlled with 4% cocaine pledgets and pressure, but if nec-essary, the surgeon can apply a laryngeal electrocautery. Blood can be kept from the lungs by keeping the tube cuff inflated and by surveillance and suctioning of the subglottic region. Postoperative bleeding should be treated by inflation of the cuff. If, after several hours, bleeding is still evident, the trachea should be reinspected with an endoscope, at which time hemostatic agents and cautery can be applied.

3. Complications regarding the T-tube procedure are described in Chapter 95.

chapter 104

Treatment of Subglottic Stenosis Using Interposition Grafts and Tracheal-Cricothyroid Anastomosis

INDICATIONS

If excision of subglottic granulations and scar tissues and dilatation, with or without stenting, are unsuccessful, the next step should be a cartilage-splitting procedure with graft enlargement of the airway or resection of the stenosis and advancement of the trachea to the cricoid remnant and thyroid laminae. The interposition graft technique is best considered for conditions of limited damage. If the injury is extensive, involving most of the circumferential ring of cricoid or the first few rings of trachea, then resection followed by direct anastomosis is the best option. Fixation of the vocal cords and/or recurrent laryngeal nerve injury can complicate the condition and affect therapeutic options.

PROCEDURE

A An anode tube should be fixed to the neck and the neck prepared and draped as a sterile field. A nasogastric tube is inserted. A low collar incision, to include the tracheostomy, is carried into the subplatysmal layer. A superiorly based neck flap is elevated to the level of the hyoid bone. The strap muscles are identified and retracted laterally, and the pretracheal fascia is incised over the trachea. The thyroid isthmus is then divided between clamps, and the hemostasis is controlled with cauterization or fine silk ligatures. The isthmus and portions of the thyroid gland are dissected free of the trachea, carefully avoiding injury to the recurrent nerves.

With the thyroid laminae, cricoid, and upper trachea exposed, a 7 × 40–cm bronchoscope is introduced transorally. The area of subglottic stenosis is again examined and measured by placing marker needles at the appropriate levels of the airway. This will determine the caudal-cephalic extent of resection.

B–D The trachea and cricoid are divided in the midline and spread laterally. Thick scar tissues should be removed. A portion of the hyoid, pedicled on the sternohyoid and omohyoid muscles (as described in Chapter 98), is rotated and inserted into the defect. Fine wire extraluminal closure is employed to hold the graft into position. To release tension, the muscle pedicle is attached to the strap muscles of the opposite side with 4-0 chromic sutures. Whether a skin or mucosal graft, along with a stent, should be applied, will depend on the degree of raw tissue present. If the approximation of mucosa is almost complete, stenting will not be required.

E For those patients in whom there is an obvious destruction of most of the cartilage of the cricoid and trachea, a resection should be carried out. The approach is identical to that used in the hyoid interposition procedure described earlier.

Using a bronchoscope to isolate the inferior and superior extent of stenosis, the surgeon should make an incision at the lower level of the involved trauma. The trachea is then transected through the cartilage and the mucosa of the posterior wall. The superior resection is usually directed just above the anterior portion of the cricoid ring and through the cricothyroid membrane. The cut is made diagonally through the ring to preserve the posterior lamina. The intervening tissues are removed, carefully avoiding injury to the recurrent nerves.

F For closure of the defect, the trachea is mobilized upward and the larynx dropped downward. The inferior relaxation is accomplished by a sharp and blunt dissection just deep to the pretracheal fascia. The larynx is released by incising the suprahyoid musculature free from the hyoid bone. The digastric and stylohyoid attachments are usually retained, whereas the body is cut free from the lesser and greater cornua.

TREATMENT OF SUBGLOTTIC STENOSIS WITH HYOID INTERPOSITION

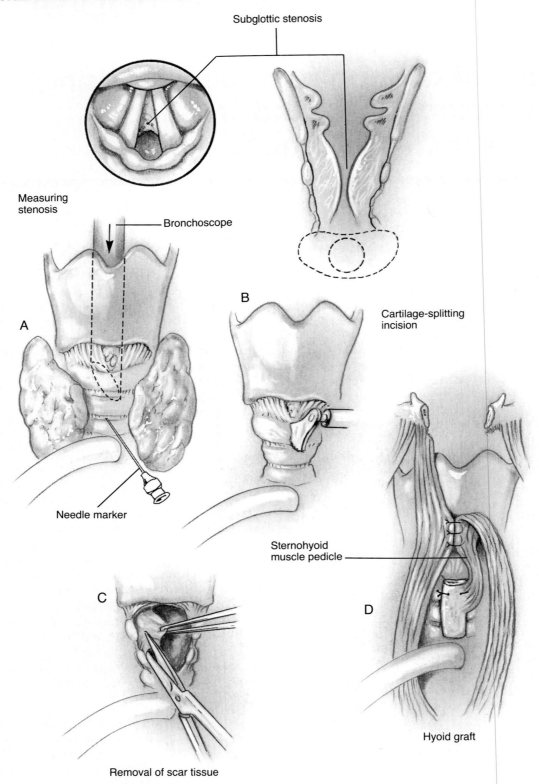

Subglottic stenosis

Measuring
stenosis

Bronchoscope

A

B

Cartilage-splitting
incision

Needle marker

Sternohyoid
muscle pedicle

C

D

Removal of scar tissue

Hyoid graft

Wm. Loechel,

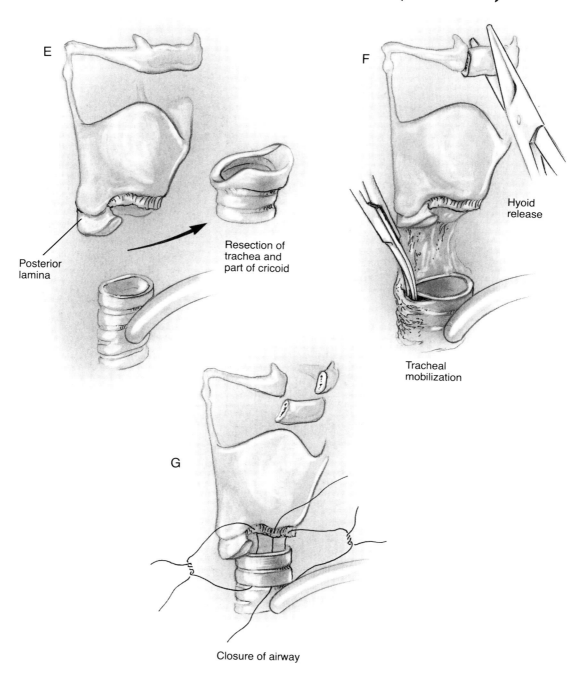

E

Posterior
lamina

Resection of
trachea and
part of cricoid

F

Hyoid
release

Tracheal
mobilization

G

Closure of airway

G After mobilization of the inferior and superior portion of the airway, the trachea is sutured to the posterior cricoid lamina and the thyroid cartilage. The first sutures are placed posteriorly and the knots directed to the extraluminal surface. The sutures are then placed anteriorly to close the trachea to the thyroid lamina. The wound is irrigated with saline, and a ½-inch Penrose drain is placed subplastymally. The wound is then closed in layers, with 4-0 chromic sutures through the platysma and 5-0 nylon sutures through the skin. The anode tube is replaced with a tracheostomy tube, and a light compression dressing is applied.

Postoperatively the patient is kept in the flexed position, which is facilitated with tapes running from the head to the chest. Antibiotics are used for 7 to 10 days. The drain is removed in 2 to 4 days and the nasogastric tube in about 10 days.

PITFALLS

1. Evaluation of the vocal cords preoperatively will help determine whether the patient has glottic stenosis and/or bilateral vocal cord paralysis. If the patient has one of these conditions, the surgeon should also consider a thyrotomy and treatment of the fixation and/or paralytic state (see Chapters 100 through 103).

2. When there is a large area of denuded mucosa, a mucosal or skin-covered stent should be employed for 5 to 7 days.

3. Relaxation procedures will usually compensate for about 2 to 3 cm of tracheal deficit. If more resection is necessary, the surgeon must consider relaxation either by incising opposite sides of the tracheal rings (annular ligaments) or by releasing the hilum and pulmonary ligaments. For large resections, a thoracic surgeon should be consulted.

4. In small children, a cricoid split and hyoid graft is a popular procedure. Alternatively, the surgeon can split the cricoid and upper trachea with zigzag cuts and reapproximate the segments over a stent.

COMPLICATIONS

1. The most common complication is recurrent stenosis. The scarring that causes the stenosis can be minimized by the practice of atraumatic techniques, reduced tension, and extraluminal sutures. If possible, stents should be avoided. If stenosis develops, the surgeon should retain the tracheostomy and treat early granulations and/or scar with endoscopic and/or laser surgery. Long-term use of T tubes or revisional surgery can also be considered.

2. Recurrent laryngeal nerve paralysis can adversely affect the results. Knowledge of the anatomy of the recurrent nerve should prevent most injury, and particular care should be taken during retraction of the thyroid gland. The resection of the stenosis should be carried out in a subperichondrial plane. If the patient shows signs of nerve paralysis postoperatively, the surgeon should then wait 6 to 9 months, and if there is no return of function, one of the techniques described in Chapters 90 and 100 should be applied.

3. Infection should be avoided, as it causes more scarring and restenosis. It can often be prevented by careful closure of the airway, drainage of the wound, and use of prophylactic antibiotics. If infection develops, the wound should be debrided and packed with antibiotic-treated gauze. Cultures should be obtained to determine specific antibiotic therapy.

section VII

Tracheal Stenosis

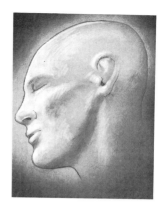

chapter 105

Treatment of Tracheal Stenosis With Segmental Resection and Anastomosis
Alternative Techniques of T-Tube Reconstruction and Wedge Resection

INDICATIONS

Tracheal stenosis is characterized by a narrowing of the trachea below the subglottic region and above the carina. Usually this is caused by intubation and/or tracheostomy, but occasionally it is the result of blunt or penetrating trauma. Pressure, necrosis at the tube tip, and scarring at the tracheostomy site are commonly implicated factors. Once the diagnosis is made, it is important to establish an airway below the area of obstruction and then, with endoscopy, computed tomographic (CT) scans, and basic swallowing and pulmonary function tests, determine the extent of injury and the degree of incapacitation.

In general, resection of the trachea is indicated in acute trauma when there has been extensive damage and in cases of chronic stenosis in which there has been a collapse or buckling of at least 3 to 5 cm of the trachea. If the stenosis is caused by granulation tissues and early soft scar, excision and dilatation and even long-term stents (T tubes) can be used. If the lesion involves the anterior wall or less than two to three rings, the surgeon can use a wedge resection with or without an interpositional graft. The segmental resection is contraindicated in patients who are severely debilitated, who require permanent tracheostomy, and in whom there is laryngeal incompetence.

PROCEDURE

A Anesthesia is administered through an anode tube placed through a prior tracheostomy. The neck is extended by placing a blanket roll under the shoulders. The neck and chest are prepared and draped as a sterile field.

B The incision is designed to remove the old tracheostomy wound. A collar incision is thus created, and a vertical incision is also drawn down to the jugular notch. The area is infiltrated with 1% lidocaine containing 1:100,000 epinephrine to assist in hemostasis.

C The dissection is carried through the platysma layer, and a superior flap is elevated to the level of the thyroid cartilage. Two inferolateral flaps are developed in a similar plane to expose the strap muscles. The sternohyoid and sternothyroid muscles are retracted laterally and the tracheostomy separated from the adjacent scar tissues. Pretracheal fascia is incised and the trachea exposed inferiorly. If the thyroid gland is obscuring vision, it should be divided and ligated to expose the upper trachea and cricoid.

D At this point, the anesthesiologist should introduce a nasotracheal tube. Under visual guidance, the anode tube is removed and the endotracheal tube passed through the stenosis. Vertical incisions through the area of stenosis will help pass the tube.

Having achieved control of the airway below the stenosis, vertical incisions are then used to assess the extent of stenosis in the area to be resected. Tracheal rings are usually removed by way of subperiosteal dissection from the adjacent scar tissues. The mucosa on the posterior wall is dissected free from the tracheoesophageal space.

E Closure is initiated by relaxation techniques. The inferior release is accomplished by a sharp and blunt dissection beneath the pretracheal fascia. This can be facilitated by a finger dissection below the clavicle and sternum. Above, the body of the hyoid is separated from the lesser and greater cornua and freed from the suprahyoid musculature as described in Chapter 104.

F,G The trachea is closed with extralumenally placed 3-0 polyglactin sutures. The sutures are first positioned posteriorly and left loose. The anterior sutures are then placed, and the sutures are tied sequentially from posterior to anterior. Additional relaxation can be obtained by removing the shoulder roll and flexing the head. The strap muscles are subsequently closed in the midline, and a medium-sized suction drain is placed between the strap muscles and platysma. The platysma is closed with 3-0 chromic sutures and the skin with 5-0 nylon sutures.

Postoperatively, the patient is maintained on prophylactic antibiotics (i.e., penicillin or erythromycin) for 7 to 10 days. The endotracheal tube should be retained until the patient is alert and breathing without difficulty. Postoperative bucking and coughing should be avoided. A bandage should be placed from the head to the chest to hold the head in a position of flexion for 2 to 3 weeks.

PITFALLS

1. The area of stenosis dictates the degree of resection. Because small lesions can be handled with limited excision and larger lesions require resection and anastomosis, the size of the lesion should be assessed with a bronchoscope before the resection is performed. The technique is described in Chapter 104.

2. Resections larger than 5.0 cm require additional relaxation techniques. For such procedures, annular ligaments between the trachea can be incised on alternate sides, and if more length is needed, the resection should be performed by relaxation of the right hilum and pulmonary ligaments.

3. Airway management is challenging. The surgeon has the option during the procedure to place an anode at the lower portion of stenosis or intubate directly by way of an oral endotracheal tube. The method of choice will be dictated by the pathologic condition. In general, the endotracheal tube is used during the anastomosis and removed soon after surgery. However, if there is concern (i.e., too much tension or poor anastomosis), a temporary tracheostomy tube can be placed below the area of resection.

4. The objectives of the procedure are to remove mucosa, cartilage, and scar tissue and bring the trachea together; recurrent nerve injury should be avoided. This can be accomplished by dissecting close to the cartilage and the mucosal surface.

5. For stenosis that does not require resection, other techniques can be employed. Portions of the anterior tracheal wall can be removed with or without T tubes. Interpositional grafts can also be employed (see Chapter 104).

6. For high lesions involving the subglottic space, part of the cricoid can be resected with the trachea. This reconstruction is described in Chapter 104.

7. Tension is relieved at the suture line by any of a number of techniques: (1) upward mobilization of the trachea; (2) relaxation of the larynx; (3) neck flexion; and (4) annular ligament incisions on opposite sides of the trachea. If these are not sufficient, an intrathoracic procedure will have to be carried out to release the traction at the pulmonary hila.

8. Postoperative care is important. The patient should be in an intensive care unit, and bucking and coughing should be avoided. When the patient is stabilized, the endotracheal tube can be removed and the patient's head and neck kept in a flexed position until the wounds have healed.

COMPLICATIONS

1. One of the causes of recurrent stenosis is wound infection. Thus the chances for infection should be

TREATMENT OF TRACHEAL STENOSIS WITH SEGMENTAL RESECTION

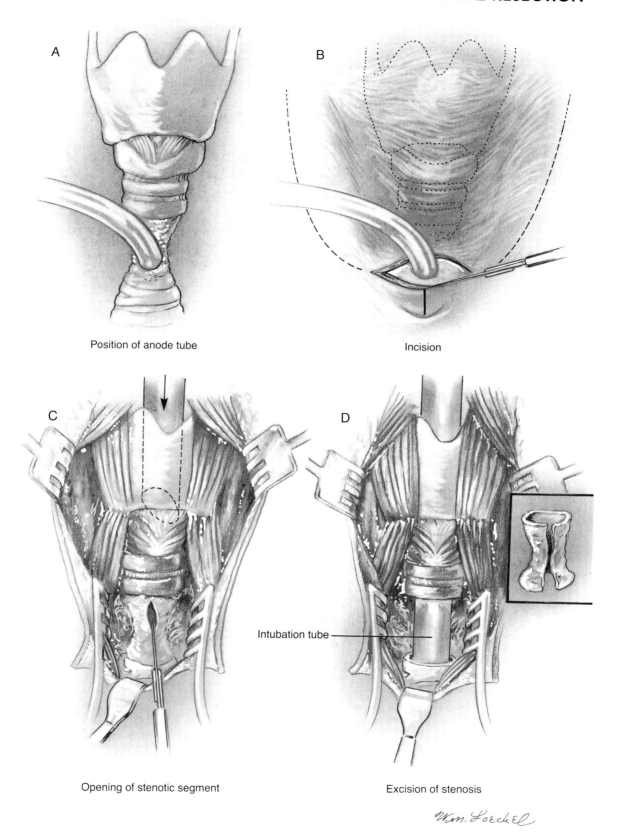

A

Position of anode tube

B

Incision

C

Opening of stenotic segment

D

Intubation tube

Excision of stenosis

Wm. Loechel

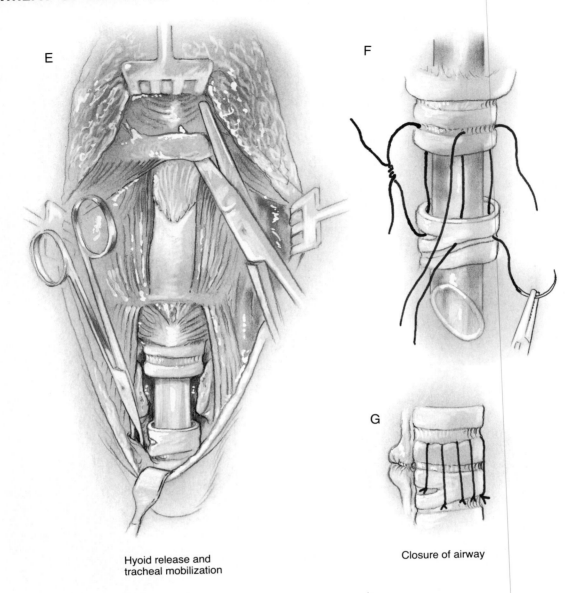

E

F

G

Hyoid release and
tracheal mobilization

Closure of airway

minimized by use of prophylactic antibiotics and drainage of the subplatysmal space. If infection develops, the wound should be opened and treated with debridement and packed with gauze. Pathogen-specific antibiotics should be employed. Limited scarring can be treated with endoscopic techniques. For recurrent significant stenosis, the surgeon should consider T-tube placement and/or permanent tracheostomy.

2. Separation at the suture line is rare, but if it occurs, the patient will develop granulation tissue and possibly respiratory distress. The tension should be relieved by one or several relaxation methods described above. Granulation tissues can be treated conservatively with endoscopic surgery or laser techniques.

3. Recurrent laryngeal nerve injury can develop and cause problems with laryngeal competence. After splitting the thyroid isthmus and thyroid laminae, the surgeon should remember the course of the nerve and its entry into the cricoarytenoid region. Injury should also be avoided by using a subperichondrial dissection and trying to remove only scarred cartilage and mucosa. If one or both nerves become impaired, one of the specialized techniques described in Chapters 99 or 100 can be employed.

4. Esophageal injury with tracheoesophageal fistula is possible, especially if the "party wall" is injured during the resection of the trachea. To avoid this problem, the dissection should be limited to the mucosa only. The nasogastric tube within the esophagus should give a clue as to the location and depth of the esophageal mucosa. However, if a fistula develops, repair with a muscle interposition must be considered.

5. Airway problems as a result of this procedure can also occur. The surgeon should thus be certain that the patient is breathing quietly and without distress on removal of the endotracheal tube. If there is any respiratory difficulty, the surgeon should inspect the airway to evaluate competency of the larynx (i.e., for recurrent laryngeal nerve injury). A formal endoscopy is necessary if a tracheal separation is suspected. In the presence of such a condition, endotracheal intubation or a new tracheostomy, or both, is indicated.

ALTERNATIVE TECHNIQUE OF T-TUBE RECONSTRUCTION

When the tracheal stenosis is soft and characterized more by malacia than by stenosis, a T tube should be considered. This procedure is also indicated when excision and dilatation (with or without stents) has failed and when there are lacerations and "weak-nesses" of the tracheal walls from acute tracheal trauma.

a–d The procedure is usually carried out using endoscopic methods and exposure through the tracheostomy site. An endotracheal or tracheostomy tube is used for control of the airway. If the stenosis is at or above the tracheostomy site, the trachea should be explored by way of a horizontal incision. Strap muscles are separated from the midline, and the thyroid isthmus is divided. Bleeding is controlled by silk ligatures and/or cauterization. The area of stenosis is exposed, the pretracheal fascia is elevated, and the trachea is incised over the affected area. After excision of the stenosis and/or granulation tissues, the defect can be left open anteriorly or optionally reconstructed with a small cartilage graft. The T tube, used as a stent, is placed through the tracheostomy so that the upper limb is just above the area of resection (see Chapter 95). The soft tissues (i.e., strap muscles) are then approximated in the midline over the defect. A Penrose drain is inserted and the platysma and skin closed in layers.

Usually the T tube is left in place for several months. Radiographs should be obtained and a hairline radiolucency noted around the tube before it is removed. Crusting can be a problem and must be controlled with humidification and suctioning. If the T tube becomes plugged, it should be removed and temporarily replaced with a tracheostomy tube. T-tube complications are discussed in Chapter 95.

ALTERNATIVE TECHNIQUE OF WEDGE RESECTION

Stenosis characterized by exuberant soft tissues probably can be corrected by one of the endoscopic techniques with or without stenting. However, if the stenosis is limited to a small area of the trachea or an anterior area of the tracheal wall, a partial wedge resection can be considered. If the patient has any form of incompetency of the larynx, the procedure is probably contraindicated.

a,'b' For the wedge resection, the tracheostomy tube is converted to an anode tube, and the tracheostomy opening is elliptically excised as part of the collar incision. The skin flaps are elevated in a subplatysmal plane, and the strap muscles are retracted from the midline. The tracheostomy site is dissected free from surrounding tissues. The level and length of stenosis should be confirmed by endoscopic methods. A transoral endotracheal tube is inserted beyond the area of stenosis, and the anode tube is removed. The anterior wall of the trachea is resected. The defect is closed with a cartilage-to-cartilage ring anastomosis using 3-0 chromic or polyglactin sutures.

TREATMENT OF TRACHEAL STENOSIS

ALTERNATIVE TECHNIQUE OF T-TUBE INSERTION

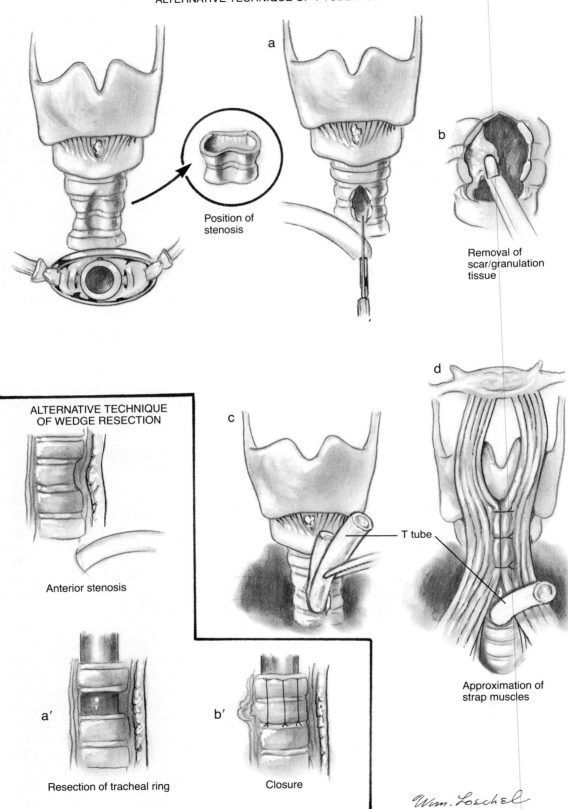

Position of stenosis

a

b

Removal of scar/granulation tissue

d

ALTERNATIVE TECHNIQUE OF WEDGE RESECTION

Anterior stenosis

c

T tube

a'

Resection of tracheal ring

b'

Closure

Approximation of strap muscles

Wm. Loschel

part
thirteen

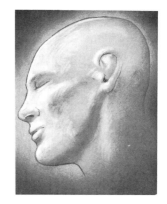

Soft Tissue
Injury

section I

Carotid Artery Injury

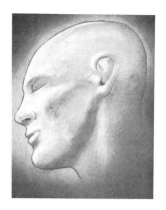

chapter 106

Treatment of Penetrating Injuries of the Carotid Artery
Alternative Technique for Blunt Trauma

In Consultation With Ramon Berguer, MD, PhD

INDICATIONS

Trauma to the carotid artery may result from a penetrating injury from a knife or firearm or, rarely, from a bony fragment from a fractured facial bone or skull. Penetrating injuries to the carotid manifest as an usually tense and expanding hematoma of the neck and/or brisk external bleeding. The most commonly associated injury is a tear of the internal jugular vein. Other frequently associated injuries are located in the pharynx, larynx, esophagus, brachial plexus, and spinal cord. The patient may be neurologically normal or may present with unilateral symptoms or coma.

Injuries to the carotid are often divided according to site into three zones: zone 1, below the clavicle; zone 2, from the clavicle to the angle of the jaw; and zone 3, above the angle of the jaw (see **A**). Injuries to zone 1 are often associated with injuries to other supraaortic trunks. To define these associated inju-

ries, patients who are hemodynamically stable should undergo arteriography after obtaining airway control. In injuries to zone 2 that are actively bleeding or have tense, expanding hematomas, immediate exploration is advised. Arteriography in stable patients with wounds in zone 2 may, in selective instances, avoid a surgical exploration, but the patient may also deteriorate rapidly in the arteriography suite and never benefit from the surgical repair. In zone 3 injuries, if the patient has no neurologic symptoms and is hemodynamically stable with control of the airway, arteriography is recommended to define the injured artery and its operability. Exploration of the skull base is far more complex and risky than that of the midneck. Thus zone 3 patients with an intact neurologic status and no evidence of bleeding are best managed with attentive watching if the arteriogram is negative.

In patients who are stable without tense expanding hematomas, the trajectory of injury may suggest the

521

coexistence of additional soft tissue injuries. If there is crepitus and/or dysphagia, an esophagogram and/or esophagoscopy is helpful in identifying and locating the site of injury. For those patients with crepitus, dyspnea, and hoarseness, indirect and direct laryngoscopy and/or bronchoscopy will define the status of the hypopharynx, larynx (or trachea). In penetrating wounds of the neck, a variety of neurologic deficits (e.g., those accompanying Horner's syndrome), brachial plexus deficits, hemiplegia, and loss of visual acuity can occur. Vascular injury can also cause carotid embolization and central nervous system ischemia.

Absolute indications for surgery include active hemorrhage from the neck wound, a history of hemorrhage with hypotension, active bleeding from the mouth, and an expanding cervical hematoma. Exploration is generally advised for wounds that extend beneath the platysma and that are associated with continuous bruits or central nervous system symptoms.

PROCEDURE

B The first order of business in patients with suspected injuries to the carotid artery is to obtain hemodynamic stability and control of the airway. In patients actively bleeding from a neck wound, the bleeding is controlled by manual pressure while endotracheal intubation is performed. Two large-bore intravenous lines are started. A subclavian line is indicated but should be avoided on the side or in the path of injury. One of the large-bore intravenous lines is usually placed in the femoral vein.

Following intubation, the patient can be taken either to the operating room for an immediate exploration or to another appropriate department for additional diagnostic studies, such as arteriography and/or endoscopy.

Once the patient is placed on the operating table, the entire neck and chest are prepared as a sterile field. While this is being done, an arterial line is started in the radial artery contralateral to the injury. A nasogastric tube is placed so that the surgeon can decompress the stomach and identify the esophagus during exploration. Both thighs are prepared to harvest saphenous vein grafts, which may be needed for repair of the carotid artery. Intravenous antibiotic therapy is started.

The neck incision follows the anterior border of the sternocleidomastoid muscle. The muscle is retracted posteriorly, and branches of the anterior jugular veins are divided and ligated. This permits entry into the carotid sheath and dissection of the common carotid, its bifurcation and external and internal carotid arteries. Control of bleeding can be obtained with digital pressure and/or application of double Silastic loops below and above the injury. Commonly associated internal jugular vein tears can be handled by a lateral repair (in the case of a knife wound) or by ligation above and below the destroyed wall (in the case of a firearm injury).

Repair of the Common Carotid

In the midneck, the dissection of the common carotid artery is kept close to its wall. In the lower portion of the neck, the surgeon should avoid the vagus nerve, which often moves from a posterior to an anterolateral position. If the injury of the common carotid artery is low in the neck and difficulty with proximal control is anticipated, the neck incision is lengthened with a median sternotomy, which exposes the supraaortic trunks.

C,D Once proximal and distal control is obtained, the repair of common carotid injuries employs standard vascular techniques. Small injuries, such as those caused by a knife, may be repaired by lateral arteriography or by resection and anastomosis. For repair of a lateral defect, the artery is cross-clamped, and the clean tear is sutured with 6-0 polypropylene sutures (after ensuring by direct inspection that there is no other intimal damage, such as a tear in the opposite wall of an intimal flap). For injuries other than a partial and clean cut that do not involve more than an inch of common carotid artery, the artery can be amply freed, cross-clamped, and repaired by an end-to-end anastomosis. In such cases, the edges of the artery should be freshened and the vessel repaired. A continuous suture (made with a double-armed needle) is placed at the midpoint of the back wall. Both ends of the suture usually meet at the midpoint of the front wall.

E An arterial repair associated with tension at the anastomosis should be managed with a common carotid artery ligation and replacement with an end-to-end saphenous vein graft that should be at least 3.5 mm in diameter. If there is a serious disparity in size between the common carotid artery and the saphenous vein, the repair can still be made by closing both ends of the common carotid artery and bridging the defect with a vein graft anastomosed end-to-side to both ends of the common carotid artery. A saphenous vein graft, less than 3.5 mm in diameter, is inadequate to bridge a common carotid artery defect. If the common carotid artery injury is extensive and there is no associated visceral injury or significant contamination, the repair of the common carotid artery can be made with an 8-mm-diameter polytetrafluoroethylene (PTFE) prosthesis.

TREATMENT OF CAROTID ARTERY INJURIES

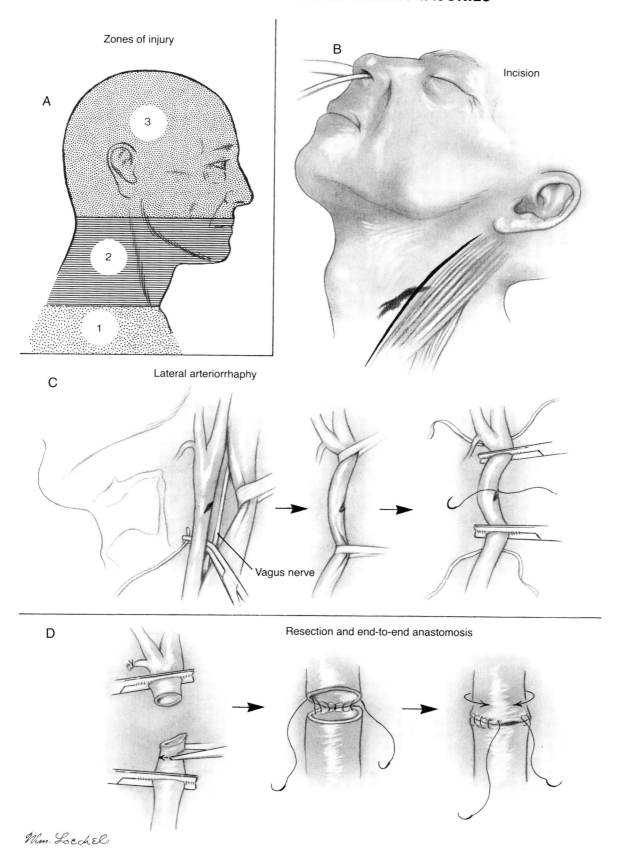

Zones of injury

A

3

2

1

B

Incision

C

Lateral arteriorrhaphy

Vagus nerve

D

Resection and end-to-end anastomosis

Wm. Loechel

F A low common carotid artery injury near its origin can also be repaired by ligating its proximal stump and anastomosing the distal common carotid artery to the second portion of the subclavian artery. This procedure is easier on the right side of the neck. To obtain exposure, the phrenic nerve is identified and dissected free of its bed, followed by division of the underlying scalenus anticus muscle. An end-to-side anastomosis is subsequently carried out. The subclavian artery has an extremely thin wall and tears easily, and this should be borne in mind when dissecting the artery and applying clamps to it. Bleeding from a damaged subclavian artery will often have to be controlled by proximal and distal ligation of the artery, a procedure in itself fraught with the risk of further tear and life-threatening hemorrhage.

Repair of External and Internal Carotid Arteries

G,H Injuries to the bifurcation of the carotid are repaired by lateral arteriorrhaphy or bypass grafting from the common carotid artery to the internal carotid artery with a saphenous vein graft. If the injury involves the external carotid artery, the artery is ligated above and below the point of injury and is not repaired.

Injuries of the internal carotid artery are managed according to the level of injury. The digastric muscle serves as a recognizable anatomic landmark to separate the two surgical approaches.

Injuries below the digastric muscle are treated with standard vascular techniques. Digital pressure over the transverse process of C1 and over the origin of the internal carotid artery will generally slow the bleeding enough to permit dissection of the injured internal carotid artery. The origin of the external carotid artery is clamped, and care is taken to avoid damage to the hypoglossal nerve and the superior laryngeal nerve. Injury to the hypoglossal nerve is avoided by a positive identification of the nerve, which may be covered by an anterior branch of the internal jugular vein. The superior laryngeal nerve does not need to be identified. It is usually injured either by blunt dissection behind the carotid bulb or by clamping the superior thyroid artery away from its origin. The internal carotid artery is then clamped. If there are no other associated injuries, 7000 units of heparin are given intravenously at that time. Repair of the internal carotid artery is then usually carried out by means of a vein graft. If a vein graft is not available and the internal carotid artery injury involves the bulb, the skeletonized external carotid artery may be transposed to the internal carotid artery to bridge the defect.

If the carotid artery is thrombosed at the site of injury but has brisk anterior and retrograde bleeding after removing the thrombus plug at the site of injury, the artery is reconstructed with a vein graft. An intimal injury present at the site of distal anastomosis is a contraindication. If bleeding is not observed, no effort should be made to obtain retrograde flow by manipulation of balloon thrombectomy catheters in the high neck or intracranial segment of the internal carotid artery. Under these circumstances, a thrombosed carotid artery is ligated.

I Injuries to the internal carotid artery above the digastric muscle are more difficult to control. If the level of injury to the internal carotid artery has been determined by arteriography to be high, it is advantageous to convert to a nasotracheal intubation; this will permit bite closure and anterior advancement of the angle of the jaw, the main obstruction met by the surgeon when trying to reach the high cervical carotid (at or above C1). Proximal common carotid or internal carotid artery control is obtained by clamping the corresponding vessel. Digital pressure over C1 may provide distal control. For exposure, the digastric muscle is divided. The occipital artery, which crosses the internal carotid artery below the posterior edge of the digastric, is also divided. Our preference is then to reconstruct the distal internal carotid artery from behind, rather than from in front of the internal jugular vein, and for this approach (which we use routinely in distal vertebral bypass operations), the dissection proceeds between the jugular vein and the sternocleidomastoid muscle. The spinal accessory nerve is identified and gently retracted with a Silastic loop. The jugular vein and vagus are reflected anteriorly to the internal carotid artery, and the latter is exposed between C3 and C1. Again, care must be taken not to injure the hypoglossal or vagus nerve during this maneuver. The superior laryngeal nerve that exits the vagus above and behind the carotid bulb must be preserved.

In those cases in which it is impossible to obtain proper distal control of high internal carotid injuries, ligation is the advisable form of therapy. If the associated injuries and general condition of the patient permit, the internal carotid artery ligation should be treated with heparin for approximately 5 days postoperatively. This is done to curtail the extension of the thrombus into the segment of the intracranial internal carotid artery and into its main branches, the anterior and middle cerebral arteries.

Postoperative antibiotic therapy is indicated when there is gross contamination of the wound or associated injury of the aeroesophageal tract and whenever a prosthetic graft is used. In an isolated reconstruction of the carotid (or other extracranial artery) where a prosthetic graft is used, intravenous anti-

TREATMENT OF CAROTID ARTERY INJURIES *(Continued)*

SAPHENOUS VEIN GRAFT REPAIR

E

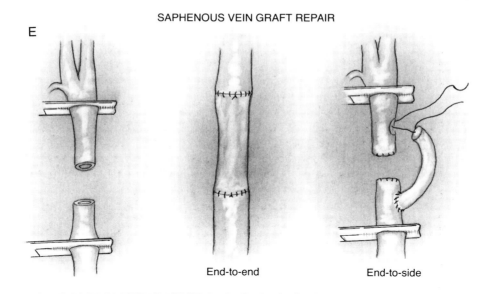

End-to-end   End-to-side

ANASTOMOSIS OF COMMON CAROTID TO SUBCLAVIAN

F

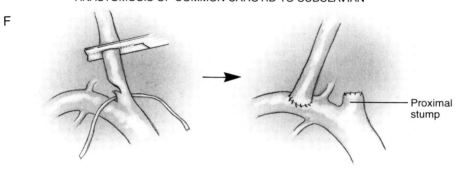

Proximal stump

BYPASS GRAFT FROM COMMON TO INTERNAL CAROTID

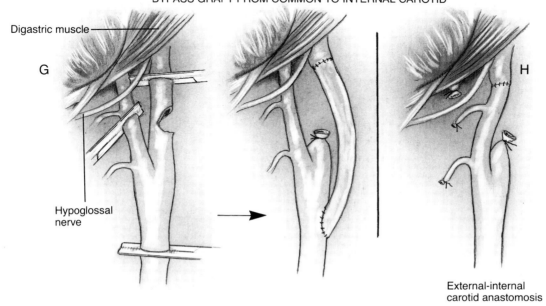

Digastric muscle

G

Hypoglossal nerve

H

External-internal carotid anastomosis

biotics are maintained for 3 to 5 days. When there is an esophageal fistula, evidence of inflammation, or sepsis, antibiotic therapy should be prolonged.

An arteriogram is not needed after repair of a carotid injury (whether the vessel has been repaired or ligated), unless the patient shows adverse signs or symptoms such as a false aneurysm; evidence of sepsis, mass, or hematoma; a transient ischemic attack; or stroke. Duplex imaging is adequate for the assessment of the patency of the reconstruction. This is done in the noninvasive laboratory about 3 weeks after repair when most of the tissue edema has subsided and visualization is improved.

In most vascular reconstructions, drains are left for 12 hours. The dressings are light and are needed for only 24 hours.

PITFALLS

1. The saphenous vein graft should be 3.5 mm in diameter to replace or bypass a common or internal carotid artery. The vein graft is placed so that the valves do not interfere with blood flow.

2. If the carotid artery injury is associated with atheroma of the carotid wall, care should be taken to include the full thickness of the wall with the suture. Under these circumstances, a lateral repair is done by placing interrupted sutures from inside out. This prevents intralumenal dissection beneath the plaque or fragmentation of the plaque into the lumen.

3. Injuries to the external carotid can be managed with ligation. The technique for repair of injuries to the internal carotid artery is determined by the level of injury.

4. If a common carotid artery injury is low or associated with a subclavian or innominate artery or a brachiocephalic vein injury, the sternocleidomastoid incision is lengthened into a median sternotomy; partial sternotomy should be avoided. The sternotomy, however, should not be used in patients who have had previous aortocoronary bypass grafting. Under these circumstances, resection of the clavicle and control of the common carotid artery from the neck is a safer approach.

5. Subclavian artery injuries may be associated with common carotid injuries. Injuries in the first portion of the right subclavian artery are controlled by midsternotomy; injuries on the left require a fourth-space thoracotomy. Injuries to the second portion of the subclavian artery require division of the scalenus anticus muscle for exposure. The phrenic nerve, which rides over the scalenus anticus, must be carefully preserved. Because the subclavian artery has a particularly thin wall, direct repair of injuries to the artery may be impossible. If this is the

case, we advise ligation proximally and distally to the site of injury and restoration of the blood supply to the arm by means of a common carotid–to–axillary artery saphenous vein bypass.

6. Concomitant vertebral injuries are not uncommon in penetrating neck trauma. Injuries to the first segment of the vertebral artery (from the origin of the subclavian to the transverse process of C6) present with active bleeding and are treated by ligation. Associated injuries of the vertebral artery in its intraspinal portion (C1–C6) have a tendency for spontaneous hemostasis and for the formation of a false aneurysm or an arteriovenous fistula. This is the result of the vertebral artery running through a tight osteomuscular compartment surrounded by a plexus of veins that are intimately associated with the artery and are therefore injured with it. In such cases, the vertebral artery should be explored and ligated or clipped above and below the point of injury.

COMPLICATIONS

1. One of the most dreaded complications is hemorrhage. Often the patient has lost large amounts of blood, which must be replaced by whole blood (or temporarily, by blood volume expanders). Large-bore access lines inserted into the femoral or the opposite subclavian artery are used. A radial artery line is placed in the arm opposite to the site of injury for monitoring of central blood pressure. Active bleeding can be controlled with digital pressure, cross-clamps, or tape looped around the arteries.

2. Postoperative hematomas present as an expanding firm mass of the deep neck tissues. The patient's airway may become compromised. In such a situation, reintubation, drainage, and control of bleeding are indicated.

3. Embolism and thrombosis are potential problems. Indicative signs are transient central nervous system deficits such as aphasia, hemiparesis, and impaired vision. These patients should have an immediate arteriogram. If the embolus is found and is accessible, it should be removed by reconstruction or excluded by ligation. Anticoagulant therapy may be the only alternative, depending on the level of the lesion and other associated conditions.

ALTERNATIVE TECHNIQUE FOR REPAIR OF BLUNT TRAUMA

Blunt trauma to the carotid artery may be the result of a direct blow from the outside or of an impact on and stretching of the vessel by the transverse process of C1 or a fragment from the fractured mandible. On rare occasions, the internal carotid artery may be contused as a consequence of intraoral trauma, as seen in children who fall with a pencil or lollipop in their mouth.

Blunt trauma often produces a characteristic clinical picture. An intimal tear and an intramural hematoma or dissection are common consequences. These lesions may eventually lead to distal embolization of the brain or thrombosis of the carotid artery. This process and the subsequent appearance of neurologic symptoms may take hours or days. The delayed appearance of symptoms is the most common presentation of blunt trauma to the carotid. In addition, mural contusion with hematoma or dissection of the carotid may result in a stenosis, which may produce neurologic symptoms years later.

The possibility of blunt trauma to the carotid artery should be suspected in patients who have undergone direct blows to the neck or have trauma of the head and neck associated with the appearance of neurologic symptoms. These patients are candidates for immediate arteriography, which is the only test that will provide an accurate diagnosis and allow a plan of therapy.

a—c Once the arteriogram has defined the arterial lesion or thrombosis suspected to be secondary to trauma, an exploration is indicated. If the damage to the carotid has resulted in sequential thrombosis and/or spasm and the distal portion of the internal carotid artery is accessible through the neck, an immediate exploration is advised, with resection and grafting of the carotid using a saphenous vein. If a saphenous vein is not available, a thin, 6-mm, PTFE graft will provide an acceptable substitute.

In patients in whom the internal carotid artery is thrombosed and the arteriogram shows the petrous and cavernous portion of the carotid to be patent by a collateral flow (from the opposite internal carotid or from the ipsilateral external carotid), an exploration is advised. The exploration is done through the standard incision anterior to the sternocleidomastoid, exposing the common carotid bifurcation and internal carotid artery. The retrojugular approach, described earlier, provides improved access to the distal cervical internal carotid artery. The internal carotid artery is then opened at the level of C1 through a longitudinal arteriotomy. Thrombus is cleared by insertion of a short length of a balloon (Fogarty) embolectomy catheter, which must not reach the intracavernous carotid. The intima of the distal cervical internal carotid is inspected. If it is intact at this level, plans are made for a common-to-distal cervical internal carotid artery saphenous vein bypass graft. At the conclusion of this grafting procedure, a clip is placed immediately below the anastomosis to exclude the proximal internal carotid artery and transform these into functional end-to-end anastomoses. In children with extensive damage requiring grafting, the surgeon may consider an end-to-end transposition of the external to the internal carotid artery or the use of a free arterial graft from a segment of superficial femoral artery that can itself be replaced with a No. 6 PTFE tube.

If the limited insertion of a Fogarty catheter does not clear the carotid satisfactorily and brisk backflow is not obtained, no distal manipulation of the intracranial carotid with a Fogarty catheter is advised. In such a case, it is better to ligate the internal carotid artery and maintain the patient on intravenous heparin for at least 5 days. This should help avoid progression of the internal carotid artery thrombus into the anterior and medial cerebral artery branches.

TREATMENT OF CAROTID ARTERY INJURIES *(Continued)*

EXPOSURE OF INJURIES ABOVE THE DIGASTRIC MUSCLE

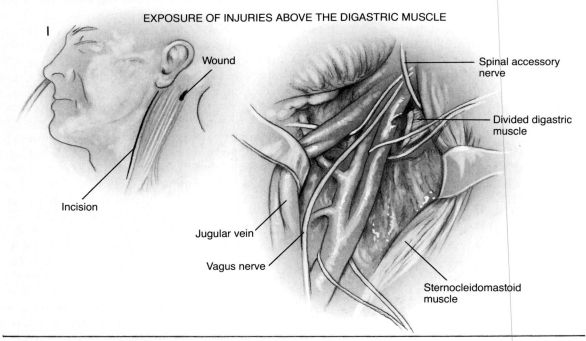

I

Wound

Incision

Spinal accessory nerve

Divided digastric muscle

Jugular vein

Vagus nerve

Sternocleidomastoid muscle

ALTERNATIVE TECHNIQUE FOR REPAIR OF BLUNT TRAUMA

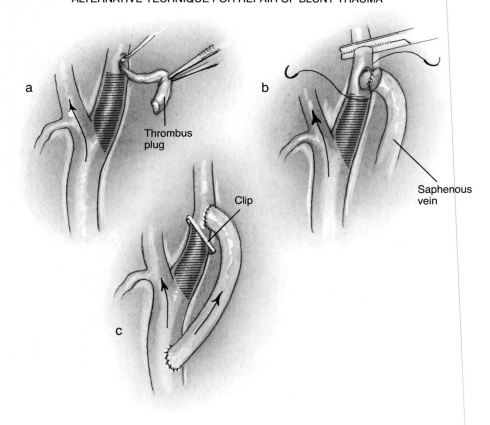

a

Thrombus plug

b

Saphenous vein

Clip

c

section II

Facial Nerve Injury

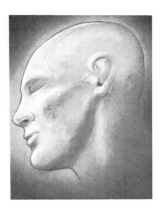

chapter 107

Neurorrhaphy for Facial Nerve Injury
Alternative Technique of Interposition Nerve Graft

INDICATIONS

Immediate facial paralysis after trauma suggests a partial or complete transection of the facial nerve. Paralysis associated with a wound lateral to the nasolabial fold carries a poor patient prognosis; more medially oriented wounds, on the other hand, are associated with transient weakness and usually good return of function.

The history, physical findings, and laboratory tests are important. An immediate loss of function usually means an interruption of the nerve, whereas a delayed onset often indicates a neurapraxia and a reversible phenomenon. For those patients in whom the onset and duration of paralysis are not clear, facial nerve stimulation and electromyographic studies should be performed. If the threshold for stimulation of the affected side exceeds that of the normal side by 3.5 mA or, on electromyography, action potentials are replaced by fibrillation potentials, then there is degeneration and the possibility of a transection. A continuation of action potentials usually denotes a good patient prognosis and probable return of function.

When findings indicate a disruption of the nerve, exploration and repair should be considered. In general, the earlier the exploration, the better the chance to find the ends of the nerves and effect an anastomosis. Loss of neural tissue requires nerve grafts, and for most patients, the great auricular nerve is the ideal donor. For injuries occurring within the temporal bone, the reader is referred to Chapter 89.

PROCEDURE

Surgery is usually performed under general anesthesia, with the head of the patient facing toward the anesthesist. Paralyzing agents are avoided, especially if intraoperative testing is anticipated. A preliminary injection of 1% lidocaine containing 1:100,000 epinephrine to the incision and operative site will assist in hemostasis.

A Our preference is to explore the facial nerve by way of a superficial parotidectomy. An incision is first marked in a preauricular crease. It is then extended below the earlobe in the form of a lazy S to join a line in the neck crease, about 3 cm below the angle of the mandible. The skin is incised, and the superficial layer of fascia (superficial musculoaponeurotic layer) is exposed. The flaps are developed in a subcutaneous plane anteriorly to the nasolabial fold, superiorly to the posterior half of the zygoma, and inferiorly to the level of the hyoid bone.

B The preauricular incision is then deepened to separate the parotid from the tragus. The triangular portion of the tragal cartilage will "point" toward the facial nerve. A plane is developed between the mastoid tip and the parotid gland and deepened to the level of the digastric muscle. Superiorly the superficial temporal artery and vein are identified, and if they are in the way, they are either ligated or retracted from the field.

Several important landmarks should be noted. The nerve lies directly beneath the tympanomastoid suture at a level about 1.5 to 2 cm below the mastoid prominence. The digastric muscle, which inserts on the deep aspect of the mastoid, is directly inferior and deep to the nerve. Several fibrous attachments are noted just lateral to the facial nerve as it exits the stylomastoid foramen.

C Once the facial nerve is identified, the nerve trunk is followed anteriorly into the parotid gland. Spoonlike retractors help keep the parotid tissues out of the way. Using a blunt and sharp dissection, the superficial lobe is separated from the deep lobe of the gland (i.e., a parotidectomy is performed). The major divisions of the nerve (superior and inferior) are traced into the area of injury. A useful technique is to spread the soft tissues along the nerve with a fine clamp and incise those fibers that lie posterior to the main nerve pedicle.

As the surgeon approaches the periphery of the gland, several landmarks should be appreciated. The mandibular branch of the facial nerve lies just above the posterior facial vein. The buccal branch of the facial nerve parallels the parotid duct. The frontal branch crosses the zygoma at a point one half the distance from the root to the orbital rim.

D-F Once the superficial lobe of the parotid gland is removed and the area of damage is isolated, both proximal and distal branches of the nerve should be identified and freshened by cutting the ends with a No. 11 knife blade over a wooden tongue blade. Using microscopic control, the nerve is then anastomosed with 7-0 nylon sutures. We prefer the "halving" technique, so that once the suture is placed through the perineurium, it is tagged with a microvascular clamp, and the nerve is rotated 180°. Another suture is then placed, followed by additional sutures between the attachments. The sutures will then be located clockwise at 12, 3, 6, and 9 o'clock,

respectively. The larger nerve trunks require four to six sutures, whereas the smaller branches can be easily repaired with three to four sutures. The repairs should be without any tension.

The wound is closed with three Penrose drains: one anterior to the tragus, a second beneath the earlobe, and a third along the cervical incision. The subcutaneous tissues are closed with 3-0 chromic sutures and the skin with interrupted 5-0 nylon sutures. A light pressure dressing of stretch gauze and fluffs is then placed over the ear in a figure-of-eight design that includes both the eye and forehead and the neck and jaw region. The eye is protected with eye ointment and an eye patch. Prophylactic antibiotics (i.e., penicillin or erythromycin) are used for 5 to 7 days. The drains are removed when drainage has ceased, and the sutures are usually removed at 7 days.

PITFALLS

1. Early exploration and repair of a neural discontinuity is desirable. Late repairs are made more difficult by the appearance of inflammatory tissues, which tend to bleed and obscure details of the reconstruction.

2. The surgeon should be aware of the facial nerve anatomy and the landmarks available to find the nerve roots and branches. Paralytic agents should be avoided, as there will be opportunity during the operative procedure to also stimulate the peripheral branches and identify their locations.

3. Nerve repair should be accomplished without tension. We prefer an epineural anastomosis using 7-0 nylon sutures. The edge of the epineurium should be held with jeweler forceps, and the needle should just penetrate the epineurium (about 2 mm from the edge). Injury to the fascicles should be avoided. The "halving" technique should be used, placing enough sutures to approximate the ends without tension.

4. Return of function should not be expected for at least 4 to 6 months, as the neural tissues grow about 1 mm per day in length. Some weakness and synkinesis should be expected.

COMPLICATIONS

1. Hematomas, seromas, and salivary gland fistulae are possible complications of the surgery. For these reasons, the entire superficial lobe of the parotid should be removed, the wound should be adequately drained, and the drains should not be removed until all drainage has ceased. A light compression dressing will help prevent accumulation of blood or serum beneath the flaps.

NEURORRHAPHY FOR FACIAL NERVE INJURY

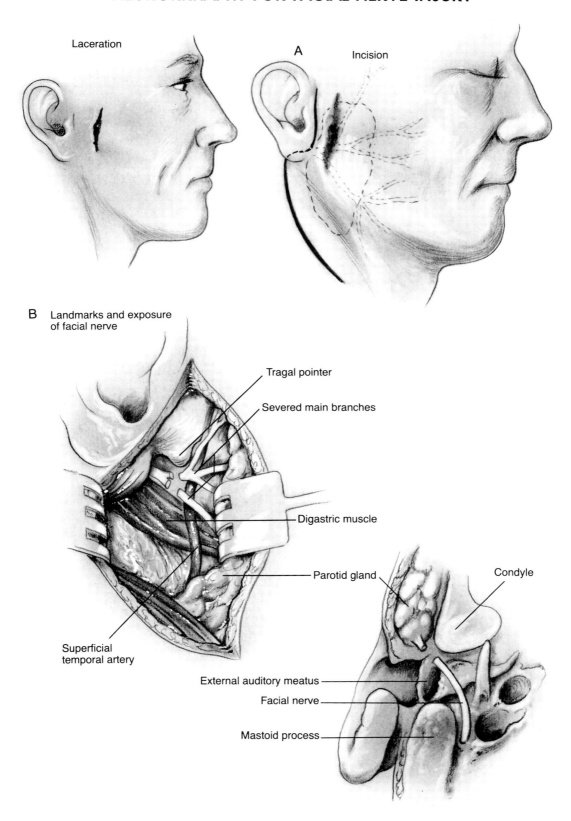

Laceration

A   Incision

B   Landmarks and exposure
of facial nerve

Tragal pointer

Severed main branches

Digastric muscle

Parotid gland

Condyle

Superficial
temporal artery

External auditory meatus

Facial nerve

Mastoid process

2. Gustatory sweating (Frey's syndrome) is a common sequela. It is believed that this condition develops as the parasympathetic fibers reinnervate the overlying skin. If the sweating becomes incapacitating (which is rare), the surgeon can place a piece fascia or Silastic sheeting between the skin and overlying tissues. Alternatively, the parasympathetic supply delivered by the chorda tympani and Jacobson's nerve can be lysed.

3. A depression of skin over the parotid gland should be expected. This can sometimes be avoided by rotating a platysma flap into the defect. A later correction is also possible, but because the nerve is very close to the skin, there is a risk of injury to the nerve.

4. Continued paresis and/or paralysis is also a possibility. The surgeon should consider a temporary tarsorrhaphy to protect the eye. If nerve function does not return, reexploration and repair or, alternatively, interposition and/or hypoglossal grafts should be considered. Once atrophy has occurred, muscle flaps and transposition procedures should be used (see Chapter 108).

ALTERNATIVE TECHNIQUE OF INTERPOSITIONAL NERVE GRAFT

If the nerve injury is characterized as penetrating and avulsive and the destruction between the neural segments exceeds 5 mm, the surgeon should consider a great auricular nerve graft interposition. The great auricular nerve is close by and in the same surgical field, and its thickness resembles that of the facial nerve. The disadvantages of using the great auricular nerve are that (1) it is a sensory nerve, and (2) the fascicles will not match.

a For the procedure, the surgeon should isolate the facial nerve and then develop subcutaneous flaps inferiorly to expose the great auricular nerve. Usually the great auricular nerve penetrates the platysma and fascia just lateral to the upper portion of the sternocleidomastoid muscle. More inferiorly, it passes from the deeper tissues behind the sternocleidomastoid muscle about 6 cm caudal to the mastoid tip. The main branch spreads out into smaller branches in the preauricular and infraauricular space. A secondary branch usually transverses the sternocleidomastoid muscle and continues across the neck. At least 8 to 10 cm of nerve should be harvested. This means that the nerve must be carefully dissected from the superficial layers of tissue and from those tissues that are deep to the sternocleidomastoid muscle. After the nerve is removed, the edges should be sharpened with a No. 11 knife blade; the nerve should be kept in physiologic solution or left to lie in the tissues until it is used for grafting.

b,c The neurorrhaphy technique resembles that used for the primary anastomosis. Tension should be avoided. The use of microscopic control, 7-0 to 10-0 nonreactive sutures, and "halving" techniques is desirable. Drains and soft compression dressings are applied, and the wounds are closed in layers. Postoperative care is essentially the same as that used for the direct anastomosis technique.

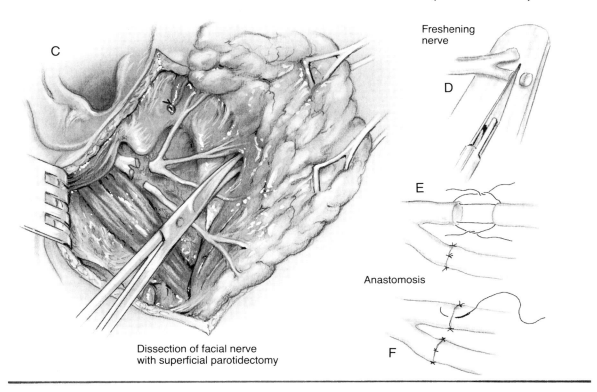

C

Freshening nerve

D

E

Anastomosis

F

Dissection of facial nerve
with superficial parotidectomy

ALTERNATIVE TECHNIQUE OF
INTERPOSITIONAL NERVE GRAFT

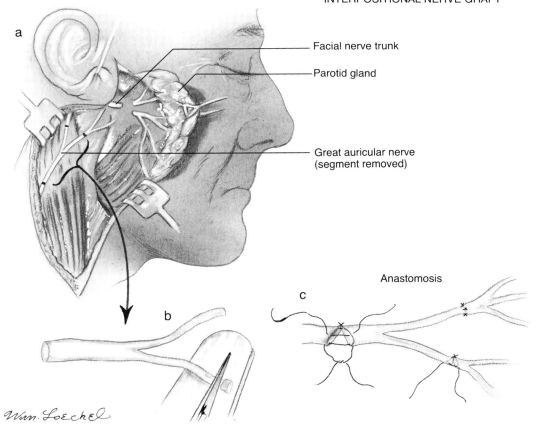

a

Facial nerve trunk

Parotid gland

Great auricular nerve
(segment removed)

b

Anastomosis

c

Wm. Loechel

chapter 108

Reanimation of the Paralyzed Face With a Temporalis Muscle Galea Flap

INDICATIONS

Interruption of the facial nerve often leads to paralysis of the face and, depending on the degree and location of muscle weakness, a dysfunction of the eye, mouth, and nares. When the nerve is completely severed, the best method of repair is an early exploration, freshening of the ends of the nerve, and a direct anastomosis. If there is a neural deficit of several centimeters, great auricular nerve grafts are indicated. These techniques are discussed in Chapter 107.

Long-standing facial paralysis, however, is different. With time, there is an atrophy of muscle and neural tissues. In such situations, the surgeon must test for residual nerve function, and if it is insufficient for reanimation, a muscle transposition technique must be considered. The temporalis muscle galea flap provides an opportunity to transfer functional muscular units to a different area of the face. The method is particularly useful when there are accompanying craniofacial defects and/or destruction of the peripheral branches of the nerve.

PROCEDURE

In preparation for surgery, the patient's scalp is shaved, and the skin is treated with a standard antiseptic solution. The face and one half of the scalp are then draped as a sterile field.

A Skin incisions are first outlined with a marking solution and then infiltrated with 1% lidocaine containing 1:100,000 epinephrine to help control hemostasis. A line is then drawn along the preauricular crease and extended upward several millimeters behind the temporal hairline. A horizontal limb is fashioned about 2.5 cm above the pinna and, starting from the anterior line, drawn toward the occiput. Additionally, the surgeon can draw another horizontal line beneath the earlobe, just beyond the cervical hairline, and connect it to the upper horizontal limb with a vertical line, but for many cases, the superior and anterior lines will be sufficient.

B The preauricular incision is used to elevate the skin in a suitable plane as in a classic rhytidoplasty procedure. The skin of the face is retracted to expose the fibers of the orbicularis oris, depressor groups, zygomaticus, levator labii superiorus, and orbicularis oculi. The plane of dissection around the eye is facilitated by additional upper and lower eyelid incisions through crease lines. This exposure will help at a later time with the attachment of the muscle flaps to the orbicularis oculi musculature.

The temporalis muscle galea flap is exposed by elevation of superficial scalp flaps at a level just beneath the hair follicles and external to the superficial temporal artery. This artery should be identified and maintained within the deeper tissues, as it will nourish primarily the galea flap. The extent of the superior and posterior part of the flap is determined by the length of the temporalis muscle and galea needed for reconstruction.

C Once the design of the muscle galea flap is complete, a curvilinear incision is made along the galea from the frontal to the occipital region. Working in a plane between the galea and pericranium, the galea is elevated to the level of the temporalis fossa, at which point the pericranium is incised, and the pericranium and temporalis muscle are elevated from the fossa. Nerve and vascular injuries are avoided by a dissection close to the skull.

D,E Rotation of the flaps should provide complete coverage of the hemiface. Additional length can be achieved by incisions strategically placed along the zygomaticofrontal process and along the pretragal root of the zygoma. The galea can then be split into three to five compartments, the lower two of which can be placed below and above the lips, the middle one at the midface, and the upper two below and above the eyelids. Excess galea should not be excised, but rather folded onto itself and sutured to the base of each compartment with 3-0 chromic sutures.

TEMPORALIS MUSCLE GALEA FLAP REANIMATION PROCEDURE

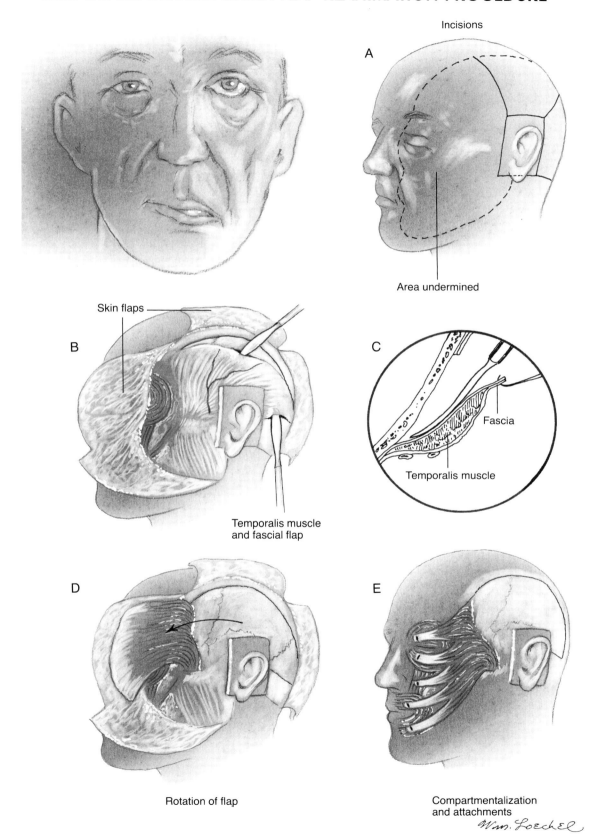

Incisions

A

Area undermined

Skin flaps

B

C

Fascia

Temporalis muscle

Temporalis muscle and fascial flap

D

E

Rotation of flap

Compartmentalization and attachments

Wm. Loechel

With the flap in appropriate position, each extension is sutured with 3-0 polyglactin to the appropriate facial muscles. Ideally the lower compartments are secured to the lateral and middle thirds of the orbicularis oris, the middle to the levator labii superioris muscle, and the upper to the inner aspect of the orbicularis oculi of the upper and lower eyelids. The tension of each flap segment should be adjusted to obtain a slight smile and almost complete closure of the palpebral fissure.

All wounds are treated with multiple small Penrose drains. Skin flaps are sutured into position with a layered closure. Prophylactic antibiotics are desirable. A light decompression bandage is applied for 24 to 48 hours.

PITFALLS

1. The temporalis muscle galea flap is best used when there is no longer any opportunity for neural repair (i.e., the muscle and/or nerve have undergone atrophy or there are large defects of the face in which it is not possible to repair nerve segments). Neurorrhaphy, if indicated, is described in Chapter 107.

2. The muscle galea technique is time consuming and requires a meticulous dissection to avoid injury to the muscle, arterial supply, and overlying hair-bearing tissues. The surgeon should study the anatomy of the superficial temporal artery and be prepared to follow the artery to the periphery. Doppler studies may be helpful.

3. Flaps should be designed to provide appropriate length and compartmentalization. Each segment can potentially operate as an independent neuromuscular unit, and if independent eye and lip movements are to be achieved, these segments must be separated from each other. To preserve viability, each segment should be 2 to 3 cm in width and no longer than 5 to 6 cm in length.

4. The tension provided by the muscle galea slings will temporarily establish facial "tone." Ideally the surgeon should strive for a half closure of the palpebral fissure and a slight smile. As the muscle begins to function, tension and relaxation should increase, and additional reanimation should become apparent.

5. The patient should be instructed to practice movements of the face. Biting down on the jaws should cause contraction of the muscles. Changes in the bite will cause certain muscle groups to become more activated than others.

COMPLICATIONS

1. Alopecia will occur if the hair-bearing follicles are injured during elevation of the flap. The dissection is therefore carried out in a plane just deep enough to avoid the follicles, but not so deep as to injure the superficial temporal artery. The wound should be drained and closed without tension. If alopecia develops, small areas of hair loss may be excised; larger areas require tissue expansion and advancement techniques.

2. Rotation of the temporalis muscle flap will cause a depression over the parietal region and a bulge along the zygomatic arch. The deformity will become less noticeable over time as the tissues atrophy. Removal of the zygoma and/or implants above the bulge may help to camouflage the irregularity.

3. Although reanimation is to be expected, it is not as "natural" as that seen with the neurorrhaphy technique. If more tension is needed in the tissues, the method can be augmented with tarsorrhaphy, springs, facial slings, and Z-plasty. However, these techniques should be applied only after the patient has had sufficient time for rehabilitation.

section III

Parotid Duct Injury

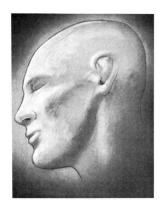

chapter 109

Open Repair of Parotid Duct Injury

INDICATIONS

Penetrating wounds of the cheek can injure the parotid (Stensen's) duct and cause a leakage of saliva into the soft tissues. Although parotid gland drainage will stop with pressure, leakage from the parotid duct will persist, often causing accumulation of fluids and/or a fistula. Early recognition and repair is desirable.

Several options for treatment of a parotid duct injury are available. For a laceration or avulsion injury that occurs between the anterior portion of the parotid gland and the anterior portion of the masseter muscle, an end-to-end anastomosis should be considered. For those injuries closer to the duct orifice, a new opening should be created into the oral cavity. Frequently the duct injury is associated with a facial nerve injury, and duct repair is carried out at the same time as a neurorrhaphy or grafting (see Chapter 107).

PROCEDURE

The location of the duct and the site of injury should be mapped out on the face. The area is then prepared and draped as a sterile field. The patient should be under light anesthesia only, as this will provide an opportunity to stimulate and find the position of the branches of the facial nerve, which will be an excellent guide to the duct system. Paralytic agents should thus be avoided.

The main parotid duct travels along the buccal branch of the facial nerve. The nerve can be located with a facial nerve stimulator, and once this branch is found, it will be easy to define the proximal and distal ends of Stensen's duct and carry out the repair.

Another method of finding the duct is with intubation. For this technique, the duct orifice is cannulated with a lacrimal probe. Pulling the cheek laterally will help straighten the duct and assist with the cannulation.

A–D After the duct is isolated, a small polyethylene tube should be placed through the proximal and distal segments. The long end of the catheter should be brought out through the oral cavity and fixed to the oral-buccal mucosa with sutures and to the corner of the mouth and cheek with adhesive tape. The duct is then closed around the tubing, using 6-0 or 7-0 silk sutures and atraumatic needles. The catheter should be retained for approximately 10 days. Pro-

537

REPAIR OF PAROTID DUCT

Anatomic considerations

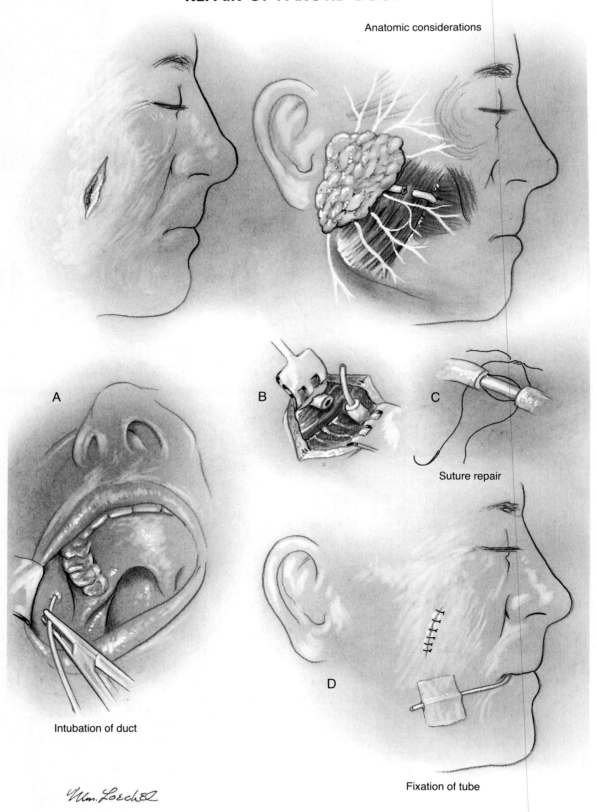

A

B

C

Suture repair

D

Intubation of duct

Fixation of tube

Wm. Loechel

phylactic antibiotics are administered for the duration of intubation.

PITFALLS

1. The duct can be tortuous and difficult to cannulate. Pulling the duct and gland laterally will straighten the duct and provide for an easier passage of the intubation tube.

2. Dislodgement of the intubation tube is common and can be avoided by securing the tube to the cheek tissues with tape and directly to the oral mucosa with sutures.

3. Avoid any additional injury to the facial nerve. The buccal branch should be identified. If the nerve has been injured, it can be treated at the same time as duct repair (see Chapter 107).

COMPLICATIONS

1. Accumulation of fluid and fistulization can occur in spite of carefully applied reconstructive techniques. If such complications develop, the surgeon can attempt packing and/or pressure dressings. Salivary flow can be diminished by lysing the chorda tympani and/or Jacobsen's nerve. If these procedures are unsuccessful, ligation of the duct and/or radiation must be considered.

2. Parotitis is always possible, especially when the flow is obstructed and associated with stasis of secretion. Antibiotic treatment and generous use of sialagogues are indicated. However, if the condition persists, the surgeon can consider denervation by way of resection of the chorda tympani. Failure of this technique should prompt removal of the gland (superficial parotidectomy).

Bibliography

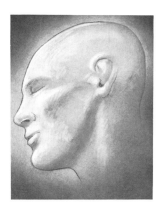

This atlas reflects the author's 25 years of experience in the treatment of craniomaxillofacial injuries. Textbooks and articles have provided much of the information that is used and sometimes modified for successful patient care. Below is a list of suggested readings that contain many of these excellent works.

GENERAL REFERENCES

Alling CC III, Osbon DB: Maxillofacial Trauma. Philadelphia, Lea & Febiger, 1988.

Andreason JO: Traumatic Injuries of the Teeth, ed 2. Philadelphia, WB Saunders, 1981.

Becker DP, Gudeman SK (eds): Textbook of Head and Neck Injury. Philadelphia, WB Saunders, 1989.

Converse JM: Kazanjian and Converse's Surgical Treatment of Facial Injuries, vols 1 and 2, ed 3. Baltimore, Williams & Wilkins, 1974.

Converse JM (ed): Reconstructive Plastic Surgery, vols 1–3. Philadelphia, WB Saunders, 1964.

Cummings CW, Sessions DG, Weymuller EA Jr, Wood P: Atlas of Laryngeal Surgery. St Louis, CV Mosby, 1984.

Dingman RO, Natvig P: Surgery of Facial Fractures, ed 2. Philadelphia, WB Saunders, 1967.

Fisch U: Facial Nerve Surgery. Birmingham, AL, Aesculapius, 1977.

Foster CA, Sherman JE (eds): Surgery of Facial Bone Fractures. New York, Churchill Livingstone, 1987.

Habal MB, Ariyan S (eds): Facial Fractures. Philadelphia, BC Decker, 1989.

Hotte HHA: Orbital Fractures. Springfield, IL, Charles C Thomas, 1970.

Keen WW: Surgery Principles and Practice. Philadelphia, WB Saunders, 1909.

Kellman RM (ed): Facial plating. Otolaryngol Clin North Am 20(3), 1987.

Killey HC: Fracture of the Middle Third of the Facial Skeleton, ed 2. Bristol, England, J Wright, 1971.

Manson PN (ed): Rigid Fixation and bone grafts in craniofacial surgery. Clin Plastic Surg Vol 16 No 1 1989.

Mathog RH (ed): Symposium on maxillofacial trauma. Otolaryngol Clin North Am 9(2), 1976.

Mathog RH (ed): Maxillofacial Trauma. Baltimore, Williams & Wilkins, 1984.

Miehlke A: Surgery of the Facial Nerve, ed 2. Philadelphia, WB Saunders, 1973.

Mustarde JC: Repair and Reconstruction of the Orbital Region. Baltimore, Williams & Wilkins, 1966.

Myers EN, Stool SE, Johnson JT (eds): Tracheotomy. New York, Churchill Livingstone, 1985.

Rowe NL, Killey HC (eds): Fractures of the Facial Skeleton, ed 2. Edinburgh, E & S Livingstone, 1968.

Rowe NL, Williams LI (eds): Maxillofacial Injuries, vols 1 and 2. New York, Churchill Livingstone, 1985.

Salyer KE: Techniques in Aesthetic Craniofacial Surgery. Philadelphia, JB Lippincott, 1989.

Saunders WH, Paparella MM: Atlas of Ear Surgery. St Louis, CV Mosby, 1968.

Schuknecht HJ: Pathology of the Ear. Cambridge, MA, Harvard University Press, 1974.

Schultz RC: Facial Injuries, ed 3. Chicago, Year Book Medical Publishers, 1988.

Shambaugh GE, Glasscock ME III: Surgery of the Ear, ed 3. Philadelphia, WB Saunders, 1982.

Smith B, Nesi F: Practical Techniques in Ophthalmic Plastic Surgery. St Louis, CV Mosby, 1981.

Spiessl B (ed): New Concepts in Maxillofacial Bone Surgery. Berlin, Springer-Verlag, 1976.

Spoor TC, Nesi FA (eds): Management of Ocular, Orbital, and Adnexal Trauma. New York, Raven Press, 1988.

Stout R: Manual of Standard Practice of Plastic and Maxillofacial Surgery. Philadelphia, WB Saunders, 1943.

541

Wheeler RC: A Textbook of Dental Anatomy and Physiology, ed 4. Philadelphia, WB Saunders, 1965.

SPECIFIC REFERENCES

Emergency Measures

Atkin JP: Current utilization of tracheotomy as a therapeutic measure. A review of the literature and an analysis of 526 cases. Laryngoscope 70:1672–1690, 1960.

Brantigan CO, Grow JB: Cricothyroidotomy: Elective use in respiratory problems requiring tracheotomy. J Thorac Cardiovasc Surg 71:72–80, 1976.

Committee on Trauma of the American College of Surgeons: Early Care of the Injured Patient. Philadelphia, WB Saunders, 1976.

Davidson JSD, Birdsell DC: Cervical spine injury of patients with facial skeletal trauma. J Trauma 29:1276–1278, 1989.

Davis HS, Kretchmer HE, Bryce-Smith R: Advantages and complications of tracheostomy. JAMA 153:1156–1157, 1953.

Dugan DJ, Sampson PC: Tracheostomy: Present day indications and techniques. Am J Surg 106:290–306, 1963.

Fearon B: Acute obstructive laryngitis in infants and children. Hosp Med 4:51–67, 1968.

Glas WW, King OJ Jr, Lui A: Complications of tracheostomy. Arch Surg 85:56–63, 1962.

Gwyn DP, Carraway JH, Horton CE, et al: Facial fractures—associated injuries and complications. Plast Reconstr Surg 47:225–230, 1971.

Head JM: Tracheostomy in the management of respiratory problems. N Engl J Med 264:587–590, 1961.

Herrin TJ, Brzustowitz R, Hendrickson M: Anesthetic management of neck trauma. South Med J 72:1102–1106, 1979.

Horton JM: Immediate care of head injuries. Anaesthesia 30:212–218, 1975.

Koopman CF, Feld RH, Coulthard SW: The effects of cricoid cartilage injury and antibiotics in cricothyroidotomy. Am J Otolaryngol 2:123–128, 1981.

Lewis VL, Manson PN, Morgan FG, et al: Facial injuries associated with cervical fractures: Recognition, patterns and management. J Trauma 25:90–93, 1985.

Mathog RH: Croup and laryngeal inflammation. Postgrad Med 52:106–110, 1972.

Mathog RH, Kenan PD, Hudson WR: Delayed massive hemorrhage following tracheostomy. Laryngoscope 81:107–119, 1971.

McCallum CA: Complication resulting from maxillofacial injuries. J Oral Surg 27:488–496, 1969.

Meade JW: Tracheotomy. Its complications and their management. A study of 212 cases. N Engl J Med 265:519–523, 1961.

Morgan BDG, Madan DK, Bergerot JPC: Fractures of the middle third of the face. A review of 300 cases. Br J Plast Surg 25:147–151, 1972.

Nelson TG: Tracheotomy: A clinical and experimental study. Am J Surg 23:660–694;750–783;941–981, 1957.

Oliver P, Richardson JR, Clubb RW, Flake CG: Tracheotomy in children. N Engl J Med 267:631–637, 1962.

Roberge RJ, Wears RC, Kelly M, et al: Selective application of cervical spine radiography in alert victims of blunt trauma: A prospective study. J Trauma 28:784–788, 1988.

Rosen Z, Romanoff H, Zelig S, Borman JB: A critical review of tracheostomy with special emphasis on the newer indications. Laryngoscope 73:1326–1355, 1963.

Ruskin JD, Tu HK: Integrated management of the maxillofacial trauma patient with multiple injuries. Oral Maxillofac Surg Clin North Am 2:15–27, 1990.

Schaefer SD, Bucholz RW, Jones RE, et al: "How I do it" head and neck. Treatment of transpharyngeal missile wounds to the cervical spine. Laryngoscope 91:146–148, 1981.

Schultz RC: Facial injuries from automobile accidents. A study of 400 consecutive cases. Plast Reconstr Surg 40:415–425, 1967.

Schultz RC, Oldham RJ: An overview of facial injuries. Surg Clin North Am 57:987–1010, 1977.

Starkhammar H, Olofsson J: Facial fractures: A review of 922 cases and special reference to medicine and aetiology. Clin Otolaryngol 7:405–409, 1982.

Strate RG, Boies LR: The emergency management of trauma. Otolaryngol Clin North Am 9:315–329, 1976.

Thompson JN, Gibson B, Kohut R: Airway obstruction in Le Fort fractures. Laryngoscope 97:275–279, 1987.

Walton RL, Hagan RF, Parry SH, Deluchi SF: Maxillofacial trauma. Surg Clin North Am 62:73–96, 1982.

Watts JMK: Tracheostomy in modern practice. Br J Surg 50:954–975, 1963.

Woo P, Kelly G, Kirschner P: Airway complications in the head injured. Laryngoscope 99:725–731, 1989.

Yarington CT, Frazer JP: Complications of tracheostomy. Arch Surg 91:652–655, 1968.

Mandible Fractures

Allgower M, Perren S, Pathew P: A new plate for internal fixation: The dynamic compression plate (DCP). Injury 2:40–47, 1970.

Bailey BJ, Gaskill JR: Fractures of the mandible. Laryngoscope 77:1137–1154, 1967.

Beckler DM, Walker RV: Condyle fracture. J Oral Surg 27:563–564, 1969.

Belvins C, Gores RJ: Fractures of the mandibular condylar process: Results of conservative treatment in 140 cases. J Oral Surg 19:393–407, 1961.

Bernstein L, McClurg FL: Mandibular fractures: A review of 156 consecutive cases. Laryngoscope 88:951–961, 1978.

Blair VP: Operative treatment of ankylosis of the mandible. South Surg Gynecol Trans 26:435–465, 1913.

Boyne PJ: Restoration of osseous defects in maxillofacial casualties. J Am Dent Assoc 78:767–776, 1969.

Boyne PJ, Upham C: The treatment of long standing bilateral fracture non- and mal-union in atrophic edentulous mandibles. Int J Oral Surg 3:213–217, 1974.

Braham RL, Roberts MW, Morris ME: Management of dental trauma in children and adolescents. J Trauma 17:857–865, 1977.

Brown AE, Obeid G: A simplified method for the internal fixation of fractures of the mandibular condyle. Br J Oral Maxillofac Surg 22:145–150, 1984.

Bruce RH, Strachan DS: Fractures of the edentulous mandible: The Chalmers J Lyons Academy study. J Oral Surg 34:973–979, 1976.

Calhoun KH, Spencer L, Clark WD, et al: Surgical care of submental gunshot wounds. Arch Otolaryngol 114:513–519, 1988.

Cameron JR: Complications in the treatment of fractures. J Oral Surg 23:14–16, 1965.

Champy M, Lodde JP, Schmitt R, et al: Mandibular osteosynthesis by miniature screwed plates via a buccal approach. J Maxillofac Surg 6:14–21, 1978.

Converse JM: Surgical release of bilateral intractable temporomandibular ankylosis. Plast Reconstr Surg 64:404–407, 1979.

Davis WH, Delo RI, Weiner JR, Terry B: Transoral bone graft for atrophy of the mandible. Oral Surg 28:760–765, 1970.

Dierks E: Transoral approach to fractures of the mandible. Laryngoscope 97:4–6, 1987.

Dingman RO: Ankylosis of the temporomandibular joint. Am J Orthod 32:120–125, 1946.

Dingman RO, Grabb WC: Reconstruction of both mandibular condyles with metatarsal bone grafts. Plast Reconstr Surg 34:441–451, 1964.

Dingman RO, Grabb WC: Intra-articular temporomandibular joint arthroplasty. Plast Reconstr Surg 38:179–185, 1966.

Eby JD: Principles of orthodontia in the treatment of maxillofacial injuries. Int J Orthod 6:273–310, 1920.

Fernandez JA, Mathog RH: Open treatment of condylar fractures with biphase technique. Arch Otolaryngol 113:262–266, 1987.

Georgiade NG: The surgical correction of temporomandibular joint dysfunction by means of autogenous dermal grafts. Plast Reconstr Surg 30:68–73, 1962.

Georgiade NG, Masters FW, Metzger JT, Pickrell KL: Fractures of the mandible and maxilla in children. J Pediatr 42:440–449, 1953.

Georgiade NG, Pickrell K, Douglas W, Altany F: External pinning of displaced condylar fractures. Plast Reconstr Surg 18:377–383, 1956.

Giordanno A, Brady D, Foster D, Adams G: Particulate cancellous marrow crib graft reconstruction of mandibular defects. Laryngoscope 90:2027–2036, 1980.

Gunning RB: The treatment of fractures of the lower jaw by interdental splints. NY State J Med 3:433–444, 1961.

Harper R, Weinberg S: Treatment of malunited, unusual displaced bilateral condylar fractures. J Oral Surg 36:716–719, 1978.

Hayward JR: Fractures involving the mandibular condyle: A post-treatment survey of 120 cases: Chalmers J Lyons Club J Oral Surg 5:45–73, 1945.

Hohman A: Management of alveolar fractures. Minn Med 50:975–977, 1967.

Hoopes J, Wolfort F, Jabaley M: Operative treatment of fractures of the mandibular condyle in children. The post-auricular approach. Plast Reconstr Surg 46:357–362, 1970.

Humphry GM: Excision of the condyle of the lower jaw. Assoc Med J (London) 160:61–62, 1856.

Irby WB: Correction of malreduced fractures of mandible at angles. Oral Surg Oral Med Oral Path 11:26–30, 1958.

Irving SP, Costa LE, Salisbury PL: The occlusal wafer: Simple technique for construction and its use in maxillofacial surgery. Laryngoscope 94:1036–1041, 1984.

Ivy RH: Operative treatment of ununited fractures of the mandible. Ann Surg 71:363–376, 1921.

Ivy RH: Practical method of fixation in fractures of the mandible. Surg Gynecol Obstet 22:620–673, 1934.

Jackson IT, Somers PC, Kjar JG: The use of champy miniplates for osteosyntheses in craniofacial deformities and trauma. Plast Reconstr Surg 77:729–736, 1986.

James RW, Fredericks C, Kent JM: Prospective study of mandibular fractures. J Oral Surg 39:275–281, 1981.

Jones K, Bauer BS, Pensler JM: Treatment of mandibular fractures in children. Ann Plast Surg 23:280–283, 1989.

Jones JK, Van Sickels JE: Rigid fixation: A review of concepts and treatment of fractures. Oral Surg 65:13–18, 1988.

Juniper RP, Awty MD: The immobilization period for fractures of the mandibular body. Oral Surg Oral Med Oral Path 36:157–163, 1973.

Kellman RM: Repair of mandibular fractures via compression plating and more traditional techniques: A comparison of results. Laryngoscope 94:1560–1567, 1984.

Kiehn CL, Des Prez JD: Total prosthetic replacement of the temporomandibular joint. Ann Plast Surg 2:5–15, 1979.

Klein JC: Intraoral open reduction. Arch Otolaryngol 103:645–647, 1977.

Koberg WR, Moorman W: Treatment of fractures of the articular process by functional stable osteosynthesis using miniaturized dynamic compression plates. Int J Oral Surg 7:256–262, 1978.

Krebs FJ: Dynamic compression plating in treatment of the fractured edentulous mandible. Laryngoscope 98:198–201, 1988.

Kreutziger K: Surgery of the temporomandibular joint. I. Surgical anatomy and surgical incisions. Oral Surg 58:637–646, 1984.

Leake DL: A new alloplastic tray for osseous contour defects. J Maxillofac Surg 2:146–149, 1974.

Leake DL, Doykos J, Habal MB, Murray JE: Long-term follow-up of fractures of the mandibular condyle in children. Plast Reconstr Surg 47:127–131, 1971.

Leake DL, Leake RD, Davie JS, Hansen R: Definitive treatment of mandibular fractures in young children. Oral Surg 36:164–169, 1973.

Lehman JA, Saddawi N: Fractures of the mandible in children. J Trauma 16:773–777, 1976.

Levine PA: Mandibular reconstruction: The use of open reduction with compression plates. Otolaryngol Head Neck Surg 90:585–588, 1982.

Levine PA, Goode RL: Treatment of fractures of the edentulous mandible. Arch Otolaryngol 108:167–173, 1982.

MacIntosh RB, Henry FA: A spectrum of application of autogenous costochondral grafts. J Maxillofac Surg 5:257–267, 1977.

Marchmont-Robinson H, Crinzi RH: A simplified technique for closure of surgical sites following intraoral open reduction of mandibular fractures. Oral Surg Oral Med Oral Path 62:138–139, 1986.

Mathog RH: Non-union of the mandible. Otolaryngol Clin North Am 16:70–84, 1983.

Mathog RH, Boies LR Jr: Non-union of the mandible. Laryngoscope 86:908–920, 1976.

Mathog RH, Crane LR, Nowak GS: Antimicrobial therapy follow-ing head and neck trauma. In Johnson JT (ed): Antibiotic Therapy in Head and Neck Surgery. New York, Marcel Dekker, 1987, pp 31–49.

Mathog RH, Leonard MS: Reconstruction of the hemimandible with rib autograft. In Bernstein L (ed): Plastic and Reconstructive Surgery of the Head and Neck, vol 2. Rehabilitative Surgery. New York, Grune & Stratton, 1981, pp 198–206.

Mathog RH, Nelson RJ, Petrilli A, Humphreys B: Self-inflicted gunshot wounds to the face. Surgical and psychiatric considerations. Otolaryngol Head Neck Surg 88:568–574, 1988.

May M, Tucker HM, Ogura JA: Closed management of mandibular fractures. Arch Otolaryngol 95:55–57, 1972.

McCoy FS, Chandler RH, Crow ML: Facial fractures in children. Plast Reconstr Surg 37:209–215, 1966.

McGuirt WF, Salisbury PL: Mandibular fractures: Their effect on growth and dentition. Arch Otolaryngol 113:257–261, 1987.

Michelet FX, Deymes J, Dessus B: Osteosynthesis with miniaturized screwed plates in maxillofacial surgery. J Maxillofac Surg 1:79–83, 1973.

Morris JH: Biphase connector: External skeletal splint for reduction and fixation of mandibular fractures. J Oral Surg 2:1382–1389, 1949.

Mulliken JB, Kaban LB, Murray JE: Management of facial fractures in children. Clin Plast Surg 4:491–502, 1977.

Neal DC, Wagner WF, Alpert B: Morbidity associated with teeth in line of mandibular fracture. J Oral Surg 36:859–862, 1978.

Niederdellmann H, Shetty V: Solitary lag screw osteosynthesis in the treatment of fractures of the angle of the mandible: A retrospective study. Plast Reconstr Surg 80:68–74, 1987.

Obeid G, Guttenberg SA, Connole PW: Costochondral grafting in condylar replacement and mandibular reconstruction. J Oral Maxillofac Surg 48:177–182, 1988.

Obwegeser HL, Sailer HF: Another way of treating fractures of the atrophic edentulous mandible. J Maxillofac Surg 1:213–221, 1973.

Perren SM, Russenberger M, Steinemanns S, et al: A dynamic compression plate. Acta Orthop Scand (Suppl) 125:29–41, 1964.

Peters RH, Caldwell JB, Olsen TW: A technique for open reduction of subcondylar fractures. Oral Surg Oral Med Oral Path 41:273–280, 1976.

Petzel JR: Instrumentarium and technique for screw-pin osteosynthesis of condylar fractures. J Maxillofac Surg 10:8–13, 1982.

Prein J, Kellman RM: Rigid internal fixation of mandibular fractures. Basics of AO technique. Otolaryngol Clin North Am 20:441–456, 1987.

Richter HE, Boyne PJ: New concepts in facial bone healing and grafting procedures. J Oral Surg 27:557–559, 1969.

Risdon F: The treatment of fractures of the jaw. Can Med Assoc J 20:260–262, 1929.

Rontal E, Hohman A: External fixation of facial fractures. Arch Otolaryngol 98:393–396, 1973.

Rontal E, Myerhoff W, Hohman A: The transoral reduction of mandibular fractures. Arch Otolaryngol 97:279–282, 1973.

Rontal E, Myerhoff W, Wilson K: Biphase external fixation: Technique and application. Laryngoscope 84:1104–1440, 1974.

Rowe NL: Fractures of the facial skeleton in children. J Oral Surg 26:505–515, 1968.

Rowe NL: Fractures of the jaws in children. J Oral Surg 27:497–507, 1969.

Rowe NL: Non-union of the mandible and maxilla. J Oral Surg 27:520–529, 1969.

Sanders B, Beumer J: Augmentation rib grafting to the inferior border of the atrophic edentulous mandible: A 5-year experience. J Prosthet Dent 47:16–22, 1982.

Sanders B, McKelvy B, Adams D: Aseptic osteomyelitis and necrosis of the mandibular condylar head after intracapsular fracture. J Oral Surg 43:665–670, 1977.

Sazima HJ, Grafft ML, Fulcher CL: Transoral reduction of mandibular fractures. J Oral Surg 29:247–254, 1971.

Schilli W: Compression osteosynthesis. J Oral Surg 35:802–808, 1977.

Schneider SS: Teeth in the line of the mandibular fracture. J Oral Surg 29:107–109, 1971.

Siegel LG, Myerhoff WL: Reduction of mandibular fractures. Otolaryngol Clin North Am 9:439–451, 1976.

Spiessl B: Rigid internal fixation of fractures of the lower jaw. Reconstr Surg Traumatol 13:124–140, 1972.

Spiessl B: A new method of anatomical reconstruction of extensive defects of the mandible with autogenous cancellous bone. J Maxillofac Surg 8:78–83, 1980.

Strelzow VV, Friedman WH: Dynamic compression plating in the treatment of mandibular fractures. Arch Otolaryngol 108:583–586, 1982.

Thomson HG, Farmer AW, Lindsay WK: Condylar neck fractures of the mandible in children. Plast Reconstr Surg 34:452–463, 1964.

Waite DR: Pediatric fractures of jaw and facial bones. Pediatrics 51:557–558, 1973.

Wald RM, Abemayor E, Zemplenyi J, et al: The transoral treatment of mandibular fractures using non-compression miniplates: A prospective study. Ann Plast Surg 20:409–413, 1988.

Walker RV: Traumatic mandibular condylar fracture dislocations. Am J Surg 100:850–863, 1960.

Walker RV: Delayed occlusal and maxillofacial deformities after trauma. JAMA 82:858–861, 1977.

Welsh LW, Welsh JJ: Fractures of the edentulous maxilla and mandible. Laryngoscope 86:1333–1341, 1976.

Wilkie C, Diecidue AA, Simses RJ: Management of teeth in the line of mandibular fracture. J Oral Surg 11:227–230, 1953.

Williams CN, Cohn M, Schultz RC: Immediate and long term management of gunshot wounds to the lower face. Plast Reconstr Surg 82:433–439, 1988.

Wilson KS, Christiansen TA, Quick C: External fixation of maxillofacial surgery. Otolaryngol Clin North Am 2:523–531, 1976.

Wilson KS, Hohman A: Dental anatomy and occlusion. Otolaryngol Clin North Am 9:24–37, 1976.

Zallen RD, Curry JT: A study of antibiotic usage in compound mandibular fractures. J Oral Surg 33:431–434, 1975.

Zatten R, Fitzgerald B: Treatment of mandibular fractures with use of malleable titanium mesh: Report of 56 cases. J Oral Surg 34:748–754, 1976.

Zide MF, Kent SM: Indications for open reduction of mandibular condyle fractures. J Oral Maxillofac Surg 41:89–98, 1983.

Maxillary Fractures

Adams WM: Internal wiring fixation of facial fractures. Surgery 12:523–540, 1942.

Antoni AA, Vandemark TB, Weinberg S, Schofield L: Surgical treatment of longstanding malunited horizontal fractures of the maxilla. Can Dent Assoc J 31:22–25, 1965.

Arden RL, Mathog RH: Maxillary fractures. In Paparella MM, Shumrick DA, Gluckman JL, Myerhoff WL (eds): Otolaryngology, vol IV, ed 3. Philadelphia, WB Saunders, 1991, pp 2927–2938.

Conway H, Smith JW, Behrman JJ: Another method of bringing the midface forward. Plast Reconstr Surg 46:325–331, 1970.

Dawson RLG, Fordyce GF: Complex fractures of the middle third of the face and their early treatment. Br J Surg 41:254–268, 1953.

Finkle DR, Ringler SL, Luttenton CR, et al: Comparison of the diagnostic methods used in maxillofacial trauma. Plast Reconstr Surg 75:32–38, 1985.

Furnas DW: Transverse maxillary osteotomy for malunion of maxillary fractures. Plast Reconstr Surg 42:378–383, 1968.

Georgiade N, Nash T: An external cranial fixation apparatus for severe maxillofacial injuries. Plast Reconstr Surg 38:142–146, 1966.

Gruss JS: Naso-ethmoid-orbital fractures: Classification and role of primary bone grafting. Plast Reconstr Surg 75:303–317, 1985.

Gruss JS, MacKinnon SE: Complex maxillary fractures: Role of buttress reconstruction and immediate bone grafts. Plast Reconstr Surg 78:9–22, 1986.

Gruss JS, MacKinnon SE, Kassel EE, Cooper PW: Role of primary bone grafting in complex craniomaxillofacial trauma. Plast Reconstr Surg 75:17–24, 1983.

Henderson D, Jackson IT: Naso-maxillary hypoplasia. The LeFort II osteotomy. Br J Oral Surg 11:77–93, 1973.

Hillstrom RP, Mathog RH, Moore GK: Medial maxillary fractures. Otolaryngol Head Neck Surg 104:270–275, 1991.

Hovinga JA: Fractures of the middle third of the face. Mod Probl Ophthalmol 14:513–522, 1975.

Jackson IT, Somers PC, Kjar JG: The use of Champy miniplates for osteosynthesis in craniofacial deformities and trauma. Plast Reconstr Surg 77:729–736, 1986.

Kellman RM, Schilli W: Plate fixation of the mid and upper face. Otolaryngol Clin North Am 20:559–572, 1987.

Kreutziger KL: Surgical management of complex maxillofacial fractures. Laryngoscope 92:192–198, 1982.

Le Fort R: Experimental study of fractures of the upper jaw. Rev Chir de Paris 23:208–217; 360–379, 1901. Reprinted in Plast Reconstr Surg 50:497–506, 1972.

Lewis JES, Losken HW: LeFort III osteotomy to correct dish face deformity resulting from trauma. S Afr Med J 49:1915–1920, 1975.

Manson PN, Crawley WA, Yaremchuk MJ, et al: Midfacial fractures: Advantages of extended open reduction and immediate bone grafting. Plast Reconstr Surg 76:1–10, 1985.

Manson PN, Hoopes JE, Su CT: Structural pillars of the facial skeleton: An approach to the management of LeFort fractures. Plast Reconstr Surg 66:54–61, 1980.

Manson PN, Shack RB, Leonard LG, et al: Sagittal fractures of the maxilla and palate. Plast Reconstr Surg 72:484–488, 1983.

Mathog RH, Crane LR, Nowak GS: Antimicrobial therapy following head and neck trauma. In Johnson JT (ed): Antibiotic Therapy in Head and Neck Surgery. New York, Marcel Dekker, 1987, pp 31–49.

Mathog RH, Leonard M, Bevis R: Surgical correction of maxillary hypoplasia. Arch Otolaryngol 105:399–403, 1979.

Mathog RH, Rosenberg Z: Complications in the treatment of facial fractures. Otolaryngol Clin North Am 9:533–553, 1976.

May M, Phipatanakul P: Fracture of the medial aspect of the maxilla. Arch Otolaryngol 97:286–287, 1973.

McGraw BL, Cole RR: Pediatric maxillofacial trauma: Age-related variables in injury. Arch Otolaryngol 116:41–45, 1990.

Merville L: Multiple dislocations of the facial skeleton. J Maxillofac Surg 2:187–200, 1974.

Mixter RC, Feldman PD: Stabilization of the midface with a cranium-to-alveolus bone graft. Plast Reconstr Surg 83:348–355, 1989.

Nahum AM: The biomechanics of maxillofacial trauma. Clin Plast Surg 2:59–64, 1978.

Nikura K, Hasuike T, Nikura K, et al: Occlusal rehabilitation combining LeFort I osteotomy and prosthetic technics in a case of maxillary fracture. Josai Shika Daisaku Kiyo 13(2):448–454, 1984.

Obwegeser HL: Surgical correction of small or retrodisplaced maxillae. Plast Reconstr Surg 43:351–365, 1969.

Schultz RC, Carbonell AM: Midfacial fractures from vehicular accidents. Clin Plast Surg 2:107–130, 1975.

Shioda S, Shinmori Y, Nasayama T, et al: Surgical correction of malunited maxillary fracture by means of LeFort I type osteotomy (Obwegeser's method); report of a case. Nippon Koku Geka Gakkai Zasshi 22(1):18–24, 1976.

Sofferman RA, Danielson PA, Quatela V, et al: Retrospective analysis of surgically treated LeFort fractures. Arch Otolaryngol 109:446–448, 1983.

Stanley RB: Reconstruction of the midface vertical dimension following LeFort fractures. Arch Otolaryngol 110:571–575, 1984.

Stanley RB, Funk GF: Rigid internal fixation for fractures involving tooth-bearing maxillary segments. Arch Otolaryngol 114:1295–1299, 1988.

Stanley RB, Nowak GM: Midfacial fractures. Importance of angle of impact to horizontal craniofacial buttresses. Otolaryngol Head Neck Surg 93:186–191, 1985.

Tessier P: Total osteotomy of the middle third of the face for faciostenosis or for sequela of LeFort III fractures. Plast Reconstr Surg 48:533–541, 1971.

Yarington CT Jr: Maxillofacial trauma in children. Otolaryngol Clin North Am 10:25–32, 1977.

Zachariades N, Vairaktaris E, Papavassiliou D, et al: Traumatic LeFort III osteotomy. Br J Oral Maxillofac Surg 24(1):69–71, 1986.

Nasal Fractures

Bailey BJ, Caruso VH: Maxillofacial injury. Adv Oto-Rhino-Laryngol 23:155–168, 1978.

Beekhuis GJ: Nasal fractures. Trans Am Acad Ophthalmol Otolaryngol 74:1058–1059, 1970.

Beyer CK, Fabian RL, Smith B: Naso-orbital fractures: Complications and treatment. Ophthalmology 89:456–463, 1982.

Bowers DG, Lynch JB: Management of facial fractures. South Med J 70:910–918, 1977.

Clark GM, Wallace CS: Analysis of nasal support. Arch Otolaryngol 92:118–123, 1970.

Clark WD: Nasal and nasal septal fractures. Ear Nose Throat J 62:25–32, 1983.

Courtiss EH: Septorhinoplasty of the traumatically deformed nose. Ann Plast Surg 1:443–449, 1978.

Drumheller GH: Nasal fractures in children. Postgrad Med 48:123–127, 1970.

Farrior RT: Modifications in rhinoplasty. Where and when. Trans Am Acad Ophthalmol Otolaryngol 78:341–348, 1974.

Farrior RT: The osteotomy in rhinoplasty. Laryngoscope 88:1449–1459, 1978.

Farrior RT: Corrective and reconstructive surgery of the external nose. In Naumann HH (ed): Head and Neck Surgery, vol 1. Stuttgart, Georg Thieme, 1980, pp 173–277.

Farrior RT, Connolly ME: Septorhinoplasty in children. Otolaryngol Clin North Am 3:345–364, 1970.

Fry H: Nasal skeletal trauma and the interlocked stresses of the nasal septal cartilage. Br J Plast Surg 20:146–158, 1967.

Goldman IB: When is rhinoplasty indicated for a correction of recent nasal fractures? Laryngoscope 74:689–700, 1964.

Goode RL, Spooner TR: Management of nasal fractures in children. A review of current practices. Clin Pediatr 11:526–529, 1972.

Harrison DH: Nasal injuries: Their pathogenesis and treatment. Br J Plast Surg 32:57–64, 1979.

Hinderer KH: Nasal problems in children. Pediatr Ann 5:488–509, 1976.

Holt GR: Immediate open reduction of nasal septal injuries. Ear Nose Throat J 57:345–354, 1978.

Jordan LW: Acute nasal and septal injuries. Eye Ear Nose Throat Monthly 3:508–512, 1974.

Kaban LB, Mulliken JB, Murray JE: Facial fractures in children. Plast Reconstr Surg 59:15–20, 1977.

Kane AP, Kane LA: Open reduction of nasal fractures. J Otolaryngol 7:183–186, 1978.

Mackay IS: The deviated nose. Plast Reconstr Surg 3:253–265, 1986.

Marshall DR, Slattery PG: Intracranial complications of rhinoplasty. Br J Plast Surg 36:342–344, 1983.

Mathog RH: Management of acute nasal fractures. In Cummings GW, Frederickson JM, Harkin LA, et al (eds): Otolaryngology—Head and Neck Surgery, vol 1. St Louis, CV Mosby, 1986, pp 611–624.

Mayell MJ: Nasal fractures: Their occurrence, management and some late results. J R Coll Surg Edinb 18:31–36, 1973.

Moran WB: Nasal trauma in children. Otolaryngol Clin North Am 10:95–101, 1977.

Murray JAM, Maran AGD: The treatment of nasal injuries by manipulation. J Laryngol Otolaryngol 94:1405–1410, 1980.

Murray JAM, Maran AGD, MacKenzie IJ: Open vs closed reduction of the fractured nose. Arch Otolaryngol 110:797–802, 1984.

Olsen KD, Carpenter RJ, Kern EB: Nasal septal injury in children. Arch Otolaryngol 106:317–320, 1980.

Schultz RC: The management of common facial fractures. Surg Clin North Am 53:3–32, 1973.

Schultz RC, deVillers YT: Nasal fractures. J Trauma 15:319–327, 1974.

Smith B: Reduction of nasal orbital fractures and simultaneous dacryocystorhinostomy. Trans Am Acad Ophthalmol Otolaryngol 82:527–530, 1976.

Stranc MF, Robertson GA: A classification of injuries of the nasal skeleton. Ann Plast Surg 2:468–474, 1979.

Stucker FJ, Bryarly RC, Shockley WW: Management of nasal trauma in children. Ann Otolaryngol 110:190–192, 1984.

Wexler MR: Reconstructive surgery of the injured nose. Otolaryngol Clin North Am 8:633–673, 1975.

Malar Fractures

Altonen M, Kohonen A, Dickhoff K: Treatment of zygomatic fractures: Internal wiring-antral packing-reposition without fixation. J Maxillofac Surg 4:107–115, 1976.

Antonyshyn O, Gruss JS, Kassel EE: Blow-in fractures of the orbit. Plast Reconstr Surg 84:10–20, 1989.

Barclay TL: Diplopia in association with fractures involving the zygomatic bone. Br J Plast Surg 11:147–157, 1958.

Bernard RW, Matusow GF, Bonnano PC: Blow-in fracture causing exophthalmos. NY State J Med 78(4):652–653, 1978.

Crewe TC: Significance of the orbital floor in zygomatic injuries. Br J Oral Surg 7:235–239, 1978.

Crumley RL, Leibsohn J, Krause CJ, Burton TC: Fractures of the orbital floor. Laryngoscope 87:934–947, 1977.

Dingman RO, Natvig P: Surgery of facial fractures. Philadelphia, WB Saunders, 1964, pp 211–245.

Eisele DW, Duckert LF: Single-point stabilization of zygomatic fractures with the minicompression plate. Arch Otolaryngol 113:267–270, 1987.

Ellis E, El-Attar A, Moos KF: Analysis of 2,067 cases of zygomatico-orbital fracture. Oral Maxillofac Surg 43:417–428, 1985.

Fain J, Peri G, Verge P, Thevonen D: The use of single frontozygomatic osteosynthesis plate and a sinus balloon in the repair of fractures of lateral middle third of the face. J Maxillofac Surg 9:188–193, 1981.

Gillies MD, Kelner TP, Stone D: Fractures of the malar-zygomatic compound. Br J Plast Surg 14:651–675, 1927.

Gordon S, McCrae II: Monocular blindness as a complication of the treatment of a malar fracture. Plast Reconstr Surg 6:228–232, 1950.

Hardt H, Steinhauser EW: Treatment results after zygomatic-orbital fractures. Schweiz Monatsschr Zahnheilkd 86:825–835, 1976.

Hinderer UT: Malar implants for improvement of the facial appearance. Plast Reconstr Surg 56:157–165, 1975.

Holmes KD, Matthews BL: Three point alignment of zygoma fractures with miniplate fixation. Arch Otolaryngol Head Neck Surg 115:961–963, 1989.

Karlan MS, Cassisi NJ: Fractures of the zygoma. Arch Otolaryngol 105:320–327, 1979.

Karlan M, Skobel BS: Reconstruction for malar asymmetry. Arch Otolaryngol 106:20–24, 1980.

Kazanjian ES, Converse JM: Surgical Treatment of Facial Injuries, vol 2, ed 3. Baltimore, Williams & Wilkins, 1974, pp 287–306.

Knight JS, North JF: The classification of malar fractures: An analysis of displacement as a guide to treatment. Br J Plast Surg 13:325–332, 1961.

Kristensen S, Tveteras K: Zygomatic fractures: Classification and complications. Clin Otolaryngol 11:123–129, 1986.

Larsen OD, Thomsen M: Zygomatic fractures II. A follow-up study of 137 patients. Scand J Plast Reconstr Surg 12:59–63, 1978.

Lederman IR: Loss of vision associated with surgical treatment of zygomatico-orbital floor fracture. Plast Reconstr Surg 68:94–99, 1981.

Lund K: Fractures of the zygoma: A follow-up study of 62 patients. J Oral Surg 29:557–560, 1971.

Martin BC, Trabue JC, Leech TR: An analysis of the etiology, treatment and complications of fractures of the malar compound and zygomatic arch. Am J Surg 92:920–924, 1956.

Mathog RH: Reconstruction of the orbit following trauma. Otolaryngol Clin North Am 16:585–607, 1983.

Mathog RH, Crane LR, Nowak GS: Antimicrobial therapy following head and neck trauma. In Johnson JT (ed): Antibiotic Therapy in Head and Neck Surgery. New York, Marcel Dekker, 1987, pp 31–47.

Mathog RH, Rosenberg Z: Complications in the treatment of facial fractures. Otolaryngol Clin North Am 9:547–550, 1976.

Matsunaga RS, Simpson W, Toffel PH: Simplified protocol for treatment of malar fractures. Arch Otolaryngol 103:535–538, 1977.

Mustarde JC: The role of Lockwood's suspensory ligament in preventing downward displacement of the eye. Br J Plast Surg 21:73–81, 1968.

Nordgaard JO: Persistent sensory disturbances and diplopia following fractures of the zygoma. Arch Otolaryngol 102:80–82, 1976.

Rinehart GG, Marsh JL, Hemmer KM, Bresina S: Internal fixation of malar fractures: An experimental biophysical study. Plast Reconstr Surg 84:21–25, 1989.

Rowe NL, Killey HC: Fractures of the facial skeleton. Baltimore, Williams & Wilkins, 1986, pp 276–344.

Schiffer HD, Austerman KH, Busse H: Ophthalmological long-term effects of malar fractures. Klin Monatsbl Augenheilkd 71:567–570, 1977.

Scrimshaw GC: Malar-orbital-zygomatic fracture causing fracture of underlying coronoid process. J Trauma 18:367–368, 1978.

Stanley RB, Mathog RH: Evaluation and correction of combined orbital trauma syndrome. Laryngoscope 93:856–865, 1983.

Stanley RB, Mathog RH: Late reconstruction of the orbit after trauma to the inferior and lateral walls. In Ward PH, Berman WC (eds.): Plastic and Reconstructive Surgery: Proceedings of the Fourth International Symposium. St Louis, CV Mosby, 1984.

Tajima S, Sugimoto C, Tanino R, et al: Surgical treatment of malunited fracture of zygoma with diplopia and with comments on blowout fracture. J Maxillofac Surg 2:201–210, 1974.

Whitaker LA: Aesthetic augmentation of the malar-midface structures. Plast Reconstr Surg 80:337–346, 1987.

Wiesenbaugh JM: Diagnostic evaluation of zygomatic complex fractures. J Oral Surg 28:204–208, 1970.

Yanigasawa E: Symposium on maxillofacial trauma. III. Pitfalls in the management of zygomatic fractures. Laryngoscope 88:527–546, 1973.

Orbital Wall Fractures

Antonyshyn O, Gruss JS, Galbraith DJ, Hurwitz JJ: Complex orbital fractures: A critical analysis of immediate bone graft reconstruction. Ann Plast Surg 22:220–235, 1989.

Bartkowski SB, Krzystkowa KM: Blow-out fracture of the orbit. Diagnostic and therapeutic considerations, and results in 90 patients treated. J Maxillofac Surg 10:155–164, 1982.

Bite V, Jackson IT, Forbes GS, Gehring DG: Orbital volume measurements in enophthalmos using three-dimensional CT imaging. Plast Reconstr Surg 75:502–507, 1985.

Briggs PC, Heckler FR: Lacrimal gland involvement in zygomaticofrontal fracture site. Plast Reconstr Surg 80:682–685, 1987.

Burres S, Cohn AM, Mathog RH: Repair of orbital blow-out fractures with Marlex mesh and Gelfilm. Laryngoscope 91:1881–1886, 1981.

Converse JM: Correction of enophthalmos by disentrapment of an orbital blowout fracture. Plast Reconstr Surg 62:788–789, 1978.

Converse JM: Orbital fractures. In English FM (ed): Otolaryngology, vol 4. Hagerstown, MD, Harper & Row, 1981, pp 1–22.

Converse JM, Cole G, Smith B: Late treatment of blowout fractures of the orbit. Plast Reconstr Surg 28:183–190, 1961.

Converse JM, Firmin T, Wood-Smith D, Friedland JA: The conjunctival approach in orbital fractures. Plast Reconstr Surg 52:656–657, 1973.

Converse JM, Smith B: Reconstruction of the floor of the orbit by bone grafts. Arch Ophthalmol 44:1–21, 1950.

Converse JM, Smith B: Enophthalmos and diplopia in fractures of the orbital floor. Br J Plast Surg 9:265–274, 1975.

Converse JM, Smith B, Obear M: Orbital blowout fractures: A ten year survey. Plast Reconstr Surg 39:20–26, 1967.

Converse JM, Smith B, Wood-Smith D: Deformities of the midface resulting from malunited orbital and naso-orbital fractures. Clin Plast Surg 2:107–130, 1975.

Converse JM, Smith B, Wood-Smith D: Malunited fractures of the orbit. In Converse JM (ed): Reconstructive Plastic Surgery, vol 2. Philadelphia, WB Saunders, 1977, pp 989–1033.

Converse JM, Wood-Smith D: Orbital and naso-orbital fractures. In Converse JM (ed): Reconstructive Plastic Surgery, vol 2. Philadelphia, WB Saunders, 1977, pp 740–776.

Coster DJ, Galbraith JEK: Diced cartilage grafts to correct enophthalmos. Br J Ophthalmol 64:135–136, 1980.

Crikelair GF, Rein JM, Potter GP, Cosman B: A critical look at the "blowout" fracture. Plast Reconstr Surg 49:374–379, 1972.

Crumley RL, Leibsohn J, Krause CJ, Burton TC: Fractures of the orbital floor. Laryngoscope 97:934–947, 1977.

Dulley B, Fells P: Long-term follow-up of orbital blowout fractures with and without contrast surgery. Mod Probl Ophthalmol 14:467–470, 1975.

Emery JM, Von Noorden GK, Schlernitzauer DA: Orbital floor fractures: Long-term follow-up of cases with and without sur-

gical repair. Trans Am Acad Ophthalmol Otolaryngol 75:802–812, 1971.

Fells P: Acute enophthalmos. Trans Ophthalmol Soc UK 102:88–89, 1982.

Fradkin AH: Orbital floor fractures and ocular complications. Am J Ophthalmol 72:699–700, 1971.

Fries R: Some problems in therapy of traumatic enophthalmos. Mod Probl Ophthalmol 14:637–644, 1975.

Fujino T: Experimental "blowout" fracture of the orbit. Plast Reconstr Surg 54:81–82, 1974.

Fujino T, Makino K: Entrapment mechanism and ocular injury in orbital blowout fracture. Plast Reconstr Surg 65:571–574, 1980.

Hawkes MJ, Dortzbach RK: Surgery on orbital floor fractures. Influence of time and repair and fracture size. Ann Acad Ophthalmol 90:1066–1070, 1983.

Heckler FR, Songcharoen S, Sultani FA: Subciliary incision and skin-muscle flap for orbital fractures. Ann Plast Surg 10:309–313, 1983.

Howtof D: The dermis fat graft for correction of the eyelid deformity of enophthalmos. Mich Med June: 331–332, 1975.

Jabaley ME, Lerman M, Sanders HJ: Ocular injuries in orbital fractures. A review of 119 cases. Plast Reconstr Surg 56:410–418, 1975.

Jones DEP, Evans JNG: "Blowout" fractures of the orbit: An investigation into their anatomical basis. J Laryngol Otol 81:1109–1120, 1967.

Kawamoto HK: Late posttraumatic enophthalmos: A correctable deformity? Plast Reconstr Surg 69:423–432, 1982.

Kersten RC: Blowout fracture of the orbital floor with entrapment caused by isolated trauma to the orbital rim. Am J Ophthalmol 103:215–219, 1987.

Kirkegaard J, Greisen O, Poul EH: Orbital floor fractures: Early repair and results. Clin Otolaryngol 11:69–73, 1986.

Koornneef L: Current concepts on the management of orbital blow-out fractures. Ann Plast Surg 9:185–200, 1982.

Lang W: Traumatic enophthalmos with retention of perfect acuity of vision. Eye 9:44–45, 1889.

Leiman B: Blowout fractures of the orbit: Diagnosis and treatment. Br J Ophthalmol 52:90–98, 1970.

Maisel RH, Acomb TE, Cantrell RW: Medial orbital blow-out fracture: A case report. Laryngoscope 85:1211–1215, 1975.

Malauskas AT, Fueges GF: Serious ocular complications associated with blowout fractures of the orbit. Am J Ophthalmol 62:670–672, 1966.

Maniglia AJ: Conjunctival approach to the orbit for repair of blow-out fracture. Laryngoscope 90:1564–1568, 1980.

Manson PN, Clifford CM, Su CT, et al: Mechanisms of global support and posttraumatic enophthalmos: I. The anatomy of the ligament sling and its relation to intramuscular cone orbital fat. Plast Reconstr Surg 77:193–202, 1986.

Manson PN, Grivas A, Rosenbaum A, et al: Studies on enophthalmos II. The measurement of orbital injuries and their treatment by quantitative computed tomography. Plast Reconstr Surg 77:203–214, 1986.

Martinez-Lage JL: Reconstruction of the orbital region. Ann Plast Surg 7:464–479, 1981.

Mathog RH: Reconstruction of the orbit following trauma. Otolaryngol Clin North Am 16:585–607, 1983.

Mathog RH: Maxillofacial orbital blowout fractures. In Pillsbury HC, Goldsmith MM (eds): Operative Challenges in Otolaryngology—Head and Neck Surgery. Chicago, Year Book Medical Publishers, 1991, pp 471–496.

Mathog RH, Archer KF, Nesi FA: Posttraumatic enophthalmos and diplopia. Otolaryngol Head Neck Surg 94:69–77, 1986.

Mathog RH, Crane LR, Nowak GS: Antimicrobial therapy following head and neck trauma. In Johnson JT (ed): Antibiotic Therapy in Head and Neck Surgery. New York, Marcel Dekker, 1987, pp 31–47.

Mathog RH, Rosenberg Z: Complications in the treatment of facial fractures. Otolaryngol Clin North Am 9:533–553, 1974.

Matsuo K, Horose T, Furata S, et al: Semiquantitative correction of posttraumatic enophthalmos with sliced cartilage grafts. Plast Reconstr Surg 83:429–437, 1989.

McCoy FJ: Management of the orbit in facial fractures. Facial Plast Reconstr Surg 19:236–245, 1957.

Messinger A, Radkowski MA, Greenwald MJ, Pensler JM: Orbital roof fractures in the pediatric population. Plast Reconstr Surg 84:213–216, 1989.

Miller GR: Blindness developing a few days after a midface fracture. Plast Reconstr Surg 42:384–385, 1968.

Miller GR, Tenzel RR: Ocular complications of midfacial fractures. Plast Reconstr Surg 39:37–42, 1967.

Nesi F, LiVecchi F, Mathog RH: Orbital blowout fractures. In Mathog RH (ed): Maxillofacial Trauma. Baltimore, Williams & Wilkins, 1983, pp 318–320.

Nicholson DH, Guzak ST: Visual loss complicating repair of orbital fractures. Arch Ophthalmol 86:370–375, 1971.

Noyek AM, Kassel EE, Wortzman G, et al: Contemporary radiologic evaluation of maxillofacial trauma. Otolaryngol Clin North Am 16:473–508, 1983.

Ord RA: Post-operative retrobulbar haemorrhage in blindness complicating trauma surgery. Br J Oral Surg 19:202–207, 1981.

Otto AJ, Borghouts JMHM: Secondary correction of posttraumatic changes in the orbit with alloplastic material. Ophthalmologica 165:519–521, 1972.

Panje WR, Gross CE, Anderson RL: Sudden blindness following trauma. Otolaryngol Head Neck Surg 87:941–948, 1981.

Parkin JL, Stevens MH, Stringham JC: Absorbable gelatin film versus silicone rubber sheeting in orbital fracture treatment. Laryngoscope 97:1–3, 1987.

Parsons GS, Mathog RH: Orbital wall and volume relationships. Arch Otolaryngol 114:743–747, 1988.

Pearl RM: Surgical management of volumetric changes in the bony orbit. Ann Plast Surg 19:349–358, 1987.

Pearl RM, Vistnes LM: Orbital blowout fractures: An approach to management. Ann Plast Surg 1:267–270, 1978.

Pfeiffer RL: Traumatic enophthalmos. Arch Ophthalmol 30:718–726, 1943.

Polley JW, Ringler SL: The use of Teflon in orbital floor reconstruction following blunt facial trauma: A 20 year experience. Plast Reconstr Surg 79:39–43, 1987.

Putterman AM: Late management of blowout fractures of the orbital floor. Trans Am Acad Otol 83:650–659, 1977.

Putterman AM, Stevens T, Urist M: Nonsurgical management of blowout fractures of the orbital floor. Am J Ophthalmol 77:232–238, 1974.

Putterman AM, Urist MJ: Treatment of enophthalmic narrow palpebral fissure after blowout fracture. Ophthalmic Surg 6:45–49, 1975.

Raflo GT: Blow-in and blow-out fractures of the orbit: Clinical correlations and proposed mechanisms. Ophthalmic Surg 15:114–119, 1984.

Rankow RM, Mignogna FV: Surgical treatment of orbital floor fractures. Arch Otolaryngol 101:19–22, 1975.

Rauch SD: Medial orbital blow-out fracture with entrapment. Arch Otolaryngol 111:53–55, 1985.

Smith B, Lisman RD, Simonton J, DellaRocca R: Volkmann's contracture of the extraocular muscles following blowout fracture. Plast Reconstr Surg 74:200–214, 1984.

Smith B, Regan WF: Blowout fractures of the orbit. Mechanism and correction of inferior orbital fracture. Am J Ophthalmol 44:733–739, 1957.

Smith B, Taiara C: Correction of enophthalmos and deep supratarsal sulcus by posterior subperiosteal glass bead implantation. Br J Ophthalmol 57:741–746, 1974.

Spira M, Gerow F, Hardy SB: Correction of posttraumatic enophthalmos. Acta Chir Plast 16:107–111, 1974.

Stallings JO, Pakiam AI, Cori CC: The late treatment of enophthalmos: A case report. Br J Plast Surg 26:57–60, 1973.

Stanley RB, Mathog RH: Evaluation and correction of combined orbital trauma syndrome. Laryngoscope 93:856–865, 1983.

Stasior OG, Roen JL: Traumatic enophthalmos. Ophthalmol 89:1267–1273, 1982.

Sullivan WG, Smith AA: The split calvarial graft donor site in the elderly. A study in cadavers. Plast Reconstr Surg 84:29–31, 1988.

Tessier P: The conjunctival approach to the orbital floor and maxilla in congenital malformation and trauma. J Maxillofac Surg 1:3–8, 1973.

Thering HR, Bogart JN: Blowout fracture of the medial orbital wall with entrapment of the medial rectus muscle. Plast Reconstr Surg 63:848–852, 1979.

Wilkins RB: Current treatment of blowout fractures. Ophthalmology 89:464–466, 1982.

Wolfe SA: Surgical treatment of exophthalmos and enophthalmos. Ann Ophthalmol 13:995–1002, 1981.

Wolfe SA: Application of craniofacial surgical precepts in orbital reconstruction following trauma and tumour removal. J Maxillofac Surg 10:212–223, 1982.

Naso-Orbital Fractures

Arden R, Mathog RH, Nesi FA: Flap reconstruction techniques in conjunctivorhinostomy. Otolaryngol Head Neck Surg 102(2):150–155, 1990.

Balle VH, Andersen R, Siim C: Incidence of lacrimal obstruction following trauma to the facial skeleton. Ear Nose Throat J 67:66–70, 1988.

Beyer CK, Smith B: Naso-orbital fractures, complications and treatment. Ophthalmologica 163:418–427, 1972.

Busse H: The Kaleff-Hollwich technique and results of external dacryocysto-rhinostomy operation. J Maxillofac Surg 7:135–141, 1979.

Callahan A: Secondary reattachment of the medial canthal ligament. Trans Am Acad Ophthal Otol 52:240–241, 1947.

Converse JM, Hogan MV: Open sky approach for reduction of naso-orbital fractures. Plast Reconstr Surg 46:396–398, 1970.

Converse JM, Smith B: Canthoplasty and dacryocystorhinostomy in malunited fractures of the medial wall of the orbit. Am J Ophthalmol 35:1103–1114, 1952.

Converse JM, Smith B: Nasoorbital fractures and traumatic deformities of the medial canthus. Plast Reconstr Surg 38:147–162, 1966.

Converse JM, Smith B, Wood-Smith D: Deformities of the midface resulting from malunited orbital and naso-orbital fractures. Clin Plast Surg 2:107–130, 1975.

Dingman RO, Grabb WC, Oneal RM: Management of injuries of the naso-orbital complex. Arch Surg 98:566–571, 1969.

Duvall AJ, Banovetz JD: Nasoethmoid fractures. Otolaryngol Clin North Am 9:507–515, 1976.

Duvall AJ, Foster CA, Lyons DP, Letson RD: Medial canthoplasty: Early and delayed repair. Laryngoscope 91:173–183, 1981.

Fox SA: Downward displacement of the medial canthus. Ann Ophthalmol 3:1082–1084, 1971.

Freihoffer HPM: Experience with transnasal canthopexy. J Maxillofac Surg 8:119–124, 1980.

Freihoffer HPM: Inner intercanthal and interorbital distances. J Maxillofac Surg 8:324–326, 1980.

Furnas DW: The pulley canthoplasty for residual telecanthus after hypertelorism repair or facial trauma. Ann Plast Surg 5:85–94, 1979.

Furnas DW, Bircoll MJ: Eyelid traction test to determine if the medial canthal ligament is detached. Plast Reconstr Surg 52:315–317, 1973.

Gruss JS: Naso-ethmoid-orbital fractures. Classification and role of primary bone grafting. Plast Reconstr Surg 75:303–317, 1985.

Gruss JS, Hurwitz JJ, Nik NA, Kassel EE: The pattern and incidence of nasolacrimal injury in naso-orbital-ethmoid fractures: The role of delayed assessment and dacryocystorhinostomy. Br J Plast Surg 38:116–121, 1985.

Hanna DC, Clairmont AA: Nasolacrimal duct reconstruction with a vein graft. A non-invasive technique. Plast Reconstr Surg 62:85–88, 1978.

Jabaley ME, Lerman M, Sanders HJ: Ocular injuries in orbital fractures. Plast Reconstr Surg 56:410–417, 1979.

Jones LT: The cure of epiphora due to canalicular disorders; trauma and surgical failure on the lacrimal passages. Trans Am Acad Ophthal Otol 66:506–524, 1962.

Lawson W: Management of soft tissue injuries of the face. Otolaryngol Clin North Am 15:35–48, 1982.

Macomber WB, Wang MKH, Linton PC: A technique of canthal ligament reconstruction. Plast Reconstr Surg 33:253–257, 1964.

Marsh JL: Blepharo-canthal deformities in patients following craniofacial surgery. Plast Reconstr Surg 61:842–853, 1978.

Mathog RH: Reconstruction of the orbit following trauma. Otolaryngol Clin North Am 16:585–607, 1983.

Mathog RH: Traumatic telecanthus. In Mathog RH (ed): Textbook of Maxillofacial Trauma. Baltimore, Williams & Wilkins, 1983, pp 303–318.

Mathog RH, Bauer W: Post-traumatic pseudohypertelorism (telecanthus). Arch Otolaryngol 105:81–85, 1979.

Mathog RH, Rosenberg Z: Complications in the treatment of facial fractures. Otolaryngol Clin North Am 9:547–550, 1976.

Mustarde JC: Epicanthus and telecanthus. Br J Plast Surg 16:345–356, 1963.

Ramselaar JM, Van der Meulen JC, Bloem JJ: Naso-orbital fractures. Mod Probl Ophthalmol 14:107–110, 1975.

Smith B: Reduction of nasal orbital fractures and simultaneous dacryocystorhinostomy. Trans Am Acad Ophthalmol Otol 82:525–530, 1976.

Smith B, Beyer CK: Medial canthoplasty. Arch Ophthalmol 82:344–348, 1969.

Stranc MF: Primary treatment of naso-ethmoid injuries with increased intercanthal distance. Br J Plast Surg 23:8–25, 1970.

Stranc MF: The pattern of lacrimal injuries in naso-ethmoid fractures. Br J Plast Surg 23:335–346, 1970.

Tessier P: Experiences in the treatment of orbital hypertelorism. Plast Reconstr Surg 53:1–18, 1974.

Van der Muelen JC, Ramselaar JM, Bloem JJ: Hypertelorism. Mod Probl Ophthalmol 14:611–617, 1975.

Whitaker LA, Katowitz JA, Jacobs WE: Ocular adnexal problems in craniofacial deformities. J Maxillofac Surg 7:55–60, 1979.

Whitaker LA, Schaffer DB: Severe traumatic oculo-orbital displacement. Diagnosis and secondary treatment. Plast Reconstr Surg 59:352–359, 1977.

Frontal Sinus Fractures

Adkins WY, Cassone RD, Putney FJ: Solitary frontal sinus fracture. Laryngoscope 89:1099–1104, 1979.

Arden RL, Mathog RH, Thomas LM: Temporalis muscle-galea flap in craniofacial reconstruction. Laryngoscope 97:1336–1342, 1987.

Bagolini B: Leakage of spinal fluid into upper lid following trauma. Arch Ophthalmol 57:454–456, 1957.

Bloem JJ, van der Meulen JC, Ramselaar JM: Orbital roof fractures. Mod Probl Ophthalmol 14:510–512, 1975.

Bordley JE, Bischofberger W: Osteomyelitis of the frontal bone. Laryngoscope 77:1234–1244, 1967.

Brawley BW, Kelly WH: Treatment of basal skull fractures with or without cerebrospinal fluid fistulae. J Neurosurg 26:57–61, 1967.

Cabbage EB, Shively RS, Malik P: Cranioplasty for traumatic deformities of the frontoorbital area. Ann Plast Surg 13:175–184, 1984.

Calcaterra TC: Extracranial surgical repair of cerebrospinal fluid rhinorrhea. Ann Otol Rhinol Laryngol 87:108–116, 1980.

Capanna AH: A new method of cranioplasty. Surg Neurol 14:385–386, 1980.

Curtin H, Wolfe D, Schramm V: Orbital roof blowout fractures. AJR 139:969–972, 1982.

Davis EDD: Discussion on injuries of the frontal and ethmoidal sinuses. Proc R Soc Med 35:805–810, 1942.

Donald PJ: Frontal sinus ablation by cranialization. Arch Otolaryngol 108:142–146, 1982.

Donald PJ, Bernstein L: Compound frontal sinus injuries with intracranial penetration. Laryngoscope 88:225–232, 1978.

Donald PJ, Ettin M: The safety of frontal sinus obliteration when sinus walls are missing. Laryngoscope 96:190–193, 1986.

Flanagan JC, McLachlan DL, Shannon GM: Orbital roof fractures. Neurologic and neurosurgical considerations. Am Acad Ophthalmol 87:325–339, 1980.

Foustanos AP, Anagnostopoulos D, Katsianos G, Rapidis AD: Cranioplasty: A review of 10 cases. J Maxillofac Surg 11:83–86, 1983.

Gates GA: The lateral facial approach to the nasopharynx and infratemporal fossa. Otolaryngol Head Neck Surg 99:321–325, 1988.

Gruss JS: Fronto-naso-orbital trauma. Clin Plast Surg 9:577–589, 1982.

Hardy JM, Montgomery WW: Osteoplastic frontal sinusotomy. Ann Otol Rhinol Laryngol 85:523–532, 1976.

Heller EM, Jacobs JB, Holliday RH: Evaluation of the frontonasal duct in frontal sinus fractures. Head Neck 11:46–50, 1989.

Horowitz JH, Persing JA, Winn HR, Edgerton MT: The late treatment of vertical orbital dystopia resulting from orbital roof fracture. Ann Plast Surg 13:519–524, 1984.

Hybels RL: Posterior table fractures of the frontal sinus II. Clinical aspects. Laryngoscope 87:1740–1745, 1977.

Hybels RL, Newman MH: Posterior table fractures of the frontal sinus. I. An experimental study. Laryngoscope 87:171–179, 1977.

Ioannides C, Freihofer HPM, Bruaset I: Trauma of the upper third of the face. Management and follow-up. J Maxillofac Surg 12:255–261, 1984.

Jackson IT, Adham MN, Marsh WR: Use of the galeal frontalis myofascial flap in craniofacial surgery. Plast Reconstr Surg 77:905–910, 1986.

Johns ME, Winn HR, McLean WC, et al: Pericranial flap for closure of defects of craniofacial resections. Laryngoscope 91:952–959, 1981.

Knox BE, Gates GA, Berry SM: Optic nerve decompression via a lateral facial approach. Laryngoscope 100:458–462, 1990.

Kurzer A, Patel PM: Superior orbital fissure syndrome associated with fractures of the zygoma and orbit. Plast Reconstr Surg 64:715–719, 1979.

Larrabee WF, Travis LW, Tabb HG: Frontal sinus fracture—their suppurative complications and surgical management. Laryngoscope 90:1810–1813, 1980.

Levine SB, Rowe LD, Keane WM, Atkins JP: Evaluation and treatment of frontal sinus fractures. Otolaryngol Head Neck Surg 95:19–22, 1986.

Lynch RC: The technique of a radical frontal sinus operation which has given me the best results. Laryngoscope 31:1–5, 1921.

Manson PN, Crawley WA, Hoopes JE: Frontal cranioplasty: Risk factors and choice of cranial vault reconstructive material. Plast Reconstr Surg 77:888–898, 1986.

Mathog RH: Frontoethmoid fractures. In Gates GA (ed): Current Therapy in Otolaryngology—Head and Neck Surgery. Philadelphia, BC Decker, 1984–1985, pp 100–104.

Mathog RH, Crane LR, Nowak GS: Antimicrobial therapy following head and neck trauma. In Johnson JT (ed): Antibiotic Therapy in Head and Neck Surgery. New York, Marcel Dekker, 1987, pp 31–47.

Maves MD, Matt BH: Calvarial bone grafting of facial defects. Otolaryngol Head Neck Surg 95:464–470, 1986.

May M, Ogura JH, Schramm V: Nasofrontal duct in frontal sinus fractures. Arch Otolaryngol 92:534–538, 1970.

Mayer R, Brihaye J, Brihaye M, et al: Reconstruction of the orbital roof by acrylic prostheses. Mod Probl Ophthalmol 4:506–509, 1975.

McClurg FL, Swanson PJ: An orbital roof fracture causing diplopia. Arch Otolaryngol 102:497–498, 1976.

McLachlan DL, Flanagan JC, Shannon GM: Complications of orbital roof fractures. Am Acad Ophthalmol 89:1274–1278, 1982.

Merville LC, Derome D, de Saint-Jorre G: Fronto-orbito-nasal dislocations. J Maxillofac Surg 11:71–82, 1983.

Merville LC, Real JD: Fronto-orbitonasal dislocation. Initial total reconstruction. Scand J Plast Reconstr Surg 15:287–297, 1981.

Messinger A, Radkowski MA, Greenwald MJ, Pensler JM: Orbital root fractures in the pediatric population. Plast Reconstr Surg 84:213–216, 1984.

Newman MH, Travis LW: Frontal sinus fractures. Laryngoscope 83:1281–1291, 1973.

O'Brien MD, Reade PC: The management of dural tear resulting from midfacial fracture. Head Neck Surg 6:810–818, 1984.

Ousterhout DK, Tessier P: Closure of large cribriform defects with a forehead flap. J Maxillofac Surg 9:7–9, 1981.

Panje WR, Gross CE, Anderson RL: Sudden blindness following trauma. Otolaryngol Head Neck Surg 87:941–948, 1981.

Pfaltz CR: The indications of infraorbital nerve decompression. ORL J Otorhinolaryngol Relat Spec 35:214–216, 1973.

Pollack K, Payne EE: Fractures of the frontal sinus. Otolaryngol Clin North Am 9:517–522, 1976.

Potter JA, Siddoway JR, Mathog RH: Injury to the orbital plate of the frontal bone. Head Neck Surg 10:78–84, 1987.

Prendergast ML, Wildes TO: Evaluation of the orbital floor in zygoma fractures. Arch Otolaryngol Head Neck Surg 114:446–450, 1988.

Prolo DJ, Oklund SA: Composite autogeneic human cranioplasty:

frozen skull supplemented with fresh iliac corticocancellous bone. Neurosurgery 15:846–851, 1984.

Psillakis JM, Nocchi LB, Zanini SA: Repair of large defect of frontal bone with free graft and outer table of parietal bones. Plast Reconstr Surg 64:827–830, 1979.

Raveh J, Vuillemen T: Subcranial management of 395 combined frontobasal-midface fractures. Arch Otolaryngol Head Neck Surg 114:1114–1122, 1988.

Sataloff RT, Sariego J, Myers DF, Richter HJ: Surgical management of the frontal sinus. Neurosurgery 15:593–596, 1984.

Schenck NL: Frontal sinus disease. III. Experimental and clinical factors in failure of the frontal osteoplastic operation. Laryngoscope 85:76–92, 1975.

Schenck NL, Rauchbach E, Ogura JE: Frontal sinus disease. II. development of the frontal sinus model: Occlusion of the nasofrontal duct. Laryngoscope 84:1233–1247, 1974.

Schultz RC: Frontal sinus and supraorbital fractures from vehicle accidents. Clin Plast Surg 2:93–106, 1975.

Schultz RC: Supraorbital and glabellar fractures. Plast Reconstr Surg 45:227–233, 1980.

Shockley WW, Stucker FJ, Gage-White L, Anthony SO: Frontal sinus fractures: Some problems and some solutions. Laryngoscope 98:18–22, 1988.

Stanley RB, Becker TS: Injuries of the nasofrontal orifices in frontal sinus fractures. Laryngoscope 97:728–731, 1987.

Stanley RB, Schwartz MS: Immediate reconstruction of contaminated central craniofacial injuries with free autogenous grafts. Laryngoscope 99:1011–1015, 1989.

Van Gool A: Preformed polymethylmethacrylate cranioplasties. J Maxillofac Surg 13:2–8, 1988.

Wallis A, Donald PJ: Frontal sinus fractures: A review of 72 cases. Laryngoscope 98:593–598, 1988.

Waring GO, Flanagan JC: Pneumocephalus. A sign of intracranial involvement in orbital fracture. Arch Ophthalmol 93:847–850, 1975.

Williamson LK, Miller RH, Sessions RB: Treatment of nasofrontal ethmoidal complex fractures. Otolaryngol Head Neck Surg 89:587–593, 1981.

Wilson BC, Davidson B, Corey JP, Haydon RC: Comparison of complications following frontal sinus fractures managed with exploration with or without obliteration over 10 years. Laryngoscope 98:516–520, 1988.

Wolfe SA: The utility of pericranial flaps. Ann Plast Surg 1:146–153, 1978.

Wolfe SA, Johnson P: Frontal sinus injuries: Primary care and management of late complications. Plast Reconstr Surg 82:781–789, 1988.

Sphenoid Fractures

Anderson RL, Panje WR, Gross CE: Optic nerve blindness following blunt forehead trauma. Ophthalmology 89:445–455, 1982.

Eriksson L, Hakansson H: Unilateral fracture of the pterygoid process. Report of a case. Oral Surg 47:127–130, 1979.

Fukado Y: Results in 400 cases of surgical decompression of the optic nerve. Mod Probl Ophthalmol 14:474–481, 1975.

Funk GF, Stanley RB, Becker TS: Reversible visual loss due to impacted lateral orbital wall fractures. Head Neck Surg 11:295–300, 1989.

Gelman HK, Janzen WR, Skolnick EM: Ocular hypertension following use of an antral balloon. Arch Otolaryngol 99:449–450, 1974.

Ghobrial W, Amstatz S, Mathog RH: Fractures of the sphenoid bone. Head Neck Surg 8:447–455, 1986.

Habal MB, Maniscalco JE: Surgical relations of the orbit and optic nerve: An anatomical study under magnification. Ann Plast Surg 4:265–275, 1979.

Harris AE, McMenamin PG: Carotid artery-cavernous sinus fistula. Arch Otolaryngol 110:618–623, 1984.

Hasso AN, Lasjaunias P, Thompson JR, Hinshaw DB: Venous occlusions of the cavernous area—a complication of crushing fractures of the sphenoid bone. Radiology 132:375–379, 1979.

Holt RG, Holt JE: Incidence of eye injuries in facial fractures: An analysis of 727 cases. Otolaryngol Head Neck Surg 91:276–279, 1983.

Hooper RS: Orbital complications of head injury. Br J Surg 39:126–138, 1951.

Hughes B: Indirect injury of the optic nerve and chiasm. Bull Johns Hopkins Hosp 111:98–126, 196.

Jabaley ME, Lerman M, Sanders HJ: Ocular injuries in orbital fractures. Plast Reconstr Surg 56:410–418, 1975.

Kennerdell JS, Amsbaugh GH, Myers EN: Transantral-ethmoidal decompression of optic canal fracture. Arch Ophthalmol 94:1040–1043, 1976.

Ketchum LD, Ferris B, Masters FW: Blindness without direct injury to the globe—a complication of facial fractures. Plast Reconstr Surg 58(2):187–191, 1976.

Krausen AS, Ogura JH, Burde RM, Ostrow DE: Emergency orbital decompression: A reprieve from blindness. Otolaryngol Head Neck Surg 89:252–256, 1981.

Lipkin AT, Woodson GE, Miller RH: Visual loss due to orbital fracture. Arch Otolaryngol 113:81–83, 1987.

Manfredi SJ, Rajii MR, Sprinkle PM, et al: Computerized tomographic scan findings in facial fractures associated with blindness. Plast Reconstr Surg 68:479–489, 1981.

Montgomery WW: Surgery of the Upper Respiratory System, vol 1, ed 1. Philadelphia, Lea & Febiger, 1971, pp 66–93.

Niho S, Niho M, Niho K: Decompression of the optic canal by the transethmoidal route and decompression of the superior orbital fissure. Can J Ophthalmol 5:22–40, 1970.

Niho S, Yasuda K, Sato T, et al: Decompression of the optic canal by the transethmoidal route. Am J Ophthalmol 51:659–665, 1961.

Obenchain TG, Killeffer FA, Stern WE: Indirect injury of the optic nerves and chiasm with closed head injury. Bull Los Angeles Neurol Soc 38:13–20, 1973.

Osguthorpe JD, Sofferman RA: Optic nerve decompression. Otolaryngol Clin North Am 21:155–169, 1988.

Panje WR, Gross CE, Anderson RL: Sudden blindness following trauma. Otolaryngol Head Neck Surg 89:941–948, 1981.

Pringle JH: Atrophy of the optic nerve following diffused violence to the skull. Br Med J 2:1156–1157, 1922.

Ramsay JH: Optic nerve injury in fracture of the canal. Br J Ophthalmol 63:607–610, 1979.

Raveh J, Vuillemin T: Subcranial management of 395 combined frontobasal-midface fractures. Arch Otolaryngol Head Neck Surg 114:1114–1122, 1988.

Resneck JD, Lederman IR: Traumatic chiasmal syndrome associated with pneumocephalus and sellar fracture. Am J Ophthalmol 92:233–237, 1987.

Sherman R, Gottlieb LJ: Carotid-cavernous sinus fistula complicating a complex shotgun facial injury. Ann Plast Surg 21:251–256, 1988.

Shoji N, Kazuhide Y, Yikasi S, et al: Decompression of the optic canal by the transethmoidal route. Am J Ophthalmol 51:659–665, 1961.

Sofferman RA: Sphenoethmoid approach to the optic nerve. Laryngoscope 91:184–196, 1981.

Spoor TC, Mathog RH: Restoration of vision after optic nerve decompression. Arch Ophthalmol 104:804–805, 1986.

Stanley RB: The temporal approach to impacted lateral orbital wall fractures. Arch Otolaryngol Head Neck Surg 114:550–553, 1988.

Unger JD, Unger GF: Fractures of the pterygoid process accompanying severe facial bone injury. Radiology 98:311–316, 1971.

Walsh FB: Pathological clinical correlations. 1. Indirect trauma to the optic nerves and chiasm. Invest Ophthalmol 5:433–449, 1966.

Weymuller EA: Blindness and LeFort III fractures. Ann Otol Rhinol Laryngol 93:2–5, 1984.

Yoshinao F: Results in 350 cases of surgical decompression of the optic nerve. Trans Fourth Asia-Pacific Congress Ophthalmol 4:96–99, 1972.

Ethmoid Fractures

Applebaum E: Meningitis following trauma to the head and face. JAMA 1973:1818–1822, 1960.

Barrs DM, Kern EB: Use of intranasal pledgets for localization of cerebrospinal fluid rhinorrhea (notes in technique). Rhinology 17:227–230, 1979.

Brandt F, Nahser HC, Hartjes H, Kunitsch G: The value of

metrizamide CT cisternography in the diagnosis of CSF fistulae. Acta Neurochir 69:37–42, 1983.

Calcaterra TC: Extracranial surgical repair of cerebrospinal fluid rhinorrhea. Ann Otol Rhinol Laryngol 89:108–116, 1980.

Charles DA, Snell D: Cerebrospinal fluid rhinorrhea. Laryngoscope 89:820–826, 1979.

Chiro GD, Ommaya AK, Ashburn WL, Briner WH: Isotope cisternography in the diagnosis and follow-up of cerebrospinal fluid rhinorrhea. J Neurosurg 28:522–529, 1960.

Chow JM, Goodman D, Mafee MF: Evaluation of CSF rhinorrhea by computerized tomography with metrizamide. Otolaryngol Head Neck Surg 100:99–100, 1989.

Crow HJ, Keogh G, Northfield DW: The localization of cerebrospinal fluid fistulae. Lancet 271:325–327, 1956.

Dukert LG, Mathog RH: Diagnosis in persistent cerebrospinal fluid fistulas. Laryngoscope 87:18–25, 1977.

Evans JP, Keegan HR: Danger in the use of intrathecal methylene blue. JAMA 174:856–859, 1960.

Goshujra K: Metrizamide CT cisternography in the diagnosis and localization of cerebrospinal fluid rhinorrhea. J Comput Assist Tomogr 4:306–310, 1980.

Hanley J, Bales J, Byrd B: Recurrent meningococcal meningitis with occult CSF leak. Arch Intern Med 139:702–703, 1979.

Hunt JG: Accidental rupture of the ethmoid roof with subsequent recovery. Arch Otolaryngol 3:452–453, 1926.

Kirchner FR, Proud GO: Method for identification and localization of cerebrospinal fluid rhinorrhea and otorrhea. Laryngoscope 70:921–930, 1960.

Klatersky J, Sadeghi M, Brihaye J: Antimicrobial prophylaxis in patients with rhinorrhea or otorrhea: A double blind study. Surg Neurol 6:111–114, 1976.

Lantz EJ, Forbes GS, Brown ML, Laws ER, Jr: Radiology of cerebrospinal fluid rhinorrhea. AJR 135:1023–1030, 1980.

Lewin W: Cerebrospinal fluid rhinorrhea in nonmissile head injuries. Clin Neurosurg 12:237–252, 1964.

Mahaley MS, Odom GL: Complication following intrathecal injection of fluorescein. J Neurosurg 25:298–299, 1966.

Markham JW: Clinical features of pneumocephalus based upon a survey of 284 cases with report of 11 additional cases. Acta Neurol 15:1–78, 1967.

Mathog RH: Frontoethmoid fractures. In Gates G (ed): Current Therapy in Otolaryngology—Head and Neck Surgery, Philadelphia, BC Decker, 1984, pp 100–104.

May M: Nasal frontal ethmoidal injuries. Laryngoscope 87:948–953, 1977.

McCabe BF: The osteomucoperiosteal flap in repair of cerebrospinal fluid rhinorrhea. Laryngoscope 86:537–539, 1976.

Montgomery WW: Cerebrospinal fluid rhinorrhea. Otolaryngol Clin North Am 6:751–771, 1973.

Moseley JI, Carton CA, Stern WE: Spectrum of complications in the use of intrathecal fluorescein. J Neurosurg 48:765–767, 1978.

North JB: The importance of intracranial air. Br J Surg 58:826–829, 1971.

Ramsden RT, Block T: Traumatic pneumocephalus. J Laryngol Otol 90:345–355, 1990.

Schaefer SD, Diehl JT, Briggs WH: The diagnosis of CSF rhinorrhea by metrizamide CT scanning. Laryngoscope 90:871–875, 1980.

Waring GO, Flanagan JC: pneumocephalus—a sign of intracranial involvement in orbital fracture. Arch Ophthalmol 93:847–850, 1975.

Yokoyama K, Hasegawa M, Shiba K, et al: Diagnosis of CSF rhinorrhea: Detection of tau-transferrin in nasal discharge. Otolaryngol Head Neck Surg 98:328–332, 1988.

Temporal Bone Fractures

Alford BR, Weber SC, Sessions RB: Neurodiagnostic studies in facial paralysis. Ann Otol 79:227–233, 1970.

Babin RW: Topognostic and prognostic evaluation of traumatic facial nerve injuries. Otolaryngol Head Neck Surg 90:610–611, 198.

Barber HO: Positional nystagmus, especially after head injury. Laryngoscope 4:891–944, 1964.

Barber HO: Head injury. Audiological and vestibular findings. Ann Otol 78:239–252, 1969.

Bellucci RJ: Traumatic injuries of the middle ear. Otolaryngol Clin North Am 16:633–650, 1983.

Benitez JT, Bouchard KR, Lane R, Szopo D: Pathology of deafness and dysequilibrium in head injury. A human temporal bone study. Am J Otol 1:163–167, 1980.

Browning GC, Swan IRC, Gatehouse S: Hearing loss in minor head injury. Arch Otolaryngol 108:474–477, 1982.

Cannon CR, Jahrsdoerfer R: Temporal bone fractures. Arch Otolaryngol 109:285–288, 1983.

Chalat NT: Middle ear effects of trauma. Laryngoscope 81:1286–1303, 1971.

Coker NJ, Kendall KH, Jenkins HA, Alford BR: Traumatic intratemporal facial nerve injury: Management rationale for preservation of function. Otolaryngol Head Neck Surg 97:262–269, 1987.

Dawkes DK: Ossicular fixation. J Laryngol Otol 94:573–593, 1980.

Derlacki EL: Office closure of central tympanic membrane perforations: A quarter century of experience. Trans Am Acad Ophthal Otol 77:53–66, 1973.

Dommerby H, Tos M: Sensorineural hearing loss in post-traumatic incus dislocation. Arch Otolaryngol 109:257–261, 1983.

Eby TL, Pollak A, Fisch U: Histopathology of the facial nerve after longitudinal temporal bone fracture. Laryngoscope 98:717–720, 1988.

Emmett JR, Shea JJ: Traumatic perilymph fistula. Laryngoscope 90:1513–1520, 1980.

Fisch U: Facial paralysis in fractures of the petrous bone. Laryngoscope 84:2141–2154, 1974.

Fisch U: Management of intratemporal facial nerve injuries. J Laryngol Otol 94:129–134, 1980.

Fisch U: Prognostic value of electrical tests in acute facial paralysis. Am J Otol 5:494–498, 1984.

Fredrickson JM, Griffith HW: Transverse fracture of the temporal bone. Arch Otolaryngol 78:54–68, 1963.

Freeman J: Temporal bone fractures and cholesteatoma. Ann Otol Rhinol Laryngol 92:558–560, 1983.

Goodhill V, Harris I, Brockman SJ, Hantz O: Sudden deafness and labyrinthine window ruptures. Ann Otol 82:2–12, 1973.

Goodwin WS, Jr: Temporal bone fractures. Otolaryngol Clin North Am 16:651–659, 1983.

Graham MD: Surgical exposure of the facial nerve. Otolaryngol Clin North Am 7:437–456, 1974.

Griffin WL: A retrospective study of traumatic tympanic membrane perforations in a clinical practice. Laryngoscope 89:261–282, 1979.

Gros JC: The ear in skull trauma. South Med J 60:705–711, 1967.

Hasso AN, Ledington JA: Traumatic injuries of the temporal bone. Otolaryngol Clin North Am 21:295–316, 1988.

Hicks GW, Wright JW Jr, Wright JW: Cerebrospinal fluid otorrhea. Laryngoscope 90(suppl 25):1–25, 1980.

Hough JVD: Restoration of hearing loss after head trauma. Ann Otol 78:210–226, 1969.

Hough JVD, Stuart WD: Middle ear injuries in skull trauma. Laryngoscope 78:899–937, 1968.

Kamerer DB: Intratemporal facial nerve injuries. Otolaryngol Head Neck Surg 90:612–615, 1982.

Kettel K: Peripheral facial palsy in fractures of the temporal bone. Arch Otolaryngol 51:25–41, 1950.

Lambert PR, Brackman DE: Facial paralysis in longitudinal temporal bone fractures: A review of 26 cases. Laryngoscope 94:1022–1026, 1984.

Laumans EPJ, Yongkees LBW: On the prognosis of peripheral facial paralysis of endotemporal origin. Ann Otol Rhinol Laryngol 72:622–636; 894–899, 1963.

Pennington CL: Incus transposition techniques. Ann Otol Rhinol Laryngol 82:518–531, 1973.

Pulec JL: Total facial nerve exposure. Arch Otolaryngol 89:179–183, 1969.

Schuknecht HF: Mechanism of inner ear injury from blows to the head. Ann Otol 78:253–262, 1969.

Shea JJ, Emmett JR: Traumatic perilymph fistula. Laryngoscope 90:1513–1520, 1980.

Strom M: Trauma of the middle ear. Adv Otorhinolaryngol 35:1–254, 1986.

Tos M: Prognosis of hearing loss in temporal bone fractures. J Laryngol Otol 85:1147–1159, 1979.

Yanagihara N: Transmastoid decompression of the facial nerve in the temporal bone fracture. Otolaryngol Head Neck Surg 90:616–621, 1982.

Ylikosky J, Sanna M: Vestibular neurectomy for dizziness after head trauma. ORL J Otorhinolaryngol Relat Spec 45:216–225, 1983.

Laryngeal Injuries

Alonso WA, Pratt LL, Zollinger WK: Complications of laryngotracheal disruption. Laryngoscope 84:1276–1290, 1974.

Bergstrom B, Ollman B, Lindholm CE: Endotracheal excision of fibrous tracheal stenosis and subsequent prolonged stenting. Chest 71:6–12, 1977.

Bogdasarian RS, Olson NR: Posterior glottic laryngeal stenosis. Otolaryngol Head Neck Surg 88:765–772, 1980.

Bryce DP: The surgical management of laryngotracheal injury. J Laryngol Otol 86:547–587, 1972.

Bryce DP: Subglottic stenosis. Laryngoscope 89:320–324, 1979.

Chandler JR: Avulsion of the larynx and pharynx as the result of a waterski rope injury. Arch Otolaryngol 96:365–367, 1972.

Cohn AM, Peppard SB: Laryngeal trauma. In English GM (ed): Otolaryngology. Hagerstown, MD, Harper & Row, 1980, pp 1–14.

Cummings CW, Sessions DG, Weymuller EA Jr, Wood P: Atlas of Laryngeal Surgery. St Louis, CV Mosby, 1984, pp 43–190.

Dedo HH, Rowe LP: Laryngeal reconstruction in acute and chronic injuries. Otolaryngol Clin North Am 16:373–388, 1983.

Dedo HH, Sooy FA: Surgical repair of late glottic stenosis. Ann Otol 77:435–441, 1968.

Fearon B, Cotton R: Surgical correction of subglottic stenosis of the larynx. Ann Otol 81:508–513, 1972.

Finnegan DA, Wong ML, Kashima HK: Hyoid autograft repair of chronic subglottic stenosis. Ann Otol Rhinol Laryngol 84:643–649, 1975.

Geffin B, Grillo HC, Cooper JC, Pontoppidant L: Stenosis following tracheostomy for respiratory care. JAMA 216:1984–1988, 1971.

Grillo HC: Circumferential resection and reconstruction of the mediastinal and cervical trachea. Ann Surg 162:374–388, 1965.

Grillo HC: Management of cervical mediastinal lesions of the trachea. JAMA 197:1085–1090, 1966.

Gussack GS, Jurkovich GJ, Luterman A: Laryngotracheal trauma: A protocol approach to a rare injury. Laryngoscope 96:660–665, 1986.

Harris HH, Ainsworth JZ: Immediate management of laryngeal and tracheal injuries. Laryngoscope 75:1103–1115, 1965.

Kennedy KS, Harley EH: Diagnosis and treatment of acute laryngeal trauma. Ear Nose Throat 67:584–599, 1988.

Kennedy TL: Epiglottic reconstruction of laryngeal stenosis secondary to cricothyroidostomy. Laryngoscope 90:1130–1134, 1980.

Krekorian EA: Laryngopharyngeal injuries. Laryngoscope 85:2069–2086, 1975.

LeJeune FE: Laryngotracheal separation. Laryngoscope 88:1956–1962, 1976.

Lewy RB: Experience with vocal cord injection. Ann Otol 85:440–450, 1976.

McKenna J, Jacob HJ: Trauma to the larynx. In Walt AJ, Wilson RF (eds): Management of Trauma: Pitfalls and Practice. Philadelphia, Lea & Febiger, 1975.

McNaught RC: Surgical correction of anterior web of the larynx. Laryngoscope 60:264–272, 1950.

Miehlke A: Rehabilitation of vocal cord paralysis. Arch Otolaryngol 100:431–441, 1974.

Miller RP, Gray SD, Cotton RT, Myer CM: Airway reconstruction following laryngotracheal thermal trauma. Laryngoscope 98:826–829, 1988.

Montgomery WW: The surgical management of supraglottic and subglottic stenosis. Ann Otol Rhinol Laryngol 77:534–546, 1968.

Montgomery WW: Surgery of the Upper Respiratory System, vol 2, ed 1. Philadelphia, Lea & Febiger, 1973, pp 315–372.

Montgomery WW, Gamble JE: Anterior glottic stenosis. Arch Otolaryngol 92:560–567, 1970.

Myer CM, Orobello P, Cotton RT, Bratcher GO: Blunt laryngeal trauma in children. Laryngoscope 97:1043–1048, 1987.

Newman MH, Work WP: Arytenoidectomy revisited. Laryngoscope 86:840–849, 1976.

Ogura JH, Biller HF: Reconstruction of the larynx following blunt trauma. Ann Otol Rhinol Laryngol 80:492–506, 1971.

Ogura JH, Powers WE: Functional restitution of traumatic stenosis of the larynx and pharynx. Laryngoscope 74:1081–1110, 1964.

Olson NR: Laryngeal suspension and epiglottic flap in laryngotracheal trauma. Ann Otol Rhinol Laryngol 85:533–538, 1976.

Olson NR: Wound healing by primary intention in the larynx. Otolaryngol Clin North Am 12:735–740, 1977.

Olson NR: Surgical treatment of acute blunt laryngeal injuries. Ann Otol Rhinol Laryngol 87:716–721, 1978.

Olson NR, Miles WK: Treatment of acute blunt laryngeal injuries. Ann Otol Rhinol Laryngol 80:704–710, 1971.

Pennington CL: Glottic and supraglottic laryngeal injury and stenosis from external trauma. Laryngoscope 77:317–345, 1964.

Pennington CL: External trauma of the larynx and trachea. Ann Otol Rhinol Laryngol 81:546–554, 1972.

Peppard SB: Transient vocal cord paralysis following strangulation injury. Laryngoscope 92:31–34, 1982.

Potter CR, Sessions DG, Ogura JH: Blunt laryngotracheal trauma. Otolaryngol 86:909–923, 1978.

Quick CA, Merwin GE: Arytenoid dislocation. Arch Otolaryngol 104:267–270, 1978.

Rethi A: An operation for cicatricial stenosis of the larynx. J Otolaryngol 72:283–293, 1956.

Schaefer SD, Close LG: Acute management of laryngeal trauma: Update. Ann Otol Rhinol Laryngol 98:98–104, 1989.

Schaefer SD, Close LG, Brown OE: Mobilization of the fixed arytenoid in the stenotic posterior laryngeal commissure. Laryngoscope 96:656–659, 1986.

Schuller DE, Parrish RT: Reconstruction of the larynx and trachea. Arch Otolaryngol Head Neck Surg 114:211–219, 1988.

Stanley RB, Coleman WF: Unilateral degloving injuries of the arytenoid cartilage. Arch Otolaryngol Head Neck Surg 112:516–518, 1986.

Stanley RB, Cooper DS, Florman SH: Phonatory effects of thyroid cartilage fractures. Ann Otol Rhinol Laryngol 96:493–496, 1987.

Thawley SE, Ogura JE: Use of the hyoid graft for treatment of laryngotracheal stenosis. Laryngoscope 91:226–232, 1981.

Trone TH, Schaefer SD: Blunt and penetrating laryngeal trauma: A 13 year review. Otolaryngol Head Neck Surg 88:257–261, 1980.

Tucker HM: Human laryngeal reinnervation: Long-term experience with the nerve-muscle pedicle technique. Laryngoscope 88:598–604, 1978.

Tucker HM, Wood BJ, Levine H, Katz R: Glottic reconstruction after near total laryngectomy. Laryngoscope 89:609–617, 1979.

Ward RH, Canalis R, Fee W, Smith G: Composite hyoid sternohyoid muscle grafts in humans. Arch Otolaryngol 103:531–534, 1977.

Soft Tissue Injury

Baker DC, Conley J: Facial nerve grafting: A thirty year retrospective review. Clin Plast Surg 6:330–343, 1970.

Beall AC Jr, Shirkey AL, DeBakey ME: Penetrating wounds of the carotid artery. J Trauma 3:276–287, 1963.

Belinkie SA, Russell JC, DaSilva J, Becker DR: Management of penetrating neck injuries. J Trauma 23:235–237, 1903.

Bradley EL: Management of penetrating carotid injuries: An alternative approach. J Trauma 13:248–255, 1973.

Brown MF, Graham JM, Feliciano DV, et al: Carotid artery injuries. Am J Surg 144:748–753, 1982.

Caboud HE: Epineural and perineural fascicular nerve repairs: A critical comparison. J Hand Surg 1:131–134, 1976.

Calcaterra TC, Hotz GP: Carotid artery injuries. Laryngoscope 82:321–329, 1972.

Campbell FC, Robbs JV: Penetrating injuries of the neck: A prospective study of 108 patients. Br J Surg 67:582–586, 1980.

Crumley RL: Interfascicular nerve repair: Is it applicable in facial nerve injuries? Arch Otolaryngol 106:313–316, 1980.

Fisch U: Facial nerve grafting. Otolaryngol Clin North Am 7:517–529, 1974.

Fitchett VH, Pomerantz M, Butsch DW, et al: Penetrating wounds of the neck. A military and civilian experience. Arch Surg 99:307–314, 1969.

Flint LM, Snyder WH, Perry MO, et al: Management of major vascular injuries in the base of the neck. Arch Surg 106:407–413, 1973.

Fogelman MJ, Stewart RD: Penetrating wounds of the neck. Am J Surg 91:581–593, 1956.

Fry RE, Fry WJ: Extracranial carotid injury. Surgery 88:581–587, 1980.

Goldsmith MM, Postma DS, Jones FD: The surgical exposure of penetrating injuries to the carotid artery at the skull base. Otolaryngol Head Neck Surg 95:278–284, 1986.

Gullane PJ: Extratemporal facial rehabilitation. J Otolaryngol 8:477–486, 1979.

Hagan WE: Microneural techniques for nerve grafting. Laryngoscope 91:1759–1766, 1981.

Harris JP, Anterasian G, Hoi SU, et al: Management of carotid artery transection resulting from a stab wound to the ear. Laryngoscope 95:782–785, 1985.

Holt GR: Wound ballistics of gunshot injuries to the head and neck. Arch Otolaryngol 109:313–318, 1983.

Jahrsdoerfer RA, Johns ME, Cantrell RW: Penetrating wounds of the head and neck. Arch Otolaryngol 105:721–725, 1979.

Jones RF, Terrell JC, Salyer KE: Penetrating wounds of the neck: An analysis of 274 cases. J Trauma 7:220–223, 1967.

Lawrence KB, Shefts LM, McDaniel JR: Wounds of the common carotid arteries. Report of 17 cases from World War II. Am J Surg 76:29–37, 1948.

Ledgerwood AM, Mullins RJ, Lucas CE: Primary repair vs. ligation for carotid artery injuries. Arch Surg 115:488–493, 1980.

Liekweg WG, Greenfield LJ: Management of penetrating carotid arterial injury. Ann Surg 188:587–592, 1978.

Mathog RH: Large facial wounds. In Gates GA (ed): Current Therapy in Otolaryngology—Head and Neck Surgery, vol 3. Philadelphia, BC Decker, 1987, pp 73–77.

May M, Chadaratana P, West JW, Ogura JH: Penetrating neck wounds: Selective exploration. Laryngoscope 85:57–75, 1975.

May M, Tucker HM, Dillard BM: Penetrating wounds of the neck in civilians. Otolaryngol Clin North Am 9:361–391, 1976.

Millesi H: Technique of free nerve grafting in the face. In Rubin L (ed): Reanimation of the Paralyzed Face. St Louis, CV Mosby, 1977, pp 124–135.

Millesi H: Nerve grafting. Clin Plast Surg 11:105–113, 1984.

Monson DO, Saletta JD, Freeark RJ: Carotid vertebral trauma. J Trauma 9:987–991, 1969.

Myssiorek D: Traumatic retropharyngeal hematoma. Arch Otolaryngol Head Neck Surg 115:1130–1132, 1989.

Padberg FT, Hobson RW, Yeager RH: Penetrating carotid arterial trauma. Am J Surg 50:277–282, 1984.

Pate JW, Casini M: Penetrating wounds of the neck: Explore or not? Am J Surg 10:38–43, 1980.

Pichtel WJ, Miller RH, Feliciano DV: Lateral mandibulotomy: A technique of exposure for penetrating injuries of the internal carotid artery at the base of the skull. Laryngoscope 94:1140–1144, 1984.

Rao M, Bhatti FK, Gaudino J, et al: Penetrating injuries of the neck: Criteria for exploration. J Trauma 23:47–49, 1983.

Robbs JV, Baker LW, Human RR, et al: Cervicomediastinal arterial injuries. Arch Surg 116:663–667, 1981.

Samson D, Boone S: Extracranial-intracranial (EC-IC) arterial bypass. Past performance and current concepts. Neurosurgery 3:79–86, 1978.

Smith MFN, Goode RL: Eye protection in the paralyzed face. Laryngoscope 89:435–442, 1979.

Stroud WH, Yarbrough DR: Penetrating neck wounds. Am J Surg 140:323–326, 1980.

Szal G, Miller T: Surgical repair of facial nerve branches. Arch Otolaryngol 101:160–165, 1975.

Tucker H: The management of facial paralysis due to extracranial injuries. Laryngoscope 88:348–356, 1978.

Unger SW, Tucker SW, Urdeza MH: Carotid arterial trauma. Surgery 87:477–483, 1980.

Watson WL, Silverstone SM: Ligature of the common carotid artery in cancer of the head and neck. Ann Surg 109:1–27, 1939.

Yamada S, Kindt GW, Youmans JR: Carotid artery occlusion due to nonpenetrating injury. J Trauma 7:333–342, 1967.

Index

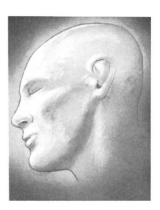

Note: Page numbers in *italics* refer to illustrations.

Canthoplasty, transnasal, for type II naso-orbital fracture, 324, *325*, 326
Canthotomy, lateral, 324, *325*
Carotid artery injury, from blunt trauma, repair of, 526–527, *528*
  from tracheostomy, 16
  penetrating, treatment of, 521–522, *523*, 524, *525*, 526
  resection and end-to-end anastomosis for, 522, *523*
  zones of, 521, *523*
Cartilage graft technique, for unilateral vocal cord paralysis treatment, 492, *493*
Cartilaginous depressions, of nose, 251
Central nervous system, intrathecal fluorescein and, 430
Cephalometric analysis, for halo frame fixation, 182
Cerebrospinal fluid leak, after inferior wall fracture repair, 379
  cribriform plate, frontoethmoidal repair approach for, 431–432, *433*
    frontotemporal approach for, 434, 436, *437*
  examination for, using intrathecal fluorescein dye, 427–428, *429*, 430
  physical examination for, 423–424
  prevention of, in transfrontal craniotomy, 410
  sites and signs of, 424, *425*
  with sphenoid fractures, transseptal repair of, 415–416, *417–418*, 419
Cervical spine, pharyngeal intubation and, 4
Children, condylar fractures of, intermaxillary fixation of, 38
  mandibular fractures of, 30, *31*
  maxillary fractures of, 146
  modified tracheostomy for, *15*, 16–17
  parasymphyseal fractures of, closed reduction of, 100, *101*, 102, *103*
  temporomandibular ankylosis of, 138
  tooth eruption of, 30, *31*
  tooth shedding of, *31*
Cholesteatoma, 452
Columella retraction, cartilage grafts for, 252, *254*
Combined orbital trauma syndrome, orbit reconstruction for, 311–312, *313*
Comminuted fractures, of anterior frontal sinus, 351, *353*
  of malar bone, 257, *258*
    open reduction and miniplate fixation of, 271, *272–273*, 274
  of mandible, 26, *27*
  of maxilla, 178
  of nose, closed treatment of, with lead plates, 234, *235*, 236
  of posterior frontal sinus, 351, *354*
  of ramus, 62
Common carotid artery injury, lateral arteriorrhaphy for, 522, *523*
Complex fracture, of mandible, 27
Complicated fracture, of mandible, 27
Compound fracture, of mandible, 25
Compression plating, of mandibular angle fractures, 65–66, *67–68*
  of mandibular body fractures, 90, *91*, 92
Computed tomography, of nasoethmoid fractures, 230
  with metrizamide, for detection of cerebrospinal fluid leak, 424
Condylar fractures, closed reduction of, indications for, 44
    Ivy loop technique for, 41, *42*
    Molar wafers for, 41, *43*
    with intermaxillary fixation, 36–38, *37*
  in edentulous patients, application of splint or denture for, 48, 50, *51–52*
    complications of, 50
    denture preparation for, 48, *49*
    pitfalls of technique for, 50
    postoperative care for, 50
    splint fabrication for, 44, *45–47*, 48
  open reduction of, complications of, 55
    indications for, 53
    interosseous wire technique for, 55, *56*
    pitfalls of, 55
    with external pin fixation, 53, *54*
  stability of, 27, *29*
Condylar head, dislocation of, 33

Condylar head (*Continued*)
  reduction procedure for, 33–34, *35*
Condyle, ankylosis of, 41, 102
Condyle dislocation, closed reduction of, 33–34, *35*
  recurrent, condyloplasty for, 34, *35*
Condyloplasty, for recurrent dislocation, 34, *35*
Conjunctivodacryocystorhinostomy, 339
Conjunctivorhinostomy, for canalicular repair, 339, *340*
Copper mold method, with methylmetacrylate plate technique, for forehead deformity repair, 392, 394, *395*
Coronal approach with cranial grafts, for malunion of malar fractures, 281, *282*
Coronal flap approach, for Le Fort III fractures, complications of, 174–175
  contraindications for, 169
  pitfalls of, 170, 174
  procedure for, 170, *171–173*
Coronal incision, beveled, for osteoplastic flap formation, 364, *365*
  for forehead deformity repair, 391, *393*
Coronal osteoplastic flap and fat obliteration, for inferior wall fracture of frontal sinus, 377, *378*, 379
  for posterior wall fracture of frontal sinus, 363–364, *365–368*, 369
Coronal skin flaps, 408
Coronoid fracture fixation, 57, 58, *59*
  indications for, 57
  pitfalls of, 57–58
Coronoidectomy, 58, *59*
Cottle elevator, 238, 283, 292
Cranial grafts, for orbital reconstruction, 308–309, *310*
Cranialization technique, for posterior wall frontal sinus fracture, 370, *371*, 372
Craniotomy, frontotemporal, for superior orbital wall fracture repair, 388, *389*
  transfrontal, for optic nerve decompression, 408, *409*, 410
  pitfalls of, 408, 410
Cribriform plate cerebrospinal fluid leak, frontoethmoidal repair approach for, 431–432, *433*
  frontotemporal repair approach for, 434, 436, *437*
Cricoid injury, from cricothyrotomy, 10
  open repair of, 483, 485, *486*
Cricothyrotomy, 10, *11*

D
Dacryocystitis, 326, 342
Dacryocystorhinostomy, complications of, 342
  indications for, 341
  pitfalls of, 342
  procedure for, 341–342, *343–344*
Decompression, of facial nerve, using transmastoid approach, 443–444, *445*, 446
  of infraorbital nerve, 283
  of optic nerve, 403–404, *405–406*, 407
  of superior orbital fissure, using frontotemporal approach, 411–412, *413–414*
Degloving approach, with interosseous wire fixation, for medial maxillary fractures, 187–188, *189–190*
Degloving gingivolabial sulcus incision, 162, *163*, 176
Dental arch, in fabrication of lingual splint for parasymphaseal fracture, 102, *103*
Denture fixation, of Le Fort I fracture, 158, *159*, 160
Denture preparation, for edentulous patient, with condylar fractures, 48, *49*
Denture suspension wiring, for edentulous patient, with Le Fort III fracture, 178, *179–180*, 181
Diplopia, after orbital reconstruction, 308
  after orbital wall fracture repair, 295
  in medial orbital wall fracture, 298
Displaced angle of medial canthus, repair of, 345–346, *347*
Dural tears, 410, 412

555